FASCIA

In Sport and Movement

FASCIA

In Sport and Movement

Editors Robert Schleip and Jan Wilke

Assistant Editor Amanda Baker

Contributors

Abraham	Kelsick
Alfredson	Kjaer
Allen	Klingler
Arampatzis	Krause
Avison	Larkam
Baar	Mayberry
Bartsch	Mersmann
Bauermeister	Mosetter
Behm	Müller-Wohlfahrt
Bohm	Müller
Brauner	Myers
Chaitow	O'Clair
Dennenmoser	Parisi
Dommerholt	Petersen
Earls	Puta
Eder	Rodríguez
Findley	Sharkey
Fischer	Shockett
Franklin	Simmel
Frederick	Stecco
Frederick	Steffen
Galán del Río	Steidten
Grilley	Sterzing
Hansen	Yucesoy
Heiduk	Zullo
Hoffmann	

Foreword by Thomas W Findley

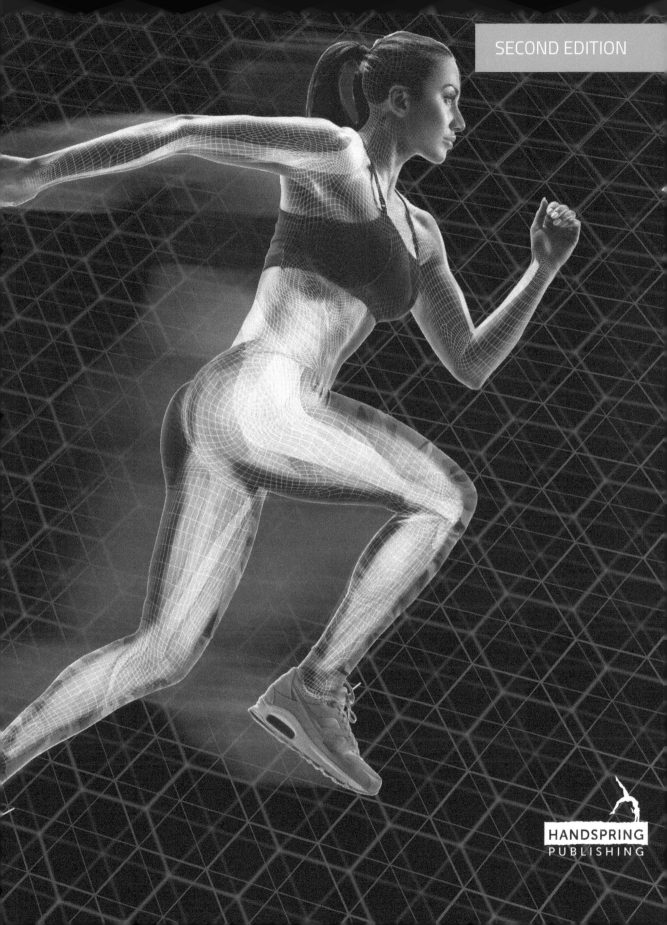

HANDSPRING
PUBLISHING

HANDSPRING PUBLISHING LIMITED
The Old Manse, Fountainhall,
Pencaitland, East Lothian
EH34 5EY, United Kingdom
Tel: +44 1875 341 859
Website: www.handspringpublishing.com

First published 2021 in the United Kingdom by Handspring Publishing
First edition published 2013 in the United Kingdom by Handspring Publishing
Second edition published 2021 in the United Kingdom by Handspring Publishing
Copyright © Handspring Publishing Ltd 2021

ISBN 978-1-912085-77-4
ISBN (Kindle ebook) 978-1-912085-78-1

British Library Cataloguing in Publication Data
A catalogue record for this book is available from the British Library

Library of Congress Cataloguing in Publication Data
A catalog record for this book is available from the Library of Congress

Commissioning Editor Sarena Wolfaard
Project Manager Morven Dean
Copy Editor Dylan Hamilton
Cover and Design Direction Bruce Hogarth
Indexer Aptara, India
Typesetter DiTech Process Solutions, India
Printer Ashford Colour Press Ltd, UK

The
Publisher's
policy is to use
paper manufactured
from sustainable forests

CONTENTS

CONTENTS

CONTENTS

ABOUT THE EDITORS

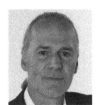

Robert Schleip directs the Fascia Research Project at Ulm University, Germany, and is Research Director of the European Rolfing Association. He is a certified Rolfing Instructor and Feldenkrais teacher. He is the author and co-editor of several books and has written numerous research articles. For his laboratory research work on active contractile properties in fascial tissues he was awarded the Vladimir Janda Award for Musculoskeletal Medicine. He was the co-initiator and organizer of the inaugural Fascia Research Congress (Boston, 2007) as well as all subsequent congresses.

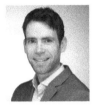

Jan Wilke leads the "Fascia in Motion" research group at Frankfurt University, Germany. He is a member of the American College of Sports Medicine, and has been invited as a Visiting Fellow by Amsterdam University (the Netherlands) and Liverpool University (the UK). His chapter on Myofascial Chains, published in *Gray's Anatomy*, represents one of the first anatomical atlas contributions explicitly focusing on fascia and movement. In addition to his academic tasks, Wilke is a conditioning coach and has worked with high-level athletes, including the former world No. 1 tennis player, Angelique Kerber.

Amanda Baker is an experienced yoga teacher and Pilates instructor working in a clinical practice. After completing her Masters degree, she became a freelance journalist in the health and fitness industry, and then qualified as a Fascial Fitness Trainer.

ABOUT THE CONTRIBUTORS

Dr Amit Abraham (PhD, MAPhty, BPT) is a musculoskeletal physical therapist specializing in dance and sport injuries and mental imagery for dancers, athletes, and people with Parkinson disease. He is an Assistant Professor in the Department of Physical Therapy, Faculty of Health Sciences at Ariel University (Israel). Dr Abraham holds a Bachelor in Physical Therapy from Tel-Aviv University (Israel), a Master's Degree in Musculoskeletal Physical Therapy from The University of Queensland (Australia), and a PhD in Physical Therapy from the University of Haifa (Israel). He completed his post-doctoral training at Emory University School of Medicine (Atlanta, USA).

Professor Håkan Alfredson (MD, PhD) is a research specialist in the field of chronic painful Achilles and patellar tendon and cartilage repair. He has published more than 150 articles in peer-reviewed scientific journals. He currently works at the Alfredson Tendon Clinic (Sweden), for Pure Sports Medicine (UK), and at the Sports Medicine Unit, University of Umeå (Sweden).

Johnathon Allen is a writer/photographer and co-author of *Fascia Training: A Whole-System Approach.* His work has appeared in *Bicycling, Outside, Adventure Journal, Decline,* and other publications. He is also author of the nonfiction books *Ray's* and *Doppelganger Effect.*

Professor Adamantios Arampatzis is Head of the Department of Training and Movement Sciences, and is Spokesperson of the Berlin School of Movement Science. His research deals with the interaction of the central nervous and peripheral systems, and how these systems develop over the lifespan and adapt to changing environmental demands.

Joanne Avison (MSS) is an advanced Yoga Teacher, Yoga Therapist (C-IAYT) and Structural Integration practitioner/teacher. Her fascination with fascia and human architecture led her to becoming a founding member of the Biotensegrity Interest Group, pioneering the application of biotensegrity for movement and manual practitioners. She is also the author of *YOGA: Fascia, Anatomy and Movement* (Handspring, 2015).

Professor Keith Baar (PhD) is a molecular exercise physiologist with a specific interest in the molecular response of the musculoskeletal system to nutrition and loading as a function of age. The Baar lab uses a series of complex animal and human models and has also developed unique 2- and 3-dimensional tissue culture assays that can be used to study the effects of genes and nutrients on muscle and tendon/ligament function. Using these models, the Baar lab performs translational research on the molecular signals that underly musculoskeletal function and how these signals are affected by age, diet, and exercise. Prof Baar collaborates closely with clinical partners at UC Davis and around the world. At UC Davis, Prof Baar works with clinicians at the School of Medicine and the School of Veterinary Medicine to optimize musculoskeletal health and performance. Three primary avenues of research are actively pursued: 1) The molecular determinants of muscle size and strength; 2) Optimizing exercise and nutrition for tendon/ligament function; and 3) Determining the role of the musculoskeletal system in the neurocognitive benefits of a ketogenic diet. Because of the applied nature of Prof Baar's work, he has worked with elite athletes, as a scientific advisor to the numerous professional and Olympic organizations. His work with these organizations is designed to maximize the effects of training for both endurance and strength while minimizing injury.

Katja Bartsch (BSc, MBA, BCSI) Formerly research assistant at Technische Universität München and Friedrich-Alexander-Universität Erlangen-Nürnberg. Certified Anatomy Trains Structural Integration Practitioner IASI Board Certified Structural Integration Practitioner Kalaman Yoga and Training, E-RYT 500 certified Yoga Teacher, Germany.

Professor Wolfgang Bauermeister (MD, PhD) works in the Department of Physical Rehabilitation and Sports Medicine at Kharkiv National Medical University (Ukraine). He is also CEO of the Pain-Institute Munich (Germany) with a particular focus on research and development in Ultrasound-Elastography, orthopedic shockwave application and outpatient care. He developed trigger point shockwave therapy and fascia and trigger point Ultrasound-Elastography for clinical applications in sports and pain medicine.

Dr David G Behm has worked at Memorial University (Newfoundland, Canada) since 1995. He has published research in more than 230 publications, including neuromuscular responses to stretching, resistance training, balance and fatigue. He has received an NSCA Outstanding Sport Scientist and CSEP Honour Award, and was awarded Memorial University President's Award for Outstanding Research and Service Excellence.

Sebastian Bohm has worked as an employee in training and movement science since 2011. After completing his studies in Sport Science at Humboldt University (Berlin) in 2011, he graduated as a PhD in 2015. His current research focus concerns muscle-tendon interaction and mechanics during regular and perturbed locomotion.

Professor Torsten Brauner teaches movement sciences and scientific methods at the College for Applied Health Sciences in Mannheim, Germany. His research focuses on the effects of mechanical loading on the musculoskeletal system with respect to sports performance, injury prevention and injury rehabilitation. Additionally, he has worked in the development and evaluation of functional footwear in numerous projects.

Leon Chaitow was known internationally as the author of over 60 publications on natural health and complementary medicine, ranging from easy-to-understand guides on health issues and treatment approaches to reference books for healthcare students, practitioners and their clients. After graduating in osteopathy and naturopathy at the British College of Osteopathic Medicine in 1960, he went on to study acupuncture, cranial osteopathy and orthomolecular nutrition prior to working at Marylebone Health Centre (London) and being appointed as a Senior Lecturer, Module leader and member of the course design team at the School of Life Sciences, University of Westminster. He died in 2018, just a few weeks before the publication of the second edition of his book *Fascial Dysfunction*.

Dr Stefan Dennenmoser is a Certified Advanced Rolfer™ and Rolf Movement® Practitioner who is renowned for his gyrotonic and gyrokinesis training. He is also a Sports Scientist, Doctor of Human Biology, and a Member of Fascia Research at Ulm University (Germany).

Dr Jan Dommerholt is President/CEO of Bethesda Physiocare®, CEO of PhysioFitness, co-founder of The Center for Transformative Care (MD, USA), and co-founder and President/CEO of Myopain Seminars. He graduated as a Master of Professional Studies with specialization in Biomechanical Trauma and Healthcare Administration from Lynn University (FL, USA) and with a Doctorate in Physical Therapy from the University of St. Augustine for Health Sciences (FL, USA). He has written more than 70 book chapters and more than 100 articles on myofascial pain, dry needling, fibromyalgia, complex regional pain syndrome and manual physical therapy.

James Earls is a writer, lecturer and bodyworker who specializes in myofascial release, structural integration and functional movement. His research led to the development of Active Fascial Release, a blend of manual techniques and functional movement, and also to the publication of *Born to Walk*, in which he describes the myofascial system's contribution to an efficient gait.

Klaus Eder is a lecturer and instructor in manual therapy, physiotherapy and osteopathic physiotherapy. He has worked as a physiotherapist for the German Olympic (1984–2016), soccer (1988–2018) and Davis Cup (1990–2018) teams. Since 2002 he has been Head of Physiotherapy at the German Olympic Sports Confederation.

Dr Thomas Findley is Professor of Physical Medicine and Rehabilitation at Rutgers University New Jersey Medical School and is an associate member of the Cancer Institute of New York. He is also a co-founder of the International Fascia Research Congress. His research is focused on fascia, exercise and cancer.

Professor Martin S Fischer has been Director of the Institute for Zoology and Evolutionary Research at the University of Jena (Germany) since 1993. He has a deep interest in functional morphology, and he integrates computer modeling, biomechanics and robotics into his research. With co-workers, he has advanced the development of high-speed X-ray fluoroscopy and applied it to a large variety of tetrapods.

Eric Franklin (BSc, BFA) is a movement teacher and an expert in imagery training and its application to dance, movement and body therapies, about which he has written 23 books. He is the founder of The Franklin Method and Dynamic Neurocognitive Imagery, and teaches at the Juilliard School in New York, Bolshoi Ballet, Rutgers University, the University of Vienna, the Royal Ballet School and Trinity Laban in London.

Ann Frederick originally created Fascial Stretch Therapy™ (FST) in 1995 with specific protocols for collegiate athletes while working in the Athletics Department of Arizona State University. She further developed FST while working at the Olympics and Trials in 1996, 2000 and 2004, and thereafter in private practice, primarily with professional athletes. During this time she developed therapeutic applications for specific indications related to function and pain, and for pre-activity preparation and post-activity recovery.

Chris Frederick is a former professional dancer, and has been a sports and orthopedic physical therapist since 1989. He is a lead instructor at the Stretch to Win Institute and is also certified in Anatomy Trains® structural integration. In addition to carrying out original research on the effects of low back pain, he is co-author of *Fascial Stretch Therapy* and *Stretch to Win*.

Fernando Galán del Río is a physiotherapist and member of the Royal Spanish Football Federation medical team. He gained a Master's Degree in Osteopathy at the Universidad Rey Juan Carlos, Madrid, where he is currently a Professor in the Physical Therapy Department. Since 2000 he has conducted research into sports injuries and the mechanical behavior of soft tissues.

Paul Grilley teaches the theory of yoga with an emphasis on how skeletal variation impacts asana practice. He is the creator of three DVDs about yoga practice and is the author of *Yin Yoga: principles and practice*. He graduated with a Master's degree from St. John's College (Santa Fe) in 2000 and received an honorary PhD from the California Institute for Human Science in 2005.

Dr Mette Hansen gained her PhD at the Institute of Sports Medicine, Bispebjerg Hospital, Copenhagen University, in 2009. Three years later she was appointed associate professor at the Department for Public Health of Aarhus University (Denmark). She has published more than 50 scientific papers on the effects of hormones and nutrients on skeletal muscle structure, function and performance, and has won several investigation awards.

Robert Heiduk works as a performance and health consultant in a wide range of fields and co-founded the Athletic Conference, an elite sport conference and exhibition for strength and conditioning coaches in Germany. He is also a lecturer and author.

Helmut Hoffmann has more than 30 years' expertise in applied biomechanics in pro-sport rehabilitation after sport injuries, and more than 30 years of experience in medical training therapy in orthopedic/traumatologic rehabilitation. He has contributed to various publications, with a focus on sport-specific adaptation profiles, function-based rehabilitation conceptions and clinical performance diagnostics.

Dr Wilbour Kelsick (BSc, DC) is a Fellow of the College of Chiropractic Sport Sciences (Canada), a Fellow of the College of Chiropractic Rehabilitative Sciences (Canada) and a faculty member in the Department of Graduate Studies at the Canadian Memorial Chiropractic University. For more than 22 years he worked as a team doctor at the Olympics, World Championships and Commonwealth Games. He is the founder and director of the Maxfit Movement Institute and Teach Me to Run workshops.

ABOUT THE CONTRIBUTORS continued

Professor Michael Kjaer works in Sports Medicine at the University of Copenhagen. He is a medical doctor, a specialist in rheumatology, as well as Head of Institute of Sports Medicine at Bispebjerg Hospital (Copenhagen). His research focuses on adaptation of muscle and connective tissue to physical activity.

Professor Werner Klingler (MD, PhD) studied medicine at Ulm University (Germany) and Guy's and St. Thomas' hospitals (London) before continuing his training in Applied Physiology at Ulm University, where he also specialized as a clinical anesthesiologist in the field of complex pain medicine. He was a founding committee member of the first fascia research conference in 2007 and has received several honors, including the World Congress on Low Back Pain Award and the Vladimir Janda Award for Musculoskeletal Medicine.

Dr Frieder Krause (PhD) completed his Magister degree in Exercise Science, Sports Medicine and Psychology at the Goethe University Frankfurt. He is currently the head sport scientist at a sports and rehabilitation center in Kronberg. His research focuses on the effects of foam rolling and myofascial force transmission.

Elizabeth Larkam is internationally recognized as an innovator in movement education and practice. Her book *Fascia in Motion: Fascia-focused movement for Pilates* (Handspring, 2017) combines over 30 years of Pilates practice with 15 years of studying the neuromyofascial system. She was awarded the Medal of the Danish Society of Military Medicine in 2010 in recognition of her efforts to improve the rehabilitation of wounded soldiers.

Nathan Mayberry (PT, DPT, OCS, CSCS, CMTPT) received his Doctorate of Physical Therapy from the University of Maryland at Baltimore School of Medicine. Currently he is an instructor for Myopain Seminars, the first dry needling program in the USA. He has co-authored several book chapters and articles on myofascial pain, hypermobility and hypomobility, and specializes in the treatment of patients with chronic pain and Ehlers-Danlos syndrome.

Falk Mersmann studied sport science at the Humboldt-Universität zu Berlin. He completed his PhD thesis on the adaptation process of morphological and mechanical properties of muscles and tendons of young athletes in 2016. He currently works as a research assistant on specific questions of muscle and tendon plasticity, muscle-tendon interaction and motor control.

Dr Kurt Mosetter studied medicine in Freiburg (Germany) before investigating the concepts of Far Eastern medicine in India, Tibet and Nepal. He proceeded to create a specific and highly effective approach to therapy called Myoreflex Therapy.

Dr Hans-Wilhelm Müller-Wohlfahrt was trained in Berlin as a specialist in orthopedics and sports medicine. From 1977 he was the club doctor of Bayern Munich and from 1995 to 2018 he was the Germany national soccer team's doctor. In 2015, he and his team were honored with the prestigious Carl Rabl Prize for Muscle Injuries in Sports, and, in 2017, the Fascia Research Society awarded him the Clinical Pioneer Award.

Divo G. Müller is a natural-medicine practitioner and body therapist. She is known internationally as a pioneer of modern movement programs. Along with a team of scientists and respected movement therapists, she developed the successful training program Fascial Fitness. In addition to several book publications and DVDs, she has been featured in numerous TV and radio programs. She gives lectures and conducts workshops in and outside Europe, and offers a unique movement program at her studio in Munich, Germany.

Thomas Myers is the author of *Anatomy Trains*, the co-author of *Fascial Release for Structural Balance*, and has also written numerous articles for trade magazines and journals. He has also produced over 15 DVDs and numerous webinars on visual assessment, fascial release technique and the applications of fascial research.

P J O'Clair has been a leader and consultant in the fitness industry for 30 years. She is a Senior Master Instructor with TRX and MERRITHEW® and was instrumental in the research and development of the STOTT PILATES® for Breast Cancer Rehab program. She has written numerous articles for industry publications and was also a recipient of the 2008 IDEA Program Director of the Year award.

Bill Parisi is the founder and CEO of the Parisi Speed School and author of *Fascia Training: A Whole-System Approach.* He is also founder of the Fascia Training Academy. With an international team of coaches and facilities in more than 100 locations worldwide, the Parisi Speed School has trained more than 650,000 athletes between the ages of 7 and 18 and produced first-round draft picks in every professional sport—including more than 145 NFL draft picks—and a host of Olympic medalists and champion UFC fighters.

Sol Petersen is a Bachelor of Education in Adaptive Physical Education. Having worked as a Tai Ji teacher for more than 40 years, he co-founded the Mana Retreat Centre in New Zealand. He is also a structural integration trainer, movement coach, psychotherapist and aquatic therapist.

Dr Christian Puta (PhD) is Head of Research at the Department of Sports Medicine and Health Promotion and Head of Center for Interdisciplinary Prevention of Diseases related to Professional Activities at the Friedrich Schiller University Jena. His research focuses on sensorimotor control and visuo-motor interactions in chronic back pain, exercise immunology and neuromuscular aspects in young athletes.

Raúl Martínez Rodríguez (PT DO) has been a physiotherapist and osteopath in sport for 25 years. As the head of physiotherapy of the National Spanish Football Team, he has participated in the last 5 World Championships, as well as being a consultant in different European and World football clubs. He is the Director of the Tensegrity Clinic, a postgraduate professor at various Universities, as well as co-director of the Course of Assessment and Treatment of the Fascial System. He is currently a member of the Real Federación Española de Futbol Medical Scientific Commission.

John Sharkey is an international educator, author and authority in the areas of clinical anatomy, fascia, biotensegrity and the manual treatment of chronic pain. He is currently a senior lecturer within the Faculty of Medicine, Dentistry and Life Sciences, University of Chester/National Training Centre (Dublin) and program leader of the biotensegrity-focused Thiel soft fix cadaver dissection courses at the Department of Anatomy and Human Identification, Dundee University.

Susan Shockett (MS, BCSI, CPT) is a manual therapist and lifestyle medicine consultant in private practice in Manhattan, New York. She is a board-certified structural integrator, licensed massage therapist and certified personal trainer. She recently completed a MS degree in Exercise Science and Rehabilitation and is currently studying for an MPH degree in Nutrition.

Liane Simmel (MD) is an osteopath and former professional dancer who specializes in the treatment of dance injuries and runs her own dance medical practice in Munich. Her books *Dance Medicine in Practice* and *Nutrition for Dancers* are regarded as standards in the literature. In 2016, she was awarded the Prize of Recognition for her pioneering work in dance medicine.

Carla Stecco (MD) is an orthopedic surgeon and Professor of Human Anatomy at the University of Padova. She is also a founder member of the Fascial Manipulation Association and of the Fascial Research Society. She is the author of more than 100 papers devoted to studying the anatomy of the human fasciae from a macroscopical, histological and physiopathological perspective, as well as the book *Functional Atlas of Human Fasciae*.

ABOUT THE CONTRIBUTORS continued

Danielle Steffen is a PhD Candidate at the University of California, Davis interested in the molecular biology underlying musculoskeletal function. Her dissertation research is on load-based treatments for tendon repair. Danielle received her BS in Biological Science from UC Davis in 2017. Her undergraduate research was at the UC Davis Neuromuscular Research Center studying the cellular/ molecular mechanisms involved in Duchenne's Muscular Dystrophy. Danielle was also a member of the UC Davis Track and Field Team where she received honors as a NCAA Division I Track & Field, All Big West Conference Honoree.

Thomas Steidten (MA) is PhD student at the Department of Sports Medicine and Health Promotion at the Friedrich Schiller University Jena. His main research topic is exercise immunology and neuromuscular aspects in young athletes.

Dr Thorsten Sterzing has been a global leader in footwear innovation initiatives for 20 years, operating at the interface of industry and academia. He has enhanced understanding of how the structural properties of athletic footwear influence the biomechanical and subjective perception responses of its wearers. His research is focused on exercise physiology and human movement sciences with an emphasis on biomechanics.

Can A Yucesoy (BSc, MSc, PhD) is an expert in biomechanics, muscular mechanics and myofascial force transmission. Since June 2004 he has been Director of the Institute of Biomedical Engineering at Boğaziçi University (Istanbul).

Dr Alberto Zullo gained a Master's Degree in Biology and a PhD in Medical Biotechnology at the University of Naples Federico II. He is a researcher and lecturer in Applied and Clinical Biochemistry at the Department of Sciences and Technologies, University of Sannio (Benevento). He also works at the CEINGE Institute of Naples, where his research is focused on molecular characterization of human disorders resulting from the dysfunction of ion channels in skeletal and cardiac muscle cells.

FOREWORD

For many years both amateur and professional athletes have looked to exercise physiologists and trainers for ways to improve and maintain their performance, and avoid injury. 40 years ago, there was research relating to building muscle strength through concentric and eccentric exercise, with isometric, isokinetic and isotonic exercises as the building blocks spaced over various repetitions and intervals. This was followed by research about muscle loss with inactivity, and exercise to combat that loss, made particularly important by the space program. Muscle biopsies showed slow twitch and fast twitch fibers, with little conversion of fiber types from one to the other. When changes in force generated by muscles were seen in a matter of days, long before there was any demonstrable change in muscle fiber size, this was attributed to changes in the innervations and activation of the muscle. At the end of the day, however, all these studies led to the same conclusion: to improve performance in a specific activity (as opposed to strength in an isolated muscle), the best training is that activity itself, which involves motion of the whole body. The greatly expanded second edition of *Fascia for Sport and Movement*, with its 23 new chapters, goes far beyond this simplistic explanation and allows one to design specific exercise for different sports based on the increasingly recognized role of fascia in human performance.

The 18 chapters in Section 1, Theory, provide a basis to understand principles of the body-wide tensional network of fascia. There is a continuity of fibrils from the extracellular matrix through the integrin receptor and the cell membrane to the nucleus. It is a useful concept to think of the body as a fascial network with connections to muscles and bones, rather than the more traditional view of a musculoskeletal system with fascia connections. This suggests that the contraction of the trunk muscles prior to use of the superficial muscle slings described in Chapter 12 may not be just stabilizing the trunk—rather, it may be taking the slack out of core fascial layers to allow "prestretch" and energy storage for release later. Golfers and martial artists know the power in proper trunk rotation.

Many aspects of fascial physiology and biochemistry are presented in Chapter 1 and the reader is advised to start their study with this chapter. This will give a broad range of factors to be taken into account to understand the basis for the broad spectrum of clinical applications presented in the next section. Some factors are specific to fascia. Others, such as work hardening, are general properties of hardening by plastic deformation which have been used with copper, steel and other metals for thousands of years.

Skeletal muscle clearly responds to loading by hypertrophy and other adaptations which increase its capacity for force generation. Chapters 4 and 5 take this concept to connective tissue and explore loading in the context of adaptation or overloading pathology. For certain occupations, specific cycles of work/rest can be identified as tolerated or leading to functional loss. Again, task specificity is paramount. Without specific training, adult tendons show little change or remodeling, unless there is wound healing to be repaired. But to put this into perspective, connective tissue turnover every two days is found in the tiny fibers connecting a muscle to the nearby arteriole, which pull open the nitric oxide receptors and increase blood flow to the contracting muscle.

As described in Chapter 7, there are clear differences in mobility of tissues around the joints—with some people being more flexible than others. However, flexibility is not always a uniform function, and the astute clinician will find patients with flexible elbows and tight hamstrings, and vice versa. Indeed there are some rare muscle disorders characterized by certain tight and other loose joints. The theme of stretching to increase range in specific parts of the body is continued in Chapter 10, where again we find that practicing a task is the best way to prepare for that task performance. If we return to the notion that fascial tissues store energy for release during activities, we come to the logical conclusion that stretching these tissues to the point where their energy absorbing properties are altered will result in reduction in energy release and decreased subsequent performance. The mechanical interactions among muscle, tendon and fascia in humans have developed over many thousands of years to allow us to adapt to a wide range of activities, and we are just beginning to understand these to be able to direct such adaptation by specific exercises and activities which differ from the final desired task.

Models of movement based on muscles and bones have been challenged by the reality of motion which could not be explained. In the low back, lumbar fascia needed to be added to the model to account for movement capabilities. The running ability of a double amputee initially excluded from the regular Olympic Games for fear that his bilateral below knee prostheses gave him an artificial advantage over athletes with normal calf muscles, shows that lower leg muscles are not sufficient or even necessary forces in propelling the human body. Studies of storage of energy in tendon and other connective tissues showed their importance in human gait—it turns out the normal myofascial locomotor system in humans is indeed just slightly better than spring-based prostheses. And in animals such as the kangaroo, energy storage in tendons is critical in maintaining the repetitive patterns of locomotion. This is discussed in Chapter 8.

More recently, studies have shown that energy storage in tissues around the shoulder allows the human to throw at speeds over 100 miles an hour, compared to a meager 20 miles per hour in our closely related primate species. Pre-contraction of the muscle stretches connective tissues, which then explosively release to accomplish a movement for which muscle power alone would be insufficient. While in the leg large tendons are found in obvious positions to store this energy, this is not the case in the shoulder. Instead, the storage is diffused across a network of as yet undefined tissues, but the "wind up" for the pitch indicates the whole body is involved. Chapter 33 is now devoted to this.

Section 2, Assessment, has been similarly expanded from 2 to 4 chapters and provides some tools and techniques for assessment to gather evidence from the clinical examination to guide initiation of treatment and monitor progress.

Section 3, Clinical Applications, includes 13 new chapters and explores more clinical applications. To a greater or lesser extent, each of the chapters refers back to some of the basic physiology underlying these activities. By alternating study between Section 1 and Section 3, the reader will develop a facility for analyzing potentially beneficial therapies which will extend beyond the specific ones presented here. This is perhaps the most useful contribution of this book, to help the reader decide which of the many competing systems of therapy they will commit to studying further, and which they will incorporate fully or partially in their own clinical approach to their patients and clients. And most importantly, to start to identify which particular approaches will work for particular patients. I expect this book will become a well-worn and dog-eared addition to the library of clinicians from many disciplines.

Thomas W. Findley MD PhD
New Jersey, USA

February 2021

PREFACE

Fascia certainly connects—not only a large variety of collagenous tissues within the human body, ranging from tendons to joint capsules to muscular envelopes—but also the rapidly growing field of fascia-oriented explorations bringing together many different professional disciplines, personalities and perspectives. These include scientists, dance and movement professionals, and sports medicine celebrities. Our book is the first interdisciplinary publication to review scientific and practical approaches investigating the importance of fascia in sports and movement therapies. This second, and substantially revised edition, that you are currently holding, contains important updates and significant additions.

We, the editors, are proud of what has been accomplished in the following pages. In an extensive, and intensive, collaboration, we have included the top scientific experts in their fields as well as leading figures from different practical approaches such as strength and conditioning, yoga, Pilates, sports rehabilitation, kettlebell training, martial arts, plyometrics, dance medicine and many others.

Note that the range of professional perspectives varies about as much as the different fibrous tissues that are connected with each other as parts of the body-wide fascial net. Based on this, the scope of this book purposely embraces different opinions. For example, the myofascial chains of our colleague, Thomas Myers, are described with their most recent and impressive advances together with detailed practical applications. However, this new edition also includes a critical review of such linear force transmission models when viewed from an anatomical and evidence-oriented perspective. As such, we present many exciting answers and a multitude of reliable and novel information. However, in addition, it also offers new inspiring questions, careful hypothetical speculations, as well as clinical observations that we consider well founded and clinically valuable.

Other new chapters in the theoretical section of the book address the influence of sex hormones on fascial connective tissues, the topics of nutrition, fluid dynamics, biotensegrity, hypo- and hypermobility, injury prevention and oncology. The section on clinical applications is now expanded by new chapters on eccentric training, foam rolling, walking, throwing, footwear, fascial strength training, mental imagery, and on periodized fascia training. And finally, a completely new section has been inserted, oriented on assessment methods and including new chapter contributions on joint mobility examination, ultrasound imaging techniques and mechanical assessment.

A huge thank you has to be expressed to our 51 authors, all of whom have endeavoured to deliver an optimal contribution from their field for this exploration of a new and promising territory. In addition, the team at Handspring Publishing has been wonderful in their enthusiastic support of our project. Their extensive publishing experience and personal familiarity with the field have been beyond anything that we could have imagined. The pioneering excitement, which is almost palpable at the ongoing congress series in 'Connective Tissues in Sports Medicine', and which continues to shape the different networking projects within this expanding field, has provided a strong motivational back-drop for all involved in this book. We trust that the reader will not only notice the exciting collaborative spirit of this new adventure but will also benefit from the resulting wealth of information and the quality of contributions from our international team.

Robert Schleip, Munich, Germany
Jan Wilke, Frankfurt, Germany
Amanda Baker, Shoreham-by-Sea, England

February, 2021

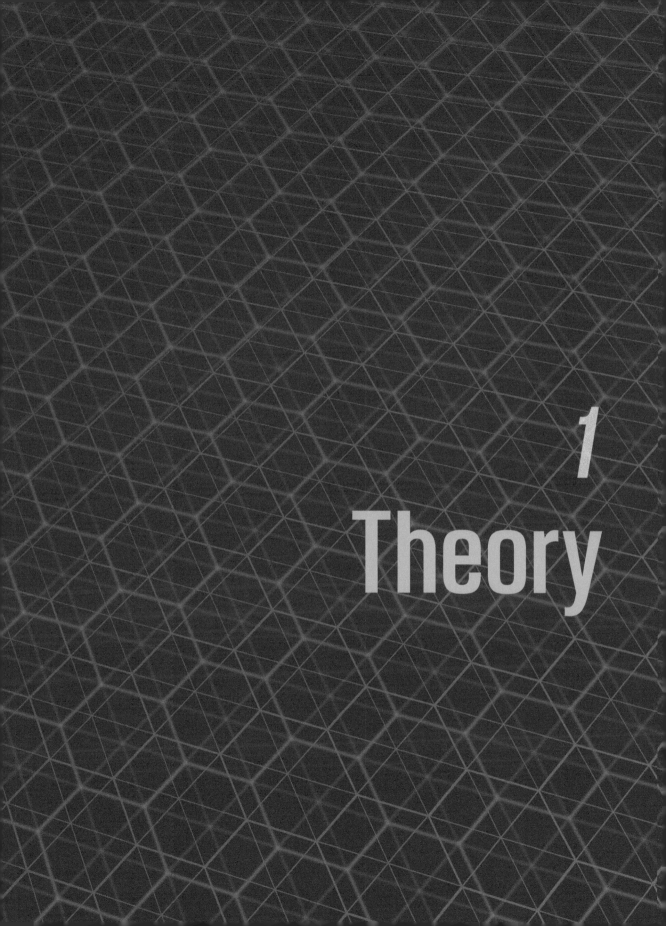

1
Theory

Highlights of fascial anatomy, morphology and function

Robert Schleip and Werner Klingler

Fascia: more than an inert packing organ

After several decades of a Cinderella-like neglect, fascia has entered the limelight within the field of human life sciences. While literally thrown away in most anatomical dissections, this colorless fibrous tissue has mostly been treated as a dull and inert packaging organ. There are several reasons for this neglect, one of which is the lack of clear distinctions, based on the ubiquitous and seemingly disordered nature of this tissue, compared with the shiny muscles and organs underneath. Another and more important reason for the severe neglect of scientific attention concerned the lack of adequate measurement tools. While x-ray imaging allowed a detailed study of bones and the electromyography of muscles, for many decades, changes in fascia were difficult to measure. For example, the fascia lata or lumbar fascia is typically less than 2 mm thick, and a local increase in thickness of 20% was too small to be seen by ultrasound (or any other affordable imaging technology in clinical practice), although it may be easily palpable to the hand of a therapist and may also be felt by the client during movement.

This unfortunate situation has changed significantly in recent years. Advances in ultrasound measurement, as well as in histology, have contributed to an increase in fascia-related studies (Chaitow et al., 2012). Examples of some of the novel insights within the rapidly advancing field of international fascia research include the role of the human thoracolumbar fascia as a potential source of low back pain (Wilke et al., 2017), the discovery of fasciacytes as a new type of connective tissue cell (see Chapter 9), and the recognition of a close link between the sympathetic nervous system and active fascial tonicity (Schleip et al., 2019). Clinical fields whose practitioners have an avid interest and participation in this process include manual therapies, physiotherapy, scar treatment, oncology (based on the matrix-dependent behavior of cancer cells), surgery and rehabilitative medicine. Similarly, sports science is embracing these developments. The first congresses on Connective tissues in sports medicine, hosted at Ulm University in 2013 and 2017, served as an important impetus for the development of this field. Today, fascia has become a favored new subject in conferences for sports sciences as well as among movement teachers.

"A fascia" and "the fascial system"

Most classical anatomy textbooks contain several descriptions of specific fasciae with clear definitions of its anatomical position and main functions. Examples include Osborne's fascia as an outer sheath of the cubital tunnel or the thoracolumbar fascia covering back muscles and spanning from spine to pelvis. However, only those membranous connective tissue structures

Chapter 1

that could easily be dissected with a conventional scalpel (and without use of a microscope) were labeled fasciae. Other collagenous structures, such as tendons, aponeuroses or the small tubular endomysium layers within the intramuscular connective tissue, were excluded. Due to the diverse form and function of fasciae, it is impossible to conclusively define the fascia. However, there are morphological and functional key elements which have been identified as common properties of a fascia. Since the use of the term fascia is non-uniform, an expert Fascia Nomenclature Committee, consisting of anatomists, physiologists, biologists and clinicians, was established in 2014.

According to this committee, the new functional terminology (see the box below) defines fascia as all components that form an interconnected collagenous three-dimensional continuum of soft collagen containing loose and dense fibrous connective tissues that permeate the body (Schleip et al., 2019).

Functional definition of the fascial system

The fascial system consists of the three-dimensional continuum of soft collagen containing loose and dense fibrous connective tissues that permeate the body.

It incorporates elements such as adipose tissue, adventitiae and neurovascular sheaths, aponeuroses, deep and superficial fasciae, epineurium, joint capsules, ligaments, membranes, meninges, myofascial expansions, periostea, retinacula, septa, tendons, visceral fasciae and all the intramuscular and intermuscular connective tissues, including endomysium/perimysium/epimysium.

The fascial system surrounds, interweaves between and interpenetrates all organs, muscles, bones and nerve fibers, endowing the body with a functional structure and providing an environment that enables all body systems to operate in an integrated manner.

While a narrower fascia terminology is still recommended for more detail-oriented descriptions in the classical fields of histology and microscopic anatomy (see the box below), the expert panel suggests using this new and wider definition for the description and discussion of functional fascia properties, such as force transmission, sensory capacities, fibrotic pathologies or wound healing. Congruently, this will be the terminology used for most of the subsequent chapters in this book. While all connective tissues—including, for example, cartilage and bone—are derivatives of the embryological mesenchyme, only some of them are considered to be part of the fascial system, and only those with very special architecture are referred to as "proper fascia" (Figure 1.1).

Histological/anatomical definition of "a fascia"

A fascia is a sheath, a sheet or any other dissectible aggregation of connective tissue that forms beneath the skin to attach, enclose and separate muscles and other internal organs.

In terms of force transmission, the expression of a collagen fiber network tends to be associated with repeated tensional strain demands. The specific shape of a fascial tissue depends on the local history of these tensional forces. If the local tensional demands are mostly unidirectional and have involved high loads, then the fascial net will express these in the shape of a tendon or ligament. In other circumstances, it may express them as a two-directional or multidirectional membrane, or as a loose fibrous areolar safron (Figure 1.2). The term "fascia" is, thus, fairly synonymous with the layperson's understanding of the term "connective tissue" (although in medical science the term

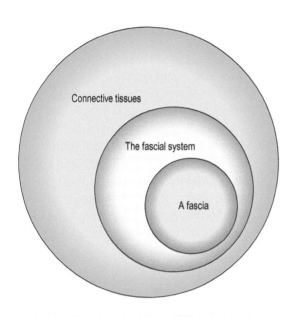

Figure 1.1

The nomenclature recommendations of the Fascial Nomenclature Committee are based on the understanding that the wider and more functional term, "the fascial net" (which some authors replace with "fascial tissues"), describes a subset of tissues belonging to the connective tissue system of the body. Similarly, the term, "a fascia" (also called "proper fascia" by some authors), describes a subset of tissues within the larger category of "the fascial system".

Illustration from Schleip et al. (2019).

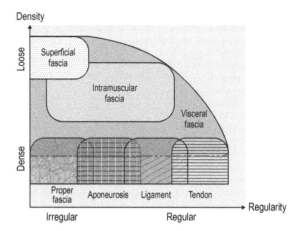

Figure 1.2 Different connective tissues as specializations of the global fascial net

In the new functional terminology, all collagenous fibrous connective tissues are considered as being part of the fascial system. These tissues differ in terms of their density and the directional alignment of collagen fibers. For example, superficial fascia is characterized by a relatively low density and mostly multidirectional or irregular fiber alignment, whereas in the denser tendons or ligaments, the fibers are mostly unidirectional. Note that the intramuscular fasciae—septi, perimysium and endomysium—may express varying degrees of directionality and density. The same is true for the visceral fasciae, like the very soft greater omentum in the belly or the much tougher pericardium. Depending on local loading history, fascia proper can express a unidirectional lattice-like or multidirectional arrangement.

Illustration courtesy of fascialnet.com.

"connective tissue" includes bones, cartilage and even blood, all of which derive from the embryonic mesenchyme tissue).

A body-wide interconnected tensional network

An advantage of this new and more encompassing terminology is that it recognizes the widespread continuities of this fibrous network, while still allowing for a detailed description of the local architecture. Note that, in contrast to the simplified anatomical textbook illustrations, the collagenous tissues around major joints in the human body express large areas of gradual transition, where a clear distinction between ligament, capsule, tendon, septum or muscular envelope is virtually impossible.

Force transmission from the muscle to the skeleton also involves more extramuscular myofascial delineations than was classically assumed. This insight constitutes a challenge to the classical biomechanical concepts in musculoskeletal medicine, in which many experts considered the mechanical importance of fascial envelopes to be roughly similar to the wrapping of an average gift in relation to its content. Just as most gifts function equally well without their wrapping, it had been considered that the function of a muscle could be understood when studying its origin, insertion and myofiber orientation in a fascia-free condition. In contrast to this common assumption, the extensive work of Huijing (2007) has shown impressively how muscles transmit up to 40% of their contraction force not into their respective tendon, but rather via fascial connections into other muscles that are positioned next to them. Interestingly, this often involves force transmission to antagonistic muscles, which are then co-stiffened and tend to increase resistance to this primary movement. An increase of this particular force transmission to antagonistic muscles has been shown to be an important complication in many spastic contractures (Huijing, 2007).

Important muscular force transmissions, via their fascial connections, have been shown between:

- latissimus dorsi and contralateral gluteus maximus via the lumbodorsal fascia (Barker et al., 2004);
- biceps femoris to the erector spinae fascia via the sacrotuberous ligament (Vleeming et al., 1995);
- biceps brachii and the flexor muscles of the lower arm via the lacertus fibrosis (Brasseur, 2012);
- gluteus maximus and lower leg muscles via the fascia lata (Stecco et al., 2013).

Ingber (1998) showed that the architecture of cells can be understood to behave like a tensegrity structure. In a tensegrity structure the compressional elements (struts) are suspended without any compressional contact towards each other, whereas the tensional elements (elastic bands or membranes) are all connected with one another in a global tension-transmitting network. This model served as a basic inspiration for the field of fascia research. Driven by the observation that healthy human bodies express a higher degree of tensegrity-like qualities in their movements, many clinicians as well as scientists have started to see the fascial web as the elastic elements of a tensegrity structure, in which bones and cartilage are suspended as spacers, rather than as classical weight-bearing structures (Levin, 2003). While this is based on the assumption that the human body is a pure tensegrity structure, it has been argued that a proper understanding of the complex force transmission dynamics in the human body should also include rheological (fluid sheer motion-orientated) properties in which sponge-like motion resistance patterns play important contributing factors as well (Bordoni et al., 2019). Nevertheless, the above examples of myofascial force transmission across several joints show that a tensegrity-inspired perspective offers an improved understanding of the fascial net and its role in musculoskeletal dynamics.

Components of fascial tissues

Fascial connective tissues basically consist of two components, cells plus the extracellular matrix (Figure 1.3). Unlike most other tissues, the cells take up a very minor part of the total volume (usually less than 5%). Most of the cells are fibroblasts, which function as construction and maintenance workers for the surrounding matrix. The matrix consists of two parts: ground substance and fibers. The ground substance consists mostly of water, which is bound by proteoglycans. Most of the fibers are collagen fibers, except for a few elastin fibers.

Highlights of fascial anatomy, morphology and function

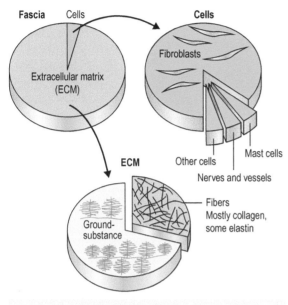

Figure 1.3 Components of fascia

The basic constituents are cells (mostly fibroblasts) and extracellular matrix (ECM), the latter of which consists of fibers plus the watery ground substance.

Illustration courtesy of fascialnet.com.

A common misconception is that ground substance and the matrix are sometimes taken as synonyms. However, the net of collagen fiber is an important matrix element. The overall architecture of the matrix can be compared with a composite structure in engineering, in which a mesh of sturdy cables is combined with a more amorphic material to provide optimum mechanical strength in multi-directional loading.

Except for water, which is extruded by the small arterioles in fascia, most of the constituents are produced, remodeled and maintained by the resident fibroblasts. These cells are responsive to mechanical stimulation as well as to biochemical stimulation. Biochemical stimulation includes the effect of inflammatory cytokines, several other cytokines, hormones, as well as changes in pH level (acidity of the ground substance). For example, human growth hormone (HGH), most of which is produced during sleep, is an important requirement for collagen production. As many bodybuilders who have experimented with HGH have discovered, muscle growth is only minimally affected by this important hormone. However, there is a clear effect on collagen production and proper collagen synthesis as renewal is dependent on a sufficient supply of HGH, which effectively acts as an important fertilizer (Kjaer et al., 2009).

Biomechanical stimulation is at least as important for tissue health as the biochemical environment. In fact, without proper mechanical stimulation, fascial fibroblasts will not create an adequate fibrous matrix, no matter how good or bad their biochemical environment is. While nutritional care can improve the biochemical milieu, sports and movement therapies are potent tools for fostering optimal biomechanical stimulation for the matrix remodeling behavior of the fibroblasts. Fibroblasts are equipped with numerous devices to sense the tensional and mechanical shear stimulation exerted upon them. In response to this, they constantly change their metabolic function.

Adaptability to mechanical loading

For a connective tissue-oriented training approach, it is key to understand that the local architecture of this network adapts to the specific history of previous strain-loading demands (Blechschmidt, 1978; Chaitow, 1988). Collagen shows an enormous adaptability to the demands in the gravitational field. For example, the human biped has developed a unique structure: the dense fascia lata on the outside of the thigh, which enables us to stabilize the hips in walking, running and hopping. No other animal, not even our genetically closest relative the chimpanzee, shows this kind of fascial feature. These fascial sheets on the lateral side of the thigh will develop a more palpable firmness than on the medial side in those who walk or run regularly. In an individual who prefers a sedentary lifestyle, or a patient in a wheelchair with almost no leg movement, this difference in tissue stiffness is scarcely found. By contrast, for regular horse riders the opposite is true: after a few months, the fascia on the medial thigh tends to become dense and strong (El-Labban et al., 1993).

Good news for tissue renewal: if the connective structures are loaded properly, the inherent networking cells, called fibroblasts, adapt their matrix remodeling activity so that the tissue architecture responds even better to daily demands. Not only does the density of bone change, as happens with astronauts who spend time in zero gravity, wherein the bones become more porous (Ingber, 2008), fascial tissues also react to their dominant loading patterns. With the help of the fibroblasts, they slowly but constantly react to everyday strain as well as to specific training (Kjaer et al., 2009). Their remodeling activity is particularly responsive to repeated challenges to the mechanical integrity of their surrounding matrix. Challenges to the tissue's strength, extensibility and ability to shear will stimulate the fibroblasts to respond in a process of constant reconstructing and rearrangement of the fascial web.

Preload for effective muscle contraction

Most notably, muscle contraction is indispensably linked to external preload given by adjacent fasciae. Skeletal muscle is a sophisticated system formed by aggregation and differentiation of satellite cells into a single muscle fiber, which is a so-called functional syncytium. The main contents of this composite are the contractile proteins, actin and myosin, which are aligned in a highly ordered manner and, together with other proteins, form the striated appearance of skeletal muscle. The basic contractile units, named sarcomeres, are arranged repetitively within the muscle fiber and have a mean resting length of ~2.2 μm. Optimum overlap of actin and myosin filaments is decisive for the generation of muscle force. *In vivo* the preload of muscle fibers is determined by the fascial system. *In vitro* this preload has to be simulated by mechanical pre-stretch of the isolated muscle fibers, otherwise muscle contractility is tremendously reduced or absent (Hoppe et al., 2014). Hence, fascial preload is necessary for effective force generation.

Fascia in sports science

In sports science, and in recent sports education, the prevailing emphasis has been on the classical triad of muscular training, cardiovascular conditioning and neuromuscular coordination (Jenkins, 2005). Comparatively little attention was given to a specifically targeted training of the connective tissues involved. This widespread practice has not taken into consideration the major role that the collagenous connective tissues play in sports associated with overuse injuries. Whether in running, soccer, baseball, swimming or gymnastics, the vast majority of associated repetitive strain injuries occur in the muscular collagenous connective tissues, such as tendons, ligaments or joint capsules. Even in so-called "muscle tears" the specific ruptures rarely occur within the red myofibers but rather within the white collagenous portions of the overall muscle structure. It seems that in these instances, the respective collagenous tissues have been less adequately prepared—and less well adapted to their loading challenge—than their muscular or skeletal counterparts (Wilke et al., 2019).

Highlights of fascial anatomy, morphology and function

Of course, any muscular training also trains the connective tissues involved, although in a non-specific and usually non-optimal manner. This is comparable with the suboptimal effect of cardiovascular endurance training on muscular strength and vice versa. Similarly, all sports training will stimulate collagen remodeling "somehow". Recent fascia-orientated training suggestions, therefore, propose that a specifically tailored connective tissue training may yield the same training enhancements as a tailored strength training, coordination training or cardiovascular fitness program does for their specific target functions.

Getting the spring back in your step

One of the most inspiring aspects for movement and sports practitioners, within this rapidly advancing field of new scientific revelations about fascia, is the ability of tendons and aponeuroses to store and release kinetic energy. This will be addressed in detail in Chapter 8. Given the right architecture of the loaded collagenous structures, and given sufficient sensorimotor refinement for sensing the appropriate resonance frequency, seemingly effortless elastic recoil motions can then be performed.

The usually higher elastic storage quality in young people is reflected in their fascial tissues showing a typical two-directional lattice arrangement, like the regular arrangement of fibers in a stocking (Staubesand et al., 1997). Aging is usually associated with a loss of elasticity, bounce and springiness in our gait, and this is also reflected in the fascial architecture (Figures 1.4 and 1.5). Here, the fibers proliferate

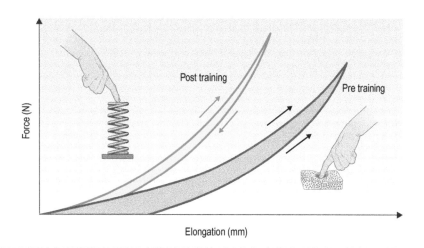

Figure 1.4 Decreased hysteresis in trained tendons

In the tendinous tissues of rats, which had to practice rapid treadmill running on a regular schedule, there were increases in elastic storage capacity, compared with their non-running peers. See the double curve on the left. The area between the respective loading versus unloading curves represents the amount of hysteresis, which is a measure for the loss of kinetic energy. The smaller hysteresis of the trained animals (left double curve) reveals their more elastic tissue storage capacity. The larger hysteresis of their non-running peers, by contrast, signifies their more viscoelastic tissue properties, also referred to as inertia. Note that compared with the original data the relative differences between the two double curves have been exaggerated for better understanding.

Illustration courtesy of fascialnet.com, modified after Reeves et al., 2006.

Chapter 1

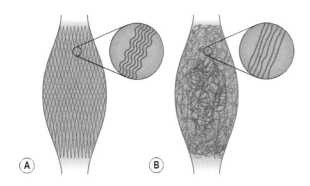

Figure 1.5 Collagen fibers respond to loading

Healthy fasciae (left image) express a clear two-directional (lattice) orientation of their collagen fiber network. In addition, the individual collagen fibers show a stronger crimp formation. Lack of exercise, on the other hand, has been shown to induce a multidirectional fiber network and a reduction in crimp formation, leading to a loss of springiness and elastic recoil (right image).

Illustration courtesy of fascialnet.com.

and take on an irregular arrangement. Animal experiments have shown that immobilization quickly leads to a dysregulation in fiber arrangement and to a multidirectional growth of additional cross-links between dense collagen fibers. Consequently, the fibers lose their elasticity as well as the smooth gliding motion against one another, and then they stick together forming tissue adhesions over time and, at worst, they become matted together (Jarvinen et al., 2002).

Taking a closer look at the microstructure of the collagen fibers reveals undulations, called crimp, which are reminiscent of elastic springs. In older people, or in those whose fascial fibers suffer from immobilization, then the structure of the fiber appears rather flattened, losing both crimp and springiness (Staubesand et al., 1997). Research has confirmed the previously optimistic assumption that proper exercise loading of the fibers, if applied regularly, can induce a more youthful collagen architecture. This regains a wavier fiber arrangement (Wood et al., 1988; Jarniven et al., 2002) and expresses a significantly increased elastic storage capacity (Figures 1.4 and 1.5) (Reeves et al., 2006; Witvrouw et al., 2007).

Given a proper elastic resilience in the fascial tissues of feet and legs, less cushioning may be required as external shock absorption in one's shoes. Habitual barefoot running, as well as running with minimalistic shoes, tends to involve an earlier forefoot contact with the ground compared with conventionally shod running. This seems to involve a higher storage capacity within the fasciae of foot and lower leg compared with shod running (Tam et al., 2014). Interestingly, this increase in elastic storage quality is more strongly expressed in barefoot running than in running with minimalistic shoes (Bonacci et al., 2013), possibly due to the role of proprioceptive stimulation involvement in barefoot contact with the ground. However, due to the slow speed of fascial adaption (see pages 12–13), transition to more "natural" footwear should be performed even more gradually than is recommended by most conservative instructions, due to the high likelihood of overuse injuries (such as bone marrow edema) during the change-over time (Ridge et al., 2013).

Mechanoadaptation and Davis' law

Wolff's law states that dense connective tissues are able to adapt their morphology to mechanical loading. While this general law was originally developed with its main focus on skeletal tissues, Davis' law applies this general principle in particular to collagenous connective tissues (Figure 1.6). It proposes that these tissues tend to adapt their architecture to the specific mechanical demands imposed upon them, provided that these demands are strong enough, and occur in a regular manner. More recently, this concept has been taken further by the mechanostat

Highlights of fascial anatomy, morphology and function

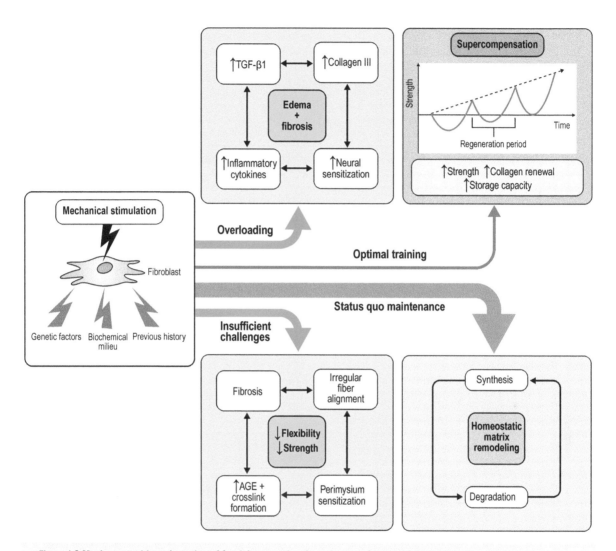

Figure 1.6 Mechanosensitive adaptation of fascial connective tissue in accordance with Davis' law

In a similar manner to bony connective tissue (described by Wolff's law), fibroblasts adapt their architectural remodeling work on collagenous connective tissue to the mechanical stimulation experienced. Both overstress and chronic underuse can trigger fibrotization. In the case of overstress, this is mostly a "wet" matting process, which is associated with inflammatory processes and the formation of edemas. The rather drier matting of underuse is characterized by a crystalline embrittlement (through what is known as advanced glycation end products) of the ground substance and the other cross-link formations. In other words, the tissue becomes crisper and less flexible. The relatively narrow stimulation range for a sustainable increase in resilience (green arrow), however, is characterized by a sufficiently high dose of challenging stress combined with appropriate regeneration times. AGE, advanced glycation end product; TGF-β1, transforming growth factor-β1.

Chapter 1

theory of Frost (1972), emphasizing that tendons, ligaments and fascia adapt their cross-sectional diameter and, correspondingly, also their stiffness in response to the muscular forces imposed upon them. However, the threshold value of mechanical loading to trigger adaptational effects for tendon is significantly higher for tendons than for muscle. While exercises performed at only 50% of maximum voluntary contraction power are sufficient to trigger an adaptational response in muscle fibers, the involved tendinous connective tissues show very little adaptational response at that impact level: they require much stronger loads in order to respond. Arampatzis et al. (2007) have shown that for the Achilles tendon and aponeurosis, a strain of 4–5% tends to be required for eliciting an adaptational response, while a strain of 2–3% is clearly insufficient. Both of these values tend to be above the magnitude of habitual daily activities. Note that the high impact loading required for an adaptational response may then be only 35% below the amount of strain at which tendon injuries do occur (Wren et al., 2001). Interestingly, the threshold for an adaptational response of intramuscular fasciae seems to be significantly lower than that for tendons (Kjaer et al., 2015).

Once the respective threshold has been reached, the adaptational response of the fibroblasts seems to be largely independent of the quantity of strain application involved in an exercise session. It is possible that only 10 or 20 elastic bounces may be required for an adaptational response, while adding 100 or more repetitions tends to have very little additional effect (Magnusson et al., 2010).

High doses of sudden tensile stress stimulate the excretion of pro-inflammatory messenger substances by the fibroblasts. Applied in the right context and with an appropriate dosage, this can be interpreted as the start of healthy repair and adaptation processes.

However, if not merely a few dozen, but rather hundreds of thousands of sudden microstrains of this kind are administered one after the other, this can then easily lead to a state of non-completion in the wound-healing dynamic (stagnating or becoming more chronically activated). This could be a frequent maladaptation dynamic in repetitive strain syndrome.

Several weeks of immobilization (such as when a cast is applied or due to a chronic lack of movement in an area of the joint), however, can lead to the formation of additional cross-links or to the matting of the collagenous architecture. The tissue then becomes brittle and less flexible. The individual collagen fibers lose their natural corrugation (known as crimp), which is typical in active and/or young people (see also Chapter 8). Apart from these remodeling activities, the fibroblasts reduce their metabolic activity and power down into standby mode.

How fast do fascial tissues change?

How rapid is the adaptation process? This seems to depend on what elements are examined. Some of the denser collagen cables in the Achilles tendon, which are composed of particularly thick collagen type 1 fiber bundles, are not replaced until the end of the skeletal growth period and show zero turnover after that age. At the other end of the spectrum, many of the proteoglycans in the water-binding ground substance are constantly remodeled in a matter of days. For the particular collagen fibers in cartilage, the half-life has been calculated as 100 years, while in skin this has been estimated as 15 years. More recent labeling techniques examining collagen proteins from Achilles and patellar tendons suggest a fractional of 1% per day for the collagen of intramuscular fasciae. The same study estimated the turnover rate of collagen tissues to be ~2–3-fold slower than the respective rate for skeletal muscle fibers (Miller et al., 2005). In summary, the remodeling speed of the body-wide fascial network is quite slow, with an average fiber renewal time of between months and years rather than days or weeks.

Fascia science put into daily practice

It is proposed that, in order to build up an injury-resistant and elastic fascial body network, it is essential to translate current insights from the field of fascia research into practical training programs. Adequately tailored training can improve the elastic storage capacity of the stimulated fascial tissues (Figure 1.4).

Recent studies have shown that during the first 2–3 days after appropriate exercise loading, collagen synthesis is increased. However, collagen degradation is also increased and, interestingly, during the first 1.5 days, the degradation outweighs the synthesis (Figure 1.7). Only afterwards does the resulting net synthesis of collagen production become positive. It is, therefore, assumed that daily strong exercise loading could lead towards a weaker collagen structure. Based on this, it is recommended that fascial tissues should be properly exercised 2–3 times per week only, in order to allow for adequate collagen renewal (Magnusson et al., 2010).

Several training recommendations for fostering an optimal remodeling of fascial tissues have been proposed, and these will be explored in the second section of this book. They attempt to translate an understanding of fascial properties into specific movement instructions or treatment recommendations. Based on their particular emphasis, they promise to foster a

stronger, faster, younger, more elastic, refined, resilient, flexible, and, above all, more injury-resistant mobility of our bodies. As this general field is fairly new within sports science, very few of these promises have, to date, been clinically proven (these are mentioned in their respective chapters). For the vast majority of these claims, only anecdotal evidence exists, which, of course may be prone to multiple biases based on evangelic expectations. Future critical research, possibly based on the measurement tools described in the last sections of this book, will reveal to what degree these promising beneficial effects are achieved.

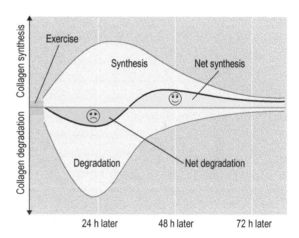

Figure 1.7 Collagen turnover after exercise

The upper curve demonstrates how collagen synthesis is increased after exercise. After 24 hours, the synthesis is increased 2-fold compared with the previous condition at rest. However, as an additional effect of exercise, the stimulated fibroblasts also increase their rate of collagen degradation. Interestingly, during the first 1–2 days, collagen degradation outweighs the collagen synthesis, whereas afterwards, this situation is reversed. Based on this, training recommendations aimed at improving connective tissue strength suggest exercising 2–3 times per week only. Data based on Miller et al. (2009).

Illustration courtesy of fascialnet.com, modified after Magnusson et al. (2010).

References

Arampatzis, A., Karamanidis, K., & Albracht, K. (2007) Adaptational responses of the human Achilles tendon by modulation of the applied cyclic strain magnitude. *J Exp Biol*. 210: 2743–2753.

Arampatzis, A., Peper, A., Bierbaum, S., & Albracht, K. (2010) Plasticity of human Achilles tendon mechanical and morphological properties in response to cyclic strain. *J Biomech*. 43: 3073–3079.

Barker, P.J., Briggs, C.A., & Bogeski, G. (2004) Tensile transmission across the lumbar fasciae in unembalmed cadavers: effects of tension to various muscular attachments. *Spine*. 29: 129–138.

Blechschmidt, E. (1978) In: Charles, C. (Ed.), *Biokinetics and Biodynamics of Human Differentiation: Principles and Applications*. Springfield, IL: Thomas.

Bonacci, J., Saunders, P.U., Hicks, A.,Rantalainen, T.,Vicenzino, B.G., & Spratford, W. (2013) Running in a minimalist and lightweight shoe is not the same as running bare-foot: a biomechanical study. *Br J Sports Med*. 47: 387–392.

Bordoni, B., Varacallo, M.A., Morabito, B., & Simonelli, M. (2019) Biotensegrity or Fascintegrity? *Cureus*. 11: e4819.

Brasseur, J.L. (2012) The biceps tendons: From the top and from the bottom. *J Ultrasound*. 15: 29–38.

Chaitow, L. (1988) S*oft-tissue Manipulation: A Practitioner's Guide to the Diagnosis and Treatment of Soft-tissue Dysfunction and Reflex Activity*. Rochester, VT: Healing Arts Press.

Chaitow, L., Findley, T.W., & Schleip, R. (Eds.) (2012) *Fascia research III – Basic science and implications for conventional and complementary health care*. Munich, Germany: Kiener Press.

El-Labban, N.G., Hopper, C., & Barber, P. (1993) Ultrastructural finding of vascular degeneration in myositis ossificans circum-scripta (fibrodysplasia ossificans). *J Oral Pathol Med*. 22: 428–431.

Frost, M.F. (1972) T*he physiology of cartilaginous, fibrous, and bony tissue*. Springfield, IL: C.C. Thomas.

Hoppe, K., Schleip, R., Lehmann-Horn, F., Jäger, H., & Klingler, W. (2014) Contractile elements in muscular fascial tissue - Implications for *in-vitro* contracture testing for malignant hyperthermia. *Anaesthesia* 69: 1002–1008.

Huijing, P.A. (2007) Epimuscular myofascial force transmission between antagonistic and synergistic muscles can explain movement limitation in spastic paresis. *J Electromyogr Kinesiol*. 17: 708–724.

Ingber, D.E. (1998) The architecture of life. *Scientific American*. January, 48–57.

Ingber, D.E. (2008) Tensegrity and mechanotransduction. *J Bodyw Mov Ther*. 12: 198–200.

Jarvinen, T.A., Jozsa, L., Kannus, P., Jarvinen, T.L., & Jarvinen, M. (2002) Organization and distribution of intramuscular connective tissue in normal and immobilized skeletal muscles. An immunohistochemical, polarization and scanning electron microscopic study. *J Musc Res Cell Mot*. 23: 245–254.

Jenkins, S. (2005) Sports Science Handbook. In: *The Essential Guide to Kinesiology, Sport & Exercise Science*, vol. 1. Essex, UK: Multiscience Publishing.

Kjaer, M., Jørgensen, N.R., Heinemeier, K., & Magnusson, S.P. (2015) Exercise and Regulation of Bone and Collagen Tissue Biology. In: Bouchard, C. (Ed.), *Molecular and Cellular Regulation of Adaptation to Exercise*. Waltham, MA: Elsevier Academic Press, 259–291.

Kjaer, M., Langberg, H., Heinemeier, K., Bayer, M.L., Hanse, M., Holm, L., Doessing, S., Kongsgaard, M., Krogsgaard, M.R., & Magnusson, S.P. (2009) From mechanical loading to collagen synthesis, structural changes and function in human tendon. *Scand J Med Sci Sports*. 19: 500–510.

Kubo, K., Kanehisa, H., Miyatani, M., Tachi, M., & Fukunaga, T. (2003) Effect of low-load resistance training on the tendon properties in middle-aged and elderly women. *Acta Physiol Scand*. 178: 25–32.

Levin, S.L., & Martin, D. (2012) Biotensegrity: The mechanics of fascia. In: Schleip, R. et al. (Eds). *Fascia – the tensional network of the human body.* Edinburgh, UK: Elsevier, 137–142.

Magnusson, S.P., Langberg, H., & Kjaer, M. (2010) The pathogenesis of tendinopathy: balancing the response to loading. *Nature Rev Rheumat.* 6: 262–268.

Miller, B.F., Olesen, J.L., Hansen M., Døssing, S., Crameri, R.M., Welling, R.J., Langberg, H., Flyvbjerg, A., Kjaer, M., Babraj, J.A., Smith, K., & Rennie, M.J. (2005) Coordinated collagen and muscle protein synthesis in human patella tendon and quadriceps muscle after exercise. *J Physiol.* 567: 1021–1033.

Reeves, N.D., Narici, M.V., & Maganaris, C.N. (2006) Myotendinous plasticity to aging and resistance exercise in humans. *Exp Physiol.* 91: 483–498.

Ridge, S.T., Johnson, A.W., Mitchell, U.H., Hunter, I., Robinson, E., Rich, B.S., & Brown, S.D. (2013) Foot bone marrow edema after a 10-wk transition to minimalist running shoes. *Med Sci Sports Exerc.* 45: 1363–1368.

Schleip, R., Hedley, G., & Yukesoy, C. (2019) Fascial nomenclature: Update on related consensus process. *Clin Anat.* 32: 929–933.

Schleip, R., & Klingler, W. (2019) Active contractile properties of fascia. *Clin Anat.* 32: 891–895.

Staubesand, J., Baumbach, K.U.K., & Li, Y. (1997) La structure fine de l'aponévrose jambière. *Phlebologie.* 50: 105–113.

Stecco, A., Gilliar, W., Hill, R., Fullerton, B., & Stecco, C. (2013) The anatomical and functional relation between gluteus maximus and fascia lata. *J Bodyw Mov Ther.* 17: 512–517.

Tam, N., Astephen Wilson, J.L., Noakes, T.D., & Tucker, R. (2014) Barefoot running: an evaluation of current hypothesis, future research and clinical applications. *Br J Sports Med.* 48: 349–355.

Vleeming, A., Pool-Goudzwaard, A.L., Stoeckart, R., van Wingerden, J.P., & Snijders C.J. (1995) The posterior layer of the thoracolumbar fascia. Its function in load transfer from spine to legs. *Spine.* 20: 753–758.

Wilke, J., Hespanhol, L., & Behrens, M. (2019) Is it all about the fascia? A systematic review and meta-analysis of the prevalence of extramuscular connective tissue lesions in muscle strain injury. *Orthop J Sports Med.* 7: 2325967119888500.

Wilke, J., Schleip, R., Klingler, W., & Stecco, C. (2017) The lumbodorsal fascia as a potential source of low back pain: a narrative review. *Biomed Res Int.* 2017: 5349620.

Witvrouw, E., Mahieu, N., Roosen, P., & McNair, P. (2007) The role of stretching in tendon injuries. *Br J Sports Med.* 41: 224–226.

Wood, T.O., Cooke, P.H., & Goodship, A.E. (1988) The effect of exercise and anabolic steroids on the mechanical properties and crimp morphology of the rat tendon. *Am J Sports Med.* 16: 153–158.

Surprising facts about fascial physiology and biochemistry

Werner Klingler and Alberto Zullo

Introduction

Myofascial tissue is composed of cellular and non-cellular elements. Both components are sensitive to physical strain, temperature, pH and humoral factors. This chapter describes the physiological and biochemical properties of fascial tissues, as well as the interaction with connected tissues, most notably skeletal muscle, and repair mechanisms after injury. Knowledge of underlying neurophysiological pathways is indispensable because "you can't depend on your eyes when your imagination is out of focus" (Mark Twain, 1889).

Neurophysiological fundamentals

Movement in sport, first and foremost, involves a sophisticated interaction of the central and peripheral central nervous system, force generating muscle and connective tissues, such as fascia, which is intrinsically tied to skeletal muscle.

Upper and lower motoneuron

The protocol of a movement (engram) is generated in the motor cortex of the brain. The electrical impulses originating from pyramidal neurons propagate along their axons, crossing over to the contralateral side on the brainstem level. This is the reason why the left hemisphere of the brain controls the right side of the body. In most cases, the left hemisphere is dominant. This is evident not only in right-handed people but, surprisingly, also in the vast majority of left-handed individuals. Aside from the brain, left predominance is found in other matched organs such as kidneys or testicles, which are slightly bigger on the left side. The heart is also localized on the left. The asymmetry of our bodies originates from the directional movements of cellular fimbriae in an early stage of fetal development.

Nerve fibers of the pyramidal tract, also denominated corticospinal tract or upper motoneurons, carry information from the brain to the spinal cord. The electrical signal from the upper motoneuron is then transmitted in the anterior horn of the spinal cord to the lower motoneuron, which finally carries the information to the skeletal muscle (Figure 2.1). By definition, an injury of the upper motoneuron leads to a spastic palsy due to disinhibition of motor reflexes. By contrast, lower motoneuron lesion results in flaccid paralysis. Connective tissue reacts to such disturbances of the reflex circuit in due course. For example, after damage to upper motoneurons, as in stroke or spinal cord injury, there is significant fascial stiffening, which in some cases may require surgical relief of the strain. The myofascial stiffening is the result of hyperreflexia due to the lesion of the central nervous system, most notably the upper motoneurons. In summary, two nerve cells, including their long axons, carry the motor information from the brain to the muscle. On the sensory side, three nerve cells are assembled. The peripheral sensory neuron transmits the information to a second neuron in the dorsal horn of the spinal cord. Here, the signal is forwarded, through the spinal cord, to a nut-like part of the brain called the thalamic nuclei. This is the central part of the sensory system, which is composed of two interconnected neurons. The thalamus is located at the center of the brain and is also known as "the door to consciousness".

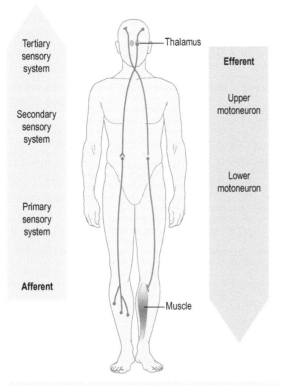

Figure 2.1 Basic neuronal elements of movement control

Two efferent nerve cells, upper and lower motor neuron, conduct specific movement information (encoded as action potential frequency) to the target organ, i.e. skeletal muscle. On the sensory side, there are three neurons interconnected. The extrapyramidal system integrates information such as optic, acoustic and sensory input and modulates the efferent coricospinal tract, i.e. the upper motoneuron. A major component of the extrapyramidal motor system is the thalamic nuclei. Formation of peripheral nerve plexus is not shown in the figure.

Extrapyramidal movement coordination

This system of motor control is subject to a variety of influences and modifications, which are collectively known as the extrapyramidal motor system. Important anatomical components of the extrapyramidal motor system are the basal ganglia, the cerebellum and numerous interneurons, which interconnect pyramidal axons recursively, side by side and with brain nuclei. The extrapyramidal system is designed to enhance or hamper signal transduction. It receives signals from the somatosensory input, and coordinates and fine-tunes movements (Chaitow & DeLany, 2000). A loss of function of this system, e.g. in Parkinson's disease, leads to a very specific akinetic and rigid movement disorder.

Interestingly, other inputs converging in the thalamic nuclei also influence the extrapyramidal movement coordination. Here, important factors are emotion and pain. Emotion is believed to be generated by a circular flow of electrical impulses along a set of anatomical brain structures known as the limbic system. Furthermore, the limbic system is a key element for memory, olfaction and evolutionary survival. It includes several anatomical brain structures, notably interfering with the thalamic nuclei and thereby giving an explanation as to why emotional state can influence movements and vice versa. In this context, it is interesting that regular sporting activity improves learning, reduces the probability of dementia, and significantly prolongs life expectancy.

Cerebral hormones such as dopamine and serotonin are key promoters for movement but also for happiness. For example, this coherence can be observed in patients with psychiatric mania, who are restlessly in motion until they are treated with neuroleptic drugs, i.e. dopamine antagonists, after which rather robotic movements may be observed. On the positive side, good mood is often associated with physical activity, such as dancing. Another example is the need for movement in children, especially as an expression of happiness. The direct effects of these hormones on fascial tissue have only been shown indirectly to date. For instance, long-term medication with potent dopamine agonists leads to fibrosis in the lungs and around the kidneys, as well as thickening and stiffening of cardiac valves.

Pain is a complex topic involving humoral factors, peripheral nervous structures and higher brain centers, e.g. thalamic nuclei. Fascia contains numerous nociceptors such as free nerve endings, whose stimulation triggers pain sensations. These nerve endings are linked to the autonomic nervous system (ANS), which comprises the sympathetic and the parasympathetic systems. ANS collects the information from the body and the external environment, and activates specific responses in the body.

In contrast to the aforementioned somatosensory neurons, which have an impulse conduction speed of 10–100 m/s, a specific type of nociceptor, the C-fibers, are not surrounded by a myelin sheet and, therefore, conduct impulses more slowly, at roughly 0.5 to 2 m/s. The resulting pain sensation is dull and less localized. Fascial tissue mostly contains unmyelinated nerves with free nerve endings serving as unspecific receptors. These free nerve endings detect several stimuli such as tension, temperature or pain, and are connected to wide dynamic range neurons for further processing of the input.

Irritation and coupling of sympathetic fibers with sensory fibers is one of the known mechanisms for the development of chronic pain, such as in the Complex Regional Pain Syndrome (also called Sudeck's disease). Moreover, fascia also contains neurons that release humoral mediators, such as substance P or calcitonin-gene related peptide, which are associated with chronic and self-sustaining pain (Tesarz et al., 2011). Further details can be found in Chapter 15.

Muscle and fascia – together strong

Skeletal muscle is composed of myofibers, which develop as a merger of several single muscle cells via multiple cell fusions. Microscopically, myofibers are readily identifiable by the regular arrangement of the contractile proteins. The subcellular contractile units are called sarcomeres, in which effective force generation requires optimum interdigitation of actin and myosin filaments. *In vitro* experiments have shown that, after surgical excision of a muscle bundle, the elastic fibers shrink by roughly one third of their length *in vivo*. Therefore, *in vitro* force measurements in a laboratory cell-dish environment require an experimental pre-stretching of the bundle.

For efficient contraction development, this pre-stretch may be dynamically regulated in the body by fascial tissue. Depending on the cross-link tension, hydration, elastic content, and even active fascial contraction, the strain on myofibers can be regulated in order to intensify or weaken muscular force generation. In other words, fascia acts as an energy-saving and intelligent servomechanism.

Myofascial tone

Muscle tone is a feature that is regularly assessed by a broad variety of medical professionals. However, diagnosis is based on the experience of the examiner, as reference standards are lacking for symptoms such as body aches or subjective stiffness. Manually assessed excessive muscle tone is also often attributed to postural pain syndromes. Systematically, it is more precise

Chapter 2

to use the term "myofascial tone" because the tensional properties originate not only from the muscle tissue itself but also from the fascial tissue (i.e. the epi-, peri- and endomysium), which can alter its mechanical properties (see below). Interestingly, the amount of connective tissue found in a specific muscle is dependent on its function. Tonic muscle contains significantly more and firmer fascial components than phasic muscle (Klingler et al., 2012). Differences are also found between species. For example, meat from mountain goats has a much higher percentage of collagenous connective tissue compared with domestic pigs. In hereditary muscle diseases, fibrosis is one of the most prominent features and may even be the first symptom of the disease. Therapeutic efforts aim to reduce the fibrosis in muscle disease, such as Duchenne myopathy. Here, corticosteroids are effective inhibitors of fibroblast proliferation and collagen synthesis. Corticosteroid treatment then significantly postpones the onset of disability, in relation to walking. Due to the adverse effects of high corticosteroid doses, alternative treatment options are currently being explored for the management of such pathologies (Klingler et al., 2012). In summary, the contribution of fascia and myofibers to muscle tone is highly variable and adaptive to external and internal factors.

Resting tone

What is resting myofascial tone? This question is not trivial and will be addressed in the following paragraph. By definition, the resting skeletal muscle is electrically silent. This means that the voluntary innervation is zero and the reflex circuit is quiescent. In theory, this is a clear condition and should be easy to assess by examining a resting muscle in terms of resistance to passive movement and firmness of the tissue (Masi and Hannon, 2008). However, from a practical point of view, it can be observed that in awake and even sleeping subjects resting muscles appear to be far from silent. In most patients who are examined by means of electromyography (EMG), signs of neural activity in the muscle tissue can be seen, even if the muscle is voluntarily slack. Indeed, the creaky sound of the EMG device can be used as a biofeedback method in order to calm and relax the patient. Another problem during clinical examination is that many people tend to innervate ("unconscious helping") the muscle/limb under investigation or suffer from disinhibition of monosynaptic reflexes, e.g. in encephalomyelitis disseminata, stroke or other pathologies of the central nervous system. A long-term neuronal overstimulation leads to a fascial remodeling, increase of collagen fibers, and more rigid and less hydrated connective fascial tissue. This fits with altered tissue microperfusion, hydration and nutrition (Chapter 9). From a purpose- or function-oriented teleological point of view, fascial hypertrophy is not only a compensation for muscle overstimulation, but also a reaction to inflammatory processes. In other words, the strategy of our bodies is based on the principle that fast healing is more important than function. This is not only visible in muscle fascia, but also in the scarring of skin lesions, or in organs, such as connective tissue replacing heart muscle after myocardial infarction, leading to a persistent loss of cardiac output. Hence, fascial hypertrophy is embedded in the survival strategy of our bodies.

A complete inhibition of innervation can be observed during general anesthesia in the hospital. Here, neuromuscular blocking agents are used for induction and tracheal intubation. For training purposes, it is helpful for any movement professional to visit an operating theatre to gain an impression of the effect of a complete neuromuscular block on myofascial tissue.

Surprising facts about fascial physiology and biochemistry

Short-term modulators

Several factors affect the function of fascia, some of which are detailed below.

Physical strain

Histological examination of fascial tissue samples shows that fascia is mainly composed of collagenous fibers embedded in a matrix. Fascial tissue also contains cellular components, such as nerves, blood vessels, fat cells, fibroblasts and myofibroblasts. These cells have contractile properties and are involved in tissue remodeling and reaction to physical strain. Fibroblasts can express contractile proteins under special conditions such as mechanical or chemical stimuli (Figure 2.2). Several growth factors are expressed in response to mechanical loading. Examples are transforming growth factor-β1 (TGF-β1), insulin-like growth factor-I (IGF-I) and connective tissue growth factor (CTGF). These factors induce the proliferation of fibroblasts, myofibroblasts and the synthesis of collagenous fibers (Table 2.1). These processes are similar to those found in skin wound healing (Klingler et al., 2012).

However, there is experimental evidence that repetitive strain leads to changing biomechanical properties independent of cellular contractility. The research shows that the variations observed in peak force and stiffness in repetitive strain originate from changes in tissue hydration due to loading and unloading of the fascial tissue. Hence, cellular aspects and temporarily changed matrix hydration play a role in the biomechanical properties of fascial tissue. The clinical implications are considered as enhanced load transfer promoting a more direct muscle–tendon interaction (Schleip et al., 2012).

The use of stretching in sports science causes debate. For fascial tissue, it can be assumed that stretching immediately before exercise increases the range of motion, possibly by influencing tissue hydration and fiber alignment.

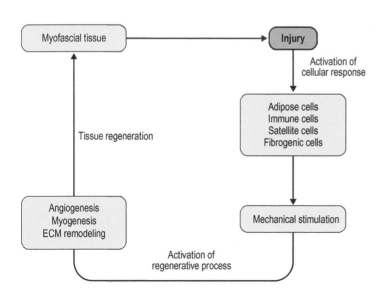

Figure 2.2 Regeneration of myofascial tissue

Following injury, a plethora of processes are activated to regenerate the lost myofascial tissue and restore its original bichemical features: immune cells are recruited to the site of injury and stimulate satellite cells, angiogenesis and remodeling of extracellular matrix (ECM); fibrogenic cells (fibroblasts and myofibroblasts) are activated and remodel ECM; satellite cells exit the quiescent state, proliferate and differentiate into mature muscle fibers; and adipose cells remove cell debris and stimulate satellite cells. In this context, mechanical stimulation promotes myogenesis, angiogenesis and ECM remodeling.

Chapter 2

Table 2.1 Factors influencing the fascial system

Factors influencing the fascial system	Example	Clinical impact
upper motoneuron	injury in stroke	spastic palsy
lower motoneuron	injury in herniated lumbar disc	flaccid palsy
extrapyramidal system	Parkinson syndrome	rigid, hypokinetic movement disorder
cerebral hormones	serotonin, dopamine	mood, need for movement
microenvironmental conditions	pH, temperature, hydration	effects on extracellular matrix and (myo)fibroblasts
humoral factors	transforming growth factor-β1 (TGF-β1), connective tissue growth factor (CTGF), relaxin, interleukins, cortisol	effects on extracellular matrix and (myo)fibroblasts
physical strain	sporting activity, stretching	effects on all discussed levels

This might be helpful in sports such as swimming (e.g. front crawl). Here, optimum propulsion significantly depends on the leverage produced by elongation of the shoulder and arm. Other sports, such as hurdling, may benefit from firm fascial structures because of more direct force transmission and reduction of ground contact time (Chapter 10).

Temperature

Temperature is highly variable in myofascial tissue and is unevenly distributed throughout the body. Moreover, myofascial tonus strongly depends on temperature. The core temperature is regulated between 36.5 and 38.5°C. Outside the body core, temperature greatly depends on environmental conditions and muscle activity. At rest, a limb can cool down to roughly 30°C, whereas during sports 40°C can be reached. Higher temperatures, for example in fever or sustained exercise, increase metabolism by roughly 10–20% per degree Celsius. Contraction in skeletal muscle is solely dependent on calcium release from internal stores, the sarcoplasmic reticulum. Calcium unmasks the binding site of the contractile enzyme myosin, which is a temperature-dependent ATPase. When adenosine-triphosphate (ATP) is consumed by myosin,

heat is produced and the muscle fibers contract. ATP is replenished by cellular respiration and glycolysis. In turn, these biochemical reactions lead to accumulation of the metabolite lactate, which promotes the synthesis of growth factors and collagen (see below).

High temperatures lead to enhanced excitability and calcium turnover in muscle cells. On excised myofibers, an increased basal tension as well as increased twitch force can be observed. Interestingly, the fascial components show a different reaction to temperature changes. Fascia shows a higher peak force and stiffness in cold conditions. In other words, an important fascial feature is heat relaxation.

At first glance, the different temperature characteristics of muscle fibers and fascial tissue appear to be conflicting. However, the opposite is true. Under resting, i.e. cool conditions, the viscoelastic properties of fascial tissue are adapted to serve stabilization and load-bearing function (Figure 2.3). When myofascial tissue is warmed up, i.e. during sport or activity, fascia demonstrates heat relaxation, allowing an expansion of movement range. Relaxation of fascial tissue, induced by low temperature, can promote injuries in some instances, probably because of a

Surprising facts about fascial physiology and biochemistry

Muscle fibers	Fascial tissue
Calcium turnover	Heat relaxation
Phasic contraction	No electrical excitability
Excitation-contraction coupling	Load bearing function in cold muscle

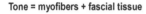

Tone = myofibers + fascial tissue

Figure 2.3 Temperature balance

During physical activity, the temperature in myofascial structures outside the body core can increase by up to 10°C. Warmth leads to enhanced skeletal muscle excitability, faster contraction and relaxation parameters, as well as increased force generation. This effect is mainly caused by an increased calcium turnover and temperature-induced facilitation of enzymatic processes, promoting contractile activity. In fascial tissue, however, higher temperature leads to heat relaxation and reduced myofascial stiffness *in vitro*. Given that there is no voluntary innervation, this effect can also be observed *in vivo*. The lesson we learn from the differential temperature effects on fasciae and myofibrils also helps us to understand passive muscle tone. At rest, i.e. in cold conditions, there is an augmentation of the load-bearing function of fascial tissue, whereas in sports, temperatures of greater than 40°C are reached, allowing fascial release and increase in the range of motion.

more rigid tissue response (Wearing et al., 2014). On the other hand, this strongly depends on the degree and type of tissue stress.

Tissue pH

pH is an indicator of acidic or alkaline conditions. It is tightly regulated in all biological systems because it is a key element of all organic processes in the body, such as oxygen uptake, coagulation and immune response. A pH-optimum is necessary for effective enzymatic functions. pH values below 7.35 indicate a high concentration of protons (H^+ ions), i.e. acidic conditions. Blood pH values above 7.45 are defined as alkalosis. Potassium is an ion that can penetrate the lipid bilayer of cell membranes and, therefore, serve as a counter ion to protons. In other words, potassium concentration increases with dropping pH.

Physical exercise leads to a drop in myofascial tissue pH. This phenomenon is due to the production of lactate and carbon dioxide by glycolysis and cellular respiration. Acidic metabolites accumulate and are exhaled by the lungs as carbonic acid and are more slowly excreted by the kidneys. To a lesser extent, acids are egested by the skin, liver and bowels. Deeper breathing after exercise is not only necessary for replenishment of oxygen but also for elimination of carbonic acid. Abnormal chronic breathing patterns, which influence pH regulation, may also have an impact on myofascial tissue (Chaitow, 2007). Muscle activation can lead to tissue acidosis, as can inflammations of various causes, whether they are traumatic, infectious or autoimmune.

This theroretical background is necessary to understand, for example, what a runner feels when moving at different levels of speed. In the first few seconds after starting a workout there is sufficient ATP available to cover the demand for energy. Approximately half a minute later, the muscular energy buffers myoglobine and creatine phosphate (CP) are activated, and they are used up until the respiratory chain and glycolysis are fully turned during the next few minutes of exercise. In other words, a 100 m runner does not depend on oxidative metabolism during their run. Of course, the energy buffers are replenished after the 100 m run, and each athlete uses oxygen for this. By contrast, a marathon runner depends heavily on their oxidative metabolism because it is a long-lasting exercise.

Chapter 2

If the energy demand exceeds the oxidative metabolism, the body will use up the afore-mentioned buffers and switch to anaerobic gly-colysis. There is a build-up of acidic metabolites, most notably lactate. Acidic metabolites physi-ologically have negative feedback on muscle excitation-contraction coupling and also medi-ate fatigue.

Lactate

Lactate plays a major role in tissue regenera-tion, not only because it promotes blood per-fusion and exchange of nutrients, but also because of its effects upon collagen synthesis and angiogenesis.

In vitro data show that acidic conditions enhance contractility of myofibroblasts (Pipelzadeh and Naylor, 1998). This feature is important in tissue repair. The opposite effects can be observed in skeletal muscle fibers. Here, increasing concentrations of protons, potassium and lactate reduce contractility and mediate fatigue by inhibition of membrane excitability and the enzymatic activity of the myosin ATPase, as well as reduction of the glycolytic rate and cal-cium turnover (Gladden, 2004).

Lactate concentration is increased nearly 2-fold in the healing of Achilles tendon rupture, indicating a key factor of the metabolic response after tissue damage. Lactate has been shown to stimulate vascular endothelial growth factor (VEGF) production. Furthermore, it induces myofibroblast differentiation via pH-depend-ent activation of transforming growth factor-ß (TGF-ß), as shown in lung fibrosis. The authors, therefore, speculate that the acidotic microenvi-ronment and the metabolite lactic acid play an important role in connective tissue remodeling (Trabold et al., 2003).

Lactate is an agonist on free nerve endings, which are numerous in fascial tissue. Hence, the "muscle soar" during and shortly after exercise is mainly due to a lactate mediated stimulation of fascial nociceptors.

Long-term modulators
Extracellular matrix

The extracellular matrix (ECM) is a dynamic complex that constantly modifies its viscoelastic properties. It adapts to changes in physiological as well as mechanical demands. It is composed of collagen fibers and a gelatinous ground substance made up of glycoproteins and proteoglycans. The latter serves as mechanical buffer system simi-lar to a water bed. Hydration can influence the mechanical properties of the ECM (Figure 2.4). TGF-ß promotes the build-up of ground sub-stance as well as regulating the expression of cat-abolic enzymes and other mediators.

From a mechanical perspective, it can be observed that, shortly after strain in the Achilles and patella tendons, the tendon's cross-sectional area decreases significantly. In transverse strain, recovery is prolonged. The authors speculate that the decrease in tendon diameter resembles a squeeze of water. The resulting rehydration in recovery may be an important contributor to a slow-acting exchange of nutrients, electrolytes and other humoral factors, such as cytokines (Wearing et al., 2014).

Notably, the excretion of humoral factors depends on the direction of strain on (myo)fibro-blasts. Irregular strain, such as in injury, leads to a significantly higher release of interleukin-6, a substance involved in regenerative processes and an increased production of nitric oxide (NO), which is a gaseous neurotransmitter and vasodi-lator (Murrell, 2007).

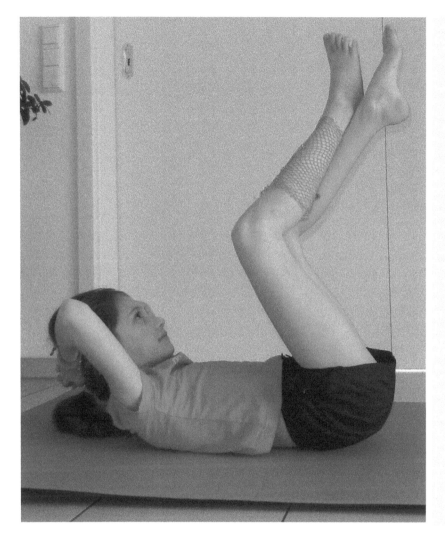

Figure 2.4 Physiology and biochemistry of myofascial tissue

Fascial tissue forms an interconnected 3-dimensional network throughout the whole body. Physiological and biochemical processes determine tissue characteristics such as collagen turnover, extracellular matrix hydration and stiffness of fascial components. The photograph shows a fictitious illustration of fascia on the lower leg. Here, a loose "fascial stocking" might contribute to the development of varicosis. On the other hand, tight fascial tissue can lead to exercise-induced pain, mismatch of blood perfusion and muscle metabolism in the calf. Indeed, compartment syndrome is a feared post-exercise complication in running athletes.

Growth factors

In fascial tissue, several growth factors are produced in response to mechanostimulation, for example, in sports, but also after tissue damage. The interaction of multiple humoral factors is a complex orchestra of biochemical processes, which does not allow simple cause-and-effect conclusions. The most prominent growth hormones in fascial tissue are TGF-ß , IGF-I, platelet-derived growth factor and CTGF. Growth factors regulate, in collaboration with several cytokines (e.g. interleukin 1, 6 and 8), the proliferation and differentiation of fibroblasts and myofibroblasts, as well as the production of collagen and extracellular matrix proteins. These humoral factors also influence blood perfusion, tissue hydration, pain generation and nutrition, as well as cell migration due to chemotactic properties (Kjaer et al., 2009).

Chapter 2

Hormones

Hormonal influences, as well as growth factors, are important to fascial tissue. Insulin has anabolic effects and enhances (myo)fibroblast proliferation *in vitro*. Estrogen and thyroid hormone receptors have also been found in fibroblasts. Preliminary experiments suggest that thyroid hormones promote fibroblast expansion and counteract apoptosis in connective tissue. Estrogen challenge leads to a greater than 40% reduction in collagen synthesis, a reduction in fibroblast proliferation *in vitro*, and a reduction of growth factor bioavailability. Female subjects on oral contraceptives had a reduced collagen synthesis in response to sporting activity. The authors speculate that this finding might explain the greater risk to female athletes of certain types of injury, for example, cruciate ligament rupture and pelvic joint instability (Hansen et al., 2009).

Endogenous cortisol is the main opponent of insulin and a regulator of tissue metabolism and inflammation. Several studies show that high doses of corticosteroid hormones and derivatives lead to a reduction in the proliferation and activity of fibroblasts and collagen synthesis, leading to delayed and hampered healing response after tissue damage. Conversely, cortisol at physiological levels is indispensable for cellular energy metabolism. Hence, the dose-dependent interaction with cells and other factors is decisive for the anabolic or catabolic effects of corticosteroid hormones. Corticosteroids can be an effective treatment for the prevention of pulmonary fibrosis, for example, in asthma. However, because of the catabolic effects at high concentrations, injections of corticosteroids in injuries or chronic pain in fascial structures should be avoided whenever possible.

Relaxin is a dimeric peptide hormone that is structurally related to the insulin family of peptides, and which is upregulated during pregnancy, for example. The most consistent biological activities of relaxin are a regulatory effect on collagen synthesis and the stimulation of collagen breakdown. Interestingly, genetically engineered mice which do not produce relaxin at all are characterized by a significant increase in type I and III collagen, resulting in severe scleroderma and interstitial fibrosis, leading to multi-organ failure. This effect could be inhibited by administration of recombinant relaxin (Samuel et al., 2005).

Fibroblasts of the fascia and connective tissue also express cannabinoid receptors (CBRs), and enzymes metabolizing endocannabinoids. The upregulation of the endocannabinoid system in fascial tissue reduces inflammation, fibrosis and pain. This evidence further supports the use and the development of CBR-targeted pharmaceutical compounds for the treatment of fascial diseases (Fede et al., 2016).

Regeneration of muscle and fascia

Intense physical exercise and normal daily activities can be harmful to myofascial structures. Indeed, sportsmen and women often experience muscle strain (Chapters 16 and 17). Once damaged, skeletal muscle and fascial tissues can regenerate. This process is achieved by the synchronized activity of many different elements, such as muscle cells (myofibers and muscle satellite cells), fascial cells (mainly fibroblasts and myofibroblasts), immune cells (mainly polymorphonuclear leukocytes and monocytes/macrophages) and components of the extracellular matrix (mainly protein fibers and growth factors) (Figure 2.2) (Schiaffino and Partridge, 2008).

The ECM in the human body does not have a permanent structure and composition. On the contrary, it varies regularly, depending on environmental and biochemical stimuli. In particular, ECM undergoes repeated cycles of breakdown and assembling. ECM degradation is due, mostly, to the activity of the metalloproteinases and a disintegrin and metalloprotease released extracellularly by different types of cells, such as fibroblasts, immune cells, and skeletal muscle cells. On the other hand, ECM production relies mainly on the secretion and assembling of fibrous proteins and macromolecules by fibroblasts and myofibroblasts. As a result, the ECM network can be restructured at any time to best fit the body's needs, and regenerated after injury (Schiaffino and Partridge, 2008).

After myofascial tissue injury, fibroblasts are recruited to the lesion site where they proliferate and build up ECM, which confers mechanical resistance to the damaged area, and secrete growth factors, which stimulate the proliferation and differentiation of myogenic cells into mature muscle fibers. In addition to the structural role of ECM, it also represents a guide and molecular switch for cells. Moreover, ECM fragments can act as chemotactic agents for the migration of cells into the injury site.

The regeneration of skeletal muscle tissue mainly depends on satellite cells (SCs), the stem cells of skeletal muscle tissue. SCs reside in a quiescent state between the sarcolemma of myofibers and the basal lamina, a fibrous layer of ECM proteins surrounding muscle fibers. As a consequence of muscle injury, SCs are activated, proliferate and differentiate into mature muscle fibers, thus replacing the lost muscle tissue.

Inflammation is a very important process in the regenerative activity of skeletal muscle and fascial tissues. Indeed, at the site of injury, immune cells such as leukocytes, monocytes/macrophages and T cells are recruited and cytokines are released. In turn, the immune response activates muscle satellite cells, stimulates the formation of new myofibers, induces angiogenesis, promotes ECM remodeling and inhibits fibrosis. Therefore,

a well-orchestrated immune response is critical for an effective regeneration of myofascial tissue, whereas a dysregulated immune reaction results in the accumulation of fibrotic tissue (Zügel et al., 2018).

There is a reciprocal influence of skeletal muscle and fascial tissues in regenerative processes of myofascia. This is due to a strict structural and functional interaction between the two tissues. According to a recent hypothesis, the regenerative potential of skeletal muscle is also influenced by adipose and nerve cells (Zullo et al., 2017).

Interestingly, adipose cells, in the form of fibro/adipogenic progenitors and adipocytes, are present in skeletal muscle tissue, where they remove cell debris and stimulate satellite cells after tissue damage and release adipokines, which have an important effect on skeletal muscle regeneration (Joe et al., 2010).

Traumatic events in myofascial tissue can also affect nerves. In this scenario, ECM guides the damaged nerves in the formation of new neuromuscular junction. In turn, growing axons modulate gene expression in the myotubes involved in the regeneration process. In the fascial and skeletal muscle tissues, protein fibers and cells retain a well-defined spatial orientation. The appropriate alignment of these elements is essential for the biomechanical properties of these tissues. During the regeneration of myofascia, mechanical force plays an important role in the regeneration process (Bove et al., 2016; Klingler et al., 2012).

Indeed, mechanical stress, in the form of muscle loading and passive therapies such as stretching, massage and manipulation, strongly influences the activity of muscle cells and fibrogenic cells, the formation of ECM, and the orientation of ECM's fibers and cells. Therefore,

Chapter 2

the application of mechanical stimuli to the myofascial tissue affects its biomechanical features and enhances the regeneration process following injury (Figure 2.2) (Zügel et al., 2018).

Regeneration of myofascial tissue is a very sensitive process. It is compromised in the presence of counteracting factors, such as an unfavorable physical or biochemical environment, or a disease, thus leading to formation of nonfunctional fibrotic tissue or to fibro-adipogenic degeneration (Klingler et al., 2012). This alteration of tissue structure and composition leads to a dysfunctional myofascia, with reduced performances, decreased mechanical resistance, and increased risk of chronic pain development (Zullo et al., 2017).

Clinical summary

- Sensory input from myofascial tissue is indispensable for nervous control of movement.

- Myofascial tone depends on neuronal excitation, activation level of intracellular myoplasmic calcium turnover, mechanical properties of myofibers and, to a great extent, on the amount and nature of interwoven, adjacent and attached fascial components.

- Sporting activity leads to significant microenvironmental changes, such as temperature increase, accumulation of metabolites, hydration shift in the extracellular matrix and alteration of protein expression including growth factors and cytokines. Adaptation processes in fascial tissue can explain parts of post-exercise phenomena such as muscle soreness.

- Knowledge about fascial tissue may help to improve movement and should be integrated in sport and exercise science and practical application. Depending on the type of sport, the fascial characteristics may be decisive for optimum performance.

References

Bove, G.M., Harris, M.Y., Zhao, H. & Barbe, M.F. (2016) Manual therapy as an effective treatment for fibrosis in a rat model of upper extremity overuse injury. *J Neurol Sci*. 361: 168–180.

Chaitow, L. & DeLany, J.W. (2000) *Clinical Application of Neuromuscular Techniques*. Vol. 1 The Upper Body. Churchill Livingstone, Edinburgh, 131–134.

Fede, C., Albertin. G., Petrelli, L., Sfriso, M.M., Biz, C., De Caro, R. & Stecco, C. (2016) Expression of the endocannabinoid receptors in human fascial tissue. *Eur J Histochem*. 60: 2643.

Gladden, L.B. (2004) Lactate metabolism: a new paradigm for the third millennium. *J Physiol*. 558: 5–30.

Hansen, M., Miller, B.F., Holm, L., Doessing, S., Petersen, S.G., Skovgaard, D., Frystyk, J., Flyvbjerg, A., Koskinen, S., Pingel, J., Kjaer, M. & Langberg, H. (2009) Effect of administration of oral contraceptives in vivo on collagen synthesis in tendon and muscle connective tissue in young women. *J Appl Physiol*. 106: 1435–1443.

Joe, A.W., Yi, L., Natarajan, A., Le Grand, F., So, L., Wang, J., Rudnicki, M.A. & Rossi, F.M. (2010) Muscle injury activates resident fibro/adipogenic progenitors that facilitate myogenesis. *Nat Cell Biol*. 12: 153–163.

Kjaer, M., Langberg, H., Heinemeier, K., Bayer, M.L., Hansen, M., Holm, L., Doessing, S., Kongsgaard, M., Krogsgaard, M.R. & Magnusson, S.P.

(2009) From mechanical loading to collagen synthesis, structural changes and function in human tendon. *Scand J Med Sci Sports*. 19: 500–510.

Klingler, W., Jurkat-Rott, K., Lehmann-Horn, F. & Schleip R. (2012) The role of fibrosis in Duchenne muscular dystrophy. *Acta Myologica*. 31: 184–195.

Masi, A.T. & Hannon, J.C. (2008) Human resting muscle tone (HRMT): Narrative introduction and modern concepts. *J Bodyw Mov Ther*. 12: 320–332.

Murrell, G.A. (2007) Oxygen free radicals and tendon healing. *J Shoulder Elbow Surg*. 16: 208–214.

Pipelzadeh, M.H. & Naylor, I.L. (1998) The *in vitro* enhancement of rat myofibroblast contractility by alterations to the pH of the physiological solution. *Eur J Pharmacol.* 357: 257–259.

Samuel, C.S., Zhao, C., Bathgate, R.A., Du, X.J., Summers, R.J., Amento, E.P., Walker, L.L., McBurnie, M., Zhao, L. & Tregear, G.W. (2005) The relaxin gene-knockout mouse: a model of progressive fibrosis. *Ann N Y Acad Sci.* 1041: 173–181.

Schiaffino, S. & Partridge, T. (2008) *Skeletal muscle repair and regeneration.* Springer.

Schleip, R., Duerselen, L., Vleeming, A., Naylor, I.L., Lehmann-Horn, F., Zorn, A., Jaeger, H. & Klingler W. (2012) Strain hardening of fascia: Static stretching of dense fibrous connective tissues can induce a temporary stiffness increase accompanied by enhanced matrix hydration. *J Bodyw Mov Ther.* 16: 94–100.

Tesarz, J., Hoheisel, U., Wiedenhöfer, B. & Mense, S. (2011) Sensory innervation of the thoracolumbar fascia in rats and humans. *Neuroscience.* 194: 302–308.

Trabold, O., Wagner, S., Wicke, C., Scheuenstuhl, H., Hussain, M.Z., Rosen, N., Seremetiev, A., Becker, H.D. & Hunt, T.K. (2003) Lactate and oxygen constitute a fundamental regulatory mechanism in wound healing. *Wound Repair Regen.* 11: 504–509.

Wearing, S.C., Smeathers, J.E., Hoo per, S.L., Locke, S., Purdam, C. & Cook, J.L. (2014) The time course of in vivo recovery of transverse strain in high-stress tendons following exercise. *Br J Sports Med.* 48: 383–387.

Zügel, M., Maganaris, C.N., Wilke, J., Jurkat-Rott, K., Klingler, W., Wearing, S.C., Findley, T., Barbe, M.F., Steinacker, J.M., Vleeming, A., Bloch, W., Schleip, R. & Hodges, P.W. (2018) Fascial tissue research in sports medicine: from molecules to tissue adaptation, injury and diagnostics: consensus statement. *Br J Sports Med.* 52: 1497.

Zullo, A., Mancini, F.P., Schleip, R., Wearing, S., Yahia, L. & Klingler, W. (2017) The interplay between fascia, skeletal muscle, nerves, adipose tissue, inflammation and mechanical stress in musculo-fascial regeneration. *J Gerontol Geriatr.* 65: 271–283.

Sex hormonal effects on tendons and ligaments

Mette Hansen

Introduction

The biomechanical properties of tendons and ligaments differ between women and men. Furthermore, sex differences in injury risk are reported that depend on the type of sport, the training status and the age of the athletes. These observations have triggered speculation among athletes, trainers and coaches, as well as doctors and researchers, about a possible influence of sex hormones on the regulation of tendon and ligament structure, biomechanical properties and the ability to adapt and repair (Leblanc et al., 2017; Chidi-Ogbolu and Baar, 2018; Hansen, 2018).

The influence of sex hormones seems to vary between different tendons and ligaments, which may be attributed to their anatomical position, diverging tissue loading profiles and tissue structures. The composition of estrogen and androgen receptors may also vary, and the expression of estrogen receptors seems differentially influenced by the presence of estrogen. These observations underline the importance of taking into account an individual person's hormonal profile. Women's sex hormonal profiles differ markedly during their lifespan. In premenopausal, healthy and regularly menstruating women, female hormones fluctuate during each menstrual cycle and reach remarkably high levels during pregnancy. In postmenopausal women, however, the levels of estrogen and progesterone are negligible. In addition, the hormonal profile changes with the use of hormonal contraception or hormone replacement therapy in young and postmenopausal women, respectively.

This chapter aims to give the reader a brief insight into current knowledge about the influence of sex hormones on ligament and tendon injury risk, structure, collagen turnover and biomechanical properties in young and aging women who are users or non-users of exogenous sex hormonal treatment (Figure 3.1).

Sex difference in tendon and ligament injury risk

The risk of sustaining anterior cruciate ligament (ACL) injury is 3- to 6-fold greater in female than in male athletes, even after taking into account socioeconomic, health and lifestyle background variables and level of sports participation (Renstrom et al., 2008). The annual incidence of ACL in female soccer and basketball players is around 5% and approximately 2- to 5-fold higher than seen in men (Prodromos et al., 2007; Renstrom et al., 2008). The risk is particularly high in high school-aged girls. Notably, an ACL injury can have serious consequences for the athlete. A retrospective study including 176 ACL patients previously engaged in organized football (soccer) showed that only half of them returned to activity and approximately one third gave up playing due to poor knee function or fear of additional injuries, which underlines the detrimental effect of this type of injury.

Chapter 3

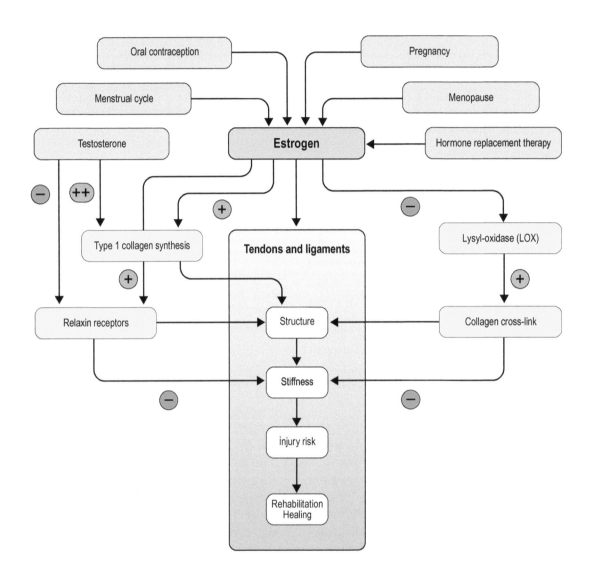

Figure 3.1

A schematic of possible modes of interaction between estrogen and T/L tissue suggested by the literature mentioned in this review. It also names common causes of changes in estrogen levels during the life of a woman. These mechanisms might affect different traits of tendon biology in diverse ways, thereby facilitating the changes observed in clinical studies.

Reprinted from Leblanc et al. (2017). Copyright © 2017 John Wiley and Sons. Used with permission.

In contrast to ACL injury risk, the odds of sustaining Achilles rupture are lower in pre-menopausal women than in men (Huttunen et al., 2014). This sex discrepancy in risk disap-pears after menopause, where the incidence of Achilles rupture in women is similar to that of age-matched men as the level of estrogen is comparable between the sexes. Similarly, the risk of developing tendinopathy is lower in pre-menopausal women than in men (Cook et al., 2000), which indicates that female hormones play a protective role. In line with this, a higher prevalence of asymptomatic rotator cuff tears is observed after menopause, when the level of estrogen decreases markedly (Abate et al., 2014).

The sex difference in injury is probably explained by a complex interaction involv-ing several risk factors (ligamentous laxity and size, limb alignment, neuromuscular control of motion and training status). The presence of sex hormone receptors in tendons and ligaments suggests that sex hormones may possibly affect tendon and ligament structure and biomechani-cal properties.

Sex differences in tendon and ligament structure and biomechanical properties

Ligaments such as the ACL improve joint stability. The stiffer a ligament, the lower the joint laxity and the risk of ligament rupture. In line here-with, joint laxity has repeatedly been reported to be larger in postpubertal women than in age-matched men (Deep, 2014), whereas no differ-ences seem to exist between prepubertal boys and girls or between postmenopausal men and women. Furthermore, the sex disparity in ACL injury risk peaks in the teenage years, when sex hormonal differences are the largest (Renstrom et al., 2008). The latter suggests the presence of a sex hormonal effect on the tissue.

A stiff tendon may be beneficial from a purely performance-related perspective as it will transmit muscle force faster to the bone and store more energy than a compliant tendon. Furthermore, the maximal load before tendon failure is greater. Nevertheless, this benefit will come at the expense of a greater risk of muscle injury. Accordingly, tendon stiffness has been reported to be lower in young women than in men during voluntary isometric contractions using ultrasonography (Magnusson et al., 2007), and women seem to incur fewer muscle injuries than men (Edouard et al., 2016).

Sex differences in tendon and ligament biomechanical properties are partly explained by a generally larger tendon size in men than in women. Even so, the Achilles and patellar tendon cross-sectional area (CSA) is larger in young male runners than in equally trained young female runners when taking their training status into account and when adjusting for body weight differences (Magnusson et al., 2007) (Figure 3.2). Furthermore, tendon CSA is reported to be larger in trained men than in untrained men, which is in agreement with some randomized controlled studies and cross-sectional studies showing a hypertrophic effect of training on patellar and Achilles tendon CSA (Couppé et al., 2008; Kongsgaard et al., 2007). By contrast, we observed no difference in tendon CSA between untrained and trained female runners who had been running >40 km/week for the past 5 years (Magnusson et al., 2007). In agreement herewith, no change in Achilles tendon CSA was observed after 34 weeks of running (in total 43 hours) in previously untrained women (Hansen et al., 2003). Nevertheless, new data from our laborato-ry show an increase in patellar tendon CSA after only 10 weeks of resistance training (Dalgaard et al., 2019); and, in experienced female hand-ball players, patellar tendon CSA is larger in the

Chapter 3

dominant jumping leg than in the contralateral leg (Hansen et al., 2013). The ability of the patellar and Achilles tendon to adapt to regular training may thus be reduced in women but not in men (Magnusson et al., 2007), or the loading threshold for adaptation may be enhanced in women. The lack of adaptation in female runners could also be attributed to hormonal disturbances related to low energy availability. Thus, amenorrhea caused by low energy availability has been reported among 60% of elite middle- and long-distance female runners and among 23% of elite female sprinters (Melin et al., 2019). These athletes are characterized by low estrogen, but also a low insulin-like growth factor I (IGF-I) level. The latter may impair the ability of their tendons to adapt to training because IGF-I has a stimulating effect on tendon collagen synthesis (Hansen et al., 2012).

The structural quality of tendons also appears to differ between young men and women. During

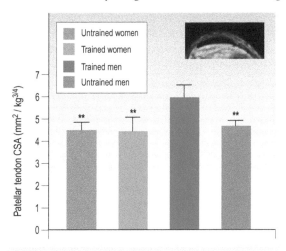

Figure 3.2

The magnetic resonance imaging-determined patellar tendon CSA for trained and untrained men and women normalized to body mass. Trained men had a greater CSA than untrained men ($P < 0.01$); however, note that trained women had a similar CSA compared with untrained women.

loading of single human patellar tendon collagen fascicles from young men and women, the ultimate stress before rupture is greater in fascicles from men than in those from women (Magnusson et al., 2007). The sex differences in fascicle mechanical properties may be related to structural differences.

The mechanical properties of both tendons and ligaments depend on collagenous fiber characteristics (type, density, diameter, orientation). The dry weight in tendons and ligaments is made up mostly of collagen (60–85%), of which type I collagen accounts for around 60% in tendons and up to 85% in ligaments. Nevertheless, the expression of type III collagen in the patellar tendon has been reported to be higher in premenopausal women than in men (Sullivan et al., 2009). Type III collagen is associated with greater elastic tissue flexibility, which is in agreement with the lower tendon and ligament stiffness observed in women. In addition, the patellar tendon dry mass and collagen content per tendon weight have been reported to be lower in women than in men (Lemoine et al., 2009).

The collagen content of ligaments and tendons is determined by the balance between the collagen protein synthesis rate and the collagen protein breakdown rate. However, tendinous collagen turnover is slow; moreover, recent data based on the carbon-14 ([14C]) bomb pulse method suggests that in healthy humans the majority of the Achilles tendon collagen matrix is developed up to the age of approximately 13 years and not renewed after this age (Heinemeier et al., 2018). This observation runs contrary to previous findings, where the tendinous collagen synthesis rate was shown to increase in response to mechanical loading, as determined by the stable isotope technique measuring changes in isotopic enrichment in human tendon biopsies. A suggested explanation is that both exercise and hormones may influence a relatively small fraction of the collagen content that has a fast turnover. Still, this may be of importance for changes in the mechanical properties and in tendon and ligament size over time. In light of this, the observation of a lower tendinous collagen synthesis rate in young women than in age-matched men both at rest and in response to exercise at the same relative intensity is remarkable (Magnusson et al., 2007). A lower tendon and ligament collagen synthesis rate may reduce the ability to adapt in response to regular loading.

Improvements in tendon mechanical properties in response to training have been reported in the majority of human studies, even in studies where tendon CSA was not significantly changed. Yet the mechanical properties of tendons and ligaments are not only determined by the collagen content but also by the presence of intra- and intermolecular crosslinks, which enhance tissue stiffness. Collagen fibers can be crosslinked either non-enzymatically (Maillard reaction between a sugar and an amino acid) or enzymatically. Lysyloxidase (LOX) facilitates enzymatic crosslinking. In engineered ligaments, it has been shown that estrogen inhibits LOX and thereby reduces the relative stiffness (elastic modulus) (Lee et al., 2015). This observation suggests that, independently of any differences in collagen content within tendons and ligaments, sex differences in tendon stiffness and joint laxity may, at least in part, be explained by the higher estrogen level, which impairs tissue crosslinking.

Influence of estrogen on the structural and biomechanical properties of tendons

Female sex hormone fluctuations during the menstrual cycle

The sex hormonal and menstrual profile varies considerably between species, which questions the transferability of results from animal studies to humans and the relevance of including animal data in a context focused on the effect of sex hormones on human beings.

In premenopausal women, 17-β estradiol is the predominant type of estrogen. Estradiol levels in women are several-fold higher than in men until menopause. In healthy premenopausal women, female hormones estradiol and progesterone fluctuate in a predictable pattern during the menstrual cycle (MC) (Figure 3.3). The mean cycle length is 28 days (range 20–45 days). During menses at the beginning of the MC (days 1–6), estradiol and progesterone are both at their lowest levels. Estradiol reaches a peak concentration in the late follicular phase (FP) (days 12–14) around the time of ovulation, when also the levels of luteinizing and follicle-stimulating hormones are peaking. In the luteal phase (LP), a second, lower rise (days 20–24) in estradiol is experienced. Progesterone gradually increases after ovulation and reaches the highest level during LP around day 19–24. Thereafter, a sharp decline in progesterone and estrogen occurs before a new cycle begins.

Use of oral contraceptives (OC) varies between countries, but in many Western European countries more than 50% of young women take OC. The primary reason for using OC is contraception, but other reasons include dysmenorrhea, controlling and manipulating the timing of menses, and reducing the symptoms experienced during a normal menstrual cycle. In OC users, the endogenous level of female hormones is suppressed, but daily OC consumption leads to increases in synthetic estradiol (ethinylestradiol) and synthetic progesterone (progestin) during the first hours after ingestion of the pill. Different types of OC are on the market. OC differ primarily with respect to the type of progestins, which bind to the progesterone

Chapter 3

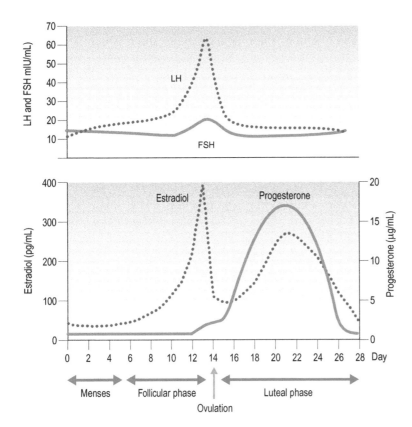

Figure 3.3

Hormonal changes during the menstrual cycle. Overview over the hormonal changes in estradiol and progesterone during the menstrual cycle in young women who do not use oral contraceptives.

Lower part reprinted from Laver et al. (2018). Copyright © 2018 Springer-Verlag GmbH, DE part of Springer Nature. Used with permission.

receptor with differential affinities and have differential androgenity. Importantly, inter-subject variability in pharmacokinetic parameters after ingestion of similar types of OC is considerable. Therefore, women may react differently to OC administration depending on the type of OC as well as on unknown individual factors.

Estrogen receptors (α and β) are localized in the cell nucleus of tendons and ligaments and belong to the nuclear receptor superfamily. When the receptors are activated by ligand binding (estrogen) or other stimuli, they function as transcriptional regulators.

Activation of the ERα and ERβ appears to induce both similar and opposing effects depending on the outcome parameter measured. The plasma membrane also contains

another type of estrogen receptor that can change intracellular cytosolic signaling pathways when activated by stimuli. Estrogen receptor distribution and the relative predominance of the different receptor isoforms vary within different tissue types, and the expression of receptors is influenced by the circulating level of estrogen.

Influence of estrogen on tendons and ligaments

It is difficult to study the isolated effect of estradiol in a human *in vivo* setting. Nevertheless, various efforts have been made to elucidate the effect of estradiol on tendons and ligaments and to clarify the effect of low versus high concentrations of estradiol during the menstrual cycle or between different groups of women.

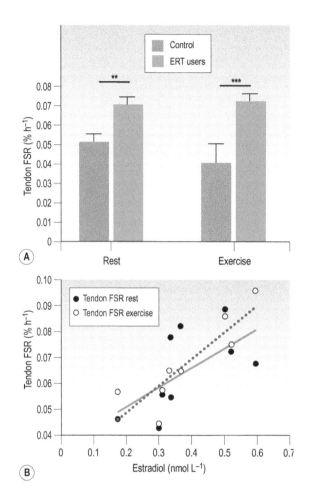

Figure 3.4

(A) Patellar tendon collagen fractional synthesis rates (FSR) at rest and 25 h after exercise in postmenopausal women who used estrogen replacement therapy (ERT) and postmenopausal women who did not use ERT (control); ** $P < 0.01$ and *** $P < 0.001$, unpaired t-test, control vs. ERT users. **(B)** The lines show relationship between tendon FSR and serum(s)-estradiol in ERT users at rest ($r^2 = 0.41$, $p = 0.06$) and postexercise ($r^2 = 0.80$, $P < 0.001$).

A systematic review from 2018 included 12 studies examining changes in knee laxity during the menstrual cycle (Herzberg et al., 2018). Six of these studies provided quantitative data for a meta-analysis, which showed significantly greater knee joint laxity (0.36 mm) around ovulation compared with the early or mid-follicular phase, but this change was not significantly different from the knee joint laxity seen in the luteal phase. In the remaining six studies, the results of three studies suggested a greater knee laxity in the ovulation phase; one study concluded that the greatest knee laxity was observed in the luteal phase, and two studies found no significant difference between phases. The authors of the metaanalysis concluded that ACL laxity may be increased in the ovulation phase of the menstrual cycle, but more high quality studies are needed to confirm this finding. However, cyclic changes in genu recurvatum and general joint laxity have also been reported, which indicates a systemic sex hormonal effect (Shultz et al., 2010). The cyclic variation in knee laxity seems to be repeated in each menstrual cycle (Shultz et al., 2010). However, the magnitude and pattern of cyclic changes in knee laxity vary significantly among women, which may be due to inter-individual variations in hormonal changes during the menstrual cycle. In support of a direct association between estrogen and tendon stiffness, an inverse relationship between circulating estradiol concentration and tendon stiffness has been observed in female handball players (Hansen et al., 2013). Furthermore, the remarkably high level of estrogen during pregnancy is associated with consistently reduced ligament stiffness and enhanced knee joint laxity in the third trimester of pregnancy compared with 5–7 weeks postpartum (Charlton et al., 2001; Cherni et al., 2019).

Confirming the greater knee laxity in the late follicular phase (ovulation), systematic reviews suggest that the risk of sustaining ACL injury during

Chapter 3

the menstrual cycle is lowest in the luteal phase and seems to peak in the late follicular phase (Herzberg et al., 2017) when estrogen, but not progesterone, is enhanced. The greater knee laxity associated with high levels of estrogen also seems to influence landing biomechanics and thereby the potential risk of non-contact ACL injury.

The mechanistic explanation for the rapid changes in ligament laxity and injury risk during the menstrual cycle is not fully elucidated. The effect of any explanatory factor needs to be rapid to explain cyclical variation in tissue laxity and injury. Evidence from animal studies shows that maximal load to failure is reduced in ACL in rabbits exposed to high estrogen levels. The collagen content probably does not change within days, but, as suggested previously, changes in the biomechanical properties of ligaments and tendons in adults are probably explained by changes in intra- and intermolecular crosslinking. In accordance with this, *in vitro* findings in engineered ligaments show that short-term (24 or 48 hours) exposure to a physiological concentration of estrogen decreases relative ligament stiffness and ultimate stress to failure, and this effect is linked to estrogen inhibiting the activity (61–77%) of the crosslinking enzyme LOX oxidase (Lee et al., 2015). If enzymatic activity is similarly reduced *in vivo* during exposure to high estrogen levels, this may explain the observations of greater knee laxity and the risk of sustaining ACL injury around the time of ovulation (Herzberg et al., 2017) as well as the reported lower tendon and ligament stiffness in women than in men.

Tendon and ligament structure and biomechanical properties may not be influenced by transient hormonal fluctuation during the menstrual cycle only. Over time, inter-individual variations in the sex hormonal profile and thus the accumulated exposure to estrogen may affect collagen turnover. A positive correlation between circulating estrogen and human tendon collagen synthesis has been reported (Hansen et al., 2009a) (Figure 3.4). Furthermore, in elderly hysterectomized women who were long-term users of estrogen replacement therapy (ERT), tendon collagen synthesis was higher and patellar tendon relative stiffness lower than in age-matched postmenopausal women with very low estrogen levels (Hansen et al., 2009a). In the estrogen-deficient state, a lower tendon collagen synthesis and slower turnover rate might enhance the risk of introducing crosslinks, which will be further stimulated by LOX, which will no longer be inhibited by estrogen. In agreement herewith, estrogen deficiency in rats correlates with down-regulation of collagen turnover and alteration in collagen fiber orientation. In addition, in oophorectomized estrogen-deficient rats exposed to Achilles tendon injury, the tenocyte proliferation rate was lower than in sham-operated rats undergoing the same exposure. A reduced tenocyte proliferation and a lower tendon collagen synthesis rate in injured tendons or ligaments may potentially reduce the regenerative capacity and be non-beneficial. Furthermore, a protective effect of estrogen in premenopausal women may explain the lower risk of Achilles tendon rupture in premenopausal women than in men.

The different effect of high levels of circulating estrogen on the Achilles tendon and ACL rupture may be due to differences in tissue composition, loading profile and relative distribution and number of estrogen receptors (α and β). Furthermore, whereas a high estrogen level during the ovulation phase of the menstrual cycle in premenopausal women enhances joint laxity to a remarkable, potentially non-beneficial high level, lack of estrogen in the postmenopausal state might be non-beneficially related to a reduced type I collagen synthesis rate. In postmenopausal women, the content of type I collagen and the type I to type III+IV ratio are lower in the arcus tendinous fasciae pelvis than in women using hormone replacement therapy (HRT). The lower type I collagen content suggests a lower tensile tissue strength, which can be linked to increased susceptibility to anterior vaginal wall prolapse in elderly women. Furthermore, in active elderly women, lack of estrogen seems to reduce the ability to cope with Achilles tendon loading compared with active elderly women using HRT. In summary, both estrogen deficiency and a very high level of estrogen may have detrimental consequences for the mechanical properties of tendons and ligaments and injury risk.

Influence of oral contraceptives on tendons and ligaments

The effects of OC on tendon and ligament structure, mechanical properties and injury risk are not fully elucidated, but preliminary results indicate that OC use influences injury risk and the mechanical properties of ligaments and tendons. As previously mentioned, the risk of sustaining an ACL rupture is higher in active premenopausal women than in men. However, case-control studies indicate that OC use is associated with an up to 20% reduction in ACL injury risk compared with non-OC users (Rahr-Wagner et al., 2014). On the other hand, OC use is linked to an increased risk of Achilles tendinopathy (Holmes and Lin, 2006), whereas premenopausal women in general have a lower risk of experiencing Achilles injury than men until the menopausal transition. Explanations for these observations may be related to tendon and ligament stiffness, which have been reported to be higher in OC users than in female controls, but evidence for this remains sparse and inconsistent. A higher tendon stiffness in OC users fits well with observations of greater muscle damage and delayed recovery of muscle strength after eccentric, non-weight-bearing exercise compared with

the response in non-OC users (Minahan et al., 2015). Hypothetically, this observation may be explained by stiffer tendons in OC users, which enhances the tensile loading on the connected muscle-tendon junctions and contractile muscle filaments during muscle contractions. If it holds true that tendon stiffness is higher in OC users, this may be because the tendons experience no periodically enhanced estrogen level, as seen in non-OC users during the ovulation phase. In support hereof, knee joint laxity does not vary during the menstrual cycle as it would during the ovulation phase in non-OC users (Lee et al., 2014). Likewise, prospective data show no periodicity in non-contact ACL injury and ankle sprains in OC users (Agel et al., 2006). Still, it needs to be confirmed that the content of collagen crosslinks is higher in OC users because they experience no marked inhibition of the crosslinking enzyme LOX, like non-OC users in the ovulation phase. Alternatively, a higher ligament stiffness in OC users could be related to the fact that circulating and local concentrations of IGF-I are reduced and the tendon collagen synthesis rate lower in OC users than in controls (Hansen et al., 2009b). A human placebo-controlled study documented that local injections of IGF-I enhance the tendon collagen synthesis rate, which underlines the stimulating effect of IGF-I on tendon collagen synthesis (Hansen et al., 2012). Although the tendon collagen synthesis rate is reported to be lower in OC users, the collagen content does not seem to be lower. This indicates a lower collagen turnover, which will enhance the possibility of introducing and maintaining crosslinks within the collagen-rich tissues and thereby resulting in greater stiffness. However, the consequence of a lower collagen turnover may be an impaired ability to cope and adapt to a progressive increase in tissue loading during training. Also, the low level of IGF-I may impair rehabilitation after tendon and ligament injury since animal findings have documented that administration of IGF-I enhances tissue healing. Future studies are needed to clarify the potentially positive and negative effects of using OC on tendon injury risk, tissue mechanical properties, and adaptability to loading and rehabilitation after injuries.

Influence of androgen and relaxin on the structural and biomechanical properties of tendons

Androgen receptors are localized in human ACL tissue, which suggests that ACL tissue is androgen-responsive. The most abundant androgen in men and women is testosterone. However, the exact regulating role of testosterone on human tendons and ligaments remains elusive.

The level of testosterone is positively correlated with ACL stiffness, whereas estrogen and the estrogen-to-testosterone ratio are negatively correlated with ACL stiffness. An anabolic effect of testosterone on tendon collagen content and tissue stiffness is supported by human data showing a higher tendon collagen synthesis rate in young men than in women at rest (Magnusson et al., 2007). In addition, animal findings show that testosterone increases the collagen content in the prostate and hip joint capsule, and reduces the passive range of motion of the patellar tendon and ligament. Furthermore, *in vitro* findings have shown that high-dose testosterone administration to human cultured tenocytes increased the tenocyte number and changed the phenotype after short-term exposure. Therefore, the reported lower knee joint laxity and greater ligament and tendon stiffness in men than in women may be coupled to the approximately 7-fold higher testosterone level in young men than in young women. However, in normally menstruating premenopausal women, the testosterone level fluctuates and is enhanced around ovulation, during which period increased knee laxity is observed. Still, in women, the testosterone level is low compared with that of men, and the findings suggest that the effect of estrogen on tendinous and ligamentous biomechanical properties in women is dominant. Nevertheless, testosterone may counteract estrogenic effects, as shown in mammary tissue. In support of the latter, animal data indicates that testosterone changes estrogen receptor α and β expression in opposite directions.

Testosterone may also have a positive influence on tendon and ligament adaptation to training. However, the human data basis is primarily based on cross-sectional data comparing men and women, showing that in response to acute exercise the tendon synthesis rate is higher in men than in women (Magnusson et al., 2007). Furthermore, after a 12-week alpine skiing program, the increase in patellar tendon stiffness was larger in elderly (aged 67 years) men (19%) than in elderly women (9%), even though training did not change tendon CSA significantly (Seynnes et al., 2011). One fact that suggests an androgenic rather than an estrogenic effect, is that the circulating estrogen level is comparable in elderly men and postmenopausal women, whereas testosterone levels are higher in men.

Similarly to estrogen, the potentially beneficial effect of testosterone on tendon and ligament injury risk probably depends on an optimal range of testosterone concentrations. In athletes who perform resistance training and use androgenic anabolic steroids, tendon stiffness and modulus are higher than in resistance-training athletes not using any androgenic anabolic steroids (Seynnes et al., 2013). However, tendon CSA was 15% higher in the athletic controls. The differences in patellar tendon morphology and mechanical properties suggest that abuse of androgens influences adaptation to training and collagen remodeling and entails higher stress on the tendon during loading. Supporting animal data shows that anabolic androgenic steroids reverse the beneficial effect of exercise on the Achilles tendon and result in inferior maximal stress values. In line with these observations, case reports indicate that abuse of testosterone or synthetic testosterone derivatives enhances the risk of tendon and ligament injuries and rupture (Kanayama et al., 2015). Superior gains in muscle mass and strength may further provoke an imbalance between training adaptations in the tendon and skeletal muscles, and explain the enhanced tendon rupture risk in abusers.

Relaxin is linked to collagenases activiation, increased tendon laxity and enhanced risk of ACL injury, but also to improved ligament healing (Dehghan et al., 2014; Dragoo et al., 2011; Pearson et al., 2011). Interestingly, animal data suggests that testosterone downregulates the expression of relaxin receptors and thereby the effects of relaxin. By contrast, animal data shows that progesterone and high doses of estrogen enhance the expression of relaxin receptors. Therefore, testosterone, progesterone and estrogen may not only influence tendons and ligaments directly, but also tendon collagen turnover, collagen content and crosslinking by changing the responsiveness to relaxin.

Clinical summary

The risk of overuse and traumatic tendon and ligament injuries differs between women and men. Sex differences in tendon biomechanical properties, tendon morphology and tendon collagen turnover suggest that sex hormones play an explanatory role in this context. However, it is difficult to identify the isolated effect of the sex hormones on tendons and ligaments in human studies due to a complex interplay between internal and external risk factors, for example, aging, training status and nutrient intake, on top of hormonal

interactions. Nevertheless, both estrogen and testosterone in balanced physiological concentrations seem to be important for tendon health and physical function, whereas very low or high concentrations of endogenously or exogenously administered sex hormones may enhance the risk of injuries and lead to inadequate adaptation to mechanical loading. Remarkably, sex hormonal differences as well as sex differences in tendon and ligament injury risk are particularly distinct during sexual maturation in the teenage years, when the tendon and ligament collagen content is primarily established. Still, during adulthood and aging, marked changes in mechanical loading and in levels of endogenous and exogenous sex hormones seem to change the mechanical properties of tendons and ligaments, thereby changing the risk of acute and overuse injuries. Nevertheless, targeted preventive exercises are able to improve the biomechanical properties of tendons and ligaments, reduce joint laxity and reduce injury risk. Improved fitness and endurance capacity are important factors to reduce the risk of non-contact injuries, since fatigue may enhance risk by impairing coordination of movements. In addition, exercises aimed at improving hamstring activation and strength, as well as balance and proper landing and cutting techniques, may help to prevent ACL rupture (Bencke et al., 2018; Monajati et al., 2016; Renstrom et al., 2008).

From a future research perspective, it is important to point out that data addressing the theme of the present chapter remains sparse, and future studies are needed to establish in detail the effect of endogenous and exogenous sex hormones during the lifespan. To date, research has primarily focused on the ACL, the Achilles tendon and the patellar tendon. Future research may elucidate whether sex hormones influence tendons and ligaments differently depending on their localization and function.

Chapter 3

References

Abate, M., Schiavone, C., Di Carlo, L. & Salini, V. (2014) Prevalence of and risk factors for asymptomatic rotator cuff tears in postmenopausal women. *Menopause.* 21: 275–280.

Agel, J., Bershadsky, B. & Arendt, E.A. (2006) Hormonal therapy: ACL and ankle injury. *Med Sci Sports Exerc.* 38: 7–12.

Bencke, J., Aagaard, P. & Zebis, M.K. (2018) Muscle activation during ACL injury risk movements in young female athletes: a narrative review. *Front Physiol.* 9: 445.

Charlton, W.P., Coslett-Charlton, L.M. & Ciccotti, M.G. (2001) Correlation of estradiol in pregnancy and anterior cruciate ligament laxity. *Clin Orthop Relat Res.* 165–170.

Cherni, Y., Desseauve, D., Decatoire, A., Veit-Rubinc, N., Begon, M., Pierre, F. & Fradet, L. (2019) Evaluation of ligament laxity during pregnancy. *J Gynecol Obstet Hum Reprod.*

Chidi-Ogbolu, N. & Baar, K. (2018) Effect of estrogen on musculoskeletal performance and injury risk. *Front Physiol.* 9: 1834.

Cook, J.L., Khan, K.M., Kiss, Z.S. & Griffiths, L. (2000) Patellar tendinopathy in junior basketball players: a controlled clinical and ultrasonographic study of 268 patellar tendons in players aged 14-18 years. *Scand J Med Sci Sports.* 10: 216–220.

Couppé, C., Kongsgaard, M., Aagaard, P., Hansen, P., Bojsen-Moller, J., Kjaer, M. & Magnusson, S.P. (2008) Habitual loading results in tendon hypertrophy and increased stiffness of the human patellar tendon. *J Appl Physiol.* 105: 805–810.

Dalgaard, L.B., Dalgas, U., Andersen, J.L., Rossen, N.B., Møller, A.B., Stødkilde-Jørgensen, H., Jørgensen, J.O., Kovanen, V., Couppé, C., Langberg, H., Kjær, M., Hansen, M. (2019) Influence of Oral Contraceptive Use on Adaptations to Resistance Training. *Front Physiol.* Jul 2;10: 824.

Deep, K. (2014) Collateral ligament laxity in knees: what is normal? *Clin Orthop Relat Res.* 472: 3426–3431.

Dehghan, F., Haerian, B.S., Muniandy, S., Yusof, A., Dragoo, J.L. & Salleh, N. (2014) The effect of relaxin on the musculoskeletal system. *Scand J Med Sci Sports.* 24: e220–e229.

Dragoo, J.L., Castillo, T.N., Braun, H.J., Ridley, B.A., Kennedy, A.C. & Golish, S.R. (2011) Prospective correlation between serum relaxin concentration and anterior cruciate ligament tears among elite collegiate female athletes. *Am J Sports Med.* 39: 2175–2180.

Edouard, P., Branco, P. & Alonso, J.M. (2016) Muscle injury is the principal injury type and hamstring muscle injury is the first injury diagnosis during top-level international athletics championships between 2007 and 2015. *Br J Sports Med.* 50: 619–630.

Hansen, M. (2018) Female hormones: do they influence muscle and tendon protein metabolism? *Proc Nutr Soc.* 77: 32–41.

Hansen, P., Aagaard, P., Kjaer, M., Larsson, B. & Magnusson, S.P. (2003) Effect of habitual running on human Achilles tendon load-deformation properties and cross-sectional area. *J Appl Physiol.* 95: 2375–2380.

Hansen, M., Boesen, A., Holm, L., Flyvbjerg, A., Langberg, H. & Kjaer, M. (2013) Local administration of insulin-like growth factor-I (IGF-I) stimulates tendon collagen synthesis in humans. *Scand J Med Sci Sports.* 23(5): 614–9.

Hansen, M., Couppé, C., Hansen, C.S., Skovgaard, D., Kovanen, V., Larsen, J.O., Aagaard, P., Magnusson, S.P. & Kjaer, M. (2013) Impact of oral contraceptive use and menstrual phases on patellar tendon morphology, biochemical composition, and biomechanical properties in female athletes. *J Appl Physiol.* 114: 998–1008.

Hansen, M., Kongsgaard, M., Holm, L., Skovgaard, D., Magnusson, S.P., Qvortrup, K., Larsen, J.O., Dahl, M., Serup, A., Frystyk, J., Flyvbjerg, A., Langberg, H. & Kjaer, M. (2009a) Effect of estrogen on tendon collagen synthesis, tendon structural characteristics, and biomechanical properties in postmenopausal women. *J Appl Physiol.* 106: 1385–1393.

Hansen, M., Miller, B.F., Holm, L., Doessing, S., Petersen, S.G., Skovgaard, D., Frystyk, J., Flyvbjerg, A., Koskinen, S., Pingel, J., Kjaer, M. & Langberg, H. (2009b) Effect of administration of oral contraceptives in vivo on collagen synthesis in tendon and muscle connective tissue in young women. *J Appl Physiol.* 106: 1435–1443.

Heinemeier, K.M., Schjerling, P., Ohlenschlaeger, T.F., Eismark, C., Olsen, J. & Kjaer, M. (2018) Carbon-14 bomb pulse dating shows that tendinopathy is preceded by years of abnormally high collagen turnover. *FASEB J.* 32: 4763–4775.

Herzberg, S.D., Motu'apuaka, M.L., Lambert, W., Fu, R., Brady, J. & Guise,

J.M. (2017) The effect of menstrual cycle and contraceptives on ACL injuries and laxity: a systematic review and meta-analysis. *Orthop J Sports Med.* 5: 2325967117718781.

Holmes, G.B. & Lin, J (2006) Etiologic factors associated with symptomatic achilles tendinopathy. *Foot Ankle Int.* 27: 952–959.

Huttunen, T.T., Kannus, P., Rolf, C., Fellander-Tsai, L. & Mattila, V.M. (2014) Acute achilles tendon ruptures: incidence of injury and surgery in Sweden between 2001 and 2012. *Am J Sports Med.* 42: 2419–2423.

Kanayama, G., Deluca, J., Meehan, W.P., Hudson, J.I., Isaacs, S., Baggish, A., Weiner, R., Micheli, L. & Pope, H.G. (2015) Ruptured tendons in anabolic-androgenic steroid users: a cross-sectional cohort study. *Am J Sports Med.* 43: 2638–2644.

Kongsgaard, M., Reitelseder, S., Pedersen, T.G., Holm, L., Aagaard, P., Kjaer, M. & Magnusson, S.P. (2007) Region specific patellar tendon hypertrophy in humans following resistance training. *Acta Physiol.* 191: 111–121.

Leblanc, D.R., Schneider, M., Angele, P., Vollmer, G. & Docheva, D. (2017) The effect of estrogen on tendon and ligament metabolism and function. *J Steroid Biochem Mol Biol.* 172: 106–116.

Lee, C.A., Lee-Barthel, A., Marquino, L., Sandoval, N., Marcotte, G.R. & Baar, K. (2015) Estrogen inhibits lysyl oxidase and decreases mechanical function in engineered ligaments. *J Appl Physiol.* 118: 1250–1257.

Lee, H., Petrofsky, J.S., Daher, N., Berk, L. & Laymon, M. (2014) Differences in anterior cruciate ligament elasticity and force for knee flexion in women: oral contraceptive users versus non-oral contraceptive users. *Eur J Appl Physiol.* 114: 285–294.

Lemoine, J.K., Lee, J.D. & Trappe, T.A. (2009) Impact of sex and chronic resistance training on human patellar tendon dry mass, collagen content, and collagen cross-linking. *Am J Physiol Regul Integr Comp Physiol.* 296: R119–R124.

Magnusson, S.P., Hansen, M., Langberg, H., Miller, B., Haraldsson, B., Westh, E.K., Koskinen, S., Aagaard, P. & Kjaer, M. (2007) The adaptability of tendon to loading differs in men and women. *Int J Exp Pathol.* 88: 237–240.

Melin, A.K., Heikura, I.A., Tenforde, A. & Mountjoy, M. (2019) Energy availability in athletics: health, performance and physique. *Int J Sport Nutr Exerc Metab.* 1–35.

Minahan, C., Joyce, S., Bulmer, A.C., Cronin, N. & Sabapathy, S. (2015) The influence of estradiol on muscle damage and leg strength after intense eccentric exercise. *Eur J Appl Physiol.* 115: 1493–1500.

Monajati, A., Larumbe-Zabala, E., Goss-Sampson, M. & Naclerio, F. (2016) The effectiveness of injury prevention programs to modify risk factors for non-contact anterior cruciate ligament and hamstring injuries in uninjured team sports athletes: a systematic review. *PLoS One.* 11: e0155272.

Pearson, S.J., Burgess, K.E. & Onambele, G.L. (2011) Serum relaxin levels affect the in vivo properties of some but not all tendons in normally menstruating young women. *Exp Physiol.* 96: 681–688.

Prodromos, C.C., Han, Y., Rogowski, J., Joyce, B. & Shi, K. (2007) A meta-analysis of the incidence of anterior cruciate ligament tears as a function of gender, sport, and a knee injury-reduction regimen. *Arthroscopy.* 23: 1320–1325.

Rahr-Wagner, L., Thillemann, T.M., Mehnert, F., Pedersen, A.B. & Lind, M. (2014) Is the use of oral contraceptives associated with operatively treated anterior cruciate ligament injury? A case-control study from the Danish Knee Ligament Reconstruction Registry. *Am J Sports Med.* 42: 2897–2905.

Renstrom, P., Ljungqvist, A., Arendt, E., Beynnon, B., Fukubayashi, T., Garrett, W., Georgoulis, T., Hewett, T.E., Johnson, R., Krosshaug, T., Mandelbaum, B., Micheli, L., Myklebust, G., Roos, E., Roos, H., Sschamasch, P., Shultz, S., Werner, S., Wojtys, E. & Engebretsen, L. (2008) Non-contact ACL injuries in female athletes: an International Olympic Committee current concepts statement. *Br J Sports Med.* 42: 394–412.

Seynnes, O.R., Kamandulis, S., Kairaitis, R., Helland, C., Campbell, E.L., Brazaitis, M., Skurvydas, A. & Narici, M.V. (2013) Effect of androgenic-anabolic steroids and heavy strength training on patellar tendon morphological and mechanical properties. *J Appl Physiol.* 115: 84–89.

Seynnes, O.R., Koesters, A., Gimpl, M., Reifberger, A., Niederseer, D., Niebauer, J., Pirich, C., Muller, E. & Narici, M.V. (2011) Effect of alpine skiing training on tendon mechanical properties in older men and women. *Scand J Med Sci Sports.* 21: S39–S46.

Shultz, S.J., Levine, B.J., Nguyen, A.D., Kim, H., Montgomery, M.M. & Perrin,

Chapter 3

D.H. (2010) A comparison of cyclic variations in anterior knee laxity, genu recurvatum, and general joint laxity across the menstrual cycle. *J Orthop Res.* 28: 1411–1417.

Sullivan, B.E., Carroll, C.C., Jemiolo, B., Trappe, S.W., Magnusson, S.P., Dossing, S., Kjaer, M. & Trappe, T.A. (2009) Effect of acute resistance exercise and sex on human patellar tendon structural and regulatory mRNA expression. *J Appl Physiol.* 106: 468–475.

Stress loading and matrix remodeling in tendon and skeletal muscle: Cellular mechano-stimulation and tissue remodeling

Michael Kjaer

Introduction—the concept of mechanical loading on tissue and cells

The loading of connective tissue is a dominant part of all body movement, from light recreational walking to high-level running and athletic activities, such as jumping or throwing. The connective tissue has to resist high levels of loading from muscular contractile activity and, clearly, very high loads will result in acute injuries of connective tissue structures like ligaments, tendons or bones. These present themselves as a tissue rupture or fracture due to a single mechanical load that surpasses the load tolerance.

With regards to repeated loading on the connective tissue there is a fine, yet undefined, line between tissue tolerance of loading and potential adaptation and the development of tissue pathology and associated clinical symptoms. It is, however, clear that very intense physical training, in elite level sports requiring repeated movements of specific body parts, does demonstrate a kind of upper limit of tolerance in the body. Table 4.1 illustrates how elite athletes within

sports, including running, swimming and rowing, experience loading of the lower extremity, shoulder or upper body of up to 40 000–50 000 repetitions per week. Clearly, genetic differences will provide a varying degree of tolerance towards repetitive loading but, in general, it is accepted among athletes that if you extend the amount of training further than that given in Table 4.1, most athletes will experience decreased performance within their sports. In general, this decrease in performance is unlikely to be a result of the total number of training hours, as athletes in several sports that require a more varied loading of the body than those listed in Table 4.1, for example, triathletes, are able to train for up to 35–38 hours per week without any resulting decrease in performance or accumulation of injuries. Thus, Table 4.1 seems to show that each specific regional connective tissue has an upper limit for repeated loading.

Connective tissue in the body is able to withstand substantial loads, varying from clear tensile loading to more compressive loading. Data, primarily from animal literature but also more

Table 4.1 Tissue tolerance in elite athletes		
	Training-dose/week	Tissue loading reps/week
Distance running	120 km/week (steps 1.5 m)	~40 000 steps/leg
Swimming	3–4 hours/day (30–40 strokes/min)	~26 000 strokes/arm
Rowing	3 hours/day (22–35 strokes/min)	~38 000 strokes

Chapter 4

recently from human experiments, shows that increased loading results in improved size and strength of tendons, ligaments, bone and cartilage (Table 4.2). It is, however, clear that the improvement is very moderate and that the adaptation requires considerable time. Compared with skeletal muscle adaptation, the response to training in matrix tissue is moderate. On the other hand, findings regarding the influence of inactivity upon different connective tissues normally indicate some kind of loss in tissue strength and mechanical characteristics (Table 4.2). These findings illustrate that connective tissue is highly dependent upon normal daily loading and is very vulnerable when not being mechanically loaded. When subjected to inactivity, the connective tissue does not diminish quickly in size, but does demonstrate a quick (within 1–2 weeks) alteration in passive mechanical properties. The explanation for this is currently unknown but indicates that molecular structures, which are of importance in regard to mechanical properties, can change quickly when unloaded. In artificial tendons it has been shown that just a few days of unloading in tendon-like structures results in a disorganization of the fibrils. In humans,

the quick changes in the mechanical properties of tendon are accompanied by a change in the expression of enzymes of importance for the formation of cross-link molecules.

Mechanotransduction—signaling and outcome

The mechanical loading of connective tissue is a complex process that involves several steps, from the initial conversion of mechanical stress upon the tissue into chemical signals. Initially, integrin receptors will be activated, and this will result in adhesion and activation of mechanotransduction pathways (Kjaer, 2004; Magnusson et al., 2010). An important pathway for mechanotransduction is the Rho-Rock pathway, and the importance of this pathway for mechanotransduction has been documented in several studies. The resulting activation of protein synthesis from the cell nucleus leads to the formation of matrix proteins, such as collagens, and subsequent tissue structure changes, either more dense tissue, larger tissue volume, or altered organization of the fibrillar and other structures, ultimately contributing to the mechanical properties of the matrix tissue (Figure 4.1).

Table 4.2 Examples of connective tissue adaptation to long-term physical training and inactivity

Function	Capacity (acute)	Training (% increase)	Inactivity (% decrease 4–8 weeks)	
Connective tissue			**Months**	
Tendon	100 MPa	10	30	(+ stiffness/cross-links)
Ligament	60–100 MPa	10	30	(+ stiffness/elastin)
Bone	50–200 MPa	5–10	30	(+ mineralization/Ca++)
Cartilage	5–40 MPa	5–10	30	(+ water/proteogl)
Skeletal muscle			**Months**	
Strength		100	60	
Muscle mass		60	20–30	

Stress loading and matrix remodeling in tendon and skeletal muscle: Cellular mechano-stimulation and tissue remodeling

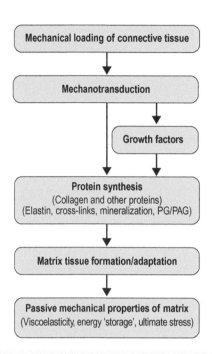

Figure 4.1 Mechanical loading of connective tissue

Mechanical loading will also lead to local upregulation (i.e. more pronounced gene expression and increased synthesis of the protein) of growth factors, such as IGF-I and TGF-β. These will probably be released from the fibroblasts of the connective tissue. Whether these growth factors will act in an autocrine or a paracrine fashion has yet to be explained, but the upregulation of these factors was found to be associated with an exercise-induced upregulation of collagen protein synthesis. This suggests a direct association between growth factor release and matrix protein formation (Figure 4.1). There is also some indication that mechanical loading and growth factors can stimulate the matrix tissue in an additive or even synergistic way (Magnusson et al., 2010).

Mechanical loading increases both collagen expression and protein synthesis in animal studies (Heinemeier et al., 2007). In humans, an upregulation of protein synthesis has been demonstrated both in peri-tendinous tissue and, determined from the incorporation of labeled amino acids, in tendon tissue (Miller et al., 2005). Furthermore, a degradation of collagen tissue has also been demonstrated in humans. Despite these rather dynamic changes of collagen turnover in tendon, this does not prove any major exchange of tendon structure with mechanical loading. Very recent data indicate that the exchange of tendon structures takes place in the first 17 years of life and that, thereafter, a more stable structure is maintained in an intact uninjured tendon (Heinemeier et al., 2013). The fact that well-trained individuals have higher cross-sectional areas of Achilles and patella tendons than untrained ones, and that within the same individual one stronger leg also shows a larger diameter tendon than on the contralateral side (Couppé et al., 2008), indicates that either the growth of tendon with training occurs in the early years, or that it represents an addition of tissue on the surface of the tendon, not unlike the addition of layers on a tree from year to year.

Cellular responses to mechanical loading: *in vitro* to *in vivo*

During the mechanical loading of connective tissue, for example, tendons, the cell within the tendon responds, as previously described, with an increase in mRNA and protein synthesis in the central elements of the matrix (collagen type I). The studies show that interstitial concentrations of collagen propeptide fragments in the peritendinous space rose after exercise. Furthermore, when infusing amino acids labeled with stable isotopes, and determining their incorporation into the relevant connective tissue, it has been shown that this incorporation into hydroxyl-proline, and thus into collagen, almost doubled in both tendon and skeletal muscle after intense exercise (Miller et al., 2005). Conversely, with inactivity over 2–3 weeks, it can be shown that such incorporation would be diminished. Therefore, it appears that collagen production in tendon and skeletal muscle matrix is affected by the degree of mechanical loading. Interestingly, both in tendon and muscle, it seems that the dose-response curve for the relationship between the intensity of loading and the responding protein synthesis outcome levels off relatively early. This means that, already at a relatively moderate loading of the tissue, a sufficient connective tissue response is observed. As adaptation of connective tissue in general is relatively slow, it represents an advantage that also relatively moderate loading will result in an increase in protein synthesis. This means that during rehabilitation after an injury, humans may stimulate their connective tissue with low levels of intensity, at a time when the tissue would otherwise be too weak to tolerate heavy muscle resistance training.

The question now is whether or not this reflects a true tissue renewal and replacement of existing fibrillar structures, or if it represents a mechanism by which mechanical loading provides collagen for potential incorporation in the case of injury. It could be that only a minor fraction of adult tendon is turned over and that a large part of the tendon is more inert and, therefore, less dynamic. To determine this, an experiment can be performed, in which the atmospheric content of the radioactive carbon isotope 14C can be used to mark the age of connective tissue. This is possible because the content of 14C peaked with atom bomb trials in the late 1950s and early 1960s, after which it was banned and the 14C content in the air dropped in subsequent years. Using this methodology, it can be shown that,

by taking into account the increased turnover of tissue in the first 17 years of life during height growth, it would appear that no major collagen turnover occurred in the adult tendon (Heinemeier et al., 2013). This implies that, despite loading, the tendon remains relatively inert during adult life and that only mechanical damage can cause changes. Therefore, it is suggested that the cells in the adult tendon are predominantly dormant and will only be activated in emergency situations.

When the adult tendon is prepared so that cells are isolated and grown in 3D culture systems where, due to attachment patterns, they will be subjected to tension, it is observed that new and artificial tendon constructs are formed. These artificial tendons are cell-rich, produce new fibrils, display an aligned fibril structure, and have the same qualitative type of mechanical properties as natural cells. They express proteins that are important for tendon structure, such as fibrillar collagens, as well as proteins that are phenotypical for tendons, like tenomodulin. Interestingly, when tension is released from these tendon constructs, they all lose their expression of collagen, tenomodulin and mechanosensitive integrin receptors. These changes do not seem to be compensated for by the excess amount of growth factors added (e.g. TGF-β). They indicate that mechanical loading is crucial for the stimulation of important proteins for matrix structure formation.

Chronic effect of mechanical loading on matrix cells and tissue

To what extent the adult tendon can adapt to physical training is not fully understood. In cross-sectional studies, it has been shown that endurance runners have thicker Achilles tendon

Stress loading and matrix remodeling in tendon and skeletal muscle: Cellular mechano-stimulation and tissue remodeling

structures than untrained weight-matched counterparts. Furthermore, when comparing athletes competing in different types of sports, it was been found that runners, who repetitively load their calves, and volleyball players, who use explosive jumping activity, display thicker Achilles tendons than kayak rowers, who load their legs less but have a similar athletic status (Magnusson et al., 2010). In elite older runners, the cross-sectional area of the patella tendon is larger than in untrained age-matched males. The fibril volume was also larger. This indicates that differences between trained and untrained tendons cannot be explained by water accumulation. This data could, therefore, imply that selection is the cause of these differences. The theory of adaptation being related to training is further supported by research into sports with different loading on two legs, such as fencing and badminton. In these examples, where the quadriceps muscle strength was greater on one leg, it was accompanied by a larger patella tendon cross-sectional area (Couppé et al., 2008). To what extent these adaptations of tendon have occurred very early in life or throughout life is not known.

In skeletal muscle, regular training is not associated with any marked increase in collagen content but extreme loading does increase collagen synthesis. This could indicate that collagen degradation increases and that the total collagen content does not, therefore, increase as a result of training. However, this does not indicate to what extent the intramuscular connective tissue will obtain altered mechanical properties with training that is unrelated to collagen content but is, rather, related to fibril arrangement or the synthesis of other molecules related to tissue mechanical properties, for example, cross links (Figure 4.2).

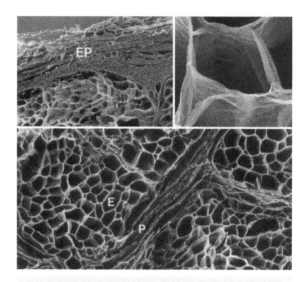

Figure 4.2 Scanning electron micrographs of intramuscular connective tissues (bovine semitendinosus muscle after removal of skeletal muscle protein)

Upper left: epimysium (EP); upper right: endomysium surrounding an individual muscle fiber; bottom picture: perimysium (P) plus endomysium (E).

Modified from Nishimura et al. (1994) with permission.

The borderline between physiological and pathological responses to loading

How much is considered to be adequate loading of connective tissue and how much is too much is an important but, to date, an unresolved question. We do know that appropriate restitution between training bouts will contribute to allow full stimulation of protein synthesis and protein degradation, in order to avoid a gradual net loss of connective tissue over time. Whether this mismatch is the major "road" leading to matrix tissue overload is not completely clear. The presence of both apoptotic cells, and the release of heat shock proteins and inflammatory substances with heavy tissue loading, could indicate that cells in an overloaded matrix tissue are changing their task from matrix protein production, and adequate maintenance

Chapter 4

and renewal of tissue, towards a role where the struggle to survive is their primary goal (Millar, 2005). It may also be that, in the case of tissue overloading, the overloaded cells are shielded from further loading and that this will, therefore, result in further degenerative local changes due to a lack of mechanical loading (Arnoczky et al., 2007). Interestingly, the histological and microstructural changes in early overloading of a tendon, for example, do not mimic the picture of an experimental rupture of a tendon. Therefore, this must represent some other changes behind the overuse of connective tissue. It is known that in some tissues, like tendons, the overuse of the tissue is associated with occurrence of neovascularization and the ingrowth of nerve structures that will result in painful symptoms from the overloaded tissue (Magnusson et al., 2010).

Influence of maturation and aging

Compared with skeletal muscle fibers, our understanding of the effects of aging on related connective tissues is scarce. Although these tissues seem to become more prone to injuries with aging, the underlying mechanisms have not been clarified. While there is not complete agreement in the literature, the current *in vitro* data indicate that aging tends to accompany a decreased potential for cell proliferation, as well as a reduction in the number of stem/progenitor-like cells. In addition, it seems that turnover in the core of the tendon after maturity is either absent or very small. By contrast, collagen content, whole tendon size and fibril diameter appear to be fairly stable during aging. The most striking feature of aging is an associated severe increase in glycation-derived cross-links.

Major mechanical, cellular and morphological changes already appear to occur during maturation. Aging appears to be associated with a reduction in failure strength and in stiffness (i.e. decreased elastic modulus; see Figure 4.3). These changes in mechanical properties may contribute to increased injury risk, although the details of this influence remain to be elucidated.

A recent magnetic resonance imaging investigation examined the muscular connective tissue

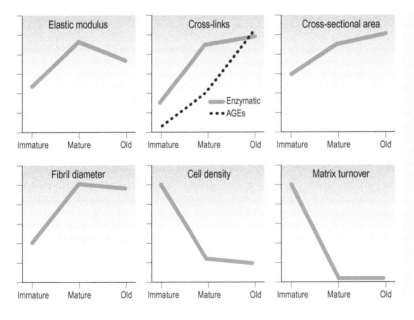

Figure 4.3 Simplified overview of changes observed in tendon tissue with maturation and aging

The graphs are not representations of specific data, but rather indicate the general trends. Highest values of each parameter are oriented towards the top of the graph while the remaining line portions represent the relative trends. AGEs, advanced glycation end products.

Illustration from Svensson et al. (2016) with permission.

Stress loading and matrix remodeling in tendon and skeletal muscle: Cellular mechano-stimulation and tissue remodeling

of the thigh in elderly (aged ~65 years) and younger (aged ~25 years) individuals who were either endurance-trained or had a sedentary lifestyle (Mikkelsen et al., 2017). The total cross-sectional area of non-contractile intramuscular tissue (fat and fibrous connective tissue) was found to be greater in older but lower in trained individuals. Subcutaneous adipose tissue was also lower in trained individuals, but was apparently not influenced by aging. The amount of fibrous connective tissues was larger in the two older groups and was lower the two trained groups (Figure 4.4). The mean proportion of these tissues in older, untrained males was 2.3-fold higher than in young, untrained males.

In vastus lateralis biopsies, no influence of age or training was found on levels of endomysial connective tissue, whereas the organization of the perimysium appeared as more complex in the two older groups. No clear difference related to training for intramuscular inflammatory signaling was seen in these samples. Gene expression of IL6 and TNFα was not different among groups, while IL1-receptor and TNFα-receptor 1 levels were lower with age.

It was concluded that the association of increased muscular connective tissues with aging seems not to be accompanied by any severe changes in intramuscular inflammatory signaling, but rather by direct regulatory factors for protein synthesis and proteolysis, which may be involved in the age-related loss of muscle mass in humans.

The finding of a higher total area of muscular connective tissues in the older subjects was seen as an indication that the "usual" age-related loss of gross skeletal muscle underestimates the true loss of the contractile muscle part, and thus of muscle force. In short, as we age, we tend to lose more and more contractile muscle fibers and gain more muscular connective tissues.

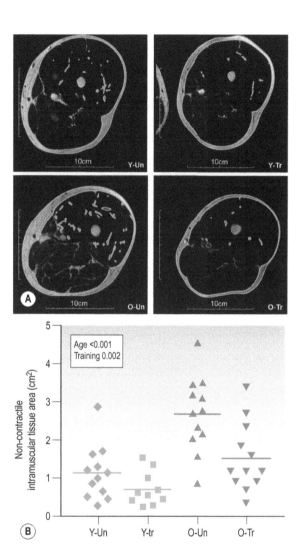

Figure 4.4 Comparison of cross-sectional area of non-contractile connective tissue (NCIT) within and around the thigh musculature (not including the subcutaneous adipose tissue)

(A) Shows representative images from each of the four groups, with NCIT marked in green. **(B)** Shows individual NCIT with line at mean. Significant effects of training and aging are given for the four groups: endurance-trained runners (O-Tr), older, untrained controls (O-Un), young males matched for current running distance (Y-Tr), and young, untrained controls (Y-Un).

Illustration from Mikkelsen et al. (2017) with permission.

Chapter 4

Clinical summary

The mechanical loading of connective tissue is important for the maintenance and adaptation of the matrix in regards to its composition, structure and passive mechanical properties. The question that remains, however, is what the cells in the connective tissue will sense. Is it strain or is it other types of stress? There is, though, no doubt that connective tissue will respond to mechanical loading, but that the response is very varied, depending upon the magnitude of the load, the type of matrix tissue, and the characteristics of the individual. Clinical work suggests that the overloading of tissue in relation to sports, for example, represents a challenge in understanding what signs and markers will provide the "warning sign" for overloading. Having said that, it is also clear that, in many clinical situations, the connective tissue is subjected to far too low a mechanical load. From the data present today, it is clear that mechanical loading provides one of the strongest stimuli, if not the strongest, towards an adaptation of matrix tissue that becomes stronger and, in an injury recovery situation, heals faster and better than if no loading were present. The mechanical stimulation associated with regular sports activity may also counteract some of the structural tissue changes of aging.

References

Arnoczky, S.P., Lavagnino, M. & Egerbacher, M. (2007) The mechanobiological aetiopathogenesis of tendinopathy: is it the over-stimulation or the under-stimulation of tendon cells? *Int J Exp Pathol.* 88: 217–226.

Couppé, C., Kongsgaard, M., Aagaard, P., Hansen, P., Bojsen-Moller, J., Kjaer, M. & Magnusson, S.P. (2008) Habitual loading results in tendon hypertrophy and increased stiffness of the human patellar tendon. *J Appl Physiol.* 105: 805–810.

Heinemeier, K.M., Olesen, J.L., Haddad, F., Langberg, H., Kjaer, M., Baldwin, K.M. & Schjerling, P. (2007) Expression of collagen and related growth factors in rat tendon and skeletal muscle in response to specific contraction types. *J Physiol.* 582: 1303–1316.

Heinemeier, K.M., Schjerling, P., Heinemeier, J., Magnusson, S.P. & Kjaer, M. (2013) Lack of tissue renewal in human adult Achilles tendon is revealed by nuclear bomb 14C. *FASEB J* 27: 2074–2079.

Kjaer, M. (2004) Role of extracellular matrix in adaptation of tendon and skeletal muscle to mechanical loading. *Physiol Rev.* 84: 649–698.

Magnusson, S.P., Langberg, H. & Kjaer, M. (2010) The pathogenesis of tendinopathy: balancing the response to loading. *Nat Revs Rheumatol.* 6: 262–268.

Mikkelsen, U.R., Agergaard, J., Couppé, C., Grosset, J.F., Karlsena, A., Magnusson, S.P., Schjerling, P., Kjaer, M. & Mackey, A.L. (2017) Skeletal muscle morphology and regulatory signalling in endurance-trained and sedentary individuals: The influence of ageing. *Exp Gerontol.* 93: 54–67.

Miller, B.F., Olesen, J.L., Hansen, M., Dossing, S., Crameri, R.M., Welling, R.J., Langberg, H., Flyvbjerg, A., Kjaer, M., Babraj, J.A., Smith, K. & Rennie, M.J. (2005) Coordinated collagen and muscle protein synthesis in human patella tendon and quadriceps muscle after exercise. *J Physiol.* 567: 1021–1033.

Nishimura, A., Hattori, A., Tkahashi, K. (1994) Ultrastructure of the intra muscular connective tissue in skeletal muscle. *Acta Anat.* 151: 250–7.

Svensson, R.B., Heinemeier, K.M., Couppé, C., Kjaer, M. & Magnusson, S.P. (2016) Effect of aging and exercise on the tendon. *J Appl Physiol.* 121: 1353–1362.

Mechanical loading and adaptive responses of tendinous tissues

Falk Mersmann, Sebastian Bohm and Adamantios Arampatzis

Mechanisms of tendon plasticity

Tendons transmit the forces generated by the muscles to the skeleton to produce movement. The elasticity of tendons, which allows tendons to deform (mostly elongate) upon load application, yet restore their original length when the load is released, importantly contributes to movement performance, since it influences the muscle fascicle behavior. As the muscle adapts well to exercise, it seems plausible that tendons feature a certain degree of plasticity as well. It has been shown already in the 1940s, by comparing tendons from rats with a different degree of habitual loading, that tendinous tissue is sensitive to mechanical stimulation (Ingelmark, 1945). However, it took some major technological and methodological developments to address the mechanisms of human tendon adaptation *in vivo*. Research from the past two decades has provided convincing evidence that the tendinous tissue of humans adapts over a whole lifespan. When a tendon is repeatedly subjected to increased mechanical loading, for instance in the course of resistance exercise, the associated increases of muscle strength are commonly accompanied by an increase of tendon stiffness (Kubo et al., 2001; Arampatzis et al., 2007). Tendon stiffness is defined as the relationship of applied force and resultant elongation and, thus, describes the capability of a tendon to resist force (Figure 5.1).

Two main mechanisms may account for the increase of stiffness in response to loading. It seems that, especially in the early stages of tendon adaptation, structural changes of the extracellular matrix influence the material properties of the tissue and increase the internal mechanical integrity of the collagenous network. These potential changes could include the type and degree of intra- and interfibrillar collagen cross-linking (Depalle et al., 2015), glycosaminoglycan content contributing to interfibrillar connections and force transfer (Cribb and Scott, 1995), and collagen area fraction (Robinson et al., 2004). Although the tendon core tissue is supposed to be relatively inert (Heinemeier et al., 2013), the elastic modulus of tendons—as a measure of their material properties based on the stress–strain relationship—might increase by up to 85% following 10–14 weeks of training (Wiesinger et al., 2015).

Hypertrophy of the tendon in response to loading, on the other hand, has been observed less frequently and is now rather considered a long-term mechanism contributing to increased tendon stiffness (Bohm et al., 2015). The radial growth probably occurs via the synthesis of new extracellular matrix in the outer layers of the tendon (Gumucio et al., 2014). It seems unlikely that a significant increase of the tendon cross-sectional area occurs much earlier than after 3 months of training, and

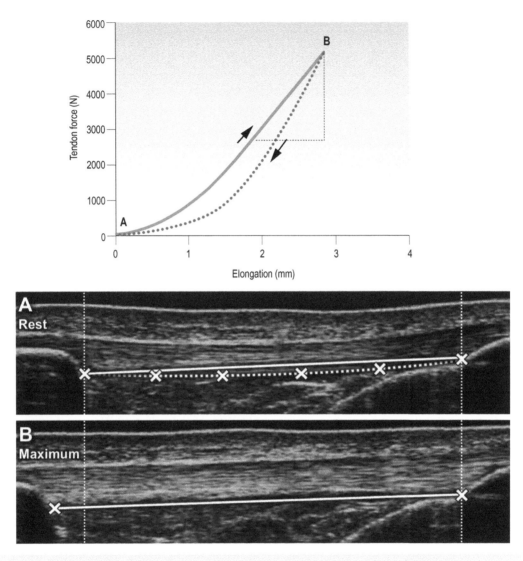

Figure 5.1 Exemplary force-elongation behavior and ultrasound images of a patellar tendon during loading from rest
(A) to a maximum voluntary muscle contraction **(B)**. The force-elongation relationship is characterized by a flat so-called "toe region", where only low forces are needed to stretch the tendon due to the wavy arrangement of the collagen fibrils and fibers, and a subsequent linear increase. The slope of this increase (indicated by the pointed triangle) is referred to as "stiffness" and describes the resistance of a tendon against elongation.

its development appears to be site-specific (i.e. in some regions of the tendon, its cross-section increases while remaining unaffected in others; Arampatzis et al., 2007; Kongsgaard et al., 2007). The radial tendon growth reported in longitudinal studies on human Achilles or patellar tendons is usually moderate in magnitude; however, years of training might lead to more marked increases of the order of up to 35% (Wiesinger et al., 2015).

Mechanical loading and adaptive responses of tendinous tissues

It is still poorly understood how the metabolic responses of tendons, structural, morphological and mechanical changes of tendinous tissue associate with one another. The temporal development of the adaptation process suggested above clearly needs further confirmation regarding the methodological challenges and simplified assumptions associated with *in vivo* investigations. Nevertheless, it is evident that tendons adapt to systematic loading with an increase of stiffness and it is likely that changes of the material properties precede tendon hypertrophy.

Relevance of tendon training

As described above, the long-term adaptation of tendon stiffness alongside the development of muscular strength may serve as a protective mechanism against injury. The ultimate strain of tendons is considered to be relatively constant (LaCroix et al., 2013), and a sole increase of muscle strength would progressively pull the tendon to levels of strain closer to and finally above its physiological threshold upon maximum effort muscle contractions. However, within a training process it might be that the balance of muscle strength and tendon stiffness gets distorted. The tissue renewal rate of tendons (turnover) is lower compared with muscle tissue (Heinemeier et al., 2013), which can result in a delayed adaptation of the tendon in early stages of training (Kubo et al., 2010; 2012) and may explain the high prevalence of overuse injuries (e.g. tendinopathy) when training loads are changed rapidly (Gabbett, 2016). Moreover, it seems that not all types of loading that induce an increase of muscle strength are equally effective for the tendon. For instance, it is well accepted that training with moderate loads until fatigue can increase muscle strength and size (Ozaki et al., 2016), while no such reports

exist for tendon stiffness. In fact, an increase of muscle strength and no change of stiffness have been observed after isometric training at 55% of the voluntary maximum (Arampatzis et al., 2007; 2010). Such asynchronous adaptation results in an increase of tendon strain and thus a higher mechanical demand for the tendon (as illustrated in the left panel of Figure 5.2), which is considered a risk factor for tendon overuse injury (Wren et al., 2003). Further, it has been demonstrated in adolescent volleyball athletes that sport-specific loading (i.e. jumping) causes a greater increase of muscle strength compared with tendon stiffness. This, in turn, leads to chronically increased levels of tendon strain during maximum effort muscle contractions (Mersmann et al., 2017b) and episodes of exceptionally high values over the course of a competitive season (Mersmann et al., 2016). Considering the dramatic prevalence of tendinopathy in athletes from jump disciplines (Lian et al., 2005), it becomes evident that it could be an important aspect of injury prevention to provide specific training stimuli to strengthen the tendon for a balanced musculotendinous development, which maintains tendon strain at physiological levels despite increased muscle strength capacity (Figure 5.2, right panel).

In addition to the prevention of overuse injury, tendon training also plays a key role in the rehabilitation of tendinopathy. Classic loading programs, such as Alfredson's eccentric training (Chapter 16), have been shown to be effective in reducing pain and improving function (Malliaras et al., 2013), yet the moderate intensity nature of loading appears insufficient to address the mechanical weakening of the tendon (Arya and Kulig, 2010) by increasing its stiffness (Foure et al., 2013). More recent approaches which use loading paradigms characterized by a high

Chapter 5

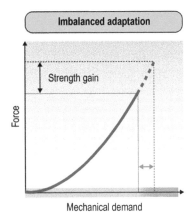

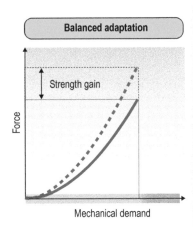

Figure 5.2

If the force that can be exerted by a muscle increases without a similar increase of tendon stiffness (left), the mechanical demand for the tendon increases to potentially detrimental levels (red zone), which could pose a risk of overuse injury. On the other hand, by adequately stimulating tendon adaptation (right), the mechanical demand for the tendon remains in physiological bounds (green), despite the greater absolute load it is subjected to.

loading intensity (e.g. heavy-slow resistance training) seem more suitable in this regard (Couppé et al., 2015).

The mechanical properties of tendons also greatly influence performance in everyday activities and sports. Since tendons can store and release elastic strain energy, they affect the operating behavior and force potential of muscles and the power output of the muscle-tendon unit (Roberts, 2016). In humans, muscle fascicle operating behavior seems optimized for metabolic economy, for example in running (Bohm et al., 2018), and for power production in jumping (Nikolaidou et al., 2017). A sole increase of muscle strength due to training could interfere with this interaction of muscle and tendon, limiting the extent to which the increased muscle capacity translates into performance. Moreover, high tendon stiffness positively affects the rate of force development and thus jump height or balance recovery, for example, after sudden perturbations (Bojsen-Møller et al., 2005; Karamanidis et al., 2008). Therefore, knowledge of effective loading paradigms to change the mechanical properties of tendons is also essential for the improvement of physical performance.

How to stimulate tendon adaptation

As described in Chapter 4, the adaptation of tendons is based on the transmission of the external tissue strain to the cytoskeleton of the embedded fibroblasts. The conformational changes of transmembrane proteins that occur during load application and the activation of stretch-sensitive ion channels in the cell membrane then trigger intracellular signaling cascades, which stimulate gene and growth factor expression for the upregulation of collagen and matrix protein synthesis (Wang, 2006).

From a mechanobiological point of view, there are four main factors which determine the transduction of the mechanical stimulus applied to the tendon into cellular signals: strain magnitude, strain rate, strain duration and strain frequency. First, the magnitude of strain applied to the tendon during loading directly determines the deformation of the fibroblasts (Arnoczky et al., 2002), which in turn seems to regulate the metabolic activity in response to loading (Lavagnino et al., 2003). It has been further suggested that the recruitment of collagen fibers is also greater during high strain compared with low strain loading (Kastelic et al., 1980), which might increase the number of effectively stimulated fibroblasts. Human *in vivo* studies on the Achilles and patellar tendon confirmed the importance of high magnitude tendon strain for the adaptive response to exercise. Arampatzis et al. (2007; 2010) compared training protocols of high intensity (i.e. 90% isometric maximum voluntary contraction [MVC] corresponding to 4.6% of tendon strain) and moderate intensity loading (i.e. 55% MVC corresponding to 2.9% of tendon strain) with equal overall training volume. Significant changes of the Achilles tendon morphological and mechanical properties were observed only following the loading regimen that induced high tendon strain during muscle contraction. Of all the factors that might determine tendon adaptation, it is now most clearly established that high loading is necessary to achieve changes of the mechanical properties of tendinous tissues (Bohm et al., 2015). A common misunderstanding is, however, that eccentric loading is most effective to stimulate a tendon. Yet the strain the tendon is subjected to during a contraction does not depend on the type of muscle contraction (i.e. isometric, concentric, eccentric) but only on the force the muscle is exerting. Accordingly, scientific evidence shows that the contraction type does not per se influence the loading response of tendons (Kjaer and Heinemeier, 2014). Nevertheless, due to the high force potential and economic force production of muscles during eccentric contractions, the exercise mode is a feasible way to provide repetitive high tendon strain with comparatively low muscle fatigue. The necessity of high tendon forces for initiating adaptive responses in the tendon also explains why stretching, against common belief, does not change the mechanical properties of tendons in the long term. As an inactive muscle has a lower stiffness compared with its tendon, the muscle belly takes over most of the length change during a passive stretch of the muscle-tendon unit and the forces and strain in the tendon are quite low (De Monte et al., 2006). The for increase in flexibility, which is commonly observed following acute or chronic stretching, seems more related to neural than mechanical changes (Freitas et al., 2018).

The strain rate (i.e. change in strain per unit of time) describes how fast strain is applied to a tendon. It has been shown that a high strain rate induces high fluid flow-related shear stress to the tenocytes, which is believed to trigger anabolic responses (Lavagnino et al., 2008). Further, the recruitment of collagen fibrils seems to increase with strain rate as well (Clemmer et al., 2010). In *in vivo* studies, high strain rates can be applied using plyometric loading through jumping exercises with short contact times. Interestingly though, the majority of these studies found no significant training effects on the mechanical properties of tendons or rather low effects. One possible explanation for these findings is the comparatively short duration of strain application with each loading cycle during plyometric loading, which seems to be another important factor for the mechanotransduction. In a series of systematic intervention studies, in which the overall loading volume (i.e. the integral of the force-time curve of the training sessions) was kept constant, high strain was applied to the Achilles tendon for <130 ms, 1 s, 3 s and 12 s per loading cycle, respectively (Arampatzis et al., 2010; Bohm et al., 2014). The strongest effects on tendon stiffness were observed following the 3 s loading protocol, which supports the idea that the duration of strain application is an important factor for tendon adaptation and that the mechanical stimulation might be too short to be effective in plyometric exercises or high frequency-short duration loading protocols. It seems possible that an increase of loading duration could lead to a more homogenous strain

Chapter 5

distribution and, thus, tenocyte stimulation within the tendon. A longer duration of tenocyte deformation might also show effects on the cellular signaling pathways, for example, the influx and propagation of calcium within and between the tenocytes (Lavagnino et al., 2015). These hypotheses (i.e. more homogeneous tenocyte stimulation and more effective signaling) do not contradict that fluid flow-induced shear stress at the cytoskeleton of the tenocytes is an important stimulus yet, under *in vivo* loading conditions, the benefit of a high compared with a low strain rate might be offset by a compromised mechanotransduction due to a reduced strain duration in certain modes of loading. However, our current understanding of the effects of specific types of mechanical stimulation of the tendon on the complex cellular machinery and signaling pathways of mechanotransduction is widely deficient, and the main conclusion that can be drawn from tendon adaptation research is that an effective stimulus for the tendon needs to exceed a certain threshold in terms of strain magnitude and, supposedly, strain duration.

Other loading determinants for tendon training are, to date, widely unclear. The effect of strain frequency, which is determined by both load and rest duration in cyclic loading, has been investigated in humans *in vivo* first by Arampatzis et al. (2010). The results suggested a lower strain frequency (0.17 Hz) to be more effective compared with a higher one (0.5 Hz). However, differences in the strain duration (3 s and 1 s in the low and high frequency protocol, respectively) might also partially account for these results. Waugh et al. (2018) compared two high intensity isometric training protocols, differing only in the rest duration between loading cycles of either 3 s (i.e. 0.17 Hz) or 10 s (i.e. 0.08 Hz), respectively. While the effect on the mechanical properties of the Achilles tendon were of similar magnitude,

some structural changes that might be interpreted as early indications of overload were detected only following the protocol with the short rest duration. However, it needs to be acknowledged that these findings might be exclusive to a training regimen of such an overall loading volume, which was markedly higher (by factor 1.9) compared with earlier work using high loading intensities (Arampatzis et al., 2010; Bohm et al., 2014). Nevertheless, it might be concluded that the results on the effects of strain frequency are in principal in accordance with reports from *in vitro* models, suggesting that intermediate levels of strain frequency between 0.1 and 0.25 Hz provide an effective stimulus (Joshi and Webb, 2008). The optimal duration of rest between training sessions, however, is even more unclear. Similarly, the effect of weekly training volume has not been investigated thus far.

Clinical summary

Although several factors influencing the effectiveness of tendon loading protocols are not well investigated, some recommendations can be given on how to increase the stiffness of a tendon (see also Figure 5.3). A tendon training program should be characterized by an intensity of ≥ 85% of the isometric or one-repetition maximum and the duration of the muscle contraction around 3 s, while the contraction mode (i.e. isometric, concentric, eccentric) does not play a major role. Isometric training should be performed in joint angles close to the optimum for force generation (i.e. ~60° knee flexion for patellar tendon training or ~10° ankle dorsiflexion and extended knee for the Achilles tendon). This has the advantage of being easy to learn and the load can be controlled precisely. During dynamic exercises (i.e., eccentric-concentric movements), high tendon forces occur only in specific ranges of joint angles during movement (e.g. between 60°

Mechanical loading and adaptive responses of tendinous tissues

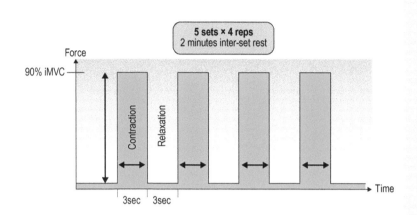

Figure 5.3

Evidence-based recommendations for a potential structure of tendon training. High intensity loading to the tendon (85–90% iMVC) should be applied in five sets of four repetitions with a contraction and relaxation duration of 3 s, and a rest between sets of 2 min. The training is to be applied 3–4 times a week for at least 12 weeks to achieve marked increases of tendon stiffness.

(Mersmann et al., 2017a. Used with permission by Frontiers Media SA.)

and 100° of knee flexion in a parallel squat; 0° = full extension). In these exercises, the overall movement duration should be increased (e.g. to ~6 s) to provide the 3 s high strain application. A low movement velocity and controlled movement behavior are essential to decrease peak forces in the joints (Bergmann et al., 2004). For exemplary exercises, the reader is referred to the supplementary material of Mersmann et al. (2017a). As the tendon already responds to adequate mechanical loading ,during childhood (Waugh et al., 2014), and the major turnover of

the tendon occurs until the end of adolescence (Heinemeier et al., 2013), it may be beneficial to start implementing specific tendon exercises in the training routines early in the athletic career. It is now well established that guided strength training even with high loads is not only safe for children and adolescents, but even reduces the risk for musculoskeletal injuries (Faigenbaum et al., 2016; Myers et al., 2017). However, as the tendon remains sensitive to exercise even at old age (McCrum et al., 2018), it never seems too late to start training one's tendons.

References

Arampatzis, A., Karamanidis, K. & Albracht, K. (2007) Adaptational responses of the human Achilles tendon by modulation of the applied cyclic strain magnitude. *J Exp Biol.* 210: 2743–2753.

Arampatzis, A., Peper, A., Bierbaum, S. & Albracht, K. (2010) Plasticity of human Achilles tendon mechanical and morphological properties in response to cyclic strain. *J Biomech.* 43: 3073–3079.

Arnoczky, S.P., Lavagnino, M., Whallon, J.H. & Hoonjan, A. (2002) In situ cell nucleus deformation in tendons under tensile load; a morphological analysis using confocal laser microscopy. *J Orthop Res.* 20: 29–35.

Arya, S. & Kulig, K. (2010) Tendinopathy alters mechanical and material properties of the Achilles tendon. *J Applied Physiol.* 108: 670–675.

Bergmann, G., Graichen, F. & Rohlmann, A. (2004) Hip joint contact forces during stumbling. *Langenbeck Arch Surg.* 389: 53–59.

Bohm, S., Marzilger, R., Mersmann, F., Santuz, A. & Arampatzis, A. (2018) Operating length and velocity of human vastus lateralis muscle during walking and running. *Sci Rep.* 8: 5066.

Bohm, S., Mersmann, F. & Arampatzis, A. (2015) Human tendon adaptation in response to mechanical loading: a systematic review and meta-analysis of exercise intervention studies on healthy adults. *Sports Med Open.* 1: 7.

Bohm, S., Mersmann, F., Tettke, M., Kraft, M. & Arampatzis, A. (2014) Human Achilles tendon plasticity in response to cyclic strain: effect of rate and duration. *J Exp Biol.* 217: 4010–4017.

Chapter 5

Bojsen-Møller, J., Magnusson, S.P., Rasmussen, L.R., Kjaer, M. & Aagaard, P. (2005) Muscle performance during maximal isometric and dynamic contractions is influenced by the stiffness of the tendinous structures. *J Appl Physiol.* 99: 986–994.

Clemmer, J., Liao, J., Davis, D., Horstemeyer, M.F. & Williams, L.N. (2010) A mechanistic study for strain rate sensitivity of rabbit patellar tendon. *J Biomech.* 43: 2785–2791.

Couppé, C., Svensson, R.B., Silbernagel, K.G., Langberg, H. & Magnusson, S.P. (2015) Eccentric or concentric exercises for the treatment of tendinopathies? *Journal of Orthopaedic and Sports Physical Therapy.* 1–25.

Cribb, A.M. & Scott, J.E. (1995) Tendon response to tensile stress: an ultrastructural investigation of collagen:proteoglycan interactions in stressed tendon. *J Anat.* 187: 423–428.

De Monte, G., Arampatzis, A., Stogiannari, C. & Karamanidis, K. (2006) *In vivo* motion transmission in the inactive gastrocnemius medialis muscle-tendon unit during ankle and knee joint rotation. *J Electromyogr Kinesiol.* 16: 413–422.

Depalle, B., Qin, Z., Shefelbine, S.J. & Buehler, M.J. (2015) Influence of cross-link structure, density and mechanical properties in the mesoscale deformation mechanisms of collagen fibrils. *J Mech Behav Biomed Mater.* 52: 1–13.

Faigenbaum, A.D., Lloyd, R.S., MacDonald, J. & Myer, G.D. (2016) Citius, altius, fortius: beneficial effects of resistance training for young athletes: narrative review. *Br J Sports Med.* 50: 3–7.

Foure, A., Nordez, A. & Cornu, C. (2013) Effects of eccentric training on mechanical properties of the plantar flexor muscle-tendon complex. *J Appl Physiol.* 114: 523–537.

Freitas, S. R., Mendes, B., Le Sant, G., Andrade, R. J., Nordez, A., & Milanovic, Z. (2018) Can chronic stretching change the muscle-tendon mechanical properties? A review. *Scandinavian Journal of Medicine & Science in Sports.* 28(3): 794–806. http://doi.org/10.1111/sms.12957

Gabbett, T.J. (2016) The training—injury prevention paradox: should athletes be training smarter and harder? *Br J Sports Med.* 50: 273–280.

Gumucio, J.P., Phan, A.C., Ruehlmann, D.G., Noah, A.C. & Mendias, C.L. (2014) Synergist ablation induces rapid tendon growth through the synthesis of a neotendon matrix. *J Appl Physiol.* 117: 1287–1291.

Heinemeier, K.M., Schjerling, P., Heinemeier, J., Magnusson, S.P. & Kjaer, M. (2013) Lack of tissue renewal in human adult Achilles tendon is revealed by nuclear bomb (14)C. *FASEB J.* 27: 2074–2079.

Ingelmark, B.E. (1945) Über den Bau der Sehnen während verschiedener Altersperioden und unter verschiedenen funktionellen Bedingungen. Eine Untersuchung der distalen Sehnen des Musculus biceps brachii und Musculus semitendineus des Menschen sowie der Achillessehnen von Kaninchen und weissen Mäusen. *Upsala Läkareförenings förhandlingar.* 50: 357–395.

Joshi, S.D. & Webb, K. (2008) Variation of cyclic strain parameters regulates development of elastic modulus in fibroblast/substrate constructs. *J Orthop Res.* 26: 1105–1113.

Karamanidis, K., Arampatzis, A. & Mademli, L. (2008) Age-related deficit in dynamic stability control after forward falls is affected by muscle strength and tendon stiffness. *J of Electromyogr Kinesiol.* 18: 980–989.

Kastelic, J., Palley, I. & Baer, E. (1980) A structural mechanical model for tendon crimping. *J Biomech.* 13: 887–893.

Kjaer, M. & Heinemeier, K.M. (2014) Eccentric exercise: acute and chronic effects on healthy and diseased tendons. *J Appl Physiol.* 116: 1435–1438.

Kongsgaard, M., Reitelseder, S., Pedersen, T.G., Holm, L., Aagaard, P., Kjaer, M. & Magnusson, S.P. (2007) Region specific patellar tendon hypertrophy in humans following resistance training. *Acta Physiol.* 191: 111–121.

Kubo, K., Ikebukuro, T., Maki, A., Yata, H. & Tsunoda, N. (2012) Time course of changes in the human Achilles tendon properties and metabolism during training and detraining *in vivo.* *Eur J Appl Physiol.* 112: 2679–2691.

Kubo, K., Ikebukuro, T., Yata, H., Tsunoda, N. & Kanehisa, H. (2010) Time course of changes in muscle and tendon properties during strength training and detraining. *J Strength Cond Res.* 24: 322–331.

Kubo, K., Kanehisa, H., Ito, M. & Fukunaga, T. (2001) Effects of isometric training on the elasticity of human tendon structures *in vivo.* *J Appl Physiol.* 91: 26–32.

LaCroix, A.S., Duenwald-Kuehl, S.E., Lakes, R.S. & Vanderby, R. (2013)

Relationship between tendon stiffness and failure: a metaanalysis. *J Appl Physiol*. 115: 43–51.

Lavagnino, M., Arnoczky, S.P., Kepich, E., Caballero, O. & Haut, R.C. (2008) A finite element model predicts the mechanotransduction response of tendon cells to cyclic tensile loading. *Biomech Model Mechan*. 7: 405–416.

Lavagnino, M., Arnoczky, S.P., Tian, T. & Vaupel, Z. (2003) Effect of amplitude and frequency of cyclic tensile strain on the inhibition of MMP-1 mRNA expression in tendon cells: an *in vitro* study. *Connect Tissue Res*. 44: 181–187.

Lavagnino, M., Wall, M.E., Little, D., Banes, A.J., Guilak, F. & Arnoczky, S.P. (2015) Tendon mechanobiology: Current knowledge and future research opportunities. *J Orthop Res*. 33: 813–822.

Lian, O.B., Engebretsen, L. & Bahr, R. (2005) Prevalence of jumper's knee among elite athletes from different sports: a cross-sectional study. *Am J Sports Med*. 33: 561–567.

Malliaras, P., Barton, C.J., Reeves, N.D. & Langberg, H. (2013) Achilles and patellar tendinopathy loading programmes: a systematic review comparing clinical outcomes and identifying potential mechanisms for effectiveness. *Sports Med*. 43: 267–286.

McCrum, C., Leow, P., Epro, G., König, M., Meijer, K. & Karamanidis, K. (2018) Alterations in leg extensor muscle-tendon unit biomechanical properties with ageing and mechanical loading. *Front Physiol*. 9: 2743.

Mersmann, F., Bohm, S. & Arampatzis, A. (2017a) Imbalances in the development of muscle and tendon as risk factor for tendinopathies in youth athletes: a review of current evidence and concepts of prevention. *Front Physiol*. 8: 1–18.

Mersmann, F., Bohm, S., Schroll, A., Marzilger, R. & Arampatzis, A. (2016) Athletic training affects the uniformity of muscle and tendon adaptation during adolescence. *J Appl Physiol*. 121: 893–899.

Mersmann, F., Charcharis, G., Bohm, S. & Arampatzis, A. (2017b) Muscle and tendon adaptation in adolescence: elite volleyball athletes compared to untrained boys and girls. *Front Physiol*. 8: 613.

Myers, A.M., Beam, N.W. & Fakhoury, J.D. (2017) Resistance training for children and adolescents. *Transl Pediatr*. 6: 137–143.

Nikolaidou, M.E., Marzilger, R., Bohm, S., Mersmann, F. & Arampatzis, A. (2017) Operating length and velocity of human M. vastus lateralis fascicles during vertical jumping. *R Soc Open Sci*. 4

Ozaki, H., Loenneke, J.P., Buckner, S.L. & Abe, T. (2016) Muscle growth across a variety of exercise modalities and intensities: Contributions of mechanical and metabolic stimuli. *Med Hypotheses*. 88: 22–26.

Roberts, T.J. (2016) Contribution of elastic tissues to the mechanics and energetics of muscle function during movement. *J Exp Biol*. 219: 266–275.

Robinson, P.S., Lin, T.W., Jawad, A.F., Iozzo, R.V. & Soslowsky, L.J. (2004) Investigating tendon fascicle structure-function relationships in a transgenic-age mouse model using multiple regression models. *Ann Biomed Eng*. 32: 924–931.

Wang, J. (2006) Mechanobiology of tendon. *J Biomech*. 39: 1563–1582.

Waugh, C.M., Alktebi, T., de Sa, A. & Scott, A. (2018) Impact of rest duration on Achilles tendon structure and function following isometric training. *Scand J Med Sci Sports*. 28: 436–445.

Waugh, C.M., Korff, T., Fath, F. & Blazevich, A.J. (2014) Effects of resistance training on tendon mechanical properties and rapid force production in prepubertal children. *J Appl Physiol*. 117: 257–266.

Wiesinger, H.-P., Kösters, A., Müller, E. & Seynnes, O.R. (2015) Effects of increased loading on *in vivo* tendon properties: a systematic review. *Med Sci Sports Exerc*. 47: 1885–1895.

Wren, T.A.L., Lindsey, D.P., Beaupré, G.S. & Carter, D.R. (2003) Effects of creep and cyclic loading on the mechanical properties and failure of human Achilles tendons. *Ann Biomed Eng*. 31: 710–717.

Nutrition and loading to improve fascia function

Danielle Steffen and Keith Baar

Introduction

Connective tissues, including bone, cartilage, tendon, ligaments, and fascia, are critical components of a functioning musculoskeletal system. These tissues serve to absorb, dissipate, and transmit the forces applied to the body during movement. Each one is specialized for one or more mechanical function based on the location in the body and the resulting amount and type of force applied to the cells within the tissue. Tendons, ligaments and fascia function primarily to transfer force within the musculoskeletal system, and fascia has the added function of facilitating movements by lubricating the interface between tissues. To facilitate the transfer of force, these connective tissues are composed of an extracellular matrix (ECM), structural proteins that give them a high tensile strength (Kjaer, 2004), and ground substance that brings water into the tissue to provide compressive strength. The primary structural proteins are collagen, laminin, and elastin, with collagen contributing ~80% of the total protein. There are 28 different collagen proteins (Ricard-Blum, 2011). Within the musculoskeletal connective tissues, type I collagen makes up more than 90% of the collagen fraction, with type III collagen comprising much of the remaining fraction. Therefore, types I and III collagen are the major fibrillar collagens that provide tensile strength to the musculoskeletal connective tissues (Kjaer, 2004).

To increase the strength of the tissues, the proteins that form the matrix are cross-linked (Figure 6.1). Cross-linking can occur in two ways: enzymatically and non-enzymatically. Enzymatic cross-links are mediated primarily by lysyl oxidase (LOX; 26, 44, 45), a copper-dependent enzyme that forms intermolecular bonds between lysine residues at the end of collagen molecules. By contrast, non-enzymatic cross-links are formed through a Maillard reaction between a sugar and an amino acid at any location within the matrix. These cross-links are called advanced glycation end-products (AGE), and, as would be expected, are higher in diabetics (Dyer et al., 1993) where blood glucose levels are chronically increased. Both enzymatic cross-linking, through LOX, and non-enzymatic cross-linking through AGEs, increase the stiffness of the matrix (Reddy, Stehno-Bittel and Enwemeka, 2002; Marturano et al., 2013). The main differences between enzymatic and non-enzymatic cross-links are their location and turnover rate, where AGEs can be made throughout the matrix and this decreases collagen turnover and over time impairs matrix function (Hammes et al., 1991; Corman et al., 1998). Further, when AGEs are high and collagen levels are low (for example in individuals who are inactive), the matrix becomes brittle (Akeson et al., 1977; Calve et al., 2005), resulting in an increase in the likelihood of catastrophic injuries in sport (Myer et al., 2011).

Chapter 6

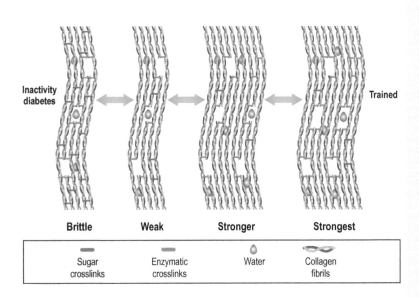

Inactivity
diabetes

Trained

Brittle   **Weak**   **Stronger**   **Strongest**

| Sugar crosslinks | Enzymatic crosslinks | Water | Collagen fibrils |

Figure 6.1

Determinants of musculoskeletal soft tissue stiffness. The major determinants of soft tissue stiffness are depicted in this cartoon. Collagen (gray) provides the mechanical backbone for the tissues; the more collagen fibers, the more robust the tissue. The collagen matrix can be stiffened by either enzymatic (red) or sugar based (advanced glycation endproducts; blue) cross-links. Water (blue drops) held within the matrix makes the tissue viscoelastic. A tissue becomes stiffer and stronger as both collagen and enzymatic cross-links increase. In contrast, a tissue with little collagen and a lot of sugar cross-links is stiff but not strong (brittle).

The major proteins of the ground substance are proteoglycans (PGs), proteins that have highly charged glycosaminoglycan (GAG) side chains. These charged GAGs serve to modulate tissue hydration and/or help organize the collagen matrix (Sasarman et al., 2016; Robinson et al., 2017). The water content of the musculoskeletal tissues is determined by the retention of free water by PGs within the matrix (Dubinskaya et al., 2007). Larger PGs are more common in compressed musculoskeletal tissues (Evanko and Vogel, 1990) and provide compressive strength by bringing large amounts of water into the tissue. By contrast, smaller PGs (biglycan and decorin) are more prevalent in tissues loaded in tension (Robinson et al., 2017). Compressive strength is utilized both during tensile loading (as the tissue is stretched), when the water within the tissue resists radial compression as the collagen molecules are squeezed together, and during compressive loading, such as when tissues wrap around bones or retinacula. Together, the dense cross-linked collagen matrix and proteoglycan-rich ground substance provide the mechanical strength of the tissues and therefore specific connective tissues use different ratios of these substances to meet their specific mechanical requirements.

In contrast to the classical view of the musculoskeletal connective tissues being relatively inert, stable tissues where the collagen has a half-life of >105 years (Heinemeier et al., 2013), more recent data suggests that connective tissues are highly dynamic. Smeets and colleagues (Smeets et al., 2019) gave subjects undergoing knee replacement surgery phenylalanine containing a heavy isotope of carbon two hours before and then throughout the operation. During surgery, all the tissues of the knee were collected and the incorporation of heavy phenylalanine into the proteins contained in those tissues was determined. As a control, the authors took a muscle biopsy at the time of surgery so that they could compare the tissues of the knee to a highly dynamic tissue.

In contrast to expectation, protein turnover in the anterior cruciate ligament (ACL) and patellar tendon was greater than the muscle tissue, cartilage protein turnover was similar to muscle, and synovial tissue turned over almost 3-times faster than muscle (Smeets et al., 2019). In support of the findings of Smeets and colleagues, Myrick et al recently showed that, over the course of an 8-month soccer season, the ACL of young women increased in size, suggesting that there was an increase in collagen in the tissue (Myrick et al., 2019). Together, these data suggest that the musculoskeletal connective tissues are highly dynamic in their response to load.

The primary forces within the musculoskeletal system are *tension*, i.e. when the Achilles tendon is loaded in one direction during plantar flexion (Figure 6.2A); *compression*, i.e. when the meniscus absorbs the impact force of a step (Figure 6.2B); and shear, i.e. when the superior extensor retinaculum allows the tendons of the tibialis anterior slide beneath it during dorsi flexion (Figure 6.2C). When the musculoskeletal system is working properly, the specific load placed on the tissue results in a stimulus that orchestrates a cascade of events within the cell that results in changes to the proteins that make up the ECM. This is most notable in embryonic development because compressive loads induce fibrocartilage formation and tensional loads produce an aligned collagen matrix within a tendon (Evanko and Vogel, 1990; Kapacee et al., 2008). This molecular response is critical to the growth, differentiation and development of the cells and dictates the resulting function of the tissue.

The connective tissues are largely made from a population of fibroblast cells that contain the high mobility group (HMG) box transcription factor SOX9 (Asou et al., 2002). Even though the cells have a similar origin, once the cells migrate into position and begin being loaded, they

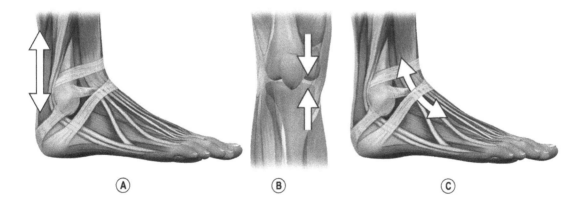

Figure 6.2

Loads within the musculoskeletal system. The three major loads in the musculoskeletal system are: **(A)** *Tension*, when a tissue is pulled in one direction; **(B)** *Compression*, when a tissue is pushed in on itself; and **(C)** *Shear*, when two tissues slide past each other.

Chapter 6

differentiate to fit their mechanical environment. In fact, fibroblast cells isolated from connective tissues at different locations in the body become transcriptionally distinct cell types (Chang et al., 2002). These data suggest that the mechanical environment is essential to driving cell fate. Therefore, understanding the mechanical environment, and the cellular response to load, is essential for maximizing musculoskeletal cell and tissue function.

Beyond the mechanical environment, connective tissues are dependent on nutritional cues. As stated above, the primary protein within connective tissues is collagen, the most abundant protein in the body. In order for the collagen made in the cells to be released into the ECM, it has to be modified by the enzyme prolyl hydroxylase (Mussini, Hutton and Udenfriend, 1967). During the hydroxylation reaction, prolyl hydroxylase consumes vitamin C. Since humans lack the enzyme L-gulono-γ-lactone oxidase (Nishikimi et al., 1988), we are unable to make vitamin C and therefore we must consume enough of this micronutrient to support normal collagen turnover. While this is the most direct nutritional input needed for healthy connective tissues, other foods are suggested to be important in connective tissue function. These foods and how they interact with loading to promote tendon, ligament and fascial structure and function will be the focus of this chapter.

Cellular and molecular response to loading

Tendons, ligaments, and fascia are formed by a dense and aligned collagen matrix. While these three tissues are structurally similar, they can undergo regional specialization based on their mechanical environment. For example, retinacular fascial tissues, that need to lubricate the constant sliding of underlying tendons, have more than 10-fold higher levels of hyaluronan, a glycosaminoglycan (GAG) that functions as a lubricant, than the epimysial fascia, that surrounds muscles where shear forces are lower (Fede et al., 2018). Similarly, the flexor digitorum profundus tendon of rabbits is structurally and functionally two distinct tendons; the tendon proper, that is loaded in tension, and a fibrocartilage portion, where the tendon is compressed as it passes through the carpal tunnel. Even though the cells of the two regions have the same origin, the total GAG content of the tendon varies from 0.2% of the dry weight in the tendon, up to 6.5% as the tissue takes on a fibrocartilage phenotype (Gillard et al., 1979). When the compressed region is experimentally released from the carpal tunnel, the GAG content within the tendon rapidly drops from 6.5 to 2.5% after only eight days and further decreases to below 1% within six months after the release surgery (Gillard et al., 1979). To determine whether compressive load was sufficient to induce a fibrocartilage phenotype, Robbins and colleagues removed deep flexor tendons from cows, subjected them to 72 hours of cyclic compressive load, and then measured markers of cartilage gene expression. Just three days of compressive loading was enough the increase expression of cartilage enriched large PGs, such as aggrecan up to 4.5-fold (Robbins, Evanko and Vogel, 1997). Therefore, in tendon compressive loading is sufficient to induce and maintain a fibrocartilage phenotype.

The type of load also influences the size and function of the PGs present within a tendon. Fibrocartilage present in compressed tendon regions is typified by larger PG. These larger PG increase water within the tissue to increase compressive strength. Smaller PGs are enriched in embryonic tendons and adult tendons under tension (Evanko and Vogel, 1990; Ehlers and Vogel,

1998). As the developmental tendon is compressed, epigenetic specialization begins and the cells within the compressed region take on a fibrocartilage phenotype, that can be recreated using *in vitro* cyclic compression (Evanko and Vogel, 1993). In the region of the tendon undergoing tensile loading, smaller PGs have a role in collagen fibrillogenesis—defining the outer surface of individual collagen fibrils. When these smaller PGs are missing, the size of the fibrils becomes disrupted and the mechanical integrity of the tendon is lost (Ameye and Young, 2002; Robinson et al., 2017).

Unlike PGs and GAGs, lubricating proteins such as Prg4/lubricin are regulated by shear stress (Nugent et al., 2006). Simply applying a shear stress to cells for 24 hours results in a 3-fold increase in lubricin secretion. Since knocking out lubricin makes tendons stick together more tightly (Hayashi et al., 2013), this suggests that shear forces are necessary to maintain the lubrication between tendons/fascial layers. Together, these data suggest that compressive and shear loads rapidly increase the expression of genes involved in cartilage formation and lubrication, respectively (Figure 6.3B, C).

Where compression and shear increase larger PGs and lubrication, tensional forces are necessary for the production of an aligned collagen matrix (Kapacee et al., 2008). The requirement for tension in the synthesis of a robust and aligned matrix is best seen when the load is removed. For example, when Majima and colleagues inserted a stainless steel wire between the tibial plateau and the base of the patella to release tension from the patellar tendon, nuclei per mm^2 increased

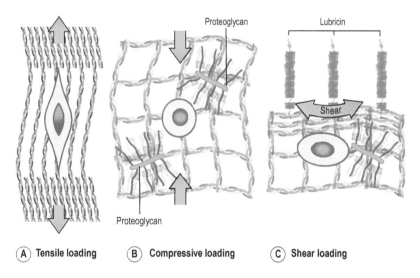

(A) Tensile loading   (B) Compressive loading   (C) Shear loading

Figure 6.3

Different loads result in different cellular responses. In response to **(A)** tensile loading, cells secrete type I collagen and make lysyl oxidase resulting in a stiff aligned collagen matrix. In contrast, **(B)** compressive loads on the same cells make proteoglycans that contain a protein like hyaluronic acid and gylcosaminoglycans like chondroitin and keratin sulfate. Over time this results in a decrease in collagen alignment and an increase in water in the tissue (held by the GAGs). Lastly, **(C)** shear loads lead to the production of proteoglycans and lubricin at the edge of the tissue, resulting in a collagen matrix that contains high amounts of fluid at the edge of the tissue to lubricate movement.

Chapter 6

~7-fold, collagen fibril diameter decreased ~40%, and collagen bundles became less well-oriented (Majima et al., 2003). These data indicate that without tensional load healthy connective tissues take on a scarred phenotype, becoming more cellular with smaller, less aligned collagen fibrils. By contrast, one hour of kicking exercise resulted in a dynamic increase in patellar tendon collagen synthesis (Miller et al., 2005). Collagen synthesis, as measured using stabile isotope infusion followed by tendon biopsies, was elevated ~40% 6 hours after the exercise bout, peaked at 80% greater 24 hours after the exercise, and was still 40% higher 72 hours after (Miller et al., 2005). Interestingly, the same group found that the one hour kicking exercise did not increase collagen synthesis in women (Miller et al., 2007); however, this could be a result of the time point of measurement (72 hours in the women), 48 hours after the peak of collagen synthesis in men (Miller et al., 2005). An even greater increase in collagen synthesis is seen in muscle with tensile loading where collagen synthesis increases ~185% 6 hours after exercise, stays at that level 18 hours later, before returning to baseline 72 hours after finishing the exercise bout (Miller et al., 2005). In chicken muscle, tensional loading increases collagen protein synthesis 5-fold, resulting in a 10-fold increase in the amount of collagen within the muscle after as little as two days (Laurent, McAnulty and Gibson, 1985). These data suggest that tensile loading increases collagen synthesis, resulting in an increase in collagen within connective tissues (Figure 6.3A).

In order to understand what about tensile loading drives an increase in collagen synthesis, we turned to an *in vitro* model of a ligament (Paxton, Grover and Baar, 2010). Three dimensional (3D) engineered ligaments are structurally and functionally very similar to embryonic ligaments. Using these cultured ligaments and a molecular marker that is necessary for the load-induced increase in collagen synthesis (the extracellular-regulated kinase; ERK; 22), we characterized what aspects of tensile loading connective tissue cells transduce into a signal that results in more collagen production (Paxton et al., 2012). These experiments demonstrated that the frequency and amplitude of the stretch on a ligament had similar effects on the cellular response, even very small loads fully activated ERK. In contrast, the duration of an exercise bout was very important; the cellular response to tensile loading peaked between five and ten minutes and then returned to baseline levels by 90 minutes (Figure 6.4A).

These data suggested that the cells were quickly becoming refractory to the tensile load. To determine how long it took to regain the capacity to signal, ligaments were loaded for ten minutes and then rested for 0.5, 1, 3, 6, and 12 hours (Figure 6.4B). Full signaling returned to the ligament cells only after resting for six hours (Paxton et al., 2012). Lastly, an intermittent tensile loading program (4 x 10 minutes separated by six hours) was compared with a continuous loading program, and the ligaments that received 40 minutes of tensile load each day in short bouts increased collagen synthesis twice as much as those being loaded 24 hours a day. These data are similar to the response in bone where cells become refractory after ~40 loads and take 6-8 hours to regain the ability to signal (Burr, Robling and Turner, 2002). Together, these data suggest that musculoskeletal connective tissues increase collagen synthesis in response to short periods (~10 minutes) of tensile load separated by load periods (~6 hours) of rest (Figure 6.4C).

Nutrition for connective tissues

As discussed above, the structure and function of tendons, ligaments, and fascia can be directly

Nutrition and loading to improve fascia function

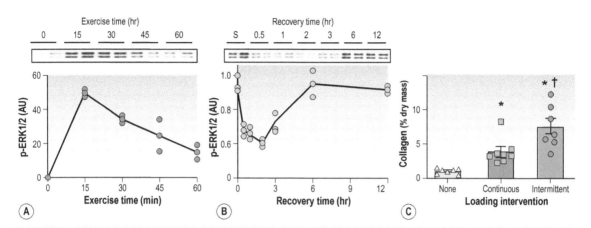

Figure 6.4 Short loads and long rest periods are optimal for musculoskeletal connective tissues.
Data are presented from engineered ligaments undergoing load (Paxton *et al.*, 2012). **(A)** The cellular response to load-ing (activation of the **E**xtracellular **R**egulated **K**inase) peaks at 10 minutes of loading (not shown) and progressively decreases even though the tissue is still being loaded. In **(B)**, ligaments were stretched for 10 minutes (S/0 time) and then rested for 0.5, 1, 3, 6, or 12 hours before another 10-minute stretch and ERK phosphorylation was determined. The data show that it takes 6 hours of rest before the cells can respond completely to a second bout of load. **(C)** Ligaments were stretched either continuously (24 hours a day) or intermittently (10 minutes of stretch, six hours of rest, 10 minutes of stretch, …) for five days and the collagen content of the ligaments was determined. Continuous loading increased col-lagen ~4-fold, whereas an intermittent loading protocol increased collagen ~7.5-fold. This indicates that short bouts of loading (~10 minutes) with long periods of rest (≥ 6 hours) is optimal for building musculoskeletal connective tissues.

affected by nutrition. In the sections below, spe-cific nutrients are discussed vis a vis their ability to improve collagen synthesis.

Vitamin C

Vitamin C is a water-soluble vitamin, meaning that we need to consume an adequate amount every day. In industrialized societies, daily con-sumption of the 46mg per day is not difficult for most people. This was not the case 250 years ago when seamen in the British Navy on long voyages would routinely get scurvy, a disease character-ized by easy bruising, tooth loss, the opening of old wounds, and the stiffening of tendons. In the first controlled nutrition study ever reported, the Scottish physician James Lind fed 12 sailors with scurvy one of six different interventions (Lind, 1753). The two sailors who ate two oranges and one lemon each recovered completely within

a week, whereas in the other sailors the symp-toms continued. It took another 200 years before Jerome Gross showed that guinea pigs on a vita-min C deficient diet did not synthesize colla-gen (Gross, 1959), finally making the molecular connection between vitamin C, collagen syn-thesis and scurvy. Vitamin C is consumed by the enzyme prolyl hydroxylase in the first post-translational reaction following the synthesis of collagen. Without vitamin C, prolyl hydroxy-lase is inactivated and the collagen triple helices become unstable and can no longer be exported (Mussini, Hutton and Udenfriend, 1967). Since vitamin C is consumed in the hydroxylation reaction, it must be replaced every day. This also means that vitamin C levels are low in the morning and need to be replenished before the body can synthesize collagen in response to loading (Lis and Baar, 2019). Even though the

Chapter 6

requirement for vitamin C in the synthesis of collagen has been recognized for 250 years, whether adding extra vitamin C increases collagen synthesis has yet to be determined.

Glycine

The proteins within tendons, ligaments and fascia contain ~40% glycine by weight (Smeets et al., 2019). Because of the amount of glycine in these tissues, some researchers have hypothesized that increasing dietary glycine would benefit tendon healing. To test this hypothesis, Vieira and colleagues injured the Achilles tendon of rats using collagenase and then fed half of the rats a diet containing 5% glycine. After three weeks, the rats on the 5% glycine diet had greater collagen and glycosaminoglycan content than those on the control diet (C. P. edroz. Vieira et al., 2015). This increase in collagen and GAGs resulted in improved mechanical strength both in this study and the follow up study where they added green tea to the nutritional supplement (C. P. edroz. Vieira et al., 2015; C. P. Vieira et al., 2015), suggesting that glycine may aide in the recovery of tendon function after injury. It is important to note that these studies have yet to be repeated in human subjects and that most people would find it difficult to consume ~25 grams of glycine a day. This is equivalent to a quarter of the bottle of most popular glycine supplements. However, given the success of the rodent data, human studies in this area are warranted.

Gelatin/hydrolyzed collagen

A natural source of glycine is dietary collagen. As of 2019, dietary collagen is the fastest growing supplement, with sales topping $45 million in the United States in 2018. As described above, collagen is ~35% glycine and therefore consuming collagen could improve collagen synthesis within the connective tissues. The two most popular

ways to consume collagen in the diet are gelatin and hydrolyzed collagen. Gelatin is released from the skin, bones, and other connective tissues of animals such as cows, pig, and fish as a result of boiling. As a result, bone broths, soups made by boiling an animal carcass, are rich in gelatin; however, the amount of gelatin in a given bone broth varies from 432–9,000 mg per serving depending on how it is made (Alcock, Shaw and Burke, 2019). For more consistent gelatin levels, commercial products from Jello® to Knox® gelatin can be found in most grocery stores. These products are normally used to make desserts since dissolving gelatin in hot water and then cooling it for ~4 hours results in the formation of jelly. For those looking to dissolve dietary collagen in a liquid, hydrolyzed collagen dissolves better than gelatin. For hydrolyzed collagen, gelatin is further processed using either acid or enzymes such as pepsin, papain, bromelain and protease (Hema et al., 2017). These proteins are proteases, enzymes that cut proteins into smaller pieces called peptides. Because processing with acids or enzymes cuts the gelatin into smaller pieces (called peptides), hydrolyzed collagen is unable to form a gel and is more soluble in room temperature water. Even though different companies use different processes that result in different collagen peptides, whether this has any biological significance has yet to be determined.

To determine whether dietary collagen could increase collagen synthesis in connective tissues, we performed a randomized double-blinded placebo-controlled crossover designed study on subjects who consumed 0, 5, or 15 grams of gelatin (Shaw et al., 2017). Over a three-day period, young men took a supplement containing 48mg of vitamin C and either a placebo, 5, or 15 grams of gelatin. The subjects took the supplement every six hours between 7am and 7pm. One hour after taking the supplement, the subjects jumped rope to stimulate bone collagen synthesis. Interestingly, consuming 15 grams of gelatin doubled the amount of collagen synthesized in either the placebo or 5 gram groups (Shaw et al., 2017). Furthermore, when blood was taken from the subjects an hour after taking the supplement and the serum was added to engineered ligaments, the engineered ligaments increased their collagen content in a dose-dependent manner. These data suggest that dietary collagen together with sufficient vitamin C increases collagen synthesis in tendons and ligaments. Repeating the study with gelatin, hydrolyzed collagen, or a gummy made with half gelatin and half hydrolyzed collagen demonstrated that the gelatin and hydrolyzed collagen increased collagen synthesis equivalently, whereas the gummy had no effect (Lis and Baar, 2019). The lack of an effect of the gummy is likely the result of boiling the juice and killing the vitamin C, since amino acid content in the blood was similar between the three feeding groups. Since dietary collagen can increase musculoskeletal collagen synthesis, it is not surprising that consumption of 10g of hydrolyzed collagen decreased knee pain from standing and walking in a randomized double-blinded placebo-controlled study in athletes (Clark et al., 2008). The decrease in knee pain could be the result of improved collagen synthesis in cartilage since cartilage thickness, measured using gadolinium labeled MRI, increases with long term consumption of hydrolyzed collagen (McAlindon et al., 2011). In support of this work, a prospective double-blinded placebo-controlled clinical trial with a cross-over design showed that runners experiencing Achilles pain benefited from collagen supplementation (Praet et al., 2019). In the study, injured runners were placed on an exercise rehabilitation program with or without supplementation with hydrolyzed collagen. Those runners in the collagen supplementation group had a significantly better outcome than those in the placebo group (Praet et al., 2019). Together, these data suggest that consuming gelatin or hydrolyzed collagen may increase collagen synthesis; however, much of the work is still preliminary and needs more research to support its widespread use.

Other nutrients

Because musculoskeletal sprains, strains, and pulls account for a third of all missed workdays and the only outcome measure in many studies is pain, a myriad of other nutrients are purported to improve tendon/ligament function. These and other nutraceuticals have recently been expertly reviewed by Fusini and colleagues (Fusini et al., 2016) and we would encourage readers to go there for details on most of these agents. Many of the nutrients reviewed by Fusini and colleagues are thought to be anti-inflammatory. These agents may therefore work by decreasing pain rather than affecting the structure and function of the musculoskeletal connective tissues. Therefore, much more work is needed to validate these purported nutraceuticals.

Combining loading and nutrition for connective tissues

Tendons and ligaments have relatively low blood flow, instead using diffusion from the environment to provide nutrients and remove waste products (Skyhar et al., 1985; Amiel et al., 1986). Most oxygen and nutrients come from the myotendinous junction (Manske and Lesker, 1982), the fat pad at the enthesis (Benjamin et al., 2004), the paratenon or the synovial sheath (Manske, Bridwell and Lesker, 1978; Lundborg, Holm and Myrhage, 1980; Whiteside and Sweeney, 1980; Amiel et al., 1986). Similar to a sponge, fluid within connective tissues moves out as

Chapter 6

the tissue is loaded and when the tissue relaxes the fluid flows back into the tissue, increasing nutrient uptake (Lundborg, Holm and Myrhage, 1980). Given that loading of connective tissue increases nutrient delivery, the timing of nutrition relative to load is an important consideration. Therefore, optimal timepoint for exercise following intake of supplement is related to the rate of digestion, adsorption and delivery of the nutrient. For 15g of vitamin C-enriched gelatin, amino acid levels in the blood peak approximately one hour after ingestion (Shaw et al., 2017). The blood isolated from subjects an hour after feeding is sufficient to increase collagen synthesis in engineered ligaments and eating the vitamin C-enriched gelatin an hour before loading results in an increase in collagen synthesis in people (Shaw et al., 2017). These data suggest that loading the target tendons at approximately the peak of appearance in the blood can increase collagen production in musculoskeletal connective tissues.

Three case/limited participant studies have utilized this combined loading and nutrition protocol to improve connective tissue function and return to play. In the first, a professional basketball player with a central core patellar tendinopathy was provided 15g of gelatin in orange juice an hour before a ten-minute exercise protocol (Baar, 2019). This rehabilitation protocol was added on top of his normal training and game schedule and contributed to the complete restoration of patellar tendon structure, as determined by MRI, and elimination of pain. In the second, nutrition and short periods of loading were used to accelerate return to play in two elite rugby players following ACL rupture (Shaw, Serpell and Baar, 2019). Soon after reconstructive surgery, the athletes performed two to three range of motion/loading sessions per day, separated by six hours, and preceded by ingestion of

10 g gelatin with 250 mg vitamin C. The rehab sessions used the idea of a minimal effect dose of load (Paxton et al., 2012) to maximally active collagen synthesis within the newly grafted ligament, and to repair the hamstring tendon that was partially used as the graft, and the timed delivery of nutrients was thought to provide necessary substrates for collagen synthesis (Shaw, Serpell and Baar, 2019). The result was a return to full hamstring strength in under 15 weeks and a return to international rugby in ~30 weeks. The last study using load and nutrition to maximize return to play was the cross-over design study on runners with Achilles pain described above (Praet et al., 2019). In this study, the 19 injured runners all performed 2 × 90 one-legged slow, eccentric drops daily for six months with the leg both straight and bent. Half of the runners were supplemented with a hydrolyzed collagen for the first three months, whereas the others got the placebo. At the halfway point, the groups were switched. In the first three months, twice as many participants returned to running from the hydrolyzed collagen group than the placebo. After the cross-over, the collagen group again had twice as many people return to running. In the end, eight subjects returned to running from the hydrolyzed collagen group, whereas only four returned to running while in the placebo group (Praet et al., 2019).

Conclusions and future focus

There is a clear relationship between load, nutrition and tendon/ligament/fascia function. In response to tension, compression, and shear loads these tissues increase collagen, cartilage, and lubrication gene expression, respectively. The positive effect of loading is best seen in recovery from injury. Starting a loading program within two days after injury decreases return to play time by 25% when compared with a group that immobilized the injured area for 9 days (Bayer, Magnusson and Kjaer, 2017). This means that the proper application of load is essential to the development of healthy musculoskeletal connective tissues. When these loads are combined with nutritional interventions such as vitamin C and gelatin or other nutrients like glycine, the result is an improvement in tissue structure and function. Even though there is strong evidence for how load alters tissue function, the role of nutrition in this process is in its infancy. Larger clinical studies are needed to determine whether dietary collagen has clinical efficacy or is simply the result of small samples sizes and a strong belief effect.

An earlier version of this article originally appeared in Fascia, Function, and Medical Applications (CRC Press 2020) by Lesondak and Akey.

References

Akeson, W.H. et al. (1977) Collagen Cross-linking alterations in joint contractures: Changes in the reducible cross-links in periarticular connective tissue collagen after nine weeks of immobilization. *Connective Tissue Research*. Informa Healthcare 5(1): 15–19. doi: 10.3109/03008207709152607.

Alcock, R.D., Shaw, G.C. & Burke, L.M. (2019) Bone broth unlikely to provide reliable concentrations of collagen precursors compared with supplemental sources of collagen used in collagen research. *International Journal of Sport Nutrition and Exercise Metabolism*, 29(3): 265–272. doi: 10.1123/ijsnem. 2018-0139.

Ameye, L. & Young, M.F. (2002) Mice deficient in small leucine-rich proteoglycans: novel in vivo models for osteoporosis, osteoarthritis, Ehlers-Danlos syndrome, muscular dystrophy, and corneal diseases. *Glycobiology*.

Amiel, D. et al. (1986) Nutrition of cruciate ligament reconstruction by diffusion: Collagen synthesis studied in rabbits. *Acta Orthopaedica Scandinavica*, 57: 201–203.

Asou, Y. et al. (2002) Coordinated expression of scleraxis and Sox9 genes during embryonic development of tendons and cartilage. *Journal of Orthopaedic Research*. 20: 827–833. doi: 10.1016/S0736-0266(01)00169-3.

Baar, K. (2019) Stress relaxation and targeted nutrition to treat patellar tendinopathy. *International Journal of Sport Nutrition and Exercise Metabolism*. pp. 1–5. doi: 10.1123/ijsnem.2018-0231.

Bayer, M.L., Magnusson, S.P. & Kjaer, M. (2017) Early versus delayed rehabilitation after acute muscle injury. *New England Journal of Medicine*. 377(133): 1300–1301. doi: 10.1056/NEJMc1708134.

Benjamin, M. et al. (2004) Adipose tissue at entheses: The rheumatological implications of its distribution. A potential site of pain and stress dissipation?. *Annals of the Rheumatic Diseases*. 63(12): 1549–1555. doi: 10.1136/ard.2003.019182.

Burr, D.B., Robling, A.G. & Turner, C.H. (2002) Effects of biomechanical stress on bones in animals. *Bone*. 30(5): 781–786. doi: 10.1016/S8756-3282(02)00707-X.

Calve, S. et al. (2005) The effect of denervation on the heterogeneous material properties of the tibialis anterior tendon. *Proceedings of the 2005 Summer Bioengineering Conference*.

Chang, H.Y. et al. (2002) Diversity, topographic differentiation, and positional memory in human fibroblasts. *Proceedings of the National Academy of Sciences of the United States of America*. doi: 10.1073/pnas.162488599.

Clark, K.L. et al. (2008) 24-Week study on the use of collagen hydrolysate as a dietary supplement in athletes with activity-related joint pain. *Current Medical Research and Opinion*. doi: 10.1185/030079908x291967.

Corman, B. et al. (1998) Aminoguanidine prevents age-related arterial stiffening and cardiac hypertrophy. *Pharmacology*. Available at: www.pnas.org. (Accessed: 1 July 2020).

Dubinskaya, V.A. et al. (2007) Comparative study of the state of water in various human tissues. *Eksperimental'noi Biologii i Meditsiny*.

Dyer, D.G. et al. (no date) Accumulation of Maillard reaction products in skin collagen in diabetes and aging.

Ehlers, T.W. & Vogel, K.G. (1998) Proteoglycan synthesis by fibroblasts from different regions of bovine tendon cultured in alginate beads. *Comparative Biochemistry and Physiology - A Molecular and Integrative Physiology*. 121(4): 355–363. doi: 10.1016/S1095-6433(98)10144-7.

Chapter 6

Evanko, S.P. & Vogel, K.G. (1990) Ultrastructure and proteoglycan composition in the developing fibrocartilaginous region of bovine tendon. *Matrix.* 10(6): 420–436. doi: 10.1016/S0934-8832(11)80150-2.

Evanko, S.P. & Vogel, K.G. (1993) Proteoglycan synthesis in fetal tendon is differentially regulated by cyclic compression *in vitro. Archives of Biochemistry and Biophysics.* 307(1): 153–164. doi: 10.1006/abbi.1993.1574.

Fede, C. et al. (2018) Quantification of hyaluronan in human fasciae: variations with function and anatomical site. *Journal of Anatomy.* 233(4): 552–556. doi: 10.1111/joa.12866.

Fusini, F. et al. (2016) Nutraceutical supplement in the management of tendinopathies: A systematic review. *Muscles, Ligaments and Tendons Journal.* 6(1): 48–57. doi: 10.11138/mltj/2016.6.1.048.

Gillard, G.C. et al. (1979) The influence of mechanical forces on the glycosaminoglycan content of the rabbit flexor digitorum profundus tendon. *Connective Tissue Research.* 7(1): 37–46. doi: 10.3109/03008207909152351.

Gross, J. (1959) Studies on the formation of collagen: IV. Effect of vitamin C deficiency on the neutral salt-extractible collagen of skin. *Journal of Experimental Medicine.* 109(6): 555–569.

Hammes, H.-P. et al. (1991) Aminoguanidine treatment inhibits the development of experimental diabetic retinopathy Wycation/hyperglycemia/microvascular disease/endotheial cells/pericytes). *Proc Nadl Acad Sci USA.*

Hayashi, M. et al. (2013) The effect of lubricin on the gliding resistance of mouse intrasynovial tendon. *PLoS ONE.* 8(12): e83836. doi: 10.1371/journal.pone.0083836.

Heinemeier, K.M. et al. (2013) Lack of tissue renewal in human adult Achilles tendon is revealed by nuclear bom (14) C. FASEB *journal : official publication of the Federation of American Societies for Experimental Biology.* 27(5): 2074–2079. doi: 10.1096/fj.12-225599.

Hema, G.S. et al. (2017) Optimization of process parameters for the production of collagen peptides from fish skin *(Epinephelus malabaricus)* using response surface methodology and its characterization. *Journal of Food Science and Technology.* 54(2): 488–496. doi: 10.1007/s13197-017-2490-2.

Kapacee, Z. et al. (2008) Tension is required for fibripositor formation. *Matrix Biology.* 27(4): 371–375. doi: 10.1016/j.matbio.2007.11.006.

Kjaer, M. (2004) Role of extracellular matrix in adaptation of tendon and skeletal muscle to mechanical loading. doi: 10.1152/physrev.00031.2003.

Laurent, G.J., McAnulty, R.J. & Gibson, J. (1985) Changes in collagen synthesis and degradation during skeletal muscle growth. *American Journal of Physiology-Cell Physiology.* 18(2): 1–4. doi: 10.1152/ajpcell.1985.249.3.c352.

Lind, J. (1753) *A Treatise of the Scurvy in Three Parts.*

Lis, D.M. & Baar, K. (2019) Effects of different vitamin C–enriched collagen derivatives on collagen synthesis. *International Journal of Sport Nutrition and Exercise Metabolism.* doi: 10.1123/ijsnem.2018-0385.

Lundborg, G., Holm, S. & Myrhage, R. (1980) The role of the synovial fluid and tendon sheath for flexor tendon nutrition. *Scandinavian Journal of Plastic and Reconstructive Surgery and Hand Surgery.* 14(1): 99–107. doi: 10.3109/02844318009105739.

Majima, T. et al. (2003) Stress shielding of patellar tendon: effect on small-diameter collagen fibrils in a rabbit model. *Journal of Orthopaedic Science : official journal of the Japanese Orthopaedic Association.* 8(6): 836–841. doi: 10.1007/s00776-003-0707-x.

Manske, P.R., Bridwell, K. & Lesker, P.A. (1978) Nutrient pathways to flexor tendons of chickens using tritiated praline. *Journal of Hand Surgery. American Society for Surgery of the Hand.* 3(4): 352–357. doi: 10.1016/S0363-5023(78)80036-7.

Manske, P.R. & Lesker, P.A. (1982) Nutrient pathways of flexor tendons in primates. *Journal of Hand Surgery. American Society for Surgery of the Hand.* 7(5): 436–444. doi: 10.1016/S0363-5023(82)80035-X.

Marturano, J.E. et al. (2013) Characterization of mechanical and biochemical properties of developing embryonic tendon. *Proceedings of the National Academy of Sciences of the United States of America.* 110(16): 6370–6375. doi: 10.1073/pnas.1300135110.

McAlindon, T.E. et al. (2011) Change in knee osteoarthritis cartilage detected by delayed gadolinium enhanced magnetic resonance imaging following treatment with collagen hydrolysate:

A pilot randomized controlled trial. *Osteoarthritis and Cartilage.* 19(4): 399–405. doi: 10.1016/j.joca.2011.01.001.

Miller, B.F. et al. (2005) Coordinated collagen and muscle protein synthesis in human patella tendon and quadriceps muscle after exercise. *Journal of Physiology.* 567(3): 1021–1033. doi: 10.1113/jphysiol.2005.093690.

Miller, B.F. et al. (2007) Tendon collagen synthesis at rest and after exercise in women. *Journal of Applied Physiology.* 102(2): 541–546. doi: 10.1152/japplphysiol.00797.2006.

Mussini, E., Hutton, J. & Udenfriend, S. (1967) Collagen proline hydroxylase in wound healing, granuloma formation, scurvy, and growth. *Science.* 157(3791): 927–929.

Myer, G.D. et al. (2011) Did the NFL lockout expose the Achilles heel of competitive sports? *Journal of Orthopaedic & Sports Physical Therapy.* 41(10): 702–705. doi: 10.2519/jospt.2011.0107.

Myrick, K.M. et al. (2019) Effects of season long participation on ACL volume in female intercollegiate soccer athletes. *Journal of Experimental Orthopaedics.* 6(1). doi: 10.1186/s40634-019-0182-8.

Nishikimi, M. et al. (1988) Occurrence in humans and guinea pigs of the gene related to their missing enzyme l-gulono-γ-lactone oxidase. *Archives of Biochemistry and Biophysics.* 267(2): 842–846. doi: 10.1016/0003-9861(88)90093-8.

Nugent, G.E. et al. (2006) Dynamic shear stimulation of bovine cartilage biosynthesis of proteoglycan 4. *Arthritis & Rheumatism.* 54(6): 1888–1896. doi: 10.1002/art.21831.

Papakrivopoulou, J. et al. (2004) Differential roles of extracellular signal-regulated kinase 1/2 and p38MAPK in mechanical load-induced procollagen α1(I) gene expression in cardiac fibroblasts. *Cardiovascular Research.* 61(4): 736–744. doi: 10.1016/j.cardiores.2003.12.018.

Paxton, J.Z. et al. (2012) Optimizing an intermittent stretch paradigm using ERK1/2 phosphorylation results in increased collagen synthesis in engineered ligaments. *Tissue Engineering Part A.* 18(3–4): 277–284. doi: 10.1089/ten.tea.2011.0336.

Paxton, J.Z., Grover, L.M. & Baar, K. (2010) Engineering an *in vitro* model of a functional ligament from bone to bone. *Tissue Engineering. Part A.* 16(11): 3515–3525. doi: 10.1089/ten.TEA.2010.0039.

Praet, S.F.E. et al. (2019) Oral supplementation of specific collagen peptides combined with calf-strengthening exercises enhances function and reduces pain in achilles tendinopathy patients. *Nutrients.* 11(1): 1–16. doi: 10.3390/nu11010076.

Reddy, G.K., Stehno-Bittel, L. & Enwemeka, C.S. (2002) Glycation-induced matrix stability in the rabbit Achilles tendon. *Archives of Biochemistry and Biophysics.* 399(2): 174–180. doi: 10.1006/abbi.2001.2747.

Ricard-Blum, S. (2011) The collagen family. *Cold Spring Harbor Perspectives in Biology.* 3(1): 1–19. doi: 10.1101/cshperspect.a004978.

Robbins, J.R., Evanko, S.P. & Vogel, K.G. (1997) Mechanical loading and TGF-β regulate proteoglycan synthesis in tendon. *Archives of Biochemistry and Biophysics.* 342(2): 203–211. doi: 10.1006/abbi.1997.0102.

Robinson, K.A. et al. (2017) Decorin and biglycan are necessary for maintaining collagen fibril structure, fiber realignment, and mechanical properties of mature tendons. *Matrix Biology.* 64: 81–93. doi: 10.1016/j.matbio.2017.08.004.

Sasarman, F. et al. (2016) Biosynthesis of glycosaminoglycans: associated disorders and biochemical tests. *Journal of Inherited Metabolic Disease.* 39(2): 173–188. doi: 10.1007/s10545-015-9903-z.

Shaw, G. et al. (2017) Vitamin C-enriched gelatin supplementation before intermittent activity augments collagen synthesis. *American Journal of Clinical Nutrition.* 105(1). doi: 10.3945/ajcn.116.138594.

Shaw, G., Serpell, B. & Baar, K. (2019) Rehabilitation and nutrition protocols for optimising return to play from traditional ACL reconstruction in elite rugby union players: A case study. *Journal of Sports Sciences.* 37(15): 1794–1803. doi: 10.1080/02640414.2019.1594571.

Siegel, R.C. (1976) Collagen cross-linking: Synthesis of collagen cross-links in vitro with highly purified lysyl oxidase. *Journal of Biological Chemistry.* Available at: http://www.jbc.org/ (Accessed: 1 April 2018).

Siegel, R.C. & Fu, J.C.C. (1976) *Collagen Cross-Linking:Purification and Substrate Specificity of Lysyl Oxidase, The Journal of Biological Chemistry.* Available at: http://www.jbc.org/ (Accessed: 1 April 2018).

Skyhar, M.J. et al. (1985) Nutrition of the anterior cruciate ligament. Effects of continuous passive motion. *American*

Journal of Sports Medicine. 13(6): 415–418. doi: 10.1177/036354658501300609.

Smeets, J.S.J. et al. (2019) Protein synthesis rates of muscle, tendon, ligament, cartilage, and bone tissue in vivo in humans. *PLOS ONE.* 14(11): e0224745. doi: 10.1371/journal.pone.0224745.

Vieira, C.P. et al. (2015) Green tea and glycine aid in the recovery of tendinitis of the Achilles tendon of rats. *Connective Tissue Research.* 56(1): 50–58. doi: 10.3109/03008207.2014.983270.

Vieira, C.P. et al. (2015) Glycine improves biochemical and biomechanical properties following inflammation of the achilles tendon. *Anatomical Record (Hoboken, N.J. : 2007).* 298(3): 538–545. doi: 10.1002/ar.23041.

Whiteside, L.A. & Sweeney, R.E. (1980) Nutrient pathways of the cruciate ligaments. An experimental study using the hydrogen wash-out technique. *Journal of Bone and Joint Surgery. American volume.* 62(7): 1176–1180. Available at: http://www.ncbi.nlm.nih.gov/pubmed/7430206 (Accessed: 10 June 2019).

Hypo- and hypermobility

Jan Dommerholt and Nathan Mayberry

Introduction

Joint mobility is a fundamental prerequisite to human movement and motor development. Commonly measured as range of motion, joint mobility is the controlled motion of a bony lever on articular surfaces (Berryman Reese and Bandy, 2017). Cardinal planes of motion and axes of rotation (frontal, sagittal, transverse) further standardize these motions. While range of motion is variable among individuals, there are suggested norms required for movement efficiency (Soucie et al., 2011). Deviation from these normative values is characterized as either hypomobility or hypermobility. Identifying and addressing impairments in joint mobility are essential components of managing aberrant movement patterns (Keer and Simmonds, 2011).

Hypomobile individuals frequently present to yoga and Pilates classes to improve their flexibility and overall physical condition but, dependent upon the underlying cause of their hypomobility, they may pose specific challenges not only for yoga and Pilates instructors, but also for other bodyworkers, physiotherapists, Feldenkrais and Alexander teachers, and neuromuscular therapists. In this chapter, we use a broad definition of "bodywork" to encompass all these and other disciplines. This chapter provides an overview of specific hypomobile syndromes and associated issues that bodyworkers should at least be familiar with. On the other hand, hypermobile persons are commonly thought of as excellent candidates for Pilates and yoga, as often they have no difficulty assuming difficult poses and stretching much further than the average yoga student. Yet hypermobility features its own specific challenges. Persons with Ehlers-Danlos Syndrome, for example, may have such loose connective tissue and lack fascial stability that maintaining certain poses or performing core training may be difficult.

Hypomobility

Hypomobility can be defined as decreased joint mobility due to inherited or acquired structural changes in the joint, joint capsule or other surrounding tissues, or because of functional alterations of the control system. It is characterized by decreased range of motion, altered movement activation patterns, shortened muscles and fascia, and possible swelling. There continues to be a paucity of studies on hypomobility and of papers describing the prevalence of hypomobility occurring at different joints. Persons who are just a bit out of shape and who have developed tight muscles and restricted fascia can do very well with bodywork interventions. Others, with more complex inherited joint hypomobility, may require significant modifications and individualized sessions addressing their unique problems.

Inherited joint hypomobility

Inherited joint hypomobility is a very complex issue. The prevalence of inherited conditions

Chapter 7

featuring joint hypomobility is probably very low, but it cannot be determined accurately without objective data. This section provides much detailed information about several inherited disorders in the hope that familiarity with these disorders will improve the quality of life for participants, and perhaps provide new business opportunities for "disease-specific" yoga classes, or Pilates mat work. Few yoga and Pilates instructors may be familiar with these disorders, and the possible benefits of bodywork have hardly been explored. Recognizing that persons with these disorders may not often present to Pilates, yoga or bodywork, we recommend consulting this section as necessary.

Inherited joint hypomobility can be related to a variety of genetic diagnoses, such as arthrogryposis multiplex congenita, which is defined by the presence of congenital non-progressive contractures across two or more major joints (Valdes-Flores et al., 2016). The prevalence of arthrogryposis multiplex congenita is 1:3000–5000 newborns (Valdes-Flores et al., 2016). The disorder is not only linked to nervous system disorders, such as focal or generalized anterior horn cell deficiency, and structural brain disorder or damage, but can also be associated with a wide range of other diagnoses, such as dysplasias (diastrophic, arastremmatic, Kniest, metatropic, and campomelic dysplasia), Schwartz syndrome, fetal alcohol syndrome with synostoses, osteogenesis imperfecta, Emery–Dreifuss muscular dystrophy, antecubital webbing syndrome, various pterygium syndromes (i.e. popliteal and multiple pterygium syndrome), and Freeman Sheldon syndrome, among others (Mennen et al., 2005). Because of the wide range of conditions linked to arthrogryposis, there are multiple possible genetic mutations and signaling pathways. Several researchers implicated mutations in X-linked zinc-finger gene ZC4H2 in

the etiology of arthrogryposis multiplex congenita (Okubo et al., 2018; Kondo et al., 2018), while others identified RYR1 mutations (Brackmann et al., 2018), TTN (Fernandez-Marmiesse et al., 2017), LG14 (Xue et al., 2017) and BICD2 mutations (Ravenscroft et al., 2016), among others. Three consanguineous families presented with different homozygous mutations in GPR126, which is required to encode G-protein-coupled receptor 126, a critical step in peripheral nervous system axonal myelination (Ravenscroft et al., 2015). In other words, the diagnosis of arthrogryposis can involve a wide range of genetic variations and, therefore, rather different presentations.

It is not necessary for bodyworkers, Pilates and yoga instructors to fully comprehend the many complexities of arthrogryposis, but they may be able to contribute to a better quality of life and at least temporary improvements in range of motion through active participation in regular individualized exercise programs. Bodywork is often offered in a non-medical environment, which may be an appealing alternative for this population. Little is known about the specific fascial restrictions in persons with arthrogryposis. It is, however, possible that the contractures feature extreme fascial webbing, whereby the main nerves and blood vessels are also shortened. In extreme cases, webbing of the knee joint may require extensive surgical release of the webbing and even shortening of the femur (Saleh et al., 1989; Ponten, 2015). In such extreme cases, bodywork approaches have limited value.

Other inherited diseases featuring joint hypomobility include congenital talipes equinovarus (clubfoot), idiopathic toe walking and symptomatic generalized hypomobility. The incidence of congenital talipes equinovarus ranges from 1–3 cases per 1000 pregnancies, with males twice as frequently affected as females.

It is less common in Asian populations, but more common among Polynesians and the Maoris in New Zealand, with an incidence of 6.5–7 per 1000 births (Drvaric et al., 1989; Chapman et al., 2000). The incidence for Indians and Pakistanis living in the UK was 7.8 per 1000 (Leck and Lancashire, 1995). One of the most used treatments is the Ponseti method, which involves serial casting followed by surgical correction for resistant deformity (Khanna and Vaishya, 2017). The method is widely used throughout the world and it is still considered the gold standard, although recently Andreoli et al. (2014) described a case of a newborn treated with serial casting combined with osteopathic manipulative treatment without having to resort to surgery. Considering that osteopathic manipulations were beneficial, perhaps there are also opportunities for modified yoga interventions, even although that would require some unorthodox, out-of-the-box thinking.

While the management of congenital talipes equinovarus is well established, not much is definitively known about the genetic predisposition and the signaling pathways. The syndrome is likely to be the result of a variety of environmental and genetic factors. Some older papers suspected an autosomal recessive inheritance, but, more likely, the development of clubfoot may be a result of one major gene effect involving interactions with additional polygenes and environmental factors (Dietz, 2002; Rebbeck et al., 1993). Basit and Khoshhal (2018) summarized the current state of affairs in a recent review. They described that genes involved in coding for contractile proteins of skeletal myofibers may be involved, but while there is no clearly identified genetic deficit, variants in TBX4, PITX1, HOXA, HOXC and HOXD clusters genes, NAT2 and others seem to play a significant role. The importance of the developmental transcriptional

pathway, known as the PITX1-TBX4 pathway, was recently confirmed (Dobbs and Gurnett, 2012). TBX4 and PITX1 are expressed in the hindlimb, which helps explain the foot phenotype observed with transcription mutations of these factors. To break this down a bit more, problems in the feet are more common than in other areas, which is explained by a genetic predisposition. Several clubfoot-like deformities are associated with craniocarpotarsal and diastrophic dysplasia, Smith-Lemli-Opitz syndrome, Pierre Robin syndrome, amyoplasia, myelomeningocele, congenital constriction bands, intrauterine poisoning by aminopterin or d-tubocurarine, some Larsen syndromes, distal arthrogryposis, and various chromosomal abnormalities (Dietz, 2002).

Idiopathic toe walking is a diagnosis by exclusion, presenting in children aged older than 3 years who exhibit an abnormal gait pattern with excessive forefoot weight bearing. It may be associated with cerebral palsy (Barber et al., 2012), Duchenne muscular dystrophy (Hyde et al., 2000), McArdle's disease (Pomarino et al., 2018), and even attention deficit and hyperactivity disorder (Soto Insuga et al., 2018). In a minority of cases a familiar predisposition is suspected (Pomarino et al., 2016). It could be related to a congenital short Achilles tendon (Shulman et al., 1997), but it is also conceivable that Achilles tendon shortening develops as a result of persistent toe walking, especially since at birth these children typically do not present with contractures (Brunt et al., 2004). Others have described a link with sensory dysfunction (Montgomery and Gauger, 1978).

Symptomatic generalized hypomobility has been described as a dysfunction with a systemic decrease in range of motion, an increased stiffness of joint ligaments and musculo-tendinous structures, lower bone density, excessive

Chapter 7

pyridinoline cross-links, and keloid scarring (Engelbert et al., 2004). There are no additional data available about symptomatic generalized hypomobility, but yoga and Pilates are likely beneficial for this population.

Acquired joint hypomobility

Acquired hypomobility can be due to a wide range of causes, such as scar tissue, kinesiophobia (fear of movement), increased age, psychological factors, inactivity and a sedentary lifestyle, and certain medical conditions, such as scleroderma, osteoarthritis, fractures, stiff person syndrome, Parkinson syndrome, cerebral palsy and spasticity, and complex regional pain syndrome, among others. Unlike for most inherited joint mobility syndromes, the role yoga and Pilates can play in the overall well-being of persons with acquired joint hypomobility is easier to grasp. Fascial restrictions associated with these disorders can be addressed by specific stretching routines and improved whole-body stability and flexibility exercises.

Within physiotherapy, chiropractic and bodywork disciplines, there seems to be a tendency to approach hypomobility from a primary biomechanical perspective, which, in many cases, may be counterproductive. For example, individuals suffering from depression may present with functional hypomobility of the shoulder joints (Okely et al., 2019). Clinicians using a strict biomechanical approach would likely miss the subtleties of the more complex presentation of depressed patients. Silva et al. (2016) described bilateral joint hypomobility of the subtalar joints in women diagnosed with fibromyalgia, whereas Brown et al. (2016) found that patients with higher levels of kinesiophobia had a greater range of motion deficits following a total knee arthroplasty. Bodyworkers should implement a comprehensive approach in dealing with persons with hypomobility issues.

With regards to altered control systems, hypomobility and hypokinetic symptoms are common in patients suffering from Parkinson syndrome. This may be linked to dysfunction of the basal ganglia, especially the subthalamic nucleus (STN) (Di Matteo et al., 2008). A decreased STN function results in hypokinetic symptoms and joint stiffness or hypomobility, commonly observed in patients with Parkinson. The innervation of the STN is strongly influenced by serotonin, which in turn is mediated by intra-STN serotonin receptors, such as the 5-HT_{1A}, 5-HT_{2A} and 5-HT_{2C} receptors (Xiang et al., 2005). The peripheral administration of the $5\text{-HT}_{2A/C}$ agonist, 2,5-dimethoxy-4-iodoamphetamine (DOI), leads to a significant reduction of mobility (Hameleers et al., 2007). Increasing STN neuronal activity results in a decrease in mobility, which can be reversed by high frequency brain stimulation (HFS). Even although there are complex underlying reasons for the noted hypomobility in Parkinson syndrome, regular participation in Pilates, yoga and other forms of bodywork may possibly slow down the degree of dysfunction and provide at least temporary improved mobility.

Another diagnosis whereby a strict biomechanical orientation is not useful is a central nervous system autoimmune disease known as the stiff-person syndrome (Ciccotto et al., 2013). The disorder has also been observed in infants, where it often is described as infantile hyperexplexia, as well as in children and adolescents (Tracy and McKeon, 2015). The syndrome features muscular rigidity and painful muscle spasms primarily in the proximal limb and axial muscles, including the paraspinal muscles. The disease is associated with auto-antibodies to glutamic acid decarboxylase, which can impair the synthesis of one of the main inhibitory neurotransmitters of the brain known as gamma-aminobutyric acid (GABA). Stiff-person syndrome must be differentiated from other rare disorders such as subacute progressive encephalomyelitis (Hutchinson et al., 2008), paraneoplastic syndrome (Sweeney and Howe, 2016), and acquired neuromyotonia (Isaacs Syndrome) (Rana et al., 2012) to assure proper individualized medical management. As with Parkinson syndrome, individuals with stiff-person syndrome may benefit from individualized bodywork.

Persons with stiff-person syndrome typically do not have pyramidal and extrapyramidal dysfunction. The pyramidal system controls voluntary movements and dysfunction of the system may lead to paralysis, for example, when someone suffers from a cerebrovascular accident, or to increased reflexes and spasticity (Tranchant et al., 2017). The extrapyramidal system controls automatic movement patterns and dysfunction of that system may cause involuntary movements such as tics, tremors, myoclonus, chorea and dystonia, among others (Cotelli et al., 2018). Examples of extrapyramidal syndromes are progressive supranuclear palsy, Parkinson's disease and corticobasal syndrome.

Range of motion

It is obvious that joint hypomobility can have far reaching consequences. For example, hypomobility of the temporomandibular joints may lead to airway obstruction, difficulty with mastication, eating and other oral functions, impaired speech and language development, and mandibular growth restrictions of the craniomandibular complex (Costello and Edwards, 2005; Sahdev et al., 2019). Hypomobility of the finger joints may negatively impact manual dexterity and precision grip force control (Campos Cde et al., 2013).

Knee, ankle and foot hypomobility can cause significant impairments of gait and overall mobility (Delafontaine et al., 2015), whereas spinal hypomobility may reduce overall functionality and mobility (Alqhtani et al., 2015; Mustur et al., 2009).

There is disagreement, however, whether restricted range of motion as the prime feature of hypomobility can be assessed accurately in the clinical setting, particularly when it concerns segmental spinal mobility. Performing a manual posterior-anterior cervical gliding test for the mid-cervical spine was comparable with the results of dynamic radiographic assessment for the diagnosis of intervertebral hypomobility (Rey-Eiriz et al., 2010). To determine whether a certain assessment method is valid and reliable, two or more examiners should reach acceptable levels of agreement regarding the findings, which is referred to as interrater reliability. Intrarater reliability refers to whether the same examiner consistently has the same findings or scores on a test. Two examiners reached good interrater reliability with palpation for stiffness in the cervical, thoracic and lumbar spine (Holt et al., 2018), which means that they reached the same conclusions following an examination. On the contrary, the interrater and intrarater reliability of passive physiological accessory movement assessment of the lumbar spine was poor when performed by novice physical therapists (Deore and May, 2012). Three experienced physical therapists also had poor interrater reliability for testing segmental mobility of the lumbar spine (Johansson, 2006), which was similar to the findings of Schneider et al. (2008), who observed poor interrater reliability for the manual assessment of lumbar segmental motion restrictions. They did establish that palpation to provoke pain responses was more reliable. Koppenhaver et al. (2014) concluded that the sensitivity and specificity estimates of judgments of hypomobility were low with no correlation between manual assessments and measures of stiffness. A systematic review found limited evidence in support of reliability and validity of clinical tests to assess cervical mobility, head posture and location of pain, and in adults with neck pain and associated disorders (Lemeunier et al., 2018). In a study of the interrater reliability of the cervicothoracic and shoulder physical examination in patients with a primary complaint of shoulder pain, most cervical and shoulder range of motion measurements had variable reliability co-efficients ranging from slight to substantial agreement; however, horizontal shoulder adduction had poor reliability (Burns et al., 2016). It is of interest that Abbott et al. (2005) established that manual clinical examination procedures do have moderate validity for detecting segmental motion abnormality, which is in line with the findings of Haneline et al. (2008), who identified several studies reporting high levels of reproducibility. Furthermore, Widerström et al. (2012) found substantial interrater reliability for pain modulation, stabilization exercise and training, but not for manipulations, which was poor.

To overcome the limitations of manual range of motion measurements, the use of three-dimensional computerized motion analysis systems may provide more accuracy and reduce inherent human errors (Karakostas et al., 2018). The most common motion analysis systems can be divided into motion sensor systems and high-speed or infrared camera systems with reflective markers. Both systems are designed to not only measure range of motion, but also to provide detailed kinetic and kinematic analyses. The utility of motion analysis system is well established for the lower extremities, but much less so for the spine and upper extremities (Piche et al., 2007; Karakostas et al., 2018). There are also other issues, such as the high costs of computerized

systems, the lack of established normative data, and the inherent variability in complexity of joint structures, making standardized assessment methods difficult.

Independent of the methods used to determine range of motion, clinicians need to consider regional interdependences (McDevitt et al., 2015), for example, the mobility of the thoracic spine influences the position of the scapula and, therefore, the mobility of the upper extremity (Theodoridis and Ruston, 2002). Patients with non-specific chronic low back pain may also present with altered positions of the scapula, which in turn may trigger movement dysfunctions of the upper extremities (Taghizadeh et al., 2017). In addition, movement dysfunction of the thoracic spine has been linked to pain in the shoulder and upper arm, which by itself will likely limit the active range of motion of the shoulder joints (Berglund et al., 2008). In other words, measuring shoulder elevation without taking the mobility of the thoracic spine into account may give inaccurate results, which inevitably would lead to less than optimal treatment strategies (Puentedura and Cleland, 2015). Similarly, cervical dysfunction may be linked to unilateral lateral epicondylalgia (tennis elbow) (Coombes et al., 2014). There are several other interdependences in the body, partially because of the interconnectedness of various fascial layers. Pilates, yoga and Feldenkrais are excellent whole-body approaches to address the interconnectedness of restrictions in range of motion. There is no question that the many fascial connections between different body regions play a key role in the regional interdependences.

Physiotherapy

Many patients with hypomobility consult with physiotherapists. As mentioned before, clinicians who adhere to a strict biomechanical approach may be too restrictive and, therefore,

Hypo- and hypermobility

it is encouraging that within the field of physiotherapy other approaches have been developed. Sahrmann et al. (2017) developed a comprehensive kinesiopathologic model of "movement system impairment syndromes", which assumes that repeated movement patterns and sustained suboptimal joint positions may lead to the development of pathology and pathoanatomical changes in tissues and joint structures. The model incorporates "the musculoskeletal system as the effector of movement, the nervous system as the regulator of movement, and the cardiovascular, pulmonary, and endocrine systems as providing support for the other systems, but that also are affected by movement". Rabey et al. (2017) concluded that manual skills, including range of motion measurements such as the assessment of passive accessory and physiological movements, are valid tools when used judiciously in the context of an individualized, multidimensional approach based on contemporary pain science and patient-centered values. Of course, bodyworkers should approach their hypomobile clients from this contextual point of view.

From a neurophysiological perspective, segmental joint hypomobility may occur due to dysfunction of neurophysiological processing, which often is linked to the experience of pain with movement and a concurrent increase in muscle tone. The interaction between extra-articular and intra-articular aspects of movement patterns plays a significant role in joint mobility, which involves both peripheral and central neural mechanisms, passive structures, including ligaments, joint capsules and intra-articular discs, and active controls from muscles and to a lesser degree from fascia.

Hypermobility

Hypermobility is defined as excessive joint movement within a normal plane of motion.

The term hypermobility is frequently used interchangeably with the terms hyperextensibility and hyperlaxity, although technically the latter refers to movement in abnormal planes (Coles et al., 2017). Hypermobility can be hereditary, constitutional, structural, or the result of functional changes in the joint and surrounding tissues. Hypermobility can be localized or generalized. Localized hypermobility may be due to trauma, such as a joint dislocation, surgery, training (i.e. excessive stretching in gymnastics), but can also be hereditary. Generalized or systemic hypermobility, involving more than five joints, is usually hereditary with individual differences based on age, sex, and ethnic background (Coles et al., 2017). Systemic hypermobility is often assessed with the Beighton Score (Figure 7.1), which has acceptable inter-rater reliability but inconclusive validity (Juul-Kristensen et al., 2017). Several other commonly used tests lack satisfactory reliability and validity (Juul-Kristensen et al., 2017). The Five-Part Questionnaire (Table 7.1) is the most commonly used questionnaire for adults with conflicting evidence of reliability and validity (Juul-Kristensen et al., 2017; Hakim and Grahame, 2003). The Bristol Impact of Hypermobility test, which aims to measure the impact of hypermobility on a person's life, showed excellent test-retest reliability (Palmer et al., 2017).

Nearly all children could be considered hypermobile with girls having greater joint mobility than boys. Range of motion tends to increase until adolescence then tapers off in adulthood and old age. Because joint mobility in children is far greater than in adults, diagnosing hypermobility in children is challenging as there are no age-related norms for range of motion in children. An Australian study of 1584 subjects showed that 61% of girls and 37% of boys were hypermobile (Morris et al., 2017), which does not necessarily indicate

Chapter 7

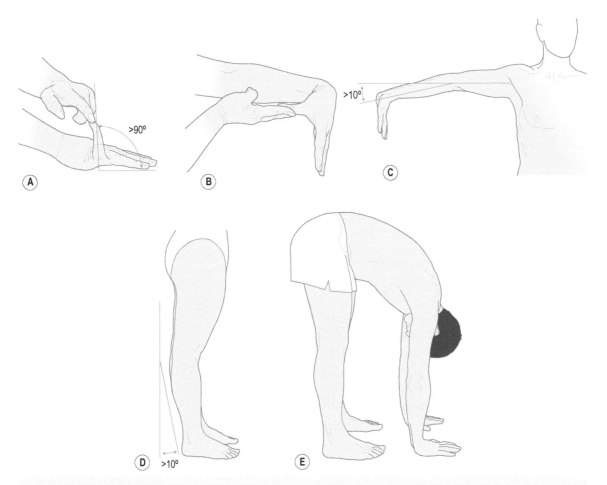

Figure 7.1 The Beighton tests

Tests **A–D** are performed bilaterally and one point is awarded for each positive test for a possible total of 0–8. Test **E** is either positive or negative; one point is awarded for a positive outcome. Although there is no universal agreement on the interpretation of the Beighton tests, many researchers agree that a score of 4–9 is indicative of systemic hypermobility.

Table 7.1 The Five-Point Questionnaire (Hakim and Grahame, 2003)
1. Can you now (or could you ever) place your hands flat on the floor without bending your knees?
2. Can you now (or could you ever) bend your thumb to touch your forearm?
3. As a child, did you amuse your friends by contorting your body into strange shapes or could you do the splits?
4. As a child or teenager, did your shoulder or kneecap dislocate on more than one occasion?
5. Do you consider yourself "double-jointed"?
A "yes" answer to two or more questions suggests joint hypermobility with 80–85% sensitivity and 80–90% specificity.

that these children had abnormal range of motion or that they experienced disproportionate pain or dysfunction. Javadi Parvaneh and Shiari (2016) modified the Beighton criteria to better identify hypermobility in children.

Pain is a very common feature of hypermobility syndromes, both in children and adults, but not all hypermobile people are necessarily symptomatic (Juul-Kristensen et al., 2017). A study of 466 hypermobile adults reported that 99% suffered from joint pain and 91% from extremity pain along with several other symptoms including chronic fatigue (82%), anxiety (73%) and depression (69%) (Murray et al., 2013). Bettini et al. (2018) concluded that joint hypermobility was a common precursor to pain hypersensitivity and central sensitization in 40 hypermobile adolescents. Managing pain in hypermobile patients can be challenging and often requires a multimodal interdisciplinary approach (Revivo et al., 2019; Zhou et al., 2018). Pain management may include manual therapy, such as trigger point therapy and soft tissue mobilizations (Tewari et al., 2017), pain science education (Louw, 2016), cognitive, emotional and behavioral therapy (Baeza-Velasco et al., 2018), and external-focus exercise therapy (Wulf and Lewthwaite, 2016; Wulf et al., 2018). Although there is little known about yoga, Pilates and other bodywork in the context of painful hypermobility syndromes, there is no question that these approaches can be very valuable for this patient population. For example, yoga has been shown to be more effective in reducing chronic low back pain compared to conventional exercise classes, a self-care book and standard medical care (Williams et al., 2003; 2009; Sherman et al., 2005). Yoga instructors may have to modify the exercises and poses to stay within a pain-free range, while keeping the focus on improving the client's whole-body and individual joint stability, muscle strength and endurance, and improved

proprioception. In addition, yoga may be able to reduce anxiety and stress by incorporating a more mental focus with breathing exercises, such as pranayama, and meditation (West et al., 2004; Kabat-Zinn, 1982). Pilates training has also been shown to improve mental health outcomes (Fleming and Herring, 2018).

Asymptomatic hypermobility can be an asset for certain activities, like yoga (Nilsson et al., 1993), ballet (Foley and Bird, 2013), modern dance (Ruemper and Watkins, 2012), gymnastics (Bukva et al., 2019), acrobatics (Purnell et al., 2010), figure skating (Tosi et al., 2019) and cheerleading (Shields and Smith, 2011). Studies found that 44–58% of dancers were systematically hypermobile (Day et al., 2011; Sanches et al., 2015). A study of elite dancers determined that over 70% met the Beighton Score criteria (Chan et al., 2018). In general, hypermobility does not necessarily increase the risk of injury (Bukva et al., 2019), although several studies did find a correlation between joint hypermobility and risk of injury (Ruemper and Watkins, 2012; McCormack et al., 2004; Tosi et al., 2019). Fifty percent of acrobatic gymnasts reported pain in their spine, hips and knees (Anwajler et al., 2005). A study of Australian yoga students did not identify any evidence of an increased risk of injury (Penman et al., 2012), but other studies revealed an increase in pain in participants with degenerative joint disease and facet arthropathy (Lee et al., 2019). The authors cautioned against extreme spinal flexion for individuals with osteopenia or osteoporosis due to a higher risk of compression fractures or deformities.

Whether hypermobility is an asset or a liability in these activities continues to be an issue of debate (Foley and Bird, 2013; Grahame and Jenkins, 1972). On one hand, being hypermobile may make such activities easier, but on the other hand, it is conceivable that the risk of micro-trauma and

Chapter 7

joint instability may increase (Harris et al., 2016; Weber et al., 2015, Ruemper and Watkins; 2012). In general, the benefits of yoga, dance and other physical activity, such as improved cardiovascular health, increased muscle strength, endurance and control, may outweigh the risks of injury (Hayes and Chase, 2010; Wiese et al., 2019). Contact sports do appear to increase the risk of injury in hypermobile athletes (Rejeb et al., 2019).

Inherent joint laxity may have directed individuals towards dance and gymnastics (Nilsson et al., 1993), but for others, increased joint laxity may be the result of regular training involving excessive stretching. Individuals with significant joint laxity, Marfan's syndrome, or Ehlers-Danlos syndrome, should be screened medically for cardiovascular abnormalities (i.e. fluctuating blood pressures, postural orthostatic tachycardia syndrome and mitral valve prolapse) and soft tissue dysfunction (i.e. tissue fragility and potential aneurysms) prior to engaging in physically challenging activities (Grahame, 1993). The focus of yoga, dance and gymnastics should shift towards maintaining and improving joint and overall body stability in symptomatic hypermobility and not emphasize flexibility. When hypermobile individuals engage in stretching exercises, typically they primarily stretch their joint capsules and ligaments and not their muscles and tendons, which will potentially increase their hypermobility and risk of subluxations and dislocations (Shields and Smith, 2011).

Hypermobile individuals can be divided into three broad groups: (1) asymptomatic hypermobility, (2) syndromic joint hypermobility, and (3) hypermobility spectrum disorders (Coles et al., 2017).

Syndromic joint hypermobility

Most hypermobility syndromes are hereditary disorders, such as the Ehlers-Danlos Syndromes (EDS) (Malfait et al., 2017), Marfan Syndrome (MFS) (Loeys et al., 2010) and Osteogenesis Imperfecta (OI) (Van Dijk et al., 2010), among others. EDS is the most common inherited connective tissue disorder with approximately 1 in 5000 births (Tinkle et al., 2017), compared with 1 in 3000–10 000 for MFS (Pyeritz, 2017) and 1 in 10 000–15 000 for OI (Lafage-Proust and Courtois, 2019; Morello, 2018).

Ehlers-Danlos Syndromes

According to the updated EDS clinical classification, published in 2017, Ehlers-Danlos Syndromes are a heterogeneous group of 13 different but overlapping connective tissue disorders, featuring joint hypermobility, skin hyperextensibility and fragile tissues (Table 7.2). Many patients with EDS experience persistent pain, autonomic dysfunction (dysautonomia) and gastrointestinal dysmotility (Beckers et al., 2017). Each subtype has its own specific major and minor criteria. For all subtypes, except the hypermobile subtype, the definitive diagnosis must be made by molecular confirmation with identification of the involved gene(s), which would also determine the particular inheritance pattern, specific risk factors, and guide the therapeutic management.

As the genetic basis of hypermobile EDS is unknown, the diagnosis is made based on history, examination and a clinical impression (Malfait et al., 2017). The autosomal dominant classical (cEDS) and hypermobile (hEDS) types are the most common. The vast majority of cEDS patients have heterozygous mutations in one of the genes encoding type V collagen (COL5A1 and COL5A2) (Bowen et al., 2017). According to the new EDS criteria, the diagnoses of hEDS and joint hypermobility syndrome are no longer considered two separate entities. Instead, both diagnoses are included in the definition of hEDS, characterized not only by hypermobility, but also

Table 7.2 Clinical classification of the Ehlers-Danlos Syndromes (EDS), genetic basis and protein type (Malfait et al., 2017)

Clinical subtype	Genetic bases	Proteins
Classical EDS	Major: COL5A1, COL5A1 Rare: COL1A1	Type V collagen Type I collagen
Classical-like EDS	TNXB	Tenascin XB
Cardiac-valvular EDS	COL1A2	Type I collagen
Vascular EDS	Major: COL3A1 Rare: COL1A1	Type III collagen Type I collagen
Hypermobile EDS	Unknown	Unknown
Arthrochalasia EDS	COL1A1, COL1A2	Type I collagen
Dermatosparaxis EDS	ADAMTS2	ADAMTS2
Kyphoscoliotic EDS	PLOD1 FKBP14	LH1 FKBP22
Brittle cornea syndrome	ZNF469 PRDM5	ZNF469 PRDM5
Spondylodysplastic EDS	B4GALT7 B3GALT6 SLC39A13	B4GalT7 B3GalT6 ZIP13
Musculocontractural EDS	CHST14 DSE	D4ST1 DSE
Myopathic EDS	COL12A1	Type XII collagen
Periodontal EDS	C1R C1S	C1r C1s

by chronic pain, dysautonomia, chronic fatigue, anxiety, and other associated symptoms. The hEDS type represents at least 80–90% of all EDS cases (Tinkle et al., 2017). Many patients with hEDS experience significant levels of disability, which is highly correlated with both physical and psychological factors (Scheper et al., 2016).

As part of the differential diagnostic process, patients must be screened for possible neurological complications resulting from tissue weakness, biophysical deformative stresses, entrapments, and tissue deformations (Henderson et al., 2017). Comorbid conditions reported with hEDS include Chiari malformations with or without tethered cord syndrome (Milhorat et al., 2007) and craniocervical instability with or without ventral brainstem compression (Henderson et al., 2018). Other common comorbidities include mast cell activation syndrome (Seneviratne et al., 2017), gastrointestinal dysfunction (Botrus et al., 2018), and postural orthostatic tachycardia syndrome (POTS) (Bonamichi-Santos et al., 2018). Many hypermobile EDS patients can benefit greatly from adjunctive bodywork approaches, such as Pilates (McNeill et al., 2018; Lewitt et al., 2019). For a successful Pilates training program, the medical classification of EDS may not be as relevant as the actual observations of the implications of hypermobility on movement patterns and motor control (Fayh et al., 2018). A qualified Pilates instructor may want to focus on establishing neuromuscular connections with slow-motion coordinated movement patterns emphasizing coordination, balance, breathing, and proprioception (McNeill et al., 2018; Bradley and Esformes, 2014). Pilates can be very effective in reducing pain and disability (Byrnes et al., 2018). Of course, the same applies to other fields, such as dance, yoga, fitness and other movement therapies.

Marfan Syndrome

Marfan syndrome (MFS) is another autosomal dominant heritable disorder of connective tissue. According to the revised Ghent Nosology for Marfan Syndrome, the cardinal clinical features are aortic root aneurysm and ectopia lentis (Loeys et al., 2010). Mutations of TGF-β are also associated with Loeys-Dietz syndrome (De Cario et al., 2018). Patients with MFS frequently experience sleep apnea associated with a narrow and high palate (Paoloni et al., 2018), cerebrovascular disease (Kim et al., 2018), thoracic aortic and other aneurysms (Faure et al., 2018). The health-related quality of life of MFS patients is below the population norm; socioeconomic factors, such as college education, marital status, higher household income, private health insurance, full-time employment and moderate alcohol use, were predictors of a better quality of life (Goldfinger et al., 2017).

Patients with MFS have a defect of the gene FBN1 responsible for encoding fibrillin-1, one of the main proteins of the extracellular microfibril, which may increase transforming growth factor beta (TGF-β) activity and lead to dilatation and aortic dissection, mitral valve prolapse, excessive bone growth, pulmonary blebs and spontaneous pneumothorax, and several other syndromes, including some forms of dwarfism. More than 1200 mutations have been identified (Pyeritz, 2017). Similar to EDS, bodywork approaches can be very helpful for patients with Marfan's Syndrome.

Osteogenesis Imperfecta

Osteogenesis Imperfecta, or brittle bone disease, is known for its genetic and clinical heterogeneity. It is an autosomal dominant inherited, generalized, connective-tissue disease with monoallelic mutations in type I collagen genes COL1A1 and COL1A2 (Reuter et al., 2013). Currently, there are 18 different types of OI based on possible genetic mutations ranging from mild (OI type 1), moderate (OI type 4), severe (OI type 3) to lethal (OI type 2) (Kang et al., 2017; Morello, 2018), but the list continues to expand (Lafage-Proust and Courtois, 2019). At least one recessive type is X-chromosome-linked. OI type 5 is due to a mutation of the IFITM5 gene. OI involves mutations in type I collagen, type I collagen synthesis and the differentiation and function of osteoblasts. It is beyond the scope of this chapter to review the many genetic mutations involved in OI.

Patients with OI have a predisposition for fractures, short stature, bone deformities, ligamentous laxity, joint hypermobility, vascular fragility, ocular and dental abnormalities, respiratory impairments due to severe scoliosis, relative macrocephaly, blue sclerae, the presence of sutural and intrasutural bones on skull radiography, progressive post-pubertal hearing loss, insertional tendinopathies, craniovertebral junction abnormalities (mostly in OI types 3 and 4), including platybasia, basilar invagination and basilar impression. Adults with unexplained bone fragility should be examined for OI, MFS, Gaucher disease, hypophosphatasia and EDS.

Treatments with bisphosphonates, such as neridronate and risedronate, teriparatide, anti-sclerostin antibody setrusumab and denosumab have not reduced the fracture risk, but they may increase bone density (Lafage-Proust and Courtois, 2019). Orthopedic fracture management is challenging, due to the craniovertebral junction abnormalities, poor bone structures, bleeding tendencies, and post-operative respiratory failure. The overall management should focus on individualized multidisciplinary care. Physiotherapy and bodywork should include treatments to strengthen muscles, reduce pain, treat tendinopathies, and to facilitate movement and optimal gait.

Hypermobility spectrum disorders

With the development of the stricter criteria for EDS, several patients with hypermobility will not meet any of the new criteria (Malfait et al., 2017) and for these individuals the term hypermobility spectrum disorders (HSDs) was coined. They usually have musculoskeletal symptoms, although some may have limited multisystem involvement. Both hEDS and HSD patients feature a myofibroblast-like phenotype with several abnormal extracellular matrix components (ECM), such as different expressions of CCN1/CYR61 and CCN2/CTGF inflammation mediators, an altered organization of -smooth muscle actin cytoskeleton, and increased levels of the ECM-degrading metallo-proteinase-9, among others (Zoppi et al., 2018). HSDs are divided into generalized (G-HSD), peripheral (P-HSD), localized (L-HSD) and historical (H-HSD) subtypes. The genetic basis, prevalence and incidence of HSDs are not known.

References

Abbott, J.H., McCane, B., Herbison, P., Moginie, G., Chapple, C. & Hogarty, T. (2005) Lumbar segmental instability: a criterion-related validity study of manual therapy assessment. *BMC Musculoskelet Disord.* 6: 56.

Alqhtani, R.S., Jones, M.D., Theobald, P.S. & Williams, J.M. (2015) Correlation of lumbar-hip kinematics between trunk flexion and other functional tasks. *J Manipulative Physiol Ther.* 38: 442–447.

Andreoli, E., Troiani, A., Tucci, V., Barlafante, G., Cerritelli, F., Pizzolorusso, G., Renzetti, C., Vanni, D., Pantalone, A. & Salini, V. (2014) Osteopathic manipulative treatment of congenital talipes equinovarus: a case report. *J Bodyw Mov Ther.* 18: 4–10.

Anwajler, J., Wojna, D., Stepak, A. & Skolimowski, T. (2005) The influence of sports acrobatic training on the range of mobility of the spine and the upper and lower extremities. *Fizjoterapia Polska.* 5: 57–64.

Baeza-Velasco, C., Bulbena, A., Polanco-Carrasco, R. & Jaussaud, R. (2018) Cognitive, emotional, and behavioral considerations for chronic pain management in the Ehlers-Danlos syndrome hypermobility-type: a narrative review. *Disabil Rehabil.* 1–9.

Barber, L., Barrett, R. & Lichtwark, G. (2012) Medial gastrocnemius muscle fascicle active torque-length and Achilles tendon properties in young adults with spastic cerebral palsy. *J Biomech.* 45: 2526–2530.

Basit, S. & Khoshhal, K.I. (2018) Genetics of clubfoot; recent progress and future perspectives. *Eur J Med Genet.* 61: 107–113.

Beckers, A.B., Keszthelyi, D., Fikree, A., Vork, L., Masclee, A., Farmer, A.D. & Aziz, Q. (2017) Gastrointestinal disorders in joint hypermobility syndrome/Ehlers-Danlos syndrome hypermobility type: A review for the gastroenterologist. *Neurogastroenterol Motil.* 29.

Berglund, K.M., Persson, B.H. & Denison, E. (2008) Prevalence of pain and dysfunction in the cervical and thoracic spine in persons with and without lateral elbow pain. *Man Ther.* 13: 295–299.

Berryman Reese, N. & Bandy, W.D. (2017) *Joint range of motion and muscle length testing.* St. Louis, MO: Elsevier.

Bettini, E.A., Moore, K., Wang, Y., Hinds, P.S. & Finkel, J.C. (2018) Association between pain sensitivity, central sensitization, and functional disability in adolescents with joint hypermobility. *J Pediatr Nurs*. 42: 34–38.

Bonamichi-Santos, R., Yoshimi-Kanamori, K., Giavina-Bianchi, P. & Aun, M.V. (2018) Association of postural tachycardia syndrome and Ehlers-Danlos syndrome with mast cell activation disorders. *Immunol Allergy Clin North Am*. 38: 497–504.

Botrus, G., Baker, O., Borrego, E., Ngamdu, K.S., Teleb, M., Gonzales Martinez, J.L., Maldonado, G., 3rd, Hussein, A.M. & McCallum, R. (2018) Spectrum of gastrointestinal manifestations in joint hypermobility syndromes. *Am J Med Sci*. 355: 573–580.

Bowen, J.M., Sobey, G.J., Burrows, N.P., Colombi, M., Lavallee, M.E., Malfait, F. & Francomano, C.A. (2017) Ehlers-Danlos syndrome, classical type. *Am J Med Genet C Semin Med Genet*. 175: 27–39.

Brackmann, F., Turk, M., Gratzki, N., Rompel, O., Jungbluth, H., Schroder, R. & Trollmann, R. (2018) Compound heterozygous RYR1 mutations in a preterm with arthrogryposis multiplex congenita and prenatal CNS bleeding. *Neuromuscul Disord*. 28: 54–58.

Bradley, H. & Esformes, J. (2014) Breathing pattern disorders and functional movement. *Int J Sports Phys Ther*. 9: 28–39.

Brown, M.L., Plate, J.F., von Thaer, S., Fino, N.F., Smith, B.P., Seyler, T.M. & Lang, J.E. (2016) Decreased range of motion after total knee arthroplasty is predicted by the Tampa scale of kinesiophobia. *J Arthroplasty*. 31: 793–797.

Brunt, D., Woo, R., Kim, H.D., Ko, M.S., Senesac, C. & Li, S. (2004) Effect of botulinum toxin type A on gait of children who are idiopathic toe-walkers. *J Surg Orthop Adv*. 13: 149–155.

Bukva, B., Vrgoc, G., Madic, D.M., Sporis, G. & Trajkovic, N. (2019) Correlation between hypermobility score and injury rate in artistic gymnastics. *J Sports Med Phys Fitness*. 59: 330–334.

Burns, S.A., Cleland, J.A., Carpenter, K. & Mintken, P.E. (2016) Interrater reliability of the cervicothoracic and shoulder physical examination in patients with a primary complaint of shoulder pain. *Phys Ther Sport*. 18: 46–55.

Byrnes, K., Wu, P.J. & Whillier, S. (2018) Is Pilates an effective rehabilitation tool? A systematic review. *J Bodyw Mov Ther*. 22: 192–202.

Chapman, C., Stott, N.S., Port, R.V. & Nicol, R.O. (2000) Genetics of club foot in Maori and Pacific people. *J Med Genet*. 37: 680–683.

Ciccotto, G., Blaya, M. & Kelley, R.E. (2013) Stiff Person Syndrome. *Neurologic Clinics*. 31: 319–328.

Coles, W., Copeman, A. & Davies, K. (2017) Hypermobility in children. *Paediatric Child Health* 28: 50–56.

Coombes, B.K., Bisset, L. & Vicenzino, B. (2014) Bilateral cervical dysfunction in patients with unilateral lateral epicondylalgia without concomitant cervical or upper limb symptoms: a cross-sectional case-control study. *J Manipulative Physiol Ther*. 37: 79–86.

Cotelli, M., Manenti, R., Brambilla, M. & Borroni, B. (2018) The role of the motor system in action naming in patients with neurodegenerative extrapyramidal syndromes. *Cortex*. 100: 191–214.

Day, H., Koutedakis, Y. & Wyon, M.A. (2011) Hypermobility and dance: a review. *Int J Sports Med*. 32: 485–489.

De Cario, R., Sticchi, E., Lucarini, L., Attanasio, M., Nistri, S., Marcucci, R., Pepe, G. & Giusti, B. (2018) Role of TGFBR1 and TGFBR2 genetic variants in Marfan syndrome. *J Vasc Surg*. 68: 225–233.

Delafontaine, A., Honeine, J.L., Do, M.C., Gagey, O. & Chong, R.K. (2015) Comparative gait initiation kinematics between simulated unilateral and bilateral ankle hypomobility: Does bilateral constraint improve speed performance? *Neurosci Lett*. 603: 55–59.

Deore, M. & May, S. (2012) The interrater and intra-rater reliability of passive physiological accessory movement assessment of lumbar spine in novice manual therapists. *J Bodyw Mov Ther*. 16: 289–293.

Di Matteo, V., Pierucci, M., Esposito, E., Crescimanno, G., Benigno, A. & Di Giovanni, G. (2008) Serotonin modulation of the basal ganglia circuitry: therapeutic implication for Parkinson's disease and other motor disorders. *Prog Brain Res*. 172: 423–463.

Dietz, F. (2002) The genetics of idiopathic clubfoot. *Clin Orthop Relat Res*. 39–48.

Dobbs, M.B. & Gurnett, C.A. (2012) Genetics of clubfoot. J Pediatr Orthop B. 21: 7–9.

Drvaric, D.M., Kuivila, T.E. & Roberts, J.M. (1989) Congenital clubfoot. Etiology, pathoanatomy, pathogenesis, and the changing spectrum of early management. *Orthop Clin North Am*. 20: 641–647.

Engelbert, R.H.H., Uiterwaal, C.S.P.M., Sakkers, R.J.B., van Tintelen, J.P., Helders, P.J.M. & Bank, R.A. (2004) Benign generalised hypomobility of the joints; a new clinical entity? Clinical, biochemical and osseal characteristics. *Pediatrics.* 113: 714–719.

Faure, E.M., el Batti, S., Abou Rjeili, M., Ben Abdallah, I., Julia, P. & Alsac, J.M. (2018) Stent-assisted, balloon-induced intimal disruption and relamination of aortic dissection in patients with Marfan syndrome: Midterm outcomes and aortic remodeling. *J Thorac Cardiovasc Surg.* 156: 1787–1793.

Fayh, A., Brodt, G.A., Souza, C. & Loss, J.F. (2018) Pilates instruction affects stability and muscle recruitment during the long stretch exercise. *J Bodyw Mov Ther.* 22: 471–475.

Fernandez-Marmiesse, A., Carrascosa-Romero, M.C., Alfaro Ponce, B., Nascimento, A., Ortez, C., Romero, N., Palacios, L., Jimenez-Mallebrera, C., Jou, C., Gouveia, S. & Couce, M.L. (2017) Homozygous truncating mutation in prenatally expressed skeletal isoform of TTN gene results in arthrogryposis multiplex congenita and myopathy without cardiac involvement. *Neuromuscul Disord.* 27: 188–192.

Fleming, K.M. & Herring, M.P. (2018) The effects of Pilates on mental health outcomes: A meta-analysis of controlled trials. *Complement Ther Med.* 37: 80–95.

Foley, E.C. & Bird, H.A. (2013) Hypermobility in dance: asset, not liability. *Clin Rheumatol.* 32: 455–461.

Goldfinger, J.Z., Preiss, L.R., Devereux, R.B., Roman, M.J., Hendershot, T.P., Kroner, B.L., Eagle, K.A. & Gen, T.A.C.R.C. (2017) Marfan syndrome and quality of life in the GenTAC Registry. *J Am Coll Cardiol.* 69: 2821–2830.

Grahame, R. (1993) Joint hypermobility and the performing musician. *N Engl J Med.* 329: 1120–1121.

Grahame, R. & Jenkins, J.M. (1972) Joint hypermobility—asset or liability? A study of joint mobility in ballet dancers. *Ann Rheum Dis.* 31: 109–111.

Hakim, A.J. & Grahame, R. (2003) A simple questionnaire to detect hypermobility: an adjunct to the assessment of patients with diffuse musculoskeletal pain. *Int J Clin Pract.* 57: 163–166.

Hameleers, R., Blokland, A., Steinbusch, H.W., Visser-Vandewalle, V. & Temel, Y. (2007) Hypomobility after DOI administration can be reversed by subthalamic nucleus deep brain stimulation. *Behav Brain Res.* 185: 65–67.

Haneline, M.T., Cooperstein, R., Young, M. & Birkeland, K. (2008) Spinal motion palpation: a comparison of studies that assessed intersegmental end feel vs excursion. *J Manipulative Physiol Ther.* 31: 616–626.

Harris, J.D., Gerrie, B.J., Lintner, D.M., Varner, K.E. & McCulloch, P.C. (2016) Microinstability of the hip and the splits radiograph. *Orthopedics.* 39: e169–e75.

Hayes, M. & Chase, S. (2010) Prescribing yoga. *Prim Care.* 37: 31–47.

Henderson, F.C., SR., Austin, C., Benzel, E., Bolognese, P., Ellenbogen, R., Francomano, C.A., Ireton, C., Klinge, P., Koby, M., Long, D., Patel, S., Singman, E.L. & Voermans, N.C. (2017) Neurological and spinal manifestations of the Ehlers-Danlos syndromes. *Am J Med Genet C Semin Med Genet.* 175: 195–211.

Henderson, F.C., SR., Henderson, F.C., JR., Wilson, W.A.T., Mark, A.S. & Koby, M. (2018) Utility of the clivo-axial angle in assessing brainstem deformity: pilot study and literature review. *Neurosurg Rev.* 41: 149–163.

Holt, K., Russell, D., Cooperstein, R., Young, M., Sherson, M. & Haavik, H. (2018) Interexaminer reliability of seated motion palpation for the stiffest spinal site. *J Manipulative Physiol Ther.* 41: 571–579.

Hutchinson, M., Waters, P., McHugh, J., Gorman, G., O'Riordan, S., Connolly, S., Hager, H., Yu, P., Becker, C.M. & Vincent, A. (2008) Progressive encephalomyelitis, rigidity, and myoclonus: a novel glycine receptor antibody. *Neurology.* 71: 1291–1292.

Hyde, S.A., Fllytrup, I., Glent, S., Kroksmark, A.K., Salling, B., Steffensen, B.F., Werlauff, U. & Erlandsen, M. (2000) A randomized comparative study of two methods for controlling Tendo Achilles contracture in Duchenne muscular dystrophy. *Neuromuscul Disord.* 10: 257–263.

Javadi Parvaneh, V. & Shiari, R. (2016) Proposed modifications to Beighton criteria for the diagnosis of joint hypermobility in children. *Indian J Rheumatol.* 11: 97–100.

Johansson, F. (2006) Interexaminer reliability of lumbar segmental mobility tests. *Man Ther.* 11: 331–336.

Juul-Kristensen, B., Schmedling, K., Rombaut, L., Lund, H. & Engelbert, R.H. (2017) Measurement properties of clinical assessment methods for classifying generalized joint hypermobility-A systematic review. *Am J Med Genet C Semin Med Genet.* 175: 116–147.

Kabat-Zinn, J. (1982) An outpatient program in behavioral medicine for chronic pain patients based on the practice of mindfulness meditation: theoretical considerations and preliminary results. *Gen Hosp Psychiatry*. 4: 33–47.

Kang, H., Aryal, A.C.S. & Marini, J.C. (2017) Osteogenesis imperfecta: new genes reveal novel mechanisms in bone dysplasia. *Transl Res*. 181: 27–48.

Karakostas, T., Watters, K. & King, E.C. (2018) Assessment of the spastic upper limb with computational motion analysis. *Hand Clin*. 34: 445–454.

Keer, R. & Simmonds, J. (2011) Joint protection and physical rehabilitation of the adult with hypermobility syndrome. *Curr Opin Rheumatol*. 23: 131–136.

Khanna, V. & Vaishya, R. (2017) Assessment of Ponseti technique for clubfoot. *Apollo Med*. 14: 31–33.

Kim, S.T., Cloft, H., Flemming, K.D., Kallmes, D.F., Lanzino, G. & Brinjikji, W. (2018) Increased prevalence of cerebrovascular disease in hospitalized patients with Marfan syndrome. *J Stroke Cerebrovasc Dis*. 27: 296–300.

Kondo, D., Noguchi, A., Takahashi, I., Kubota, H., Yano, T., Sato, Y., Toyono, M., Sawaishi, Y. & Takahashi, T. (2018) A novel ZC4H2 gene mutation, K209N, in Japanese siblings with arthrogryposis multiplex congenita and intellectual disability: characterization of the K209N mutation and clinical findings. *Brain Dev*. 40: 760–767.

Koppenhaver, S.L., Hebert, J.J., Kawchuk, G.N., Childs, J.D., Teyhen, D.S., Croy, T. & Fritz, J.M. (2014) Criterion validity of manual assessment of spinal stiffness. *Man Ther*. 19: 589–594.

Lafage-Proust, M.H. & Courtois, I. (2019) The management of osteogenesis imperfecta in adults: state of the art. *Joint Bone Spine*. 86(5): 589–593. doi: 10.1016/j.jbspin.2019.02.001.

Leck, I. & Lancashire, R.J. (1995) Birth prevalence of malformations in members of different ethnic groups and in the offspring of matings between them, in Birmingham, England. *J Epidemiol Community Health*. 49: 171–179.

Lee, M., Huntoon, E.A. & Sinaki, M. (2019) Soft tissue and bony injuries attributed to the practice of yoga: a biomechanical analysis and implications for management. *Mayo Clin Proc*. 94: 424–431.

Lemeunier, N., Jeoun, E.B., Suri, M., Tuff, T., Shearer, H., Mior, S., Wong, J.J., da Silva-Oolup, S., Torres, P., d'Silva, C., Stern, P., Yu, H., Millan, M., Sutton, D., Murnaghan, K. & Cote, P. (2018) Reliability and validity of clinical tests to assess posture, pain location, and cervical spine mobility in adults with neck pain and its associated disorders: Part 4. A systematic review from the cervical assessment and diagnosis research evaluation (CADRE) collaboration. *Musculoskelet Sci Pract*. 38: 128–147.

Lewitt, M.S., McPherson, L. & Stevenson, M. (2019) Development of a Pilates Teaching Framework from an international survey of teacher practice. *J Bodyw Move Ther*. 23(4): 943–949. doi: 10.1016/j.jbmt.2019.02.005.

Loeys, B.L., Dietz, H.C., Braverman, A.C., Callewaert, B.L., de Backer, J., Devereux, R.B., Hilhorst-Hofstee, Y., Jondeau, G., Faivre, L., Milewicz, D.M., Pyeritz, R.E., Sponseller, P.D., Wordsworth, P. & de Paepe, A.M. (2010) The revised Ghent nosology for the Marfan syndrome. *J Med Genet*. 47: 476–485.

Louw, A. (2016) Treating the brain in chronic pain. In: Fernández de las Penas, C., Cleland, J. & Dommerholt, J. (eds) *Manual Therapy for Musculoskeletal Pain Syndromes – An evidenced and clinical-informed approach*. Edinburgh, UK: Churchill Livingstone (Elsevier).

Malfait, F., Francomano, C., Byers, P., Belmont, J., Berglund, B., Black, J., Bloom, L., Bowen, J. M., Brady, A.F., Burrows, N.P., Castori, M., Cohen, H., Colombi, M., Demirdas, S., de Backer, J., de Paepe, A., Fournel-Gigleux, S., Frank, M., Ghali, N., Giunta, C., Grahame, R., Hakim, A., Jeunemaitre, X., Johnson, D., Juul-Kristensen, B., Kapferer-Seebacher, I., Kazkaz, H., Kosho, T., Lavallee, M.E., Levy, H., Mendoza-Londono, R., Pepin, M., Pope, F. M., Reinstein, E., Robert, L., Rohrbach, M., Sanders, L., Sobey, G.J., van Damme, T., Vandersteen, A., van Mourik, C., Voermans, N., Wheeldon, N., Zschocke, J. & Tinkle, B. (2017) The 2017 international classification of the Ehlers-Danlos syndromes. *Am J Med Genet C Semin Med Genet*. 175: 8–26.

McCormack, M., Briggs, J., Hakim, A. & Grahame, R. (2004) Joint laxity and the benign joint hypermobility syndrome in student and professional ballet dancers. *J Rheumatol*. 31: 173–178.

McDevitt, A., Young, J., Mintken, P. & Cleland, J. (2015) Regional interdependence and manual therapy directed at the thoracic spine. *J Man Manip Ther*. 23: 139–146.

McNeill, W., Jones, S. & Barton, S. (2018) The Pilates client on the hypermobility spectrum. *J Bodyw Mov Ther*. 22: 209–216.

Mennen, U., Van Heest, A., Ezaki, M.B., Tonkin, M. & Gericke, G. (2005) Arthrogryposis multiplex congenita. *J Hand Surg Br.* 30: 468–474.

Milhorat, T.H., Bolognese, P.A., Nishikawa, M., McDonnell, N.B. & Francomano, C.A. (2007) Syndrome of occipitoatlantoaxial hypermobility, cranial settling, and Chiari malformation type I in patients with hereditary disorders of connective tissue. *J Neurosurg Spine.* 7: 601–609.

Montgomery, P. & Gauger, J.(1978) Sensory dysfunction in children who toe walk. *Phys Ther.* 58: 1195–1204.

Morello, R. (2018) Osteogenesis imperfecta and therapeutics. *Matrix Biol.* 71–72: 294–312.

Morris, S.L., O'Sullivan, P.B., Murray, K.J., Bear, N., Hands, B. & Smith, A.J. (2017) Hypermobility and musculoskeletal pain in adolescents. *J Pediatr.* 181: 213–221.

Murray, B., Yashar, B.M., Uhlmann, W.R., Clauw, D.J. & Petty, E.M. (2013) Ehlers-Danlos syndrome, hypermobility type: A characterization of the patients' lived experience. *Am J Med Genet A.* 161A: 2981–2988.

Mustur, D., Vesovic-Potic, V., Stanisavljevic, D., Ille, T. & Ille, M. (2009) Assessment of functional disability and quality of life in patients with ankylosing spondylitis. *Srp Arh Celok Lek.* 137: 524–528.

Nilsson, C., Wykman, A. & Leanderson, J. (1993) Spinal sagittal mobility and joint laxity in young ballet dancers. A comparative study between first-year students at the Swedish Ballet School and a control group. *Knee Surg Sports Traumatol Arthrosc.* 1: 206–208.

Okely, J.A., Cukic, I., Shaw, R.J., Chastin, S.F., Dall, P.M., Deary, I.J., Der, G., Dontje, M.L., Skelton, D.A., Gale, C.R. & Seniors, U.S.P.T. (2019) Positive and negative well-being and objectively measured sedentary behaviour in older adults: evidence from three cohorts. *BMC Geriatr.* 19: 28.

Okubo, Y., Endo, W., Inui, T., Suzuki-Muromoto, S., Miyabayashi, T., Togashi, N., Sato, R., Arai-Ichinoi, N., Kikuchi, A., Kure, S. & Haginoya, K. (2018) A severe female case of arthrogryposis multiplex congenita with brain atrophy, spastic quadriplegia and intellectual disability caused by ZC4H2 mutation. *Brain Dev.* 40: 334–338.

Palmer, S., Manns, S., Cramp, F., Lewis, R. & Clark, E.M. (2017) Test-retest reliability and smallest detectable change of the Bristol Impact of Hypermobility (BIoH) questionnaire. *Musculoskelet Sci Pract.* 32: 64–69.

Paoloni, V., Cretella Lombardo, E., Placidi, F., Ruvolo, G., Cozza, P. & Lagana, G. (2018) Obstructive sleep apnea in children with Marfan syndrome: Relationships between three-dimensional palatal morphology and apnea-hypopnea index. *Int J Pediatr Otorhinolaryngol.* 112: 6–9.

Penman, S., Cohen, M., Stevens, P. & Jackson, S. (2012) Yoga in Australia: Results of a national survey. *Int J Yoga.* 5: 92–101.

Piche, M., Benoit, P., Lambert, J., Barrette, V., Grondin, E., Martel, J., Pare, A. & Cardin, A. (2007) Development of a computerized intervertebral motion analysis of the cervical spine for clinical application. *J Manipulative Physiol Ther.* 30: 38–43.

Pomarino, D., Martin, S., Pomarino, A., Morigeau, S. & Biskup, S. (2018) McArdle's disease: A differential diagnosis of idiopathic toe walking. *J Orthop.* 15: 685–689.

Pomarino, D., Ramirez Llamas, J. & Pomarino, A. (2016) Idiopathic toe walking: tests and family predisposition. *Foot Ankle Spec.* 9: 301–306.

Ponten, E. (2015) Management of the knees in arthrogryposis. *J Child Orthop.* 9: 465–472.

Puentedura, E.J. & Cleland, J.A. (2015) Towards a greater appreciation of manual therapy challenges in the thoracic spine. *J Man Manip Ther.* 23: 121–122.

Purnell, M., Shirley, D., Nicholson, L. & Adams, R. (2010) Acrobatic gymnastics injury: occurrence, site and training risk factors. *Phys Ther Sport.* 11: 40–46.

Pyeritz, R.E. (2017) Etiology and pathogenesis of the Marfan syndrome: current understanding. *Ann Cardiothorac Surg.* 6: 595–598.

Rabey, M., Hall, T., Hebron, C., Palsson, T.S., Christensen, S.W. & Moloney, N. (2017) Reconceptualising manual therapy skills in contemporary practice. *Musculoskelet Sci Pract.* 29: 28–32.

Rana, S.S., Ramanathan, R.S., Small, G. & Adamovich, B. (2012) Paraneoplastic Isaacs' syndrome: a case series and review of the literature. *J Clin Neuromuscul Dis.* 13: 228–233.

Ravenscroft, G., Di Donato, N., Hahn, G., Davis, M.R., Craven, P.D., Poke, G., Neas, K.R., Neuhann, T.M., Dobyns, W.B. & Laing, N.G. (2016) Recurrent de novo BICD2 mutation associated with arthrogryposis multiplex congenita and bilateral perisylvian polymicrogyria. *Neuromuscul Disord*. 26: 744–748.

Ravenscroft, G., Nolent, F., Rajagopalan, S., Meireles, A.M., Paavola, K.J., Gaillard, D., Alanio, E., Buckland, M., Arbuckle, S., Krivanek, M., Maluenda, J., Pannell, S., Gooding, R., Ong, R.W., Allcock, R.J., Carvalho, E.D., Carvalho, M.D., Kok, F., Talbot, W.S., Melki, J. & Laing, N.G. (2015) Mutations of GPR126 are responsible for severe arthrogryposis multiplex congenita. *Am J Hum Genet*. 96: 955–961.

Rebbeck, T.R., Dietz, F.R., Murray, J.C. & Buetow, K.H. (1993) A single-gene explanation for the probability of having idiopathic talipes equinovarus. *Am J Hum Genet*. 53: 1051–1063.

Rejeb, A., Fourchet, F., Materne, O., Johnson, A., Horobeanu, C., Farooq, A., Witvrouw, E. & Whiteley, R. (2019) Beighton scoring of joint laxity and injury incidence in Middle Eastern male youth athletes: a cohort study. *BMJ Open Sport Exerc Med*. 5: e000482.

Reuter, M.S., Schwabe, G.C., Ehlers, C., Marschall, C., Reis, A., Thiel, C. & Graul-Neumann, L. (2013) Two novel distinct COL1A2 mutations highlight the complexity of genotype-phenotype correlations in osteogenesis imperfecta and related connective tissue disorders. *Eur J Med Genet*. 56: 669–673.

Revivo, G., Amstutz, D.K., Gagnon, C.M. & McCormick, Z.L. (2019) Interdisciplinary pain management improves pain and function in pediatric patients with chronic pain associated with joint hypermobility syndrome. *PM R*. 11(2): 150 -157.

Rey-Eiriz, G., Alburquerque-Sendin, F., Barrera-Mellado, I., Martin-Vallejo, F.J. & Fernandez-de-las-Penas, C. (2010) Validity of the posterior-anterior middle cervical spine gliding test for the examination of intervertebral joint hypomobility in mechanical neck pain. *J Manipulative Physiol Ther*. 33: 279–285.

Ruemper, A. & Watkins, K. (2012) Correlations between general joint hypermobility and joint hypermobility syndrome and injury in contemporary dance students. *J Dance Med Sci*. 16: 161–166.

Sahrmann, S., Azevedo, D.C. & Dillen, L.V. (2017) Diagnosis and treatment of movement system impairment syndromes. *Braz J Phys Ther*. 21: 391–399.

Saleh, M., Gibson, M.F. & Sharrard, W.J. (1989) Femoral shortening in correction of congenital knee flexion deformity with popliteal webbing. *J Pediatr Orthop*. 9: 609–611.

Sanches, S.B., Oliveira, G.M., Osorio, F.L., Crippa, J.A. & Martin-Santos, R. (2015) Hypermobility and joint hypermobility syndrome in Brazilian students and teachers of ballet dance. *Rheumatol Int*. 35: 741–747.

Scheper, M.C., Juul-Kristensen, B., Rombaut, L., Ramekers, E.A., Verbunt, J. & Engelbert, R.H. (2016) Disability in adolescents and adults diagnosed with hypermobility-related disorders: a meta-analysis. *Arch Phys Med Rehabil*. 97: 2174–2187.

Schneider, M., Erhard, R., Brach, J., Tellin, W., Imbarlina, F. & Delitto, A. (2008) Spinal palpation for lumbar segmental mobility and pain provocation: an interexaminer reliability study. *J Manipulative Physiol Ther*. 31: 465–473.

Seneviratne, S.L., Maitland, A. & Afrin, L. (2017) Mast cell disorders in Ehlers-Danlos syndrome. *Am J Med Genet C Semin Med Genet*. 175: 226–236.

Sherman, K.J., Cherkin, D.C., Erro, J., Miglioretti, D.L. & Deyo, R.A. (2005) Comparing yoga, exercise, and a self-care book for chronic low back pain: a randomized, controlled trial. *Ann Intern Med*. 143: 849–856.

Shields, B.J. & Smith, G.A. (2011) Epidemiology of strain/sprain injuries among cheerleaders in the United States. *Am J Emerg Med*. 29: 1003–1012.

Shulman, L.H., Sala, D.A., Chu, M.L., McCaul, P.R. & Sandler, B.J. (1997) Developmental implications of idiopathic toe walking. *J Pediatr*. 130: 541–546.

Silva, A.P., Chagas, D.D., Cavaliere, M.L., Pinto, S., de Oliveira Barbosa, J.S. & Batista, L.A. (2016) Kinematic analysis of subtalar eversion during gait in women with fibromyalgia. *Foot*. 28, 42–46.

Soto Insuga, V., Moreno Vinués, B., Losada del Pozo, R., Rodrigo Moreno, M., Martínez González, M., Cutillas Ruiz, R. & Mateos Carmen, C. (2018) Caminan de manera diferente los niños con trastorno por déficit de atención hiperactividad (TDAH)? Relación entre marcha de puntillas idiopática y TDAH. *An Pediatr*. 88: 191–195.

Soucie, J.M., Wang, C., Forsyth, A., Funk, S., Denny, M., Roach, K.E., Boone, D. & Hemophilia Treatement Center (2011) Range of motion measurements: reference values and a database for comparison studies. *Haemophilia*. 17: 500–507.

Sweeney, L. & Howe, T. (2016) Paraneoplastic syndromes. *Medicine*. 44: 69–72.

Taghizadeh, S., Pirouzi, S., Hemmati, L., Khaledi, F. & Sadat, A. (2017) Clinical evaluation of scapular positioning in patients with nonspecific chronic low back pain: a case-control study. *J Chiropr Med*. 16: 195–198.

Tewari, S., Madabushi, R., Agarwal, A., Gautam, S.K. & Khuba, S. (2017) Chronic pain in a patient with Ehlers-Danlos syndrome (hypermobility type): The role of myofascial trigger point injections. *J Bodyw Mov Ther*. 21: 194–196.

Theodoridis, D. & Ruston, S. (2002) The effect of shoulder movements on thoracic spine 3D motion. *Clin Biomech*. 17: 418–421.

Tinkle, B., Castori, M., Berglund, B., Cohen, H., Grahame, R., Kazkaz, H. & Levy, H. (2017) Hypermobile Ehlers-Danlos syndrome (a.k.a. Ehlers-Danlos syndrome Type III and Ehlers-Danlos syndrome hypermobility type): Clinical description and natural history. *Am J Med Genet C Semin Med Genet*. 175: 48–69.

Tosi, M., Maslyanskaya, S., Dodson, N.A. & Coupey, S.M. (2019) The female athlete triad: a comparison of knowledge and risk in adolescent and young adult figure skaters, dancers, and runners. *J Pediatr Adolesc Gynecol*. 32: 165–169.

Tracy, J.A. & McKeon, A. (2015) The Stiffman syndrome in children and adolescents. In: Darras, B.T., Royden Jones, H., Ryan, M.M. & de Vivo, D.C. (eds) *Neuromuscular Disorders of Infancy, Childhood and Adolescence; A Clinician's Approach*. London, UK: Academic Press.

Tranchant, C., Koob, M. & Anheim, M. (2017) Parkinsonian-pyramidal syndromes: A systematic review. *Parkinsonism Relat Disord*. 39: 4–16.

Valdes-Flores, M., Casas-Avila, L., Hernandez-Zamora, E., Kofman, S. & Hidalgo-Bravo, A. (2016) Characterization of a group of unrelated patients with arthrogryposis multiplex congenita. *J Pediatr*. 92: 58–64.

van Dijk, F.S., Pals, G., van Rijn, R.R., Nikkels, P.G. & Cobben, J.M. (2010) Classification of osteogenesis imperfecta revisited. *Eur J Med Genet*. 53: 1–5.

Weber, A.E., Bedi, A., Tibor, L.M., Zaltz, I. & Larson, C.M. (2015) The hyperflexible hip: managing hip pain in the dancer and gymnast. *Sports Health*. 7: 346–358.

West, J., Otte, C., Geher, K., Johnson, J. & Mohr, D.C. (2004) Effects of Hatha yoga and African dance on perceived stress, affect, and salivary cortisol. *Ann Behav Med*. 28: 114–118.

Widerström, B., Olofsson, N., Arvidsson, I., Harms-Ringdahl, K. & Larsson, U.E. (2012) Inter-examiner reliability of a proposed decision-making treatment based classification system for low back pain patients. *Man Ther*. 17: 164–171.

Wiese, C., Keil, D., Rasmussen, A.S. & Olesen, R. (2019) Injury in yoga asana practice: Assessment of the risks. J *Bodyw Move Ther*. 23(3): 479–488.

Williams, K., Abildso, C., Steinberg, L., Doyle, E., Epstein, B., Smith, D., Hobbs, G., Gross, R., Kelley, G. & Cooper, L. (2009) Evaluation of the effectiveness and efficacy of Iyengar yoga therapy on chronic low back pain. *Spine (Phila Pa 1976)*. 34: 2066–2076.

Williams, K., Steinberg, L. & Petronis, J. (2003) Therapeutic application of Iyengar yoga for healing chronic low back pain. *Int J Yoga Ther*. 13: 55–67.

Wulf, G. & Lewthwaite, R. (2016) Optimizing performance through intrinsic motivation and attention for learning: The OPTIMAL theory of motor learning. *Psychon Bull Rev*. 23: 1382–1414.

Wulf, G., Lewthwaite, R., Cardozo, P. & Chiviacowsky, S. (2018) Triple play: Additive contributions of enhanced expectancies, autonomy support, and external attentional focus to motor learning. *Q J Exp Psychol*. 71: 824–831.

Xiang, Z., Wang, L. & Kitai, S.T. (2005) Modulation of spontaneous firing in rat subthalamic neurons by 5-HT receptor subtypes. *J Neurophysiol*. 93: 1145–1157.

Xue, S., Maluenda, J., Marguet, F., Shboul, M., Quevarec, L., Bonnard, C., Ng, A.Y., Tohari, S., Tan, T.T., Kong, M.K., Monaghan, K.G., Cho, M.T., Siskind, C.E., Sampson, J.B., Rocha, C.T., Alkazaleh, F., Gonzales, M., Rigonnot, L., Whalen, S., Gut, M., Gut, I., Bucourt, M., Venkatesh, B., Laquerriere, A., Reversade, B. & Melki, J. (2017) Loss-of-function mutations in LGI4, a secreted ligand involved in Schwann cell myelination, are responsible for arthrogryposis multiplex congenita. *Am J Hum Genet*. 100: 659–665.

Zhou, Z., Rewari, A. & Shanthanna, H. (2018) Management of chronic pain in Ehlers-Danlos syndrome: Two case reports and a review of literature. *Medicine*. 97: e13115.

Zoppi, N., Chiarelli, N., Binetti, S., Ritelli, M. & Colombi, M. (2018) Dermal fibroblast-to-myofibroblast transition sustained by alphavss3 integrin-ILK-Snail1/Slug signaling is a common feature for hypermobile Ehlers-Danlos syndrome and hypermobility spectrum disorders. *Biochim Biophys Acta Mol Basis Dis*. 1864: 1010–1023.

Elastic storage and recoil dynamics

Robert Schleip and Katja Bartsch

The catapult mechanism: Elastic recoil of fascial tissues

During the 1980s, those studying the field of muscular physiology were intrigued by the capacity of kangaroos to perform powerful jumps of up to 13 m in length. Because these animals do not have bulky leg muscles, the general assumption was that their leg musculature would contain some unusual muscle fibers that enabled them to perform explosive contractions.

In fact, some researchers were convinced that they would find "super-fast twitch fibers" in the kangaroos' hind limbs. However, no matter how hard the researchers looked, they could not find any unusual muscle fibers. This left them puzzled: if muscles create the force for these impressive jumps, why do these animals contain the same muscle fibers as a koala? Eventually, they looked for the answer where nobody had looked previously, in the properties of the tendons. It was here that they found an amazing capacity, which was subsequently called the "catapult effect". Similar to an elastic spring of stainless steel, the long tendons were able to store and release kinetic energy with amazing efficiency (Kram and Dawson, 1998).

When the kangaroo hits the ground their tendons, as well as the fascial aponeuroses of their hind legs, are tensioned like elastic bands. The subsequent release of this stored energy

is what enables these amazing jumps. Shortly afterwards, the same mechanism was also discovered in gazelles. These animals are capable of impressive leaping as well as running, although their musculature is not particularly strong. Because gazelles are generally considered to be rather delicate, it made the elastic springiness all the more interesting. Similar impressive elastic storage capacities were later confirmed to exist in horses.

Homo sapiens: The elastic "gazelle" within the primate family

It was only when the technology of high-resolution ultrasound examination achieved a sufficiently high level of resolution to observe single sarcomeres in muscles that a similar orchestration of loading between muscle and fascia was discovered in human locomotion. In fact it was found, rather surprisingly, that human fasciae have a similar kinetic storage capacity to that of kangaroos and gazelles (Sawicki et al., 2009). This capacity is not only used when we run or jump but also when walking, as a significant part of the energy of the movement comes from the same elastic springiness of the collagenous tissues described above.

Neither chimpanzees, bonobos, orangutans nor any other primate seems to have developed a similar elastic storage capacity within the fascial tissues of their legs compared with

Chapter 8

their long-legged homo sapiens relatives. This is reflected in the shorter muscle fascicles and thinner tendons in the distal legs of humans compared with non-human primates, making them much better adapted to the elastic storage and release of kinetic energy (Alexander, 1991). The human species' elastic capabilities are not limited to the lower limbs (Figure 8.1). Humans can throw projectiles at much higher speed compared to other primates. Anatomical features that enable elastic energy storage and release in the shoulder contribute to this unique capacity in homo sapiens (Roach *et al., 2013*).

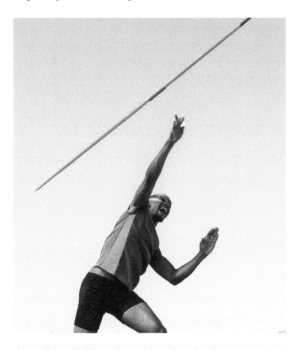

Figure 8.1

Humans are able to throw projectiles at much higher speed than other primates. However, repeated overuse of this motion can result in injuries in modern athletes. Paloeolithic hunters almost certainly threw far less frequently than modern athletes (Roach et al., 2013).

These discoveries have led to an active revision of long-accepted principles in the field of movement science. According to their previously unquestioned classical model of muscular dynamics, it was assumed that in a muscular joint movement, the skeletal muscle fibers involved shorten. This energy then passes through passive tendons, resulting in the movement (Figure 8.2). This classic form of energy transfer is still true, according to these recent measurements, for slow as well as more rapid movements with a steady limb speed, such as cycling. Here, the muscle fibers actively change their length, while the tendons and aponeuroses scarcely lengthen. The fascial elements mostly fulfil a passive role in this movement orchestration. This is in contrast to oscillatory movement with an elastic spring quality, such as hopping, running or skipping, in which the length of the muscle fibers scarcely changes. While the muscle fibers contract in an almost isometric fashion, they stiffen temporarily without any significant change of their length, the fascial elements function in an elastic way with a movement similar to that of a resonating elastic spring made of stainless steel. It is mainly this lengthening and shortening of the fascial elements that "produces" the actual movement. Think of a catapult: the person putting their muscular energy into the tensioning of the elastic band is like the muscle fibers, which store the kinetic energy in the fascial tissues. Usually the direction of the muscular preparatory work goes into an opposite orientation to the intended explosive power movement. For an archer, this would mean that their muscles pulled backwards on the bow to increase the potential movement energy. When the force is released, it is the collagen (or elastic band) that

Elastic storage and recoil dynamics

propels the object (or arrow) in the intended direction, while the muscular elements step out of the way and take a rest.

Key concept: Elasticity of elastin and collagen fibers

- Early anatomists were of the opinion that tendons did not exhibit elastic properties.
- While today the elasticity of collagenous tissue is beyond any doubt, practitioners and clinicians sometimes mistake elastin fibers to be elastic and collagenous fibers to be non-elastic.
- Elastin and collagen are not more or less elastic; the difference is rather that elastin and collagen have different quantities of elastic stiffness (quantified by Young's modulus).
- Collagen is about 100 times stiffer than elastin, meaning it can store the same amount of energy while stretching only one hundredth the amount. (Zorn and Hodeck, 2011).

Imagine an archer, who tries to shoot faster by propelling the arrow forward with their muscles. This would be too slow. When properly loaded, collagen can shorten at a much faster speed than any muscle fiber could contract. However, this only works if the loaded collagen tissue has a high elastic storage capacity. Imagine an archer

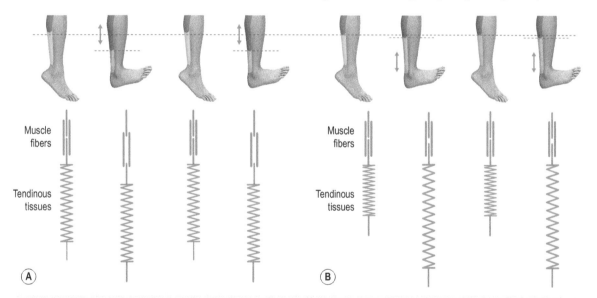

Figure 8.2 Comparison of length changes of muscular and collagenous elements in conventional "muscle training" (A) and in a more fascially oriented movement with elastic recoil properties (B)

The elastic tendinous (or fascial) elements are shown as springs, the muscle fiber as straight lines. Note that during a conventional movement **(A)**, the elastic collagenous elements do not change their length significantly, while the contractile muscle fibers change their length significantly. **(B)** However, during rhythmically oscillatory movements, like running or hopping, the muscle fibers contract almost isometrically, while the fascial collagenous elements lengthen and shorten like an elastic yo-yo spring.

(Illustration adapted from Kawakami et al. (2002) reproduced with kind permission of www.fascialnet.com).

Chapter 8

trying to shoot with a bow made of concrete and a non-elastic rope.

> ## Key concept: Elastic storage capacity and crimp pattern
>
> - Many tendons can recoil elastically when a stretching force is removed (Benjamin et al., 2008).
> - This elastic recoil property seems to be related to the so-called crimp pattern.
> - In particular tendons, the fibers are made up of fibrils that have wavy forms called crimps (Shim et al., 2012). Recent animal studies revealed that collagen crimp characteristics are strongly tendon type specific, which indicates that crimp specialization is crucial in the respective mechanical function (Spiesz et al., 2018; Zuskov et al., 2020).
> - The stiffness of tendons can vary with age. The higher storage capacity of collagenous tissues in young people is associated with a stronger crimp expression within their collagen fibers. Tailored exercise in older rats has been shown to reintroduce a similar crimp formation as is present in younger ones (Wood et al., 1988).
> - Tendon stiffness can also vary with sex: The Achilles tendon in women tends to be less stiff than in men (Kubo et al., 2003).

Resonant frequency: Length and stiffness as crucial factors

In order to understand fascial recoil, try experimenting with a weight that is suspended on an elastic band or stainless steel spring. With eyes open or closed, within a few cycles, most people intuitively figure out the optimal resonant frequency of the system. This is usually achieved when finding a rhythm in which a tiny lift action of the holding finger, starting just a split second before the turning point, increases the stretch loading of the elastic spring. Interestingly, in a completely elastic system, the ideal resonant frequency depends mostly on two factors: (1) the length of the swinging element and (2) the stiffness of the strained tissues. When trying to dance or bounce on wet sand, most people will find that slower music is more suitable, whereas a more rapid rhythm tends to suit dancing barefoot with the forefeet on a hard dance floor with tightly contracted calf muscles.

Improvement of elastic recoil properties through training

Tissues tend to adapt their architecture to the specific mechanical demands imposed on them. This also holds true for soft connective tissues such as tendons.

While aging alters the mechanical properties, it has been shown that the elastic storage capacity in human tendons can be significantly improved by regularly repeated strong mechanical loading through resistance training (Reeves, 2006).

In addition to resistance training leading to a beneficial adaptation of the tendon, repetitive hopping training has also been shown to improve its mechanical properties (Figure 8.3). A group of physically active elderly men practiced a carefully orchestrated hopping training exercise three times per week for 11 weeks. After a warm-up, the training sets comprised only 15–20 hops with short contact time and as little knee bending as possible. Jumping height and tendon utilization improved (Hoffren-Mikkola et al., 2015).

For the Achilles tendon and aponeuroses, a strain of 4–5% tends to be required for eliciting an adaptational response, while a lower load of 2–3% does not appear to be sufficient

Elastic storage and recoil dynamics

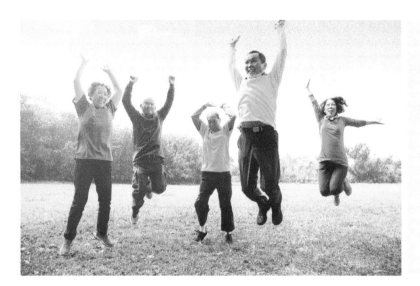

Figure 8.3 Repetitive hopping training can improve mechanical properties and tendon utilization.

A study with elderly active people showed that 15 to 20 hops with short contact time and little knee bending lead to beneficial adaptations.

(Arampatzis et al., 2007). However, the thresholds for adaptational responses appear to be significantly lower for intramuscular fascia than for tendons (Kjaer et al., 2015).

Once the adaptational threshold is reached, it is possible that only 5 or 10 elastic bounces might be required for an adaptational response, while adding many more repetitions tends to have little additional effect (Magnusson et al., 2010).

As described earlier, the rhythm of a movement should also be considered. For rhythmic movements that involve temporarily leaving the ground with both feet, such as running, hopping and skipping, rhythms of between 150 and 170 beats per minute (BPM) usually work best. When trying to find music to support effortless swinging and bouncing movements that do not involve leaving the ground, most people find that a slower rhythm of between 120 and 140 BPM is optimum. But what do you do if the music is too slow or too fast? Besides options such as only choosing every second beat, it may work to change the length of the swinging boy portion and/or to adapt the stiffness of the

loaded fascial tissues by increasing or decreasing the active tonus of some of the attached muscle portions.

Kangaroo hopping versus frog jumping

In elastically oscillating movements, such as hopping in kangaroos, the energy production of the involved muscles is mainly concerned with pacing the best rhythm. This is comparable with the movements of a conductor's baton or the sticks of a slalom skier. It is, therefore, not surprising that the muscles involved when a kangaroo hops generate the same force at all speeds (Kram and Dawson, 1998). Similarly, a study examining the gait of women of the African Luo and Kikuyu tribes carrying loads of up to 20% of their body weight on their heads found that their oxygen consumption was largely independent of the weight, provided they were allowed to walk at a speed comfortable for them. When well-trained British soldiers carrying up to 20% of their body weight on their backpacks were examined, their energy consumption increased in proportion to the

Chapter 8

weight carried. Interestingly, when the African women were asked to walk at an uncomfortably faster or slower pace, they exhibited the same weight-dependent (and probably more muscular-driven) pattern in their energy expenditure as the soldiers (Alexander, 1986; Zorn and Hodeck, 2011).

Compared with these rhythmically oscillating movements, a different orchestration between muscles and elastic tissue properties is at work during single explosive movements. For example, when a frog leaps, sometimes up to 10 m, it also utilizes the elastic recoil properties in its leg fasciae. However, here the contraction speed of the muscle fibers is of prime importance. The orchestration between muscular contractile dynamics and the rebound dynamics of collagenous tissues is similar to casting a long elastic fishing rod. A rapid muscular motion then starts to exert a strong pulling force on the distal limb as well as on related collagenous tissues. While initially some of that force seems "lost" in the elastic compliance of tendons and aponeuroses, these tissues subsequently release the stored muscular energy via a rapidly accelerating motion, the speed of which surpasses the potential maximal muscle contraction velocity by several times. Note that in such "singular" motions, a sense of rhythm or resonant frequencies is not as crucially involved as in oscillatory rhythmic motions. In addition, the magnitude of the initial muscular contraction is of major importance: the more rapidly and strongly the muscles start to contract, the more powerful the resulting elastic recoil action of the fascial tissues will become.

Of course, various complex combinations may exist between these two extremes. As mentioned above, throwing a baseball or a javelin has been shown to exert acceleration speeds that significantly surpass those of all other primates (Roach *et al.*, 2013). This is partly accomplished by a muscularly driven "stretching backwards" motion (i.e. in the opposite direction to the intended forward throwing motion), in which kinetic energy is stored in various collagenous membranes and tendons. This initial phase simulates some of the hopping kangaroo dynamics, as explored earlier, in which a sense of rhythm and resonant frequencies play important roles. The subsequent phase, consisting of a forward swinging motion, then utilizes similar storage and release dynamics to those found in the powerful frog jump.

Plyometrics: Two different mechanisms

For competitive athletes, plyometric training is considered old hat. The field of plyometrics, also known as jump training, was first introduced to the Western sports scene in the early 1980s. It involves training routines that move the total length of a "muscle-tendon complex" from a state of extension to a shortened state in a rapid or "explosive" way, such as in repetitive jumping. This is also called the "stretch-shortening cycle". The eccentric contraction of involved muscle fibers during the initial lengthening phase has been shown to play an essential role: the more rapid and powerful these preparatory eccentric contractions are, the more force is subsequently exerted in the final contraction phase. Plyometric training has been shown to increase jumping height, as well as many other athletic performances (Figure 8.4).

The general explanation for the proposed mechanisms is a combination of two factors (Figure 8.5): (1) a change in mechanical properties and (2) an optimization of neural properties (Kubo et al., 2007). While it was unclear to

Elastic storage and recoil dynamics

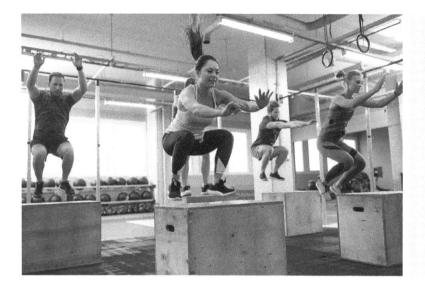

Figure 8.4

Plyometric training, if done properly, can increase jumping height and induce a gradual remodeling of tendinous tissues towards an increased kinetic storage capacity.

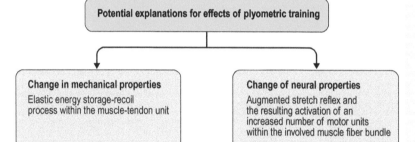

Figure 8.5

Recent investigations revealed that the performance improvement in Plyometric training goes along with a 'lazier' muscle activation in trained jumpers together with an augmented use of passive elastic recoil properties (Fouré, 2011).

what respective degree each of those very different mechanisms are involved in the total outcome, most authors, and athletes, considered the improved neuromuscular orchestration and the assumed augmentation of myogenic contraction power as the dominant player. By contrast, the proposed utilization of passive biomechanical storage and release properties was considered to play a secondary "supporting role" compared with the active muscular contraction component.

Modern ultrasound technology allowed a team of French sports scientists to investigate the relative proportion of those two mechanisms (Foure et al., 2011). By measuring length changes in the triceps surae muscles and the Achilles tendon, they observed that plyometric training, consisting of 34 sessions of 1 hour over 14 weeks, resulted in an increased utilization of passive tissue properties and a decreased utilization of active contractile muscular elements. After this systematic training process, the increased acceleration and jumping performance was accompanied by more 'lazy' muscle fibers during the shortening phase but with an increased passive "elastic recoil property" of the spring-loaded elements within the muscle-tendon unit. The authors discussed an increase in cross linkages between collagen

Chapter 8

fibrils as possible explanations for this increase, rather than changes in gross geometrical parameters of the tendons.

If the storage-release mechanism is occurring somewhere within the total muscle-tendon complex, then the question is worth exploring, whether it happens mostly within the collagenous elements (the tendon, epimysium and intramuscular connective tissues), or whether it also occurs within the muscle fibers themselves. Muscle fibers are composed of smaller tubular myofibrils, the basic functional unit of which is called a sarcomere. Several sarcomeres arranged in series constitute a myofibril. The most appealing candidates for elastic energy storage within the sarcomeres are the titin proteins (Linke, 2000). These are the largest known proteins in the human body and they form a more recently discovered third filament system within a sarcomere, apart from the previously known thick (mostly myosin) and thin (mostly actin) filaments. While these unique proteins are capable of impressive elastic recoil properties, their contribution to the stretch-shortening cycle in a rapidly accelerating single movements, such as in jumping or throwing, constituted a matter of dispute. However, a detailed examination of isolated myofibers from frogs revealed that the potential elastic recoil power of these titin proteins tends to be considerably dampened by other intramuscular contraction dynamics. They may, therefore, be prevented from contributing to the elastic recoil properties in a significant manner. The researchers concluded that titin elastic recoil is able to support the active muscular shortening under low load only or during prolonged shortening from greater physiological sarcomere lengths (Minajeva et al., 2002). In other words, with the high loads applied during most plyometric training routines, the intramuscular titin elements seem to play only a minor

role in the passive recoil dynamics of the total muscle-tendon complex. Furthermore, previous studies report that the titin isoforms of human muscles did not change after plyometric training (Pellegrino et al., 2016). These current results suggest that the collagenous (i.e. fascial) tissues are, most likely, providing the main energy storage and release mechanisms that are synonymous with the increased athletic performance achieved using plyometric exercise training.

But what about the potential contribution of the intramuscular titin elements to oscillatory rhythmic recoil movements such as in kangaroo hopping and human running? Here, the length changes of the affected myofascial tissues involve only minor length changes within the muscular sarcomeres, in contrast to the collagenous tendinous elements (Figure 8.2). Since the titin elements are embedded within the sarcomeres, this clearly suggests that most of the elastic recoil dynamics in such movements are achieved within the collagenous elements and not within the muscular titin components. In other words, the training of elastic storage capacities, whether in single motions such as throwing or in oscillatory movements such as jogging, mainly involves an increase of collagenous elastic properties, rather than intramuscular sarcomeric adaptations. This conclusion is in line with a recent examination of the adaptive response of Achilles tendons and patellar tendons in two groups of athletes who use a lot of elastic recoil (ski jumpers and runners) in comparison with other athletes (here, water polo players) and also to sedentary people (Wiesinger et al., 2017). It was found that the energy return in the tendons of the ski jumpers and runners was between 40% and 50% higher in the "bouncy sports athletes" compared with the other groups. The authors therefore concluded that this difference indicates a better energy conservation in athletes whose tendons mainly work as springs.

Clinical summary

- Fascial tissues are capable of storing and releasing kinetic energy similar to an elastic spring.
- While this catapult mechanism was first examined in a detailed manner in Australian kangaroos, subsequent research revealed that it also plays a major role in human oscillatory movements such as running, hopping or walking.
- Adequate training to improve the elastic capabilities of fascial tissues includes repeated strong mechanical loading through resistance training, repetitive hopping training and rapid accelerating movements.
- The threshold for adaptational responses is significantly lower for intramuscular fascia than for tendons.
- As was examined in the energy efficient gait of some African women, there are significant inter-individual differences as to how much this elastic recoil mechanism is utilized.
- A key factor in the orchestration is adequate timing: the precise matching of the muscular activation with the resonant frequency of the swinging system.

References

Alexander, R.M. (1986) Human energetics: Making headway in Africa. *Nature.* 319: 623–624.

Alexander, R.M. (1991) Elastic mechanisms in primate locomotion. *Zeitschrift für Morphologie und Anthropologie.* 78: 315–320.

Arampatzis, A., Karamanidis, K. & Albracht, K. (2007) Adaptational responses of the human Achilles tendon by modulation of the applied cyclic strain magnitude. *J Exp Biol.* 210: 2743–2753.

Benjamin, M., Kaiser, E. & Milz, S. (2008) Structure-function relationships in tendons: a review. *J Anat.* 212: 211–228.

Foure, A., et al. (2011) Effects of plyometric training on both active and passive parts of the plantarflexors series elastic component stiffness of muscle-tendon complex. *Eur J Appl Physiol.* 111: 539–548.

Hoffrén-Mikkola, M., et al. (2015) Neuromuscular mechanics and hopping training in elderly. *Eur J Appl Physiol.* 115: 863–877.

Kjaer, M., et al. (2015) Exercise and regulation of bone and collagen tissue biology. *Prog Mol Biol Transl Sci.* 135: 259–291.

Kram, R. & Dawson, T.J. (1998) Energetics and biomechanics of locomotion by red kangaroos *(Macropus rufus). Comp Biochem Physiol B Biochem Mol Biol.* 120: 41–49.

Kubo, K., Kanehisa, H. & Fukunaga, T. (2003) Gender differences in the viscoelastic properties of tendon structures. *Eur J Appl Physiol.* 88: 520–526.

Linke, W.A. (2000) Titin elasticity in the context of the sarcomere: force and extensibility measurements on single myofibrils. *Adv Exp Med Biol.* 481: 76–179.

Magnusson, S.P., Langberg, H. & Kjaer, M. (2010) The pathogenesis of tendinopathy: balancing the response to loading. *Nat Rev Rheumatol.* 262–268.

Minajeva, A., et al. (2002) Titin-based contribution to shortening velocity of rabbit skeletal myofibrils. *J Physiol.* 540: 177–188.

Pellegrino, J., Ruby, B.C. & Dumke, C.L. (2016) Effect of plyometrics on the energy cost of running and MHC and titin isoforms. *Med Sci Sports Exercise.* 48: 49–56.

Reeves, N.D. (2006) Adaptation of the tendon to mechanical usage. *J Musculoskel Neuron Interact.* 6: 174–180.

Roach, N.T., et al. (2013) Elastic energy storage in the shoulder and the evolution of high-speed throwing in Homo. *Nature.* 498: 483–486.

Sawicki, G.S., Lewis, C.L. & Ferris, D.P. (2009) It pays to have a spring in your step. *Exerc Sport Sci Rev.* 37: 130–138.

Shim, V., et al. (2012) Investigation of the role of crimps in collagen fibers in tendon with a microstructually based

Chapter 8

finite element model. *Conf Proc IEEE Eng Med Biol Soc.* 2012: 4871–4874.

Spiesz, E.M., et al. (2018) Structure and collagen crimp patterns of functionally distinct equine tendons, revealed by quantitative polarised light microscopy (qPLM). *Acta Biomater.* 70: 281–292.

Wiesinger, H.P., et al. (2017) Sport-specific capacity to use elastic energy in the patellar and Achilles tendons of elite athletes. *Front Physiol.* 8: 132.

Wood, T.O., Cooke, P.H. & Goodship, A.E. (1988) The effect of exercise and anabolic steroids on the mechanical properties and crimp morphology of the rat tendon. *Am J Sports Med.* 16: 153–158.

Zorn, A. & Hodeck, K. (2011) Walk with elastic fascia. In: Dalton, E. (ed.) *Dynamic body - Exploring form, expanding function.* Oklahoma, OK: Freedom From Pain Institute, 96–123.

Zuskov, A., et al. (2020) Tendon biomechanics and crimp properties following fatigue loading are influenced by tendon type and age in mice. *J Orthop Res.* 38(1): 36–42.

Water and fluid dynamics in fascia

Robert Schleip

Hydration keeps fascia alive

The human body consists mainly of water. In fact, the average adult person consists of up to 60% water. The amount of water, however, is not constant throughout the lifespan. When we are born, water constitutes approximately 90% of our body mass and as we age we gradually become less hydrated, until at over 80 years the water content may be as small as 50% (Watson et al., 1980). The main fluid of the body can be found in virtually any tissue: even in dense ligaments and tendons, the water content is >50%. We have observed this amazing fact many times in our laboratory when measuring the wet weight of ligaments from animals and then comparing this with the same weight after the tissue had been completely dried. The majority of our body water (~65%) is interstitial water, which is dissolved in our extracellular matrix . Most water enters the ground substance via the small arterioles, in which it was expressed as blood plasma. Once in the ground substance, the water usually binds in one way or another with the hydrophilic surfaces of the proteoglycans, until it may depart again, back into the central bloodstream via small lymphatic or venous vessels (Figure 9.1).

Note that only 10% of that return happens via the lymph vessels, while the remaining 90% occurs via the small venules (Schwartz et al., 2019). This may have clinical implications for fascia-oriented treatments like foam rolling, massage or vacuum treatment via suction cups.

While in healthy tissue a multidirectional motion may be the most efficient renewal approach for the ground substance water, in inflammatory conditions—such as in oedemas—it usually works best to apply the majority of strokes in a

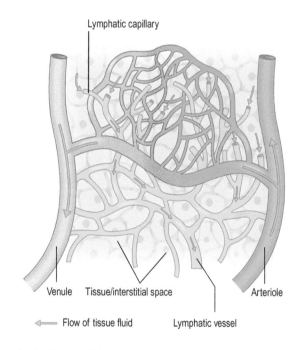

Lymphatic capillary

Venule   Tissue/interstitial space   Arteriole

⟵ Flow of tissue fluid   Lymphatic vessel

Figure 9.1

Diagram showing the flow of water from the ground substance to the ends of the lymph capillaries. Note that the majority of the ground substance water departs via the small venules, rather than the lymph pathway.

Illustration: U.S. National Cancer Institute's Surveillance, Epidemiology and End Results (SEER) Program.

Chapter 9

proximal direction towards the larger lymph vessels. This is because a large proportion of the inherent water is bound to inflammatory cells, cellular debris or pro-inflammatory cytokines, which then makes it difficult for those structures to enter the much smaller openings of the venules. In fact, several pathological tissue conditions, such as in systemic sclerosis and rheumatic diseases, have been associated with dysfunctional lymph flow dynamics. A beneficial therapeutic effect has been demonstrated for these conditions with lymphatic drainage applications (Schwartz et al., 2019).

An easy and free passage of water from the small arterioles into the ground substance, and from there back into the central bloodstream (via the small venules or lymph vessels) is an indication of healthy tissue condition (Figure 9.2). By contrast, an increasing inertia and stagnation of this fluid dynamic has been associated with a lower state of health, such as in metabolic syndrome or aging. Besides the previously mentioned lymphatic activation techniques, an enhancement of microcirculation has been recommended. This may occur via tool-assisted passive applications or via active exercise.

A novel aspect in this field are the "conduits" through the ground substance, as described by Weigelin et al. (2012). With the aid of third generation harmonic microscopy, which permits observation of cell migration *in vivo*, these researchers demonstrated that migrating cells tend to use the path of least resistance and thereby follow and widen specific pathways (conduits) through the ground substance. These conduits seem to be identical to the Primo Vascular System, previously called Bonghan channels, due to their size, distribution and high content of hyaluronan inside. While early discoverers of these channels associated them with acupuncture meridians,

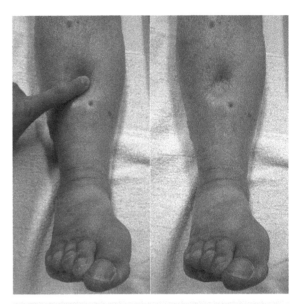

Figure 9.2

Peripheral oedema is characterized by "pitting", i.e. the persistance of indentation after a moderate pressure is applied to a small area and then released. This persistance expresses a restricted water renewal in the ground substance.

Photograph with the permission of James Heilman.

this topographical and functional association seems less clear today. However, the existence of these pathways as a third fluid transport system, next to blood and lymph vessels, is increasingly recognized (Soh et al., 2012). Increasing free and unobstructed movement through these conduits via active movement or therapeutic manipulation has been suggested to enhance immune system functioning (Swartz, 2018).

The miraculous capacities of hyaluronan

The ground substance is mainly composed of proteoglycans, most of which are hydrophilic (i.e. water loving), and of bound water. Similar to the structure of a bottle brush, or of plant mosses, the proteoglycans are arranged in a geometrical manner, thus offering the largest possible surface area for water molecules to attach to. Within the proteoglycan aggregates, hyaluronan often serves as a core protein, to which glycosaminoglycans are connected (Figure 9.3A). Hyaluronan is one of the most hydrophilic molecules in nature: it can trap up to 1000 times its own weight in water! Therefore, a high concentration of hyaluronan tends to increase the water content of a tissue.

One of the most exciting discoveries in the field of fascia science in recent years has been the reported existence of a new connective tissue cell type, which seems to be primarily focused on a rapid production of hyaluronan. A team of researchers at Padova University suggested the name "fasciacyte" for these cells, which they describe as expressing a rather round cell shape, in contrast to the spindle-like shape of regular fibroblasts. They also showed that this cell type is frequently found in the upper and lower portions of loose connective tissue layers, i.e. at their transition to denser fascial layers adjacent to them (Stecco et al., 2018).

Hyaluronan is usually considered to be a lubricant, indicating that it decreases friction between adjacent tissue layers. This function is supported by a recent histological study, in which it was shown that the concentration of fascial tissues, which are exposed to a large degree of shearing/sliding motions, express hyaluronan concentrations of up to 10-fold higher compared with fascial tissues that are exposed to very little deformation (Figure 9.3B). This suggests that providing a fascial region with regular shearing

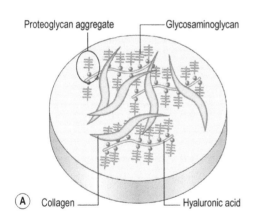

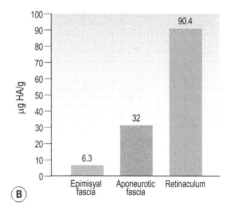

Figure 9.3A

Hyaluronan (also called hyaluronic acid) often serves as a core protein for the attachment of glycosaminoglycans within the ground substance.

© Mfigueiredo, wikicommons, CC-BY-SA 3.0.

Figure 9.3B

Mean concentrations of hyaluronan (HA) in different fascial tissues in the human body. The concentration in epimysial fasciae (here around trapezius and deltoid muscles) is lower compared with aponeurotic fasciae (fascia lata and rectus abdominis sheet), while the retinaculum (here in the ankle) expresses by far the highest concentrations.

Illustration based on data from Fede et al., 2018.

Chapter 9

motions could induce a higher hyaluronan concentration in this region. To date, no studies have compared the value of regular stretches of the muscles and fasciae in the face with the reportedly beneficial effect of external cosmetic hyaluronan injections. However, given these general interactions between shearing motion and the production of hyaluronan within the tissue itself, it would not be surprising if the "internal treatment" could at least compare with the external one.

Interestingly, hyaluronan can also function as a "sticky glue", preventing easy sliding between adjacent tissue layers. This apparently happens when hyaluronan takes on the form of super molecules, which are multiple times larger than in the usual molecular condition of this substance. There are indications that this glue-like condition, also described as an increase in viscosity, tends to happen more frequently when there is an acidic condition in the ground substance. It also happens when the tissue is exposed to repetitive mechanical overloading, such as in exercise or in repetitive strain injuries. While these changes may lead to a local stiffening and a decrease in range of motion in everyday living, an increase in tissue temperature tends to break down the large molecular structure into smaller fragments, which then express a much lower viscosity than in the previous condition (Pavan et al., 2014).

Similarly, it has been shown that the glue-like viscosity can be easily reduced with appropriate mechanical loading. While the application of sudden pressure tends to be "ignored" by the tissue, it has been shown that shearing motions, which induce a twisting/bending inside of the fibrous architecture, together with gradual redistribution of internal pressures, tend to induce a significant decrease of viscosity. This might

explain why immobility reduces fascial gliding and, consequently, range of motion. It may also explain the beneficial effects of many therapeutic myofascial release treatments (Pavan et al., 2014). A similar mechanism may also be at work when experiencing a beneficial effect in terms of a reduced tissue rigidity induced by regular movement practices in daily life. The beneficial response of such "warming up" exercises may then be partly comparable to the well-known response of shaking a ketchup bottle, which induces a decreased viscosity (or increased fluidity) in its content.

Soaking up the water

A healthy body will prevent the hyaluronan (and other hydrophilic elements within the ground substance) soaking up excessive amounts of water, since this would go along with a dramatic expansion of the total volume of the respective tissue. This healthy restraint is achieved by a constantly pre-stretched condition of the local collagen fiber network, which prevents the proteoglycan inducing an exaggerated tissue expansion (Figure 9.4). A simplified description is that in a healthy body condition, the proteoglycans are always "thirsty". It is only in the case of injury, or other pathological changes, that they can soak up as much water as they would like to and then expand beyond their previous restrained condition. This can be easily observed in a fresh ankle sprain injury: here, the clearly visible tissue swelling often occurs during the first few minutes.

Based on this consideration, it appears rather unlikely that one could influence the water content (and pre-stretch) within dense fascial tissues just by drinking more water during the day. In other words, the water content in your ankle retinaculum will be primarily regulated by the

Water and fluid dynamics in fascia

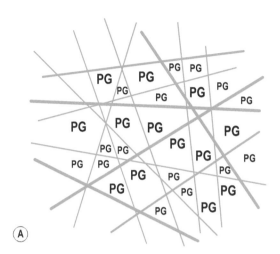
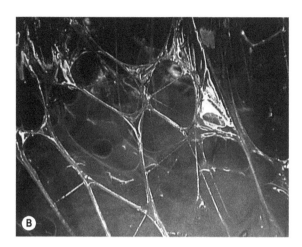

Figure 9.4

(A) Simplified model of the restraining action of collagen fibers (in pink) on the water uptake of the proteoglycans (PG) in the ground substance. In an uncontrolled condition, the proteoglycans would soak up a water volume several times their own size, which would result in tissue swelling. However, in healthy tissue, the potential swelling (and water uptake) is restrained by the constant pre-stretch of the fibrous network surrounding these "constantly thirsty" proteoglycans. **(B)** Photographic imaging of fresh fascia taken during endoscopic surgery reveals a similar pre-stretched relationship of the visible collagen fibers.

© JC Guimberteau, www.endovivo.com.

pre-stretch of the local collagen network. Once that network expands, as in a fresh injury, the proteoglycans will soak up as much water from the arterioles as they want to, independently of how much water the person had been drinking that day. Another consequence of the described pre-stretched situation in healthy tissues is that any additional uptake of water into the ground substance will probably happen via an altered fluid-pull (suction) from within the ground substance, not by an increasing supply (push) of water from the outside into the pre-stretched tissue.

Squeezing a sponge: Dynamics of dehydration and rehydration

When exposed to mechanical loading, the water content in a fascial tissue tends to be decreased: similar to the deformation of a wet sponge, once it is either stretched or compressed, some of the internal water content will be squeezed out during the loading condition. Similarly, after the loading is stopped, the sponge is expected to rehydrate again, with either the same water or with new water from within the vicinity. Our laboratory at Ulm University demonstrated this sponge-like dehydration and rehydration effect multiple times in an organ bath condition (Schleip et al., 2011). We also showed that the loading-induced dehydration tends to go along with a temporary loss of tissue stiffness (at least in ligamentous tissues), and that the subsequent rehydration tends to restore the previous tissue stiffness again (Figure 9.5). A similar effect has been documented with a foam roller-like myofascial treatment on the plantar fascia (Frenzel et al., 2015) and with therapeutic application of a Rolfing myofascial release technique on the lumbar fascia (Dennenmoser et al., 2016).

Chapter 9

Interestingly, our organ bath experiments indicated that a "supercompensation" effect can be achieved if the magnitude of the tissue loading is large and the subsequent rest period is sufficiently long. This "strain hardening" could be observed in some cases, when a subsequent increase of stiffness beyond the original condition was induced. If the supercompensation could also be shown *in vivo*, it might provide future applications for preconditioning routines in athletic performance conditions (Schleip et al., 2011). Because hydration changes can impact the failure stress of at least some fascial tissues (Werbner et al., 2019), a more detailed investigation of the various interactions between different mechanical loading protocols, resultant hydration changes and subsequent effects of biomechanical tissue properties provides a very promising area in current research.

Liquid crystals within us

Ubiquitous on earth, water is present in all life forms. However, recent research has revealed that the water inside of living bodies exposes very surprising properties, which are certainly different to what has so far been known about regular bulk water.

The basic idea that "interfacial water layers"—i.e. the arrangement of water molecules in the vicinity of biological surfaces—play a fundamental role in biological systems was proposed in a visionary paper by Szent-Györgyi (1971). As Gruebele, one of the leading scientists in this area, explains: "Water in our bodies has different physical properties from ordinary bulk water, because of the presence of proteins and other biomolecules. Proteins change the properties of water to perform particular tasks in different parts of our cells. Water can be viewed as a 'designer fluid' in living cells" (University of Illinois at Urbana-Champaign, 2008). Apparently, the interaction of water molecules with hydrophilic and hydrophobic biomolecules in their vicinity influences their behavior in very surprising manners. Gruebele states: "We previously thought proteins would affect only those water molecules directly stuck to them ... Now we know proteins will affect a volume of water comparable to their own. That's pretty amazing" (University of Illinois at Urbana-Champaign, 2008).

Pollack (2013) examined the behavior of what he calls "vicinal water" within the temporomandibular joint and described it as a crystalline architecture. While the water molecules in this state still vibrate very rapidly in this condition, they do so within very stable conditions, which are called "liquid crystal" in physics (Pollack, 2013). Because of the previously described "bottle brush architecture" of the proteoglycans in the ground substance of fascial tissues, a large proportion of the water molecules apparently take on this special crystalized condition. As Pollack (2013) states, "The combined data from three different methods lead to the conclusion that all or almost all of the water in the intact disc is bound water and does not have properties consistent with free or bulk water."

The crystalized water exposes very different properties to regular bulk water in terms of a significantly different density, an increased viscosity, different light transmission and a different electrical conductance (Sommer et al., 2011). Note that while most of the proteoglycans are hydrophilic, the small elastin fibers are hydrophobic. Their strong water repulsion then induces a coating-like accumulation of specially arranged water molecules around them, in which these molecules' binding sites face away from the fibers, and thereby take on a crystalized condition not unlike the vicinal water around hydrophilic surfaces. While it is a common assumption that morphological differences in aging skin are due to a change in the elastin fibers, Sommer et al. (2008) demonstrated that the amount of water coating around these fibers plays a major role. While the elastin in young fibers is surrounded (and buffered) with a very thick zone of crystalized water, this coating tends to get thinner and thinner as we age, due to the accumulation of free radicals and other metabolic waste products in the small vacuum-like zone between the fibers and their coatings. In an intriguing experiment, Sommer and Zhu (2008) showed that after an attempt to push the "dirty bulk water" away

from this zone using a special laser, the elastin fibers were apparently surrounded again with thicker coatings of crystalized water and the skin in these regions took on an obviously more juvenile appearance (Figure 9.5).

In a personal discussion with our department, Dr Andrej Sommer and his Rolfer colleague, Kai Hodeck, expressed an assumption that a mechanical sponge-like myofascial treatment, in which the inherent water is steadily pushed into different directions, could potentially exert a similar (or even stronger) renewal effect on these water coatings than the one reported in

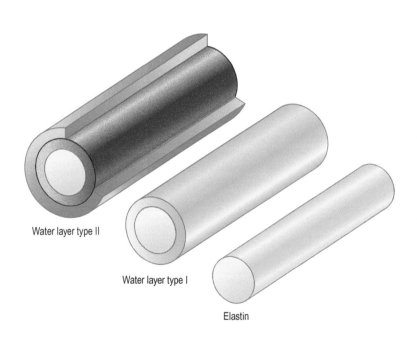

Water layer type II

Water layer type I

Elastin

Figure 9.5

Elastin fibers are hydrophobic, i.e. water repellent (right). In their native condition, the elastic fibers are surrounded by a thick layer of crystalized water layer around it (middle), which protects the structural integrity and stretch-ability of the fibers. During the process of physiological aging (left), elastin fragmentation and disintegration are probably induced by metabolic waste products (black), which inhibit the formation of the crystalized water coating. The process of aging can therefore be understood as a decrease of the protective water coating. Therapeutic intervention—via a special laser application—was apparently able to reverse some of that aging process, i.e. to shift the water environment from the situation shown on the left more towards the "younger condition" shown in the middle.

Illustration modified after Sommer and Zhu (2008).

Chapter 9

their study. If this speculation were supported and validated by future investigations, it would mean that regular stretching, foam rolling or similar treatments could induce a higher proportion of crystalized water in the ground substance and, thereby, induce and exert an anti-aging effect on the tissues. It will be exciting to follow the ongoing research of these pioneers and their colleagues in the next few years.

Clinical summary

Water constitutes the majority of the volume of our fascia. Any change in this element can be expected to exert significant effects on the whole tissue. For movement therapists, it is helpful to think of the sponge-like changes of their interventions. A skilful interplay of temporary dehydration and subsequent rehydration promises not only a renewal of the tissue, but may also change the stiffness of the treated area. Applying mechanical pressure may also induce a change of the viscosity via a molecular change of hyaluronan. Lack of motion, on the other side, will lead towards a more rapid aging effect, which probably is associated with a decrease of crystalized water within the tissue.

References

Chaitow, L. (2009) Research in water and fascia. Micro-tornadoes, hydrogenated diamonds & nanocrystals. *Massage Today*. 9: 1–3.

Dennenmoser, S., Schleip, R. & Klingler, W. (2016) Clinical mechanistic research: Manual and movement therapy directed at fascia electrical impedance and sonoelastography as a tool for the examination of changes in lumbar fascia after tissue manipulation. *J Bodyw Movem Ther*. 20: 145.

Fede, C., Angelini, A., Stern, R., Macchi, V., Porzionato, A., Ruggieri, P., De Caro, R. & Stecco, C. (2018) Quantification of hyaluronan in human fasciae: variations with function and anatomical site. *J Anat*. 233: 552–556.

Frenzel, P., Schleip, R. & Geyer, A. (2015) Responsiveness of the plantar fascia to vibration and/or stretch. *J Bodyw Movem Ther*. 19: 670.

Helmer, K.G., Nair, G., Cannella, M. & Grigg, P. (2006) Water movement in tendon in response to a repeated static tensile load using one-dimensional magnetic resonance imaging. *J Biomech Eng*. 128: 733–741.

Pavan, P.G., Stecco, A., Stern, R. & Stecco, C. (2014) Painful connections: densification versus fibrosis of fascia. *Curr Pain Headache Rep*. 18: 441.

Pollack, G.H. (2013) *The Fourth Phase of Water: Beyond Solid, Liquid, and Vapor*. Seattle, WA: Ebner and Sons.

Schleip, R., Duerselen, L., Vleeming, A., Naylor, I.L., Lehmann-Horn, F., Zorn, A., Jaeger, H. & Klingler, W. (2011) Strain hardening of fascia: static stretching of dense fibrous connective tissues can induce a temporary stiffness increase accompanied by enhanced matrix hydration. *J Bodyw Mov Ther*. 16: 94–100.

Schwartz, N., Chalasani, M.L.S., Li, T.M., Feng, Z., Shipman, W.D. & Lu, T.T. (2019) Lymphatic function in autoimmune diseases. *Front Immunol*. 10: 519.

Soh, K.-S., Kang, K.A. & Harrison, D.K. (eds) (2012) *The Primo Vascular System — Its Role in Cancer and Regeneration*. New York, NY: Springer Verlag.

Sommer, A.P. & Zhu, D. (2008) From microtornadoes to facial rejuvenation: implication of interfacial water layers. *Cryst Growth*. 8: 3889–3892.

Sommer, A.P., Zhu, D., Franke, R.P. & Fecht, H.J. (2008) Biomimetics: Learning from diamonds. *J Materials Res*. 23: 3148–3152.

Stecco, C., Fede, C., Macchi, V., Porzionato, A., Petrelli, L., Biz, C., Stern, R. & De Caro, R. (2018) The fasciacytes: a new cell devoted to fascial gliding regulation. *Clin Anat*. 31: 667–676.

Szent-Györgyi, A. (1971) Biology and pathology of water. *Perspect Biol Med*. 14: 239.

University of Illinois at Urbana-Champaign (2008) Water Is 'Designer Fluid' That Helps Proteins Change Shape. Science Daily Press Release, August 6, 2008. www.sciencedaily.com/releases/2008/08/080806113314.htm. [Accessed 19 April 2021].

Watson, P.E., Watson, I.D. & Batt, R.D. (1980) Total body water volumes for adult males and females estimated from simple anthropometric measurements. *Am J Clin Nutrition*. 33: 27–39.

Weigelin, B., Bakker, G.-J. & Friedl, P. (2012) Intravital third harmonic generation microscopy of collective melanoma cell invasion. *IntraVital*. 1: 32–43.

Werbner, B., Spack, K. & O'Connell, G.D. (2019) Bovine annulus fibrosus hydration affects rate-dependent failure mechanics in tension. *J Biomech*. 89: 34–39.

What is it good for? An evidence-based review of stretching in sport and movement

Jan Wilke

Introduction

Although its exact origins have not been scientifically validated, stretching is one of mankind's oldest health- and sport-related movements. Archeological excavations exposed millenia-old seals depicting yoga positions which substantially elongate the body's soft tissue (Lardner, 2001). Furthermore, the ancient Greeks performed flexibility exercises as a vital part of their conditioning programs when preparing themselves for the massive loads of the prestigious Olympic Games. To date, stretching continues to represent one of the most applied but, at the same time, most controversial maneuvers used to warm-up for, or recover from, physical activity.

In its most basic form, stretching is a natural and instinctive movement. After having a nap or resting for a longer period of time, cats and dogs frequently perform whole-body stretches before taking their first steps (Figure 10.1). Similarly, most people yawn and extend their joints prior to getting out of bed in the morning. Typical objectives of stretching in sports are injury prevention, performance enhancement and the acceleration of recovery. This chapter will describe the basic physiology, proven effects and limitations of related techniques in this context.

Basic assumptions of stretching interventions

Stretching always aims to elongate the soft tissue of the human body. If an applied force is large enough to increase the length of a structure, two types of deformation can be distinguished. Elastic deformation is temporary and the original length is recovered shortly after the stretching force has disappeared. As an example, a

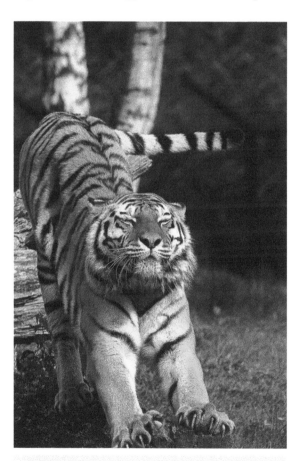

Figure 10.1

Big cats stretch too: a tiger gets ready for action

Chapter 10

rubber band returns to its original shape when it is now longer strained. By contrast, plastic deformation describes the permanent length change of an object. Wet chewing gum can be elongated to a tremendous degree but does not recover its original shape. It thus deforms plastically.

The reaction of the connective tissue to an elongating force can best be illustrated by means of the stress-strain curve of a tendon. The initially observed length changes during a stretch do not lead to a significant increase in strain because the collagen fibers, which are slightly wavy at rest, straighten. In this so-called toe region, there is no "real" tissue stretch and hence, little force is needed to achieve a length change. However, in the subsequent elastic or linear phase, the collagen is no longer crimped and starts to stretch progressively. More force is needed to induce tendon lengthening, which is associated with substantial increases in strain. When finally entering the zone of plastic deformation, the tendon may undergo irreversible length changes, potentially leading to rupture. While the stress-strain curve of other collagenous connective tissues such as ligaments or the deep fascia is similar to the tendon (Wang et al., 2009), the shape can vary substantially in the muscle depending on whether it is actively or passively lengthened.

Muscle stretching: a misnomer

In most situations, stretching interventions affect both muscular and connective tissues. However, the most basic question practitioners and therapists need to ask themselves is which tissue is intended to be effectively stretched and if this is actually possible with the selected exercise. Contrary to traditional assumptions, stretching in joint end ranges does not always predominantly affect the muscle because other structures may represent the major limiting factor. For instance, inversion of the lower ankle joint stretches its lateral ligaments more than the peroneal muscles and elbow extension is limited by the bony structures of the joint rather than the biceps brachii muscle. Different types of stoppage are given in Table 10.1. In sum, stretching will always affect a variety of tissues and the main site of effect is dependent on the particular construction of the joint. The following section gives an overview about the differential effects of stretching on relevant soft tissue components of the locomotor system.

Table 10.1 Different types of stoppage	
Type of stoppage	**Example (structure stopping movement)**
Muscle	Hip flexion with extended knees (hamstring muscles) Ankle dorsal extension with extended knees (gastrocnemius muscle)
Bone	Elbow extension (olcecranon of the ulna)
Soft tissue	Elbow flexion (biceps brachii muscle) Hip and knee flexion in obese people (posterior thigh/abdominal fat)
Ligament	Hip extension (iliofemoral ligament) Supination/inversion of the lower ankle joint (lateral ankle ligaments) Finger extension (diverse finger ligaments)
Capsule	Humeral rotation (capsule of the glenohumeral joint)

What is it good for? An evidence-based review of stretching in sport and movement

119

Effects on the muscle

Looking at the micro-level, tissue elongation stretches the cytoskeleton of the sarcomere, the smallest functional unit of the muscle. Within the sarcomere, two contractile proteins, the thick myosin and the thinner actin, extend between its borders, the z disks. Under normal conditions, the myosin and actin filaments always overlap to a certain degree and the cross-bridges between both contribute not only to force production during contraction, but also to the resistance to stretch. Stretching can temporarily reduce the overlap of both filaments. However, an interesting mechanism ensures that sarcomere length is quickly restored: titin, a highly elastic protein connects myosin to the z disk. It acts like a spring, being unfolded upon tissue lengthening and pulling back the myosin filament into the resting state as soon as the stretching force has disappeared.

Immediately following stretching, changes in the muscle's mechanical properties can be observed. Static interventions with a total net duration of 2 to 8 min acutely reduce the stiffness of the gastrocnemius muscle (Ryan et al., 2008; Nakamura et al., 2011; Maeda et al., 2017; Bouvier et al., 2017) and the hamstrings (Hatano et al., 2017). By contrast, no such effect has been shown in the quadriceps muscle of the anterior thigh (Bouvier et al., 2017). Regarding the type of stretching, static lengthening seems to elicit larger decreases, despite dynamic stretching also being effective (Maeda et al., 2017). Between 10 to 20 min post-treatment, the stiffness values return to the baseline level (Ryan et al., 2008; Nakamura et al., 2011; Hatano et al., 2017). Interestingly, functional (enhanced range of motion, reduced peak torque) and subjective (increased stretch tolerance) alterations are maintained longer than the changes in mechanical tissue stiffness (Hatano et al., 2017). This observation suggests that neuronal factors, such as a reduced cortical and/or spinal reflex excitability, contribute significantly to the effects of stretching.

The impact of chronic stretching exercise regimes on the muscle's mechanical properties has been investigated in a systematic review with meta-analysis. Including long-term interventions with durations of between 2 and 8 weeks (a minimum of two sessions per week), the authors concluded that stretching does not modify outcomes such as muscle architecture or stiffness (Freitas et al., 2018). It is hence noteworthy that the acute and chronic effects of stretching on the mechanical muscle properties are substantially different, although the high importance of sensory/neuronal adaptations (e.g. changed excitability and increased stretch tolerance) is a common feature of both applications.

Effects on the tendon

In addition to the muscle, the tendon can also undergo significant length changes. Upon passive stretching of the tibialis anterior muscle, Herbert and Gabriel (2002) found the contractile elements to account for only about 50% of the myotendinous unit (MTU) elongation. In the gastrocnemius, this share even decreased to 27%, suggesting that the tendon was lengthened considerably more than the muscle itself. These findings were confirmed by Morse et al. (2008), who reported a 53% proportion for the Achilles tendon. While both the tendon and the muscle are involved in MTU lengthening, the stretch duration seems to modify the ratio of their contribution. Kato et al. (2010) examined the effect of a static 20-min calf stretch on muscle and tendon length. Initially, both structures collectively caused the observed elongation of the myotendinous unit. However, only the tendon continued to lengthen after 10 min, whereas the muscle remained unchanged from then onwards.

Chapter 10

In contrast to the muscle, whose stiffness has been shown to decrease after or during a single bout of stretching, to date the immediate effects on the mechanical properties of the tendon are unclear. While Kubo et al. (2001) reported a 10% decrease following static stretching, Nakamura et al. (2011) detected an increase in the same outcome, and Kay and Blazevich (2009) did not find any change at all. Possibly, the acute response is time-dependent, as Kubo et al., with 10 min, used the longest stretch duration compared with the other trials' 5 min (Nakamura et al., 2011) and 3 min (Kay and Blazevich, 2009), respectively.

If chronic stretching interventions are considered, similar to the reaction of muscle tissue, there are no morphological changes in the tendon's mechanical properties following chronic stretching interventions of up to 2 months (Freitas et al., 2017). If structural effects are hence possible, exercises would have to be performed over a longer time frame.

Effects on the fascia

To date, the effect of stretching on the connective tissue surrounding the skeletal muscle has not been examined under human *in vivo* conditions. Notwithstanding, findings from fundamental research point towards a mechanical response of the fascia. When subjected to repeated isometric stretches, cadaver samples of the lumbar fascia initially reduce their stiffness. After a while, the values return to the baseline level and subsequently even increase above the pre-stretch state (Yahia et al., 1993). It was initially speculated that the activity of contractile cells may have caused this effect. In fact, fibroblasts and/or myofibroblasts can be found in the crural, plantar and lumbar fascia (Staubesand and Li, 1997; Schleip et al., 2019; Bhattacharya et al., 2010). However, two reasons suggest that factors other

than contractility represent the driving factor in acute, stretch-induced stiffness increases. The myofibroblasts located in the rat lumbar fascia reach their maximal contractile force only about 60 min following stimulation with mepyramine, a first-generation antihistamine (Hoppe et al., 2014). Furthermore, other animal experiments demonstrate that the strain hardening response of the tissue also occurs if the contractile cells are rendered unviable prior to the stretching intervention (Schleip et al., 2012). Contractility is therefore unlikely to represent the dominant mechanism of the rapid stiffness change. Instead, alterations of the water content seem to be a more important moderator: upon stretch, water is removed from the tissue and subsequently, similar to a sponge taking up new fluid, hydration increases during the rest period (Schleip et al., 2012).

Stretching and injury prevention: A fairy tale?

To stretch or not to stretch? This question is often discussed almost philosophically when it comes to the optimal preparation for physical activity. Frequently, flexibility exercise is implemented into warm-up and general prevention programs aiming to reduce injury risk. Notwithstanding, in contrast to wide-held beliefs, current evidence does not appear to support its application for this purpose. According to a series of systematic reviews, acute stretching interventions cannot decrease the overall occurrence of musculoskeletal traumas (Hart 2005; Small et al., 2008; Thacker et al., 2004). Herbert and Gabriel (2002) found only an almost trivial beneficial effect, pointing out that "the average subject would need to stretch for 23 years to prevent one injury". While these findings are discouraging at first glance, they may conceal an interesting effect of

121

What is it good for? An evidence-based review of stretching in sport and movement

pre-exercise stretching. To date, most published research has focused on the absolute number of injuries sustained during sports participation. However, even opponents of stretching will agree that stretching cannot prevent unrelated disorders such as bone fractures. By contrast, it would be plausible to assume that athletes with a more compliant soft tissue following stretching are less likely to sustain a muscle strain injury (for the role of the connective tissue in this disorder, see Chapter 16). To adequately judge the helpfulness of stretching programs, it is, hence, imperative to focus exclusively on those health problems which may be affected by the performed intervention (e.g. muscle strain injuries only). Corresponding literature analyses have yielded contrasting results. For instance, Shrier (1999) reported no effect of stretching on the risk of muscle injury, but Small et al. (2008) suggested preliminary evidence for the effectiveness in the prevention of muscle-tendon disorders. McHugh and Cosgrave (2010) also examined the question as to whether or not stretching decreases muscle injury risk, including seven trials in their review. While the three studies (one of them in runners, where strain injuries would not be expected to be dominant) providing negative results registered only very few or no muscle strains, prevalence was higher in the four studies revealing a protective effect of the intervention. If a prevalence study does not register a high number of injuries from a specific type, it cannot be evaluated if an intervention would be effective in preventing them. It may thus be inferred that the studies not demonstrating a preventive value of stretching had only limited power to detect such effect. Finally, Behm et al. (2016) examined the findings of seven trials, which mainly included athletes performing running and sprinting activities. Pooling the results of the included studies, they found a risk reduction of 54% if stretching was

performed. The prophylactic effect of the intervention seemed to be particularly pronounced in the trials using longer stretch durations of 5 min or more. In summary, it can be concluded that stretching does not reduce the overall injury risk but may slightly reduce the incidence of muscle injuries. Determining the (time) cost-effect relationship of stretching for an individual is, hence, the most important task for therapists and trainers.

Although more a sensory correlate of training-induced adaptation than a musculoskeletal injury, delayed onset muscle soreness (DOMS) is frequently intended to be prevented by the use of stretching exercises. According to a systematic review of 12 studies enrolling a total of 2377 participants, stretching, on average, leads to an insignificant soreness reduction of half a point (pre-exercise) or 1 point (post-exercise) on a 100-point scale (Herbert et al., 2011). It can therefore be concluded that it does not represent an appropriate method to clinically decrease DOMS.

Stretch to win? Exercise effects on sports performance

Besides aiming to reduce injury risk, pre-exercise stretching is used to enhance performance. Depending on the chosen technique as well as the characteristics and goals of the respective sports, it can have both beneficial and detrimental effects for the athlete. If a large range of motion (ROM) represents a decisive criterion (e.g. in yoga, pilates or some elements of gymnastics), then the long- and short-term flexibility increases following stretching, which have been unequivocally documented (Behm et al., 2016), can be classified as performance-enhancing. Basically, all stretching methods (static, dynamic, antagonist-contract, contract-relax) are similarly effective, although the proprioceptive neuromuscular

Chapter 10

facilitation (PNF) methods appear to be slightly superior (Page, 2012). Regardless of the stretching type (static, dynamic or PNF stretching), the effects develop acutely and last about 30 min. The magnitude of the increases shows considerable variation (Table 10.2) and is dependent on several factors, such as the targeted joint and treatment duration. Stretch intensity (e.g. achieving no, mild or substantial discomfort/pain during the exercise) may also be a significant effect modifier; however, very few studies have explicitly tested or precisely reported this variable (e.g. Apostolopoulos et al., 2015). Data from two systematic reviews suggest that the combined application of stretching and heat (e.g. by means of ultrasound, laser or hot packs) are superior to a unimodal intervention (Nakano et al., 2012; Bleakley and Costello, 2013). By contrast, evidence is insufficient to recommend for or against the use of cold thermal agents such as ice (Bleakley and Costello, 2013).

Despite its beneficial impact on ROM, coaches and exercise professionals have to recall the potentially negative consequences of stretching in other performance-related outcomes. As soon as an athlete requires maximal or explosive strength (e.g. powerlifters or sprinters), static stretching can have detrimental effects, causing performance decreases of up to 2% for sprints, 8% for jumps and 28% for absolute voluntary strength (McHugh and Cosgrave, 2010). Although compelling evidence clearly underpins the counter-productivity, many athletes used to performing stretches for many years do not want to break old habits. This is understandable when considering that it may also be of psychological value in the context of pre-exercise preparation. In these cases, there are different ways to modify but not forbid stretching. If the duration of a static stretch is reduced (particularly to less than 30 s), the decrements in performance shrink while ROM can still be enhanced, although to a smaller degree. A similar effect can be observed if stretch intensity is reduced (Behm and Chaouachi, 2011). In some cases, athletes will need both a large ROM and a high rate of force development. Consider a sprinter whose speed is dependent on explosive strength to create propulsion and a long stride to cover distance, which requires adequate hamstring flexibility. Reducing stretch duration and intensity may decrease the force loss but also the potential gains in stride length. In

Table 10.2 Mean range of motion improvements following stretching. The table lists data from systematic reviews					
	Static stretching	**Dynamic stretching**	**PNF stretching**	**Diverse methods**	**Time frame**
Radford et al., 2006	2.1 to 3.0° (ankle)				acute/ chronic
Harvey et al., 2002				8° (diverse joints)	chronic
Medeiros and Martini, 2018	5.2° (ankle)	3.8° (ankle, n.s.)	4.3° (ankle)		chronic
Decoster et al., 2005	5.7 to 28° (hip/knee)		5.3 to 33.6° (hip/knee)		acute/ chronic
Medeiros et al., 2016	8.4 to 12° (hip/knee)				acute/ chronic
Thomas et al., 2018	20.9% (diverse joints)	11.7% (diverse joints)	15.0% (diverse joints)		chronic
n.s. = non-significant change					

123

What is it good for? An evidence-based review of stretching in sport and movement

other words, if ROM is as important as explosive power, then the described modifications could thwart the potential benefits. As many sports do require both qualities, the solutions of reducing intensity and duration are not optimal. In addition to static stretching, extensive research has therefore been dedicated to its dynamic form, which does not substantially reduce and in some cases even slightly improves functional performance (McHugh and Cosgrave, 2010; Behm and Chaouachi, 2011). In sports involving quick powerful actions based on stretch shortening cycles, such as football (soccer), basketball or some athletic disciplines, this form of stretching seems preferable.

Out of balance? Stretching and muscular asymmetry

A frequent health-related goal of trainers treating elite and regular athletes is the reduction of muscular imbalance. The classic concept of asymmetry can be best compared to a sailing vessel. In order to properly function, its mast has to remain uprightly centered in perfect balance, thanks to the rigging ropes holding it from different sides. In our body, the mast would correspond to the bony structures, i.e. the spine, while the ropes represent the muscles and other soft tissues. If no imbalance is present, the muscles help to ensure the maintenance of the typical and optimal curvatures (lumbar lordosis, thoracic kyphosis and cervical lordosis). However, if one component, the pectoral muscles or the forestay (the cable which pulls the mast in the anterior direction) are too strong relative to the opposite side (our upper back muscles or the cable pulling the mast backwards), the spine/mast will bend in their direction. Over time, this can lead to overuse and structural damage. Besides the upper spine, where the dominance of the pectoral muscles leads to hyper-kyphosis,

another classical example of muscle imbalance relates to the lumbopelvic region. Here, weak abdominal/gluteus maximus muscles and overactive hip flexor/lumbar extensor muscles create an excessive lumbar lordosis. In some sports, lumbar lordosis is particularly frequent. Nine out of ten dancers and gymnasts exhibit moderate or strong lordosis, which is necessary for some recurrent movements (Ambegaonkar et al., 2014). However, if pain develops in the low back region, the use of corrective "de-lordosing" exercise should be considered.

The traditional treatment of muscular imbalance includes two pillars. First, the weakened muscles are strengthened/activated to counteract the bending forces. Second, the overactive/excessively strong muscles are stretched in order to decrease their tone, which should assist the strengthened antagonists in pulling the joint back in balance. However, as outlined in this chapter, a permanent stretch-induced reduction of resting tension is not possible due to the spring-like function of the titin-filaments, which restore original tone in the minutes following a stretch. Does this mean that stretching should no longer be performed if a person has bad posture caused by muscle imbalances? The answer is both yes and no. This is best illustrated by an example. If an athlete has protracted shoulders and a kyphotic thoracic spine, a basketball player, for example, they will not be able to fully extend the latter. If going up for a rebound or shot, they have to compensate in the neighboring joints (the lumbar and cervical spine, possibly also in the shoulder joint), which may cause problems and performance deficits. In the long term and under static conditions, stretching will not help because the effect of the prescribed pectoralis stretching always diminishes after a while. The preferred chronic correction strategy is, therefore, rather the strengthening of the weakened

Chapter 10

antagonists (upper back muscles). However, in the short term, stretching can still make a lot of sense: after acute bouts of stretching the pectorals, the athlete may benefit from their temporarily reduced tone to play their stint on the field without excessive protraction before being substituted. Off court, they could use the briefly corrected posture to train without and into less compensatory movement patterns.

Stretching in the rehabilitation of musculoskeletal disorders in sports

Despite its widespread use in the rehabilitation of sports-related musculoskeletal disorders, few studies have explicitly examined the value of therapeutic stretching, and in most studies, related techniques were used solely as an additional treatment. The following overview should therefore be interpreted with caution. According to one trial, stretching exercises can increase the treatment success of eccentric training in patellar tendinopathy, which develops particularly in athletes who participate in jumping and running sports. Dimitrios et al. (2012) randomly allocated 43 patients to two groups exercising five times per week. While the individuals performing eccentrics for the quadriceps femoris only increased the scores of the VISA-P questionnaire (higher scores reflect lower pain levels) from 46 at baseline to 74 after 4 weeks and 77 after 6 months, additional static stretching of the anterior thigh was shown to be significantly more effective (44 to 86 to 94 points). Similarly, stretching can be used as an adjunct therapeutic element in myofascial pain syndrome. Being characterized by the presence of active myofascial trigger points, the pathology often affects overhead athletes and manifests as neck pain. Following prior deactivation of the trigger points, for example, by means of acupuncture, it has been found that stretching further increases the analgesic treatment effect

when compared with a placebo intervention (Wilke et al., 2014). In contrast to these studies, compelling evidence is available for effectiveness in treating posterior shoulder tightness (ST) and glenohumeral internal rotation deficit (GIRD), both of which may predispose for upper extremity injury in sports or chronic impingement syndrome (Harshbarger et al., 2013; Johnson et al., 2018). Athletes typically affected by ST and GIRD include throwers (e.g. in baseball), swimmers or tennis players. According to two systematic reviews, a cross-body arm adduction stretch has a positive impact and can be recommended (Harshbarger et al., 2013; Mine et al., 2017). By contrast, the often applied sleeper stretch does not necessarily improve ST and GIRD (Mine et al., 2017).

How to do it: the different stretching methods

Over the years, different types of stretching have evolved (see Table 10.3). The most traditional methods include static and dynamic stretching. In static stretching, a constant joint position, which elongates the targeted soft tissue, is maintained without any further movement. Dynamic stretching describes repetitive movements providing cyclic lengthening stimuli, most frequently at the end range of motion (then called ballistic stretching).

In addition to static and passive stretching, newer methods aim to specially engage the central nervous system using PNF (Figure 10.2). A common feature of PNF stretches is that the deliberate stimulation of sensory receptors is suggested to trigger muscle inhibitions, which then allow a higher increase in flexibility.

- **Antagonist contraction (AC) stretching**: To actively flex the knee, the hamstring muscles need to be contracted. Simultaneously,

125

What is it good for? An evidence-based review of stretching in sport and movement

for a fluent and energy-efficient movement, it is necessary to relax the quadriceps femoris muscle, because major activity of this antagonist would decelerate or stop the flexion motion. Reciprocal inhibition represents the mechanism helping to put this principle into practice: if the hamstrings are contracted, this information is sent back to the central nervous system, which then inhibits the drive to the quadriceps muscle. AC stretching is based on reciprocal inhibition. When stretching the ventral thigh (and with this the quadriceps femoris), the hamstrings are simultaneously contracted with the aim to trigger the process described above.

- **Contract relax (CR) stretching**: As one of the most important proprioceptors, the

Golgi tendon-like organ continuously registers the contraction state of a skeletal muscle. When the quadriceps femoris is activated, the receptor fires, activating an inhibitory neuron in the spinal cord. As a consequence, the contraction of the quadriceps is released. This process is called autogenic inhibition. In CR stretching, the target muscle (in our example again the quadriceps femoris) is strongly contracted for a few seconds. During the subsequent stretch, the quadriceps can be lengthened to a stronger degree thanks to autogenic inhibition.

- **AC-CR stretching** combines the two PNF methods described above. Again, the quadriceps femoris serves as an example. Initially, the quadriceps is contracted to

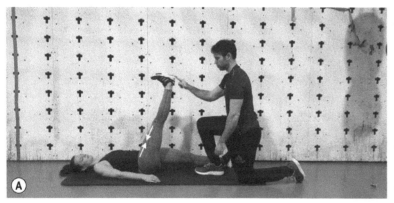

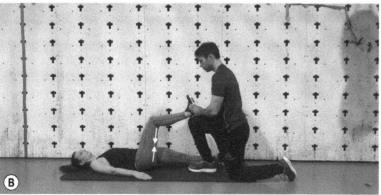

Figure 10.2

Besides static and dynamic stretching, proprioceptive neuromuscular facilitation (PNF) methods can be used by more experienced clients. In **(A)** antagonist contraction (AC) stretching, the antagonist (white arrows) is contracted during the exercise. For **(B)** contract relax (CR) stretching, the target muscle is isometrically activated (white arrows) immediately before the actual stretch. AC-CR stretching combines both methods.

Chapter 10

Table 10.3 Technique-effect matrix for different stretching methods. The table shows synthesized results from systematic reviews						
	Static		**Dynamic**		**PNF**	
	acute	chronic	acute	chronic	acute	chronic
Range of motion	↑	↑	↑	↑	↑	↑
Maximum strength	↓	↑	↔/↑	↔/↑	↓	↔
Explosive strength (jump height/sprint)	↓	↔/↑	↔	↔	↔	↔
Injury risk	↔/(↓)	↔/(↓)	↔/(↓)	↔/(↓)	↔/(↓)	↔/(↓)

Key: ↑ = increase, ↓ = decrease, ↔ = no change or unknown

elicit an autogenic inhibition releasing its tension. Immediately following this step, a stretch with simultaneous contraction of the antagonist (the hamstrings) is performed, which causes a reciprocal inhibition of the quadriceps. In summary, AC-CR stretching therefore uses two PNF pathways to more strongly decrease the activation of the target muscle.

The pros and cons of using PNF stretching in clients and patients need to be carefully weighed against each other. Due to their complexity, the techniques are more difficult to apply in some populations (particularly in elderly persons or individuals with limited sport-related experience) and can require more time. However, despite these drawbacks, they may also offer variety, refreshing an old training routine or helping an elite-level athlete to increase performance by a few but decisive percent (Table 10.3).

Summary

Stretching is a vital component of general fitness programs as well as strength and conditioning routines. However, its value is highly ambivalent and context-specific: while stretching substantially improves joint range of motion regardless of the technique used, it does not, or only to a minor degree, prevents sports injuries and, furthermore, cannot reduce muscle imbalance permanently. When warming up for explosive and powerful movements, athletes should use dynamic over static exercises as the latter may have detrimental effects. Despite extensive efforts, the mechanisms behind stretching have not been fully elucidated. Acutely, changes of the mechanical properties in the muscle, tendon and fascia become manifest. However, they may not be preserved in the long term. Besides morphological adaptations of the stretched tissues, the role of the central nervous system (e.g. by reducing stretch tolerance) continues to play an important role in the genesis of the effects.

127

What is it good for? An evidence-based review of stretching in sport and movement

References

Ambegaonkar, J.P., Caswell, A.M., Kenworthy, K.L., Cortes, N. & Caswell, S.V. (2014) Lumbar lordosis in female collegiate dancers and gymnasts. *Med Probl Perform Art*. 29: 189–192.

Apostolopoulos, N., Metsios, G.S., Flouris, A.D., Koutedakis, Y. & Wyon, M.A. (2015) The relevance of stretch intensity and position - a systematic review. *Front Physiol*. 6: 1128.

Behm, D.G., Blazevich, A.J., Kay, A.D. & McHugh, M., (2016) Acute effects of muscle stretching on physical performance, range of motion, and injury incidence in healthy, active individuals: a systematic review. *Appl Physiol Nutr Metab*. 41: 1–11.

Behm, D.G. & Chaouachi, A. (2011) A review of the acute effects of static and dynamic stretching on performance. *Eur J Appl Physiol*. 111: 2633–2651.

Bhattacharya, V., Barooah, P.S., Nag, T.C., Chaudhuri, G.R. & Bhattacharya, S. (2010) Detail microscopic analysis of deep fascia of lower limb and its surgical implication. *Ind J Plast Surg*. 43: 135–140.

Bleakley, C.M. & Costello, J.T. (2013) Do thermal agents affect range of movement and mechanical properties in soft tissues? A systematic review. *Arch Phys Med Rehabil*. 94: 149–163.

Bouvier, T., Opplert, J., Cometti, C. & Babault, N. (2017) Acute effects of static stretching on muscle-tendon mechanics of quadriceps and plantar flexor muscles. *Eur J Appl Physiol*. 117: 1309–1315.

Decoster, L.C., Cleland, J., Altieri, C. & Russell, P. (2005) The effects of stretching on range of motion: a systematic review of the literature. *J Orthop Sports Phys Ther*. 35: 377–387.

Dimitrios, S., Pantelis, M. & Kalliopi, S. (2012) Comparing the effects of eccentric training with eccentric training and static stretching exercises in the treatment of patellar tendinopathy. A controlled clinical trial. *Clin Rehabil*. 26: 423–430.

Freitas, S.R., Mendes, B., Le Sant, G., Andrade, R.J., Nordez, A. & Milanovic, Z. (2018) Can chronic stretching change the muscle-tendon mechanical properties? A review. *Scand J Med Sci Sports*. 28: 794–806.

Harshbarger, N.D., Bardly, L., Eppelheimer, L., McLeod, T.C. & McCarty, C.W. (2013) The effectiveness of shoulder stretching and joint mobilizations on posterior shoulder tightness. *J Sport Rehabil*. 22: 313–319.

Hart, L. (2005) Effect of stretching on sport injury risk: a review. *Clin J Sport Med*. 15: 113.

Harvey, L., Herbert, R. & Crosbie, J. (2002) Does stretching induce lasting increases in joint ROM? A systematic review. *Physiother Res Int*. 7: 1–13.

Hatano, G., Suzuki, S., Matsuo, S., Kataura, S., Yokoi, K., Fukaya, T., Fujiwara, M., Asai, Y. & Iwata, M. (2017) Hamstring stiffness returns more rapidly after static stretching than range of motion, stretch tolerance, and isometric peak torque. *J Sport Rehabil*. 18: 1–23.

Herbert, R.D., da Noronha, M. & Kamper, S.J. (2011) Stretching to prevent or reduce muscle soreness after exercise. *Cochrane Database Syst Rev*. 6: CD004577.

Herbert, R.D. & Gabriel, M. (2002) Effects of stretching before and after exercising on muscle soreness and risk of injury: systematic review. *BMJ*. 325: 468.

Hoppe, K., Schleip, R., Lehmann-Horn, F., Jäger, H. & Klingler, W. (2014) Contractile elements in muscular fascial tissue—implications for *in-vitro* contracture testing for malignant hyperthermia. *Anaesthesia*. 69: 1002–1008.

Johnson, J.E., Fullmer, J.A., Nielsen, C.M., Johnson, J.K. & Moorman, C.T. (2018) Glenohumeral internal rotation deficit and injuries: a systematic review and meta-analysis. *Orthop J Sports Med*. 6: 2325967118773322.

Kato, E., Kaneshisa, H., Fukunaga, T. & Kawakami, Y. (2010) Changes in ankle joint stiffness due to stretching: The role of tendon elongation of the gastrocnemius muscle. *Eur J Sport Sci*. 10: 111–119.

Kay, A.D. & Blazevich, A.J. (2009) Moderate-duration static stretch reduces active and passive plantar flexor moment but not Achilles tendon stiffness or active muscle length. *J Appl Physiol*. 106: 1249–1256.

Kubo, K., Kanseshisa, H., Fukunaga, T. & Kawakami, Y. (2001) Influence of static stretching on viscoelastic properties of human tendon structures in vivo. *J Appl Physiol*. 90: 520–527.

Lardner, R. (2001) Stretching and flexibility: its importance in rehabilitation. *J Bodyw Mov Ther*. 5: 254–263.

Maeda, N., Urabe, Y., Tsutsumi, S., Sakai, S., Fujishita, H., Kobayashi, T., Asaeda,

Chapter 10

M., Hirata, K., Mikami, Y. & Kimura, H. (2017) The acute effects of static and cyclic stretching on muscle stiffness and hardness of medial gastrocnemius muscle. *J Sports Sci Med*. 16: 514–520.

McHugh, M.P. & Cosgrave, C.H. (2010) To stretch or not to stretch: the role of stretching in injury prevention and performance. *Scand J Med Sci Sports*. 20: 169–181.

Medeiros, D.M., Cini, A., Sbruzzi, G. & Lima, C.S. (2016) Influence of static stretching on hamstring flexibility in healthy young adults: Systematic review and meta-analysis. *Physiother Theory Pract*. 32: 438–445.

Medeiros, D.M. & Martini, T.F. (2018) Chronic effect of different types of stretching on ankle dorsiflexion range of motion: Systematic review and meta-analysis. *Foot*. 34: 28–35.

Mine, K., Nakayama, T., Milanese, S. & Grimmer, K. (2017) Effectiveness of stretching on posterior shoulder tightness and glenohumeral internal-rotation deficit: a systematic review of randomized controlled trials. *J Sport Rehabil*. 26: 294–305.

Morse, C.I., Degens, H., Seynnes, O.R., Maganaris, C.N. & Jones, D.A. (2008) The acute effect of stretching on the passive stiffness of the human gastrocnemius muscle tendon unit. *J Physiol*. 586: 97–106.

Nakamura, M., Ikezoe, T., Takeno, Y. & Ichihashi, N. (2011) Acute and prolonged effect of static stretching on the passive stiffness of the human gastrocnemius muscle tendon unit in vivo. *J Orthop Res*. 29: 1759–1763.

Nakano, J., Yamabayashi, C., Scott, A. & Reid W.D. (2012) The effect of heat applied with stretch to increase range of motion: a systematic review. *Phys Ther Sport*. 13: 180–188.

Page, P. (2012) Current concept in muscle stretching for exercise and rehabilitation. *Int J Sports Phys Ther*. 7: 109-119.

Radford, J.A., Burns, J., Buchbinder, R., Langdorf, K.B. & Cook, C. (2006) Does stretching increase ankle dorsiflexion range of motion? A systematic review. *Br J Sports Med*. 40: 870–875.

Ryan, E.D., Beck, T.W., Herda, T.J., Hull, H.R., Hartman, M.J., Costa, P.B., Defreitas, J.M., Stout, J.R. & Cramer, J.T. (2008) The time course of musculotendinous stiffness responses following different durations of passive stretching. *J Orthop Sports Phys Ther*. 38: 632–639.

Schleip, R., Duerselen, L., Vleeming, A., Naylor, I.L., Lehmann-Horn, F., Zorn, A., Jaeger, H. & Klingler, W. (2012) Strain hardening of fascia: static stretching of dense fibrous connective tissues can induce a temporary stiffness increase accompanied by enhanced matrix hydration. *J Bodyw Mov Ther*. 16: 94–100.

Schleip, R., Gabbiani, G., Wilke, J., Naylor, I., Hinz, B., Zorn, A., Jäger, H., Schreiner, S. & Klin-gler, W. (2019) Fascia is able to actively contract and thereby influence musculoskeletal dynamics: a histochemical and mechanographic investigation. *Front Physiol*. doi: 10.3389/fphys.2019.00336

Shrier, I. (1999) Stretching before exercise does not reduce the risk of local muscle injury: a critical review of the clinical and basic science literature. *Clin J Sport Med*. 9: 221–227.

Small, K., Mc Naughton, L. & Matthews, M., (2008) A systematic review into the efficacy of static stretching as part of a warm-up for the prevention of exercise-related injury. *Res Sports Med*. 16: 213–231.

Staubesand, J. & Li, Y. (1997) Begriff und Substrat der Fasziensklerose bei chronisch-venöser Insuffizienz. *Phlebologie*. 26: 72–79.

Thacker, S. B., Gilchrist, J., Stroup, D.F. & Kimsey, C. D. (2004) The impact of stretching on sports injury risk: a systematic review of the literature. *Med Sci Sports Exerc*. 36: 371–378.

Thomas, E., Bianco, A., Paoli, A. & Palma, A. (2018) The relation between stretching typology and stretching duration: the effects on range of motion. *Int J Sports Med*. 39: 243–254.

Wang, H.Q., Wei, Y.Y., Wu, Z.X. & Luo, Z.J. (2009) Impact of leg lengthening on viscoelastic properties of the deep fascia. *BMC Musculoskel Disord*. 10: 105.

Wilke, J., Vogt, L., Niederer, D., Hübscher, M., Rothmayr, J., Ivkovic, D., Rickert, M. & Banzer, W. (2014) Short-term effects of acupuncture and stretching on myofascial trigger point pain of the neck: a blinded, placebo-controlled RCT. *Complement Ther Med*. 22: 835–841.

Yahia, L.H., Pigeon, P. & DesRosiers, E.A. (1993) Viscoelastic properties of the human lumbodorsal fascia. *J Biomed*. 15: 425–429.

Biotensegrity in sport and movement

John Sharkey

"We snatch in vain at Nature's veil
She is mysterious in broad daylight,
No screws or levers can compel her to reveal
The secrets she has hidden from our sight."

Faust by Johann Wolfgang von Goethe

Introduction: tensegrity versus biotensegrity

Dr Donald E. Ingber outlined his findings from 30 years of research on tensegrity and mechanotransduction at the 1st International Fascia Research Congress (IFRC), at Harvard Medical School Conference Center. Ingber revealed that "[M]olecules, cells, tissues, organs, and our entire bodies use 'tensegrity' architecture to mechanically stabilize their shape, and to seamlessly integrate structure and function at all size scales."

However, one could ask the question "What consequences does this have for individuals working in sport and movement"? The answer is clear. Scientific evidence was finally established supporting the notion that mechanical forces produce change in our biochemistry, gene expression, metabolism and our overall physiology (Ingber, 2008). No longer would genes, chemicals and DNA hold exclusive domain over our internal physiology.

Mechanical properties, behavior and movement were now understood to be serious contenders worthy of consideration in the scientific investigation concerning the health of our cells. Pioneering research from Ingber led to a proposition to replace accepted engineering principles that were firmly established as the methodology used to solve medical problems. The model of tensegrity was put forward as a means to enlighten bioengineering.

This, in effect, represented a role reversal, whereby nature would inform engineering (bioinspired) rather than non-biological engineering-inspired solutions for interventions such as hip replacements or drug delivery applications. The implications of tensegrity in sport and movement are now beginning to be appreciated.

Orthopedic surgeon Stephen Levin created the term "biotensegrity", a word comprising three parts, bio, tension and integrity. An examination and appreciation of Buckminster Fuller's ideas and Levin's unique interpretation of Kenneth Snelson's sculptures gave rise to this new concept. It became apparent that Newtonian, Hookean and linear mechanical properties are the basis for the building of all things non-biological (Levin, 1995). Buckminster Fuller (1895–1983), an architect of fame in the mid-twentieth century, coined the term "tensegrity" by blending the words tension and integrity to create a portmanteau of tensegrity. It was a genius move, encapsulating the essence of what makes tensegrity and biotensegrity so distinctive.

Fuller would later describe tensegrities as "islands of compression in an ocean of tension". In that simple phrase exists the appealing nature of tensegrity (and hence biotensegrity) for the sport and movement specialist.

Chapter 11

As a metaphor (not reality for a biotensegrity), one can instantly imagine the "ocean of tension" representing the fasciae while "islands of compression" could be represented by bones (i.e. the skeletal components invested in the fascia matrix). The fascial oceans become seas, lakes, rivers, streams and brooks embracing and becoming the sandy shores of the osseofascial tissues (Sharkey, 2018a). This description supports the more recently accepted image of a continuous tissue, ubiquitous in nature, connecting left to right, front to back, top to bottom, embracing and permeating the entire body. The visceral organs integrate structurally and physiologically into this system.

The upper and lower limbs are semi-rigid, non-linear bony segments. These segments are interconnected by non-linear connectors. These include cartilage, joint capsules and ligaments with an integrated non-linear, active motor system including the muscles, tendons and fascia. There are no limb segment boundaries. The smaller bones and joints of the hands and feet fully integrate into the biotensegrity model. The spine is a tensegrity turret that integrates with the limbs, head and tail, and also to the visceral system.

A change of tension anywhere within the system is instantly signaled to everywhere else in the body both mechanically and chemically. There is a total body response by mechanical transduction. Transduction involves a biological membrane receiving and transducing or changing a mechanical force (including light and sound) into a chemical signal or neural impulse.

However, there is a bigger, more accurate, picture. At first glance tensegrity seems like an easy model to grasp, especially as many authors use simple tensegrity models to help explain biotensegrity (Figure 11.1). It is important that the reader recognizes the varied limitations of a tensegrity model as this will help to avoid over-simplification. The tensegrity icosahedron reflects the natural process by which forces orchestrated by the environment dictate form and function. The tensegrity icosahedron is a force vector model that helps to explain what seems to be unexplainable.

Fuller first realized the significance of the tensegrity model, as a new structural design principle, in 1948 when examining a bespoke model constructed by one of his students, the artist Kenneth Snelson (1927–2016). Fuller later described Snelson's "tensegrity" model by, as previously mentioned, blending the words tension and integrity as a syntactic. A move that encapsulated the essence of what makes tensegrity so distinctive and so immediately understood at the basic level. The tensegrity has no breath or conscience and no life force. It is, in essence a model which we can use to understand the architecture of living structures from cells to whole organ systems.

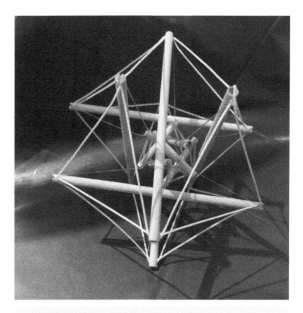

Figure 11.1 Tensegrity with a tensegrity
Model by Graham Scarr.

Biotensegrity in sport and movement

The tensegrity model has generated substantial international excitement. Its relevance in aiding sport scientists and movement practitioners to better understand the human body is gaining traction. Tensegrities contain an intriguing simplicity that, in keeping with the laws of nature, is comparable with all living structures: efficiency and the minimization of energy (Avison, 2014). It is fortunate that research pertaining to biotensegrity and fascia has reached new levels of interest almost in parallel. While the fascial system can be viewed as the fabric of continuity and communication, biotensegrity can be seen as the model for explaining the architecture underpinning continuity and communication.

Holding a tensegrity (Figure 11.1), one immediately notices the following:

1. The tensegrity structure is self-stressed and avoids collapse due to the opposing effects of its continuous elasticated member and its discontinuous compressional struts (Figure 11.1). (Note that in bodywork and movement science the opposite of collapsing would be expansive.)

2. Attempts to compress the entire structure will result in the tensegrity collapsing. It will regain its original shape and integrity once the external force is removed, returning to a position of stability and equilibrium.

3. Movement at any point, or location, of the tensegrity results in those forces being distributed throughout the entire tensegrity structure.

4. The struts (or bones) do not touch.

5. There are no joints (i.e. pin joints).

6. There is no friction (i.e. no sliding).

7. There are no bending or shear moments.

8. Attempts to pull on any aspect of the tensegrity causes an increase in "stiffness" and expansion throughout the entire structure.

9. Tensegrity is light in weight, strong and very resilient and can change shape with minimal demand on energy.

10. Tensegrities exhibit linear properties while a biotensegrity is non-linear.

What is less immediately noticeable is that tensegrities or biotensegrities do not need gravity (Eyskens, 2020). Biotensegrities can operate in any position on earth or on the space station when floating (e.g. hand-stands, cartwheels, side-lying, summersaults, high board diving and gymnastics).

Fuller had long been searching for architectural solutions in nature comparable to tensegrity because it is structurally and functionally efficient, lightweight, dynamic, and adjusts itself to its surroundings. He observed that all natural forms were the consequence of matter being dictated by forces. He proposed them as finite energy systems consisting of the forces of tension and compression acting together (Scar, 2018).

Fuller began working on a theory that respected the shape of space as central to the dynamics of nature. He even gave it a name: synergetics, the study of nature's coordinate system. Fuller used geometry to exhibit a dynamic architecture that was based on first principles (Fuller, 1975).

Nature's way—C'mon let's twist again

René Descartes (1596–1650), a French philosopher, mathematician, and scientist, put forward the model that living anatomy reflects the structure expected of an automated machine. In that regard the skeletal system was seen as separate to muscles and internal organs. A bone was considered to be a separate structure from all other bones and so the foundation was set for the model of parts rather than a model of the whole. Pin joints were the order of the day, leading to the modern day vision where surgery for hip, knee and vertebral wear and tear (or pathology) provides the evidence that we can replace these structures with materials that, while not the same, were considered mechanically similar to a knee and a hip.

In 1794, when visiting the University of Jena, Alexander Von Humboldt was working on experiments with his close friend, Johann Wolfgang von Goethe, Germany's beloved poet and author on the topic of comparative anatomy. Johann Friedrich Blumenbach had been Humboldt's professor when a student at university. Blumenbach developed theories concerning forces that shaped organisms, which he called "formative drive and vital forces".

Goethe and Humboldt collaborated so as to integrate Blumenbach's ideas into their own theories. Goethe wrote, "The snake, for example, has an endlessly long neck because 'neither matter nor force' had been wasted on arms or legs. By contrast, the lizard has a shorter neck because it has no legs, while the frog has an even shorter neck because its legs are longer."

Goethe went on to explain his belief that, contrary to Descartes's theory, animals were machines made up of autonomous parts, that a living organism was in effect a functional unified whole. One of the epistemological principles of biotensegrity is the explicit nature of our continuity. Contrary to Descartes, Goethe explained that while a machine could be dismantled and assembled again, the parts of a living organism work only in relation to each other. In a mechanical system the parts shape the whole, while in an organic system the whole shapes the parts. Humboldt interpreted the natural world as a unified whole that is animated by interactive forces (Wulf, 2016). Great minds of antiquity were coming to the tensegral reality of nature, forces, resulting proportions, symmetry, patterns, spirals, curves, heterarchy and hierarchy.

In his seminal book, *On Growth and Form*, the Scottish mathematical biologist D'arcy Wentworth Thompson described how "the forms of living things and the parts of living things can be explained by physical considerations and to realise that in general no organic forms exist save as are in conformity with physical and mathematical laws" (Thompson, 1917). In his recent, thought-provoking book, *Seeking Symmetry*, Dr Niall Galloway explains that "our human bodies are one of those living things, also 'so many portions of matter', and conformed in accordance with those same general physical laws" (Galloway and McLaren, 2018).

Today, we are coming to terms with the biotensegral nature of our continuity and the force vectors that are dictating morphological outcomes, metabolism and the physiology of all bio-systems, a reality pointed to by Goethe, Humboldt and D'arcy Thompson, among others.

In keeping with these dictates, nature has determined that everything from the cosmos to microbes is assembled upon a self-generated helical architecture. Human movement is predicated upon closed kinematic chains (Levin et al., 2017), reflecting the fractal nature of our cytoskeleton from its molecular to tissue-level organization, demonstrating the continuous nature of our heterarchy. Open kinematic chain mechanisms exhaust energy and are demanding, unidirectional, disjointed structures that are linear-based. According to Scarr (2018) the geometry of motion expressed in kinematic terms provides explanations concerning the forces of compression and tension continuously linked in a manner that alters the shape of the entire system (i.e close kinematic system).

The helical arrangement of monomers made of H- and G-proteins constitute contractile actin proteins. The more complex collagen fibers are wrapped up in a chain of left- and right-handed helices forming a cross-helical arrangement (chirality) and circumferential wrap architectural configuration. This creates shape-changing tubes within tubes. An example of the helical nature of our form is the so-called ventricular myocardial band concept of the Spanish cardiologist, Torrent Guasp, although the true anatomy of the heart is currently under debate. The helical ventricular myocardial band is an attempt to explain the heart's dynamic actions of "narrowing, shortening, lengthening, widening, twisting, and uncoiling" (Buckberg et al., 2018).

Same, same but different

Bone brittleness is approximately the same in marsupials as in a rhinoceros because the stiffness and strength of bones is approximately the same in all animals. Based on classical biomechanics, animals bigger than lions, such as horses, should break and fracture their bones with a single leap when running or jumping on their slim limbs. Based on linear mechanical laws, including Galileo's square-cube law (which are the foundation of biomechanical models), animal mass must be cubed as their surface area is squared. This should mean that animals as big as a rhinoceros will collapse under their own weight.

Working elastically at strains that are 10 x 10 x 10 times greater than strains that ordinary technological solids can withstand, demonstrates that biological tissues behave differently when compared to non-biological materials. If this was not the case, Levin (1982) informs us that "the skull should explode with each heart beat due to the blood vessels expanding and crowding out the brain. As they reach fullness the urinary bladder should thin and burst. During pregnancy the uterus should burst with the contractions of delivery."

Not exclusively mechanical, physiologic processes would be inconsistent with linear physics. Pressure within a balloon decreases as a balloon empties. Humans are omnidirectional in order that the tension elements function at all times in tension, regardless of the direction of applied force. In turn, the compression elements in biological structures "float" in a tension network. In a continuous compression model, "the shoulder has little relationship to the foot, the sub-occipital structures work autonomously with no concern for the sacrum" (Sharkey, 2018b).

The basic force-generating components for a tensegrity structure include compression and tension combining to distribute and balance mechanical stresses. Compression and tension are often described as "invisible forces" (Scarr, 2018).

It has been proposed that tension and compression represent the common, or global, language of the human body (Sharkey 2018b). At the cellular level this language needs to be translated into metabolism and physiology otherwise referred to as mechanotransduction.

Simplicity and efficiency are the building blocks for making the most complex organic or inorganic materials or organisms. This language can change depending on the scale; for example, at the molecular level, tension could be replaced with "repulsion" while compression could be replaced with "attraction".

Although not a perfect fit, we can, as a language of convenience, look at the struts of a basic tensegrity as representing our bones. The cables, be they rubber or metal, would represent the

Chapter 11

soft tissue tensional members, including muscle fibers, tendons, ligaments, cartilage, menisci, incompressible organs, nerves, vascular, lymphatic and integument.

According to Scarr (2018), "[A] strut should be considered as any structural entity that maintains a separation between one point and another - a bone, muscle, blood vessel, fascial compartment and even a single cell - and which collectively become the volumetric 'space generators' of the body."

Building a biotensegrity

To construct a biologic organism on the principles of biotensegrity, it must first have the potential to build itself. The structure would be one integrated tensegrity truss that evolved from infinitely smaller trusses, which could be both structurally independent and interdependent at the same time (Figure 11.2). Ingber (2000) described this truss as the icosahedron. Biologic tissues, such as muscles and other soft tissue, have non-linear stress/strain curves.

In classical biomechanics, the original principle that muscles, fascia and any biologic material can be compelled by the rules of hard matter physics is faulty according to the scientific evidence (Ingber, 2008) emanating from laboratories worldwide involved in investigating and researching condensed soft matter.

Ligaments and fascia, bones and cartilage would do little to support our upright forms if not for the collective activity of an integrated osseofascial/myofascial system. Pre-stress is a vital aspect of biotensegrity, with a level of tension present always within the myofascial (or neuromuscular) system. Unfortunately, scientific endeavors investigating muscle tone seldom, if ever, take bone into consideration. Malleable, bending and rotating are words we can use to describe the function of bones. Concerning the osseofascial system, this point is crucial, as the bony points researchers use to calculate the contractile elements and the elastic elements (i.e. tendonous) would obviously move. Bony points of reference, in this regard, would not be ideal for such measurements, and any conclusions derived would fall short of the robust reality required for gold standard, peer-reviewed research.

Resting tone

There are no resting muscles in living anatomy and physiology. The non-linearity of collagen does not allow for zero tension in human contractile tissue. In other words, contractile tissue never rests. We must also consider Lombard's paradox (Andrews, 1987), which is present in all two joint muscle pairings throughout the body and in closed kinematic chains. Based on classical neuroanatomical laws, it may seem ridiculous to suggest that the upper portion of the hamstring muscle group contracts while the bottom half of the quadriceps contracts simultaneously (i.e. a co-contraction). However, the paradox becomes clear when we consider the action of sitting to standing (Figure 11.2).

When sitting, rectus femoris, the largest of the quadriceps muscle group, is hypothetically in a shortened phase as the hip is in a flexion phase. Rectus femoris runs over the anterior aspect of the flexed knee enveloping the patella and associating with the tibial tuberosity by means of the patellar ligament. It is, therefore, hypothetically lengthened at the knee when sitting but shortened at the hip. Meanwhile, the hamstrings are lengthened at the hip and shortened at the posterior knee. When we move from sitting to standing our hip must extend and our knee must also extend. Rectus femoris therefore hypothetically elongates at the hip and shortens at the knee.

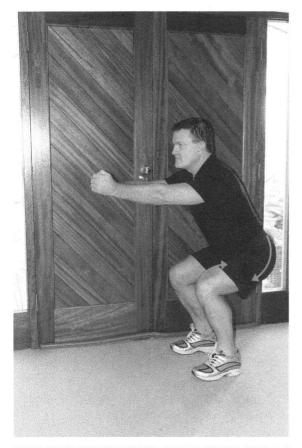

Figure 11.2 Sitting to standing.
Co-contraction of quadriceps and hamstrings—
Lombard's paradox. The arrows show direction of
movement relative to the joints.

Dr John Cleland was Professor of Anatomy and Physiology at Queen's College, Galway, Ireland, from 1863 until 1877. He stated that "I have made the measurements of the distance from the superior to the inferior attachment of the gastrocnemius muscle, when both knee and ankle were completely flexed, and when they were both completely extended, and have found that the distance remains unchanged. If we sink upon bended knees, flexing the limbs completely and remaining balanced on the toes then to rise to our full height on tip-toe, the length of the gastrocnemius remains unchanged in the movement" (Cleland, 1870).

From the biotensegrity viewpoint these are classical examples of how tissues neither lengthen nor shorten but rather shape change throughout range of motion, similar to prismatic architectural materials changing shape and reconfiguring their morphology without any individual part necessarily becoming shorter, longer, wider or narrower (Purslow, 2010). This calls into question the idea of "agonist" and "antagonist" from the classical neurological description (i.e. when an agonist contracts its antagonist relaxes). This simple example of muscular co-contraction does not include consideration of the pelvis or the tibia. Considering that the pelvis is not fixed in space, it would therefore seem reasonable to suggest that current research is working off faulty models at best. So how does this paradox allow for efficient movement?

Cadaveric investigations concerning the role of fasciae in force transmission and mechanical transduction have motivated further investigations into the possibility of this paradoxical muscle-fascial activity (Loukas et al., 2007). Observational dissection investigation on Thiel soft fixed cadaveric specimens has provided insights concerning the non-linear load distributing myofascial synergistic mechanisms of force vector dispersing of loads and conversion to movement. Fascial septal tissue provides connections, allowing force vectors in a hierarchical helical arrangement from anterior inferior (in both medial and lateral directions) to superior posterior, or vice versa (Buckberg and Gerard, 2002).

Fractals

In 2012, scientists discovered the so-called "God particle", otherwise known as the Higgs Boson.

Chapter 11

Now that we know the Higgs Boson theoretically exists, we can state that it must be made of something smaller. Everything we are made of can be seen, hypothetically, as either a cable or a strut, with each cell being made up of smaller cables and struts of different size scales (i.e. of a fractal nature), with "the relations among their parts dynamic, contextual and interdependent" (Saetzler et al., 2011). Biotensegrities are truly bottom-up and top-down structures whose parts are related to and interdependent upon the whole (Figure 11.3).

The whole is related to and interdependent upon the parts resulting in emergent properties that would not be obvious when investigating only a part (Ritter and Bailey, 1928).

Levin (2018) states that "[T]ensegrity is a multiscale, heterarchical structure and that any events at one level will, necessarily, have a structural

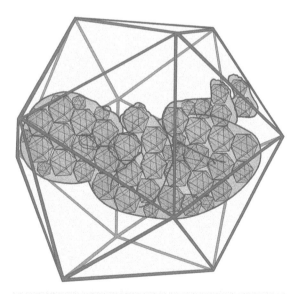

Figure 11.3

Icosahedron baby. Tensegrity within tensegrity within tensegrity. Our fractal nature (Sharkey, 2017)

Artist: Amanda Williams.

affect on all other component parts of the organism. This also applies to the dynamical mechanical events occurring within the organism, as the kinematics and kinetics of the organism are intertwined within the tensegrity structure."

A "structural effect" simply means that movement at the foot will have, for example, structural impact elsewhere in the body, perhaps at the contralateral shoulder or ipsilateral hip (or vice versa). While one can argue correctly regarding a hierarchical view concerning human anatomy and physiology, including a heterarchical model allows for an accurate whole body vision which embraces the contribution and distribution of forces throughout the body (Turvey and Fonseca, 2014). Hierarchy and heterarchy are both possible and permissible in biotensegrity.

Human movement is ultimately concerned with changes in shape in space over time. The concept of closed kinematic chains explains how movement in one body region (such as the foot) leads to movement at a distant body location (the opposite shoulder) (Findley et al., 2015).

Closed-chain kinematics of less than four bars result in no movement, or at best results in stable but rigid structures. The addition of a fourth and additional bar is necessitated to provoke and sustain controlled full-body motion. Kinematic chains, compiled of multiple bars, provide force couples which utilize combinations of three, four or multiple bar complexities. Such complexity provides energy efficient stability and motion throughout the entire biotensegrity (Levin et al., 2017).

Shedding light on fascia and biotensegrity in sport and movement

Sport scientists and movement specialists aim to provide training and movement strategies that improve performance maintain range of motion and reduce risk of injury. Unfortunately, the very nature of sport and the intense levels of training required, especially at an elite level, make this a difficult task. However, positive steps can be taken based on our current understanding of fascia-related science coupled with biotensegral principles to ensure better-informed choices and more appropriate recovery strategies.

Such strategies are applicable for the elite level athlete, the weekend warrior, or the less intense physical activities of members of all ages within our communities focusing their training on daily functionality and health-related benefits.

When we need to identify the root of a problem (e.g. an injury) we risk getting lost in the forest of "everything is connected to everything else".

A torn calcaneal tendon will require localized attention and intervention to assist in healing.

The question that biotensegrity answers and the ethos that "everything is connected" raises is "What exactly is that connection?" Did the calcaneal injury occur as a result of a more pressing problem elsewhere in the body? Is the calcaneal injury simply the messenger and, if so, how do we locate the true source of the problem?

To begin to take a step closer to answering these questions, we must accept the first principle reality that all biotensegrities are non-linear.

This fact emphatically rules out linear approaches to movement, no matter how alluring. Linear-based fascial maps provide a model that is immediately simplistic in helping to bridge the reality of the fascia-muscle fiber continuity (Figure 11.4). While this model is appealing, it does not solve the issue of non-linearity. Training regimes need to be fascia science-based and biotensegrity-informed. Sport scientists must balance high-intensity physical routines,

prescribed to improve elite athletic performance, with appropriate recovery time to reduce the risk of fascial and connective tissue injury. Differences between biotensegrity-informed movement, to achieve goals which are sport-specific, as opposed to dealing with the functional activities required when dealing with a member of the public, need to be recognized.

It has been proposed that biotensegrity-based training principles may significantly reduce the risk of injury while increasing athletic performance (Kelsick, 2015).

The principle of specificity requires the need to repeat the specific movements or actions of any given sport, such as golf, rowing, tennis or javelin-throwing. In this regard, consideration for muscle fibers is critically important.

Figure 11.4 shows an image of deep fascial compartments of a human leg. This image, coupled with Figure 11.5, highlights the role of fascia

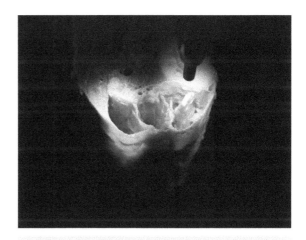

Figure 11.4 Shedding light on fascia and the biotensegrity model.

Image: Stecco, C., Sharkey, J. & Schleip, R. (2018). Human Fascial Net Plastination Project. Fascia Research Society

Credit: Thomas Stephan Photography.

Chapter 11

in the transfer of forces generated by muscle fibers, a process known as mechanotransduction (Ingber, 2008).

It is not muscle fibers that typically get damaged during intense exercise (Schleip, 2015) but rather the fascial tissue within which the muscle cells are embedded (Chapter 5).

Muscle fibers are an essential continuity of the myofascial and osseofascial systems. As there are only curves, helices and spirals in the human body, one must think in terms of 360° as the fascia enters, spirals, enfolds, penetrates, enmeshes and emerges from the various compartments. Fascia acts "to imprison its contents (vascular, neural, interstitial, lymphatic) and restrain, contain, separate, invaginate, and share forces generated within muscle fibers" (Sharkey, 2018a).

Forces generated in the fibers of any muscle are shared throughout the entire biotensegrity, locally and globally, via the softest and hardest fasciae. This changes our "one muscle, one movement" ideology. Motion is finely tuned

through synergistic, multi-bar mechanisms facilitated by the multidimensional fascial fabric (Figures 11.4 and 11.6). This is comparable to a synchronized orchestra providing not one note, not one chord but rather a symphony of sound. Similar to sound, which travels in waves, muscle forces resonate and vibrate at specific electromagnetic frequencies shared through the osseofascial system, providing the cell-specific energy for metabolism, physiology and movement (Oschman, 2015).

Foams and froth require neighboring bubbles to move and adjust in response to mechanical

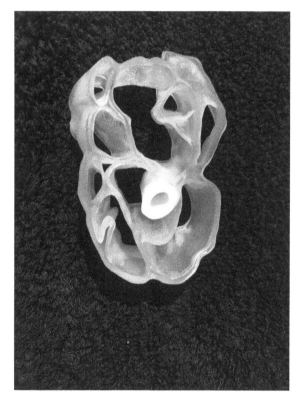

Figure 11.6

A historical image of the world's first 3D printed (mini-model version) of the deep fascial compartments of thigh. Sharkey, J. (2018).

Thanks to 3D Life Prints, NTC, Ireland, and the Fascia Research Society

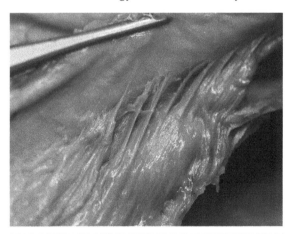

Figure 11.5

Beautifully capturing the continuity of muscle fibers within the fascia profunda.

Image: Stecco, C., Sharkey, J. & Schleip, R. (2018). Human Fascial Net Plastination Project. Fascia Research Society

changes, reflecting a multi-bar, closed-chain organization.

Our true human fascial anatomy is more closely related to the froth on your morning coffee than it is to the mechanics of an automobile, a high-rise building, or any manmade, hard matter compression-based structure.

The language of biotensegrity is tension and compression with continuity. The premise of biotensegrity is non-linear continuous matter that is self-generated (autopoiesis), self-organizing, self-stressing, hierarchical, load-distributing and low energy-consuming. There are no shear moments, no bending moments, no lever arm and no pin-joints. Sport science and movement therapies have entered an exciting new era of research with biotensegrity as the logical model underpinning future scientific investigation.

References

Andrews, J.G. (1987) The functional roles of the hamstrings and quadriceps during cycling: Lombard's Paradox revisited. *J Biomech.* 20: 565–575.

Avison, J. (2014) *Yoga: Fascia, Anatomy and Movement.* Edinburgh, UK: Handspring Publishing.

Buckberg, G. (2002) Basic science review: The helix and the heart. *J Thorac Cardiovasc Surg.* 124: 863–883.

Buckberg, G., Nanda, N., Nguyen, C., & Kocica, M. (2018) What is the heart? Anatomy, function, pathophysiology and misconceptions. *J Cardiovasc Dev Dis.* 5(2): 33.

Cleland, J. (1870) On the actions of muscles passing over more than one joint. *Journal of Anatomy and Physiology.* 1(1): 85–93.

D'arcy Thompson, W. (1917) *On Growth and Form.* Cambridge, UK: Cambridge University Press.

Eyskens, J., Sharkey, J., Appleton, J., De Nil, L. (2020) *Quest For Space: Towards a Novel Approach in Treating Pain and Fatigue on Earth* – in press.

Findley, T., Chaudhry, H. & Dhar, S. (2015) Transmission of muscle force to fascia during exercise. *J Bodyw Mov Ther.* 19(1): 119–23.

Galloway, N. & McLaren, T. (2018) *Seeking Symmetry. Finding Patterns in Human health.* Edinburgh, UK: Handspring Publishing.

Ingber, D.E. (2000) Opposing views on tensegrity as a structural framework for understanding cell mechanics. *J Appl Physiol.* 89: 1663–1670.

Ingber, E.D. (2018) Tensegrity and mechanotransduction. *J Bodyw Mov Ther.* 12: 198–200.

Kelsick, W. (2015) Functional training methods for the runners fascia. In: *Fascia in Sport and Movement.* Edinburgh, UK: Handspring Publishing.

Levin, S.M. (1982) Continuous tension, discontinuous compression, a model for biomechanical support of the body. *Bulletin of Structural Integration.* Bolder, CO: Rolf Institute, 31–33.

Levin, S.M. (1995) The importance of soft tissues for structural support of the body. *Spine.* 9.

Levin, S. (2018) From viruses to vertebrates – *A biological mechanical model using multiscale tensegrity structures* (in press).

Levin, S., Lowell de Solórzano, S. & Scarr, G. (2017) The significance of closed kinematic chains to biological movement and dynamic stability. *J Bodyw Mov Ther.* 21: 664–672.

Loukas M., Tubbs, R.S., Louis, G. Jr, Pinyard, J., Vaid, S. & Curry, B. (2007) The cardiovascular system in the pre-Hippocratic era. *Int J Cardiol.* 120: 145–149.

Oschman, J. (2015) *Energy Medicine.* 2nd edition. Elsevier.

Purslow, P.P. (2010) Muscle Fascia and force transmission. *J Bodyw Mov Ther.* 14(4): 411–417.

Ritter, W.E. & Bailey, E.W. (1928) The organismal conception: its place in science and its bearing on philosophy. *Univ Calif Pub Zool.* 31: 307–358.

Saetzler, K., Sonnenschein, C. & Soto, A.M. (2011) Systems biology beyond networks: generating order from disorder through self-organization. *Semin Cancer Biol.* 21: 165–174.

Scarr, G. (2018) *Biotensegrity: The Structural Basis of Life.* 2nd Edition. Edinburgh, UK: Handspring Publishing.

Schleip, R. (2015) *Fascia in Sport and Movement.* Edinburgh, UK: Handspring Publishing.

Chapter 11

Sharkey, J. (2018a) In: *Scars, Adhesions and the Biotensegral Body*. Edinburgh, UK: Handspring Publishing.

Sharkey, J. (2018b) Biotensegrity – anatomy for the 21st century. Informing yoga and physiotherapy concerning new findings in fascia research. *JYP*. 6: 555680.

Sharkey, J. (2017b) *The Concise Book of Dry Needling: A Practitioner's Guide to Myofascial Trigger Point Applications*. North Atlantic Press.

Wulf, A. (2016) *The Invention of Nature: The adventures of Alexander von Humboldt. The Lost Hero of Science*. London, UK: John Murray.

Credit: special thanks to photographer Thomas Stephan (https://thomas-stephan.com).

Myofascial continuity: Towards a new understanding of human anatomy

Jan Wilke

Introduction

Since time immemorial, people have strived to understand the fascinating anatomy of the human body. From Herophilus of Chalcedon (325–255 BC), who performed the first systematic dissections in Alexandria, until today, categorization and isolation represent the most important intellectual tools used to explain our inherent complexity: for instance, we distinguish a series of organ systems, all suggested to exert a specific set of functions. With regard to the locomotor system, diligent cadaver dissections have identified a total of 556 skeletal muscles. Medical students learn their names as well as their discrete origins and insertions, observing them in pictures in anatomy textbooks. However, when instructed to expose a specific tissue and its boundaries in dissection courses, they often discover that the human body, in reality, looks different to the brightly colored illustrations. Indeed, pinpointing the beginning and the end of a structure is hardly possible for the unaided eye: the scalpel needs to artificially create these points.

The isolated consideration of the skeletal muscles has severe consequences for the assumed biomechanics. As an example, the latissimus dorsi muscle, following the classical conventions, originates in the lumbar spine and inserts in the crista tuberculi minoris humeri, a prominence of the upper arm bone. If this were true, the cranial forces developed upon contraction or stretching of the latissimus would exclusively be transmitted to the humerus. However, cadaveric studies clearly demonstrate that the distal attachment of the muscle is far more complex. In addition to the bony insertions, some muscular fibers fuse strongly with the posterior aspect of the brachial fascia, which wraps around the muscles of the upper arm (Stecco et al., 2007; 2008), and in turn connects to the antebrachial fascia of the lower arm (Stecco et al., 2007). This example illustrates that contractile forces developed in the latissimus—based on its true anatomical course—may even affect the soft tissue of the hand (for an overview of the evidence regarding myofascial force transmission, see Chapters 13 and 14).

Concepts of myofascial chains

Decades ago, a number of practitioners raised doubts about the structural independence of neighboring body regions, and suggested the existence of so-called myofascial chains. A common feature of the different systems is the proposed morphological linkage between the skeletal muscles: in opposition to the idea of muscle chains or muscle slings (Tittel, 2003), where muscles are grouped based on a common function within a certain movement (e.g. extensor chain of the leg: gastrocnemius, quadriceps femoris and gluteus maximus), the components of myofascial chains are structurally connected. As the term "myofascial" indicates, a variety of tissues ("myo" for muscle, "fascial" for the diverse components of the fascial system) can form the involved continuities.

Chapter 12

Françoise Mézières (1909–1991) can be considered one of the earliest and most important pioneers who presented a system of myofascial chains (chaînes musculaires). The French therapist described four major lines of soft tissue continuity. Her most important, the chaîne postérieure, was first reported in 1949 and included a deep and a superficial plane extending dorsally from the head to the toes. In addition, Mézières proposed a deep anterior chain consisting of the continuity between the iliopsoas and the diaphragm, a brachial chain (biceps brachii, brachialis, brachioradialis, pronator teres/quadratus, flexor carpi ulnaris/radialis) and the anterior neck chain (longus colli, longus capitis and rectus capitis anterior). Although she did not provide an all-encompassing system for all parts of the body (e.g. there is no lateral chain) and her lines had either an astonishingly high (posterior) or small (deep anterior, anterior neck) number of components, Mézières' works paved the way to what can be called the age of myofascial chains. In the 1990s, several other authors presented their ideas about how the body might be connected (e.g. Busquet, 1992; Denys-Struyf, 1995; Myers, 1999). The different suggested concepts overlap significantly in a series of aspects. The connection between the psoas muscle and the diaphragm, first proposed by Mézières, is also included in the superficial front line of Myers. Likewise, both Busquet and Myers designed similarly constructed diagonal chains on the dorsal and ventral side of the body, connecting the arms to the opposite legs. However, the authors also introduced their own innovations. Besides five myofascial chains, Léopold Busquet additionally described a visceral and a neurovascular chain. Godelieve Denys-Struyf, a Belgian physiotherapist and osteopath, presented a mix of myofascial chains alongside postural patterns. Finally, Thomas Myers, who suggested a system

of 11 muscle-fascia lines, was particularly interested in linear connections between the components of chains. For instance, his superficial back line includes a structural linkage from the back extensor muscle/the lumbar fascia to the hamstrings but not to the gluteus maximus muscle because with the latter included, the direction of continuity would deviate more strongly from the cranio-caudal course of the chain. This is of relevance from a mechanical perspective because on a linear course, compared with a curved one, more force can be transferred.

Evidence for the existence of myofascial chains

The recent discoveries from fascia research have popularized treatments according to myofascial chains. Practitioners working according to the proposed concepts aim to evoke effects remote to the area of symptom localization, assuming that local dysfunctions and problems such as flexibility impairments, increased stiffness or muscle hypertonicity may (1) radiate towards or (2) originate from distant structures via the body-wide network of tissue continuity. These ideas are intriguing and revolutionary as they offer the possibility to explain and alleviate many pain conditions where local treatments have failed. Nonetheless, scientific proof for the existence of myofascial chains was, for a long time, not forthcoming, and thus all treatments performed were solely based on the clinical experience, self-reported dissection work, and beliefs of the opinion leaders who were developing the different concepts. During the last decade, however, the research output regarding this topic has increased substantially.

A comprehensive systematic review (Wilke et al., 2016) examined the question as to whether basic anatomical cadaver studies support the existence

Myofascial continuity: Towards a new understanding of human anatomy

of six of the eleven myofascial chains described by Myers (see Figure 12.1). The authors found convincing evidence for the posterior longitudinal chain, which consists of the plantar aponeurosis, Achilles tendon, gastrocnemius, hamstrings, sacrotuberous ligament, lumbar fascia and back extensor muscle. In addition, two diagonal connections between the upper and lower limb were verified. On the frontal side of the body (anterior diagonal chain), fascial tissue connects the arm via the pectoralis major and the rectus abdominis with the opposite leg (adductor longus). A similar line (posterior diagonal chain) extends on the back side, including the latissimus dorsi, the lumbar fascia and the contralateral gluteus maximus muscle. Despite these findings, not all of the lines were confirmed: while only parts of the lateral and spiral-like chain were shown to exist, there was no evidence for an anterior longitudinal chain.

Although recent research has corroborated the existence of at least some (parts) of the muscle-fascia lines (Table 12.1), there are various important key points to consider. First, imagining myofascial chains as the only pathways

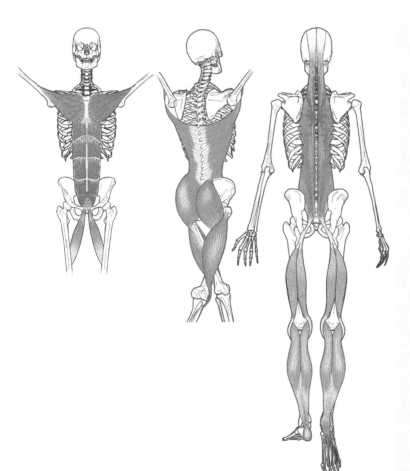

Figure 12.1

Evidence is solid for the existence of three myofascial chains: the anterior diagonal chain (left), posterior diagonal chain (center) and the posterior longitudinal chain (right). Note: the diagonal chains are bilateral, extending (1) from the left arm to the right leg and (2) vice versa.

Chapter 12

Table 12.1 Examples of myofascial chains and their assumed function (only verified continuities are listed)		
Myofascial chain	**Soft tissue components**	**Clinical comments**
Lateral longitudinal chain	• Crural fascia • Iliotibial tract • Gluteus maximus muscle/tensor fasciae latae muscle • External/internal obliquus abdominis muscle	Helps to stabilize the body (ankle, knee, hip and spine) in the frontal plane. Hypothesized continuation between ribcage and head is not yet confirmed
Spiral chain	• External/internal obliquus abdominis muscle • Serratus anterior muscle • Rhomboideus muscles	Engaged in rotatory movements (e.g. throwing). Hypothesized continuations in cranial and caudal direction not yet confirmed
Posterior longitudinal chain	• Plantar aponeurosis • Achilles tendon • Gastrocnemius muscle • Hamstring muscles • Sacrotuberous ligament • Lumbar fascia and erector spinae muscle	Provides resistance against gravity and helps to maintain upright posture. Of potential relevance in linear vertical movements (e.g. jumps)
Posterior diagonal chain	• Vastus lateralis muscle • Gluteus maximus muscle • Lumbar fascia • Contralateral latissimus dorsi muscle • Brachial fascia	Dorsal connection of both body sides. May be important in unilateral movements requiring arm-leg coupling
Anterior diagonal chain	• Adductor longus muscle • Rectus abdominis muscle • Contralateral pectoralis major muscle • Brachial fascia	Ventral connection of both body sides. May be important in unilateral movements requiring arm-leg coupling (e.g. throwing, serving when playing tennis, kicking a football)

potentially transmitting relevant mechanical forces is a fallacy. Tissue continuity is not restricted to the connected structures grouped together; it also affects other parts not included in a certain chain. For instance, the superficial back arm line from Myers describes a connection between the deltoideus muscle and the trapezius muscle. Although this morphological linkage has in fact been verified by cadaveric research, there is also a continuity from the deltoid fascia to that of the rhomboideus muscle (Day et al., 2008). It is hence evident that myofascial chains can take different tracks on their way through the body. Second, besides displaying connections in an in-series arrangement, extensive research (although mainly carried out in animals) has demonstrated most muscles to additionally fuse with others located parallel to them. As an example, in the lower leg, the fascia of the tibialis anterior merges with the connective tissue surrounding synergists such as the extensor hallucis longus and even mechanically interacts with distant antagonists such as the triceps surae complex (Rijkelijkhuisen et al., 2007; Yucesoy, 2010).

Myofascial continuity therefore represents a global construction principle of the body rather than a specific hallmark of muscle-fascia chains. Finally, the strength of a myofascial continuity is not constant and can vary depending on several factors: this is best established for the connection between the plantar aponeurosis (PA) and the Achilles tendon (AT). In a cadaver study, Snow et al. (1995) investigated the feet of adults, neonatals and fetuses. Analyses of the heel region revealed a strong fiber continuity between the aponeurosis and the tendon when considering only the youngest specimens. However, in people in their 20s, only superficial fibers of the periosteum formed the tissue bridge between both structures. No direct continuity was observed in the elderly as the PA and the AT presented only a bony insertion at the calcaneus. The age-dependency found by Snow et al. was confirmed in subsequent studies. Ballal et al. (2014) dissected 12 adult feet: only in the two youngest (aged 59 and 66 years) and a 79-year-old cadaver, were the AT and the PA clearly fused. Kim et al. (2010) investigated a total of 60 lower extremities of cadavers with a mean age of 68 (43–98) years. Morphological fusion of the AT and the PA (found in 8% of the cases) correlated with the age of the specimens. In a follow-up study using magnet resonance imaging (MRI), the same authors examined the insertion of the tendon as a function of age in younger specimens. Interestingly, they found a progressive migration into the proximal direction: the older the individuals, the more superior the insertion (Kim et al., 2011). The most recent study describing the connection between the aponeurosis and the tendon was published by Stecco et al. (2013). Contrary to previous reports, the authors, who were the only ones to use fresh cadavers without fixation, detected a direct morphological linkage in all of the 12 examined cadavers: at the heel, the PA was reported to continue as a thin band (thickness: 1–2 mm), blending with the paratenon of the AT.

In sum, the results regarding the myofascial continuity at the calcaneus are conflicting. The majority of studies suggest an age-related decrease or disappearance of the tissue linkage. However, it is also possible that in this subsample, the MRI technique (Kim et al., 2010; 2011) was not sensitive enough to detect small degrees of continuity and that the use of embalmed cadavers (Ballal et al., 2014; Snow et al., 1995) may partly have made it impossible to identify these due to adhesions between periosteal fibers and bones.

Summary

The frequently conveyed concept of skeletal muscles as being independent actuators does not sufficiently reflect the complexity of human anatomy. Both the skeletal muscles, as well as the surrounding and neighboring connective tissues, are directly fused with each other, creating a body-wide web of structural continuity. Current evidence has verified several connections that can be grouped to myofascial chains. Such muscle-fascia lines may explain the radiation of pain and dysfunction to remote body locations. However, reaching in multiple directions, structural linkage is by no way restricted to these tracks. Reducing the construct of tissue continuity to the proposed chains would therefore create the same artificial boundaries as those portrayed by classical anatomy books defining the discrete origins and insertions of the skeletal muscles. Consequently, when evaluating the mechanical interactions between adjacent tissues (Chapters 13 and 14), it is imperative to focus on both the potential clinical relevance of force transmission in series and to structures located in parallel.

Chapter 12

References

Ballal, M.S., Walker, C.R. & Molloy, A.P. (2014) The anatomical footprint of the Achilles tendon: a cadaveric study. *Bone Joint J.* B10: 1344–1348.

Busquet, L. (1992) Les chaînes musculaires. Vols 1–4. Maîtres et Clefs de la Posture Frères, Mairlot.

Day, J.A., Stecco, C. & Stecco, A. (2009) Application of fascial manipulation technique in chronic shoulder pain – anatomical basis and clinical implications. *J Bodyw Mov Ther.* 13: 128–135.

Denys-Struyf, G. (1995) Cadeias musculares e articulares: o método G.D.S. Summus Editorial.

Kim, P.J., Richey, J.M., Wissman, L.R. & Steinberg, J.S. (2010) Variability of the Achilles tendon insertion: a cadaveric examination. *J Foot Ankle Surg.* 49: 417–420.

Kim, P.J., Martin, E., Ballehr, L., Richey, J.M. & Steinberg, J.S. (2011) Variability of insertion of the Achilles tendon on the calcaneus: an MRI study of younger subjects. *J Foot Ankle Surg.* 50: 41–43.

Myers, T.W. (1997) The 'anatomy trains'. *J Bodyw Mov Ther.* 1: 91–101.

Rijkelijkhuizen, J.M., Meijer, H.J., Baan, G.C. & Huijing, P.A. (2007) Myofascial force transmission also occurs between antagonistic muscles related within opposite compartments of the rat lower limb. *J Electromyogr Kinesiol.* 17: 690–697.

Snow S.W., Bohne, W.H., DiCarlo, E. & Chang, V.K. (1995) Anatomy of the Achilles tendon and plantar fascia in relation to the calcaneus in various age groups. *Foot Ankle Int.* 16: 418–421.

Stecco, C., Gagey, O., Machi, V., Porzionato, A., De Caro, R., Aldegheri R. & Delmas, V. (2007) Tendinous muscular insertions onto the deep fascia of the upper limb. First part: anatomical study. *Morphologie* 91: 29–37.

Stecco, C., Porzionato, A., Machhi, V., Stecco, A., Vigato, E., Parenti, A., Delmas, V., Aldegheri, R. & De Caro, R. (2008) The expansions of the pectoral girdle muscles onto the brachial fascia: morphological aspects and spatial disposition. *Cells Tissues Organs* 188: 320–329.

Stecco, C., Corradin, M., Macchi, V., Morra, A., Porzionato, A., Biz, C. & De Caro, R. (2013) Plantar fascia anatomy and its relationship with Achilles tendon and paratenon. J Anat. 223: 665–676.

Tittel, K. (2003) *Beschreibende und funktionelle Anatomie des Menschen.* Munich, Germany: Urban & Fischer.

Wilke, J., Krause, F., Vogt, L. & Banzer, W. (2016) What is evidence-based about myofascial chains: a systematic review. *Arch Phys Med Rehabil.* 97: 454–461.

Yucesoy, C.A. (2010) Epimuscular myofascial force transmission implies novel principles for muscular mechanics. *Exerc Sport Sci Rev.* 38: 128–134.

Mechanical force transmission across myofascial chains

Jan Wilke

Introduction

The skeletal muscles cannot be considered as independent actuators (see Chapter 12). Instead, due to their intimate connections to the adjacent soft tissue, they may be influenced by forces originating from neighboring or even distant body locations. Some authors have refined this idea, suggesting the existence of highly specified mechanical pathways: it is assumed that myofascial chains transmit particularly large amounts of force owing to the in-series arrangement of their components (Figure 13.1). If this were true, not only the active component of the locomotor system but also the connective tissues linking the incorporated skeletal muscles (e.g. tendons, ligaments or the deep fascia) would have to possess higher force transmission capacities in the longitudinal rather than in the transversal direction.

Basic prerequisites and assumptions of myofascial force transmission

A quick view into the micro-anatomy of the connective tissue apparently supports the above hypothesis. Tendons and ligaments exhibit almost parallel collagen fibers oriented in one direction, which enables them to withstand and transfer high elongating forces. The collagen of the deep fascia has a lattice-like arrangement with a fiber-crossing angle of 80 degrees (Benetazzo et al., 2011). This construction allows for a flexible adaptation to both stretching and contraction of the underlying muscle.

Nevertheless, a particularly high longitudinal strength, similar to tendons and ligaments, can be expected because the fibers are rather oriented towards the muscle's line of pull. Indeed, findings from histological and biomechanical studies confirm the anisotropic features of the deep fascia. The fascia lata, which ensheathes the muscles of the thigh, has similar material properties to the patellar tendon (Butler et al., 1984). Its maximal stiffness is up to 7-fold higher in the longitudinal (283 Newton per millimeter) than in the transversal plane (41.9 Newton per millimeter) (Otsuka et al., 2018). Stress tests of tissues from other body regions which compared the maximal resilience in both directions showed that the loading capacity in the longitudinal plane is 5-fold higher for the crural fascia (Eng et al., 2014; Stecco et al., 2014) and 3-fold higher for the fasciae of the abdominal wall (Kirilova et al., 2011). In summary, these data show that not only ligaments and tendons, but also the deep fasciae, are stronger strain transmitters in the longitudinal direction, which often corresponds to the primary direction of muscle force development.

The mere existence of myofascial chains, as well as a high longitudinal loading capacity of the tissues connecting the included skeletal muscle components, do not necessarily imply functional relevance per se. Only if relevant forces can be transmitted across the continuities, are exercise and treatment according to them justifiable.

From a mechanical perspective, local alterations of tissue stiffness are a prerequisite of force

Chapter 13

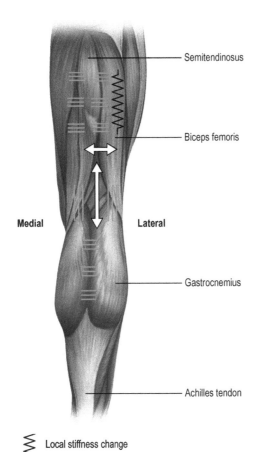

Semitendinosus

Biceps femoris

Medial   Lateral

Gastrocnemius

Achilles tendon

≷ Local stiffness change

≡ Linking fibers

⇒ Force transmission

Figure 13.1 Schematic illustration of myofascial force transmission in the lower leg

Due to direct tissue continuity, local forces produced in the biceps femoris may be transferred to muscles located in parallel (e.g. the semitendinosus) and to muscles arranged in-series (e.g. the gastrocnemius). Concepts of myofascial chains assume higher degrees of force transmission between serially connected muscles.

models, the developing radial stress is substantial, amounting to ~50% of the longitudinal stress (Findley et al., 2015). Otsuka et al. (2019) used ultrasound elastography (Chapter 20) to quantify fascial stiffness changes upon muscle contraction. Isometric knee extension at 60% of maximal voluntary strength led to large alterations of the connective tissue properties: compared with the resting state, the stiffness of the fascia lata was ~2.4-fold higher over both the rectus femoris muscle and the vastus lateralis muscle. While these increments were registered for the longitudinal direction, much lower (but still significant) contraction-induced stiffness increases occurred in the transversal plane of the fascia, which further solidifies the above evidence for the higher strain transmission capacity in the direction of the muscle's line of pull. In addition to the passive interaction through muscle expansion, mutual interactions with the surrounding connective tissue also occur, due to a special architectural feature. Some muscles present direct fibrous expansions into the fascia, which allow a selective tensioning of the connective tissue. This can, for instance, be observed in the latissimus dorsi, whose muscular fibers tighten the triceps brachii fascia (Stecco et al., 2008), and also in the pectoralis major muscle, whose fibers reach into the brachial fascia of the arm (Stecco et al., 2009).

In addition to being tensioned by the skeletal muscle, the fascia has two of its own mechanisms to regulate its stiffness. Several studies have demonstrated the occurrence of myofibroblasts, an intermediate contractile cell type between fibroblasts (known from wound healing) and smooth muscle cells in the fasciae of the limbs (e.g. the gastrocnemius, the fascia lata and the plantar aponeurosis) and the lumbar fascia of the back (Bhattacharya et al., 2010; Schleip et al., 2019). It can be assumed that myofibroblast contraction, which seems to be governed by the

transmission to other structures. They can occur via different mechanisms (Figure 13.2): as a first option, the muscle may represent the origin. Both acute contractions and chronic hypertonicity increase its diameter and, doing so, stiffen the surrounding fascia. According to mathematical

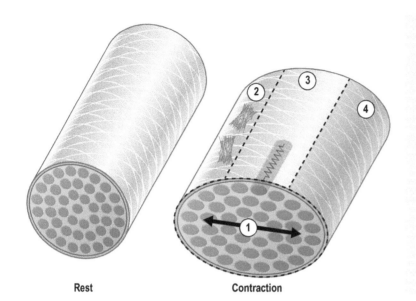

Figure 13.2 Schematic representation of four pathways modifying local fascia stiffness

Muscle contraction (right) changes its volume, transmitting radial stress to the extramuscular connective tissue (1). At the same time, direct insertions of muscle fibers allow tensioning of specific parts of the fascia (3). Without muscle contribution, fascial stiffness can increase due to myofibroblast activity (2) and changes in the water content (4).

Rest   Contraction

vegetative nervous system (Schleip et al., 2019), creates a basal fascial tension in the long term, which may be excessively increased in some cases. The second mechanism, which explains short-term rises of stiffness, consists of altered matrix hydration, which has been shown to manifest following stretching.

Load me up Scotty: What do cadaveric studies and laboratory experiments tell us about force transmission?

In view of the particularly high resilience of fascia in the longitudinal direction and the variety of mechanisms by which its stiffness can be modified, researchers have made extensive efforts to quantify the degree of in-series myofascial force transmission. Typically, related experiments were carried out in dissected cadavers, applying traction to one chain component and measuring the resulting strain or morphological displacement in a connected neighboring structure. Most available work focused on the posterior longitudinal myofascial line extending

between the plantar foot and the neck (plantar aponeurosis, Achilles tendon, gastrocnemius, hamstrings, sacrotuberous ligament, lumbar fascia, erector spinae).

- Two studies (Carlson et al., 2000; Erdemir et al., 2004) indicate a substantial degree of force transmission between the plantar aponeurosis and the Achilles tendon. Up to 50% of the forces measured in the tendon can be transmitted to the aponeurosis during simulated walking (Erdemir et al., 2004).

- One study (Cruz-Montecinos et al., 2015) has investigated the mechanical behavior of the continuity between the gastrocnemius and the hamstrings. Upon pelvic motion (which stretches the dorsal thigh muscles), a cranial displacement of the gastrocnemius fascia is visible.

- The findings of three trials (van Wingerden et al., 1993; Vleeming et al., 1989; 1995) point towards mechanical interactions between the hamstrings and the lumbar spine region. Van Wingerden et al. (1993) and Vleeming et al. (1989) showed traction of the biceps

Chapter 13

femoris to tense the sacrotuberous ligament (which connects to the lumbar fascia), although the strength of this effect was highly variable. Vleeming et al. (1995) did not measure forces but found that the pull of the biceps femoris muscle led to local movement in the thoracolumbar fascia.

In addition to the posterior longitudinal line, force transmission has also been verified for some parts of the posterior diagonal chain (latissimus dorsi, lumbar fascia, contralateral gluteus maximus, vastus lateralis).

- Two studies (Barker et al., 2004; Vleeming et al., 1995) applied traction to the latissimus dorsi and gluteus maximus muscles and observed significant displacements in the lumbar fascia, which, to some extent, were also visible on the contralateral body side. One study (Carvalhais et al., 2013) performed dynamic stretching of the latissiumus muscle and observed an altered resting position as well as an increase in passive stiffness of the opposite hip.

- Hitherto, the mechanical relevance of the continuity between the gluteus maximus and the vastus lateralis of the quadriceps femoris muscle has not been investigated.

Finally, initial evidence is available for the anterior diagonal chain, which includes the adductor longus, rectus abdominis, as well as the contralateral pectoralis major muscle.

- One trial (Norton-Old et al., 2013) has investigated the mechanical interaction between the adductor longus and the rectus abdominis. The authors of the study found that force applied to the adductor muscle leads to small and highly variable deformations of the rectus sheath.

- To date, no evidence is available for the continuity between the rectus abdominis and the pectoralis major muscle.

Despite the plethora of studies pointing towards the occurrence of in-series myofascial force transmission, several factors limit the validity of their findings. Above all, as identified, the vast majority of the experiments were conducted with cadavers. If not using fresh-frozen specimens, dissection is frequently performed on embalmed bodies. Fixation in formalin, a typically used agent in cadaveric research, causes the formation of collagenous cross-links and a reduction in the concentration of hyaluronic acid (Abe et al., 2003; Lin et al., 1997). Both processes may render the tissue more sticky and, together with the changes in the muscle fiber pennation angle also observed (Martin et al., 2001), reduce the amount of mechanical force transmitted. Notwithstanding, it cannot be concluded that the effects measured in cadaveric experiments necessarily underestimate the true magnitude: in the living organism, muscle activity can support but also counteract force transmission.

Now you see me: Visualizing myofascial force transmission may open new frontiers in research

In view of the limitations of cadaveric biomechanical testing, recent studies have attempted to translate the early findings into *in vivo* settings. In a pioneering but explorative study, Cruz-Montecinos et al. (2015) tested the potential interaction between two major components of the posterior longitudinal chain: the hamstrings and the gastrocnemius muscle. The authors instructed their participants to perform repeated pelvic motions while simultaneously assessing the position of the gastrocnemius fascia using live ultrasound. In sitting position and with the knees extended, anterior pelvic tilt (mean maximum: 6.6 degrees) caused small cranial displacements of the fascia of ~1.5 mm. In an even more standardized subsequent trial conducted by our workgroup (Wilke et al., 2020), which additionally used electromyography to control for confounding muscle activity, similar findings were made. Upon passive motion of the upper ankle joint, substantial movements of the medial hamstrings can be detected: the more the foot approaches end-range dorsal extension, the more the semitendinosus muscle and its fascia are displaced into the caudal direction. Both trials can be regarded as the first *in vivo* investigations proving in-series myofascial force transmission in humans. Further research needs to elucidate if the effects found in the lower limb occur to a similar degree in the trunk and the upper limb.

Remote exercise effects *in vivo*: Magic or a proof of myofascial force transmission?

Compelling evidence suggests that a local treatment can evoke functional changes at distant locations pertaining to the same myofascial chain. Such remote exercise effects have particularly been described for the posterior longitudinal chain. Self-myofascial release (see Chapter 27) is a popular method that is assumed to affect the stiffness of the targeted tissue. Following an intensive rolling massage of the plantar aponeurosis, sit and reach testing revealed clinically relevant increases in hamstring extensibility, which may be the result of a mechanical force transmission (Grieve et al., 2012; Wilke et al., 2019). However, the treatment response displays considerable variation. While young individuals mostly achieve a clinically relevant improvement of hamstring extensibility, trivial or no effects are more likely to occur with increasing age (Wilke et al., 2019). This can possibly be explained by the progressive loss of tissue continuity between the plantar aponeurosis and the Achilles tendon (see Chapter 12), which significantly reduces the amount of transmittable force.

Stretching is another popular intervention, which has been used to study non-local treatment effects. After three 30-s static stretching bouts of the gastrocnemius and the hamstring muscles, Wilke et al. (2016) observed a remote increase in sagittal cervical spine mobility. Again, it can be hypothesized that this effect evolves from the continuity between the targeted leg muscles and the neck extensor muscles. In a follow-up experiment, the same authors (Wilke et al., 2017) found the treatment to be as effective as local stretching of the neck muscles. Furthermore, range of motion was also examined in the frontal (lateral flexion) and transversal (rotation) plane. Interestingly, increases of flexibility not only affected the sagittal plane but also the other two movement directions. As the neck extensors (being the cranial part of the long dorsal myofascial chain) primarily limit flexion-extension movements, this may suggest that force transmission does not occur predominantly in-series. Irrespective of this, the finding of non-inferiority of remote stretching could be highly relevant in the treatment of unspecific neck pain, which is often associated with restricted range of motion. As local treatments, for example spine manipulation, can lead to severe adverse effects such as cervical arterial dissection (Puentedura et al., 2012), non-local interventions represent a safer, viable alternative.

Like cadaveric research, *in vivo* studies on myofascial force transmission also have some limitations that require further consideration. The most important of these is that the vast majority of the available trials used functional outcomes, which are an excellent way of simulating realistic training/therapeutic settings. However, without the direct measurement or visualization (and with this a proof) of force transmission, it cannot be inferred that the stretching or self-myofascial release

Chapter 13

interventions definitely caused the observed increases in range of motion. In addition to the connective tissue, peripheral nerves also cross multiple joints, and could mechanically affect distant body locations when stretched. Furthermore, it is well established that stretching has both mechanical and neuronal effects as it increases stretch tolerance. It is possible that this supraspinal reaction is not specific to the treated joint but leads to a general change in the stretch perception threshold. Despite encouraging findings, there is, hence, an urgent need for additional studies examining the cause-effect relationship of interventions based on myofascial chains. In essence, it is crucial to combine (1) the proof-of-principle imaging approaches used by Cruz-Montecinos et al. (2015) and our research group and (2) the application of a treatment in a clinically realistic scenario.

Treatments of musculoskeletal disorders based on myofascial chains

Frequently, therapists, coaches and other health professionals working with the concept of myofascial chains apply remote exercise treatments aiming to resolve musculoskeletal disorders at distant body locations. Although the preceding sections of this chapter have highlighted some open questions, initial evidence appears to support this approach.

Plantar fasciitis (also called fasciosis because inflammation is not always present) is a common cause of heel pain and may be affected by non-local abnormalities in the posterior longitudinal chain. In fact, patients with plantar fasciitis exhibit increases in the stiffness of the gastrocnemius and even the hamstrings (Bolívar et al., 2013; Harty et al., 2005; Labowitz et al., 2011). Retrospective analyses of chirurgical treatments revealed that the release of the proximal medial gastrocnemius is superior to local fasciotomy

(Monteagudo et al., 2013). Before surgery, stretching is a popular treatment among practitioners. According to a survey with therapists in the UK, more than half of the respondents always include non-local exercise for the hamstrings and/or the gastrocnemius into their routine treatment. However, Garrett and Neibert (2013) performed a literature review examining the efficacy of this approach. Their analysis of four studies showed that calf-stretching as a stand-alone treatment is not superior to a comparative or sham treatment.

Clinical example
Myofascial continuity can be easily experienced with a simple experiment. In standing, lift one leg, flexing the knee by ~60 to 90 degrees. Now move your foot between plantar flexion and dorsal extension. This should not be difficult and your ankle should display a large range of motion (ROM). Now extend the knee and repeat the same movement. Probably the ROM has decreased a bit, which can be ascribed to the bi-articularity of the gastrocnemius (knee extension pre-stretches the muscle as its origin is at the femur bone). In a third step, position your leg on a chair or a desk. While keeping your knee straight, test your ankle ROM. Again, it should have decreased slightly. If you now flex your hip (lower your upper body towards the leg on the table without flexing the lumbar spine), a further reduction will occur and in some cases, no more movement is possible (do not cheat by moving your pelvis back and forth or by flexing your toes!). What has happened? All the described steps have successively tightened the posterior longitudinal chain, which in the end restricted movement in the ankle.

Besides plantar fasciitis, individuals suffering from low back pain (LBP) could benefit from a treatment based on the posterior longitudinal chain. While it is unclear if this is always due to higher stiffness, patients with an unspecific disorder exhibited decreased hamstring extensibility (Fasuyi et al., 2017; Halbertsma et al., 2001;

Tafazzoli and Lamontagne, 1996). In a prospective study with adolescents, tight hamstrings were shown to predict the occurrence of LBP to a small degree (Feldman et al., 2001). To date, trials assessing the effectiveness of hamstring stretching to alleviate LBP are sparse. Franca et al. (2012) compared a 6-week treatment (two weekly sessions of 30 minutes) based on the posterior longitudinal chain (stretching of the calf, hamstrings and erector spinae) with segmental stabilization exercises. After the intervention period, both groups had reduced their pain level and improved physical function, but the differences were more pronounced for segmental stabilization. Additionally, there was no inactive control group and no group that performed remote stretching only.

Non-local abnormalities of back pain patients do also affect the posterior diagonal chain. Joseph et al. (2014) recruited a sample of individuals with sacroiliac joint dysfunction. Using ultrasonography, they determined the resting position of the humeral head on the body side contralateral to symptom localization. Compared with an age- and sex-matched control group, the patients exhibited a significantly increased anterior translation of the humeral head, which may indicate an insufficiency of the latissiumus dorsi muscle. As the latter is connected to the contralateral gluteus maximus via the thoracolumbar fascia, clinicians and therapists should be aware that shoulder issues and back pain may be linked or caused by each other. Other studies examining the potential relevance of the posterior diagonal chain in back pain used electromyographic muscle activity as an outcome. When performing a unilateral hip extension in the prone position, women with chronic LBP displayed increased firing of the ipsilateral gluteus maximus and the contralateral latissimus muscle (Kim et al., 2014). In a similar way, during walking, participants with sacroiliac

joint dysfunction demonstrated altered activity of the gluteus maximus on the involved side and increased activity of the opposite latissimus dorsi. After performing a strengthening torso rotation program, physiological conditions were restored (Mooney et al., 2001). While this finding is intriguing, two issues remain debatable. First, it has not yet been investigated if the electromyographic changes within the muscle-fascia lines are due to a force transmission effect and, second, regarding the study of Mooney et al. (2001), it is unclear if their corrective exercises also induced an alleviation of the back pain symptoms.

Finally, groin pain represents another pathology that may be treated by means of non-local exercise. Its prevalence is particularly high in football (soccer) players, causing pain during running, changes of direction and kicking motions. Both the adductor longus and the rectus abdominis muscle can be affected (Valent et al., 2010). As they are directly connected within the anterior diagonal chain, this observation is not surprising. However, while a combined treatment of both muscles seems prudent, to date, no study has examined its effectivity.

What to do next: an outlook

Mechanical force transmission across myofascial chains certainly represents one of the most promising fields of movement-related connective tissue research. It seems plausible that local dysfunctions (e.g. pain or restricted range of motion) have an impact on remote tissues, as changes of the mechanical tissue properties may radiate via the muscle-fascia lines. However, it has to be underlined that (1) the current state of evidence is indeed sufficient to justify a multidimensional approach in the design of exercise programs, which may include the use of non-local exercise interventions as an adjunct, but (2) a paucity of research exists regarding their effectiveness as a stand-alone treatment.

Chapter 13

References

Abe, M., Takahasi, M., Horiuchi, K. & Nagano, A. (2003) The changes in cross-link contents in tissues after formalin fixation. *Anal Biomechm*. 318: 118–123.

Barker, P.J., Briggs, C.A. & Bogeski, G. (2004) Tensile transmission across the lumbar fasciae in unembalmed cadavers: effects of tension to various muscular attachments. *Spine*. 29: 129–138.

Benetazzo, L., Bizzego, A., De Caro, R., Frigo, R., Guidolin, D. & Stecco, C. (2011) 3D reconstruction of the crural and thoracolumbar fasciae. *Srug Radiol Anat*. 33: 855–862.

Bhattacharya, V., Barooah, P.S., Nag, T.C., Chaudhuri, G.R. & Bhattachary, S. (2010) Detail microscopic analysis of deep fascia of lower limb and its surgical implication. *Indian J Plast Surg*. 43: 135–140.

Bolívar, Y.A., Munuera, P.V. & Padillo, J.P. (2013) Relationship between tightness of the posterior muscles of the lower limb and plantar fasciitis. *Foot Ankle Int*. 34: 42–48.

Butler, D.L., Grood, E.S., Noyes, F.R., Zernicke, R.F. & Brackett, K. (1984) Effects of structure and strain measurement technique on the material properties of young human tendons and fascia. *J Biomech*. 17: 579–596.

Carlson, R.E., Fleming, L.L. & Hutton, W.C. (2000) The biomechanical relationship between the tendoachilles, plantar fascia and metatarsophalangeal joint dorsiflexion angle. *Foot Ankle Int*. 21: 18–25.

Carvalhais, V.O., Ocarino, Jde.M., Araujo, V.L., Souza, T.R. & Fonseca, S.T.

(2013) Myofascial force transmission between the latissimus dorsi and gluteus maximus muscles: an in vivo experiment. *J Biomech*. 46: 1003–1007.

Cruz-Montecinos, C., González Blanche, A., López Sánchez, D., Cerda, M., Sanzana-Cuche, R. & Cuesta-Vargas, A. (2015) In vivo relationship between pelvis motion and deep fascia displacement of the medial gastrocnemius: anatomical and functional implications. *J Anat*. 227: 665–672.

Eng, C.M., Pancheri, F.Q., Lieberman, D.E., Biewener, A.A. & Dorfman, L. (2014) Directional differences in the biaxial material properties of fascia lata and the implications for fascia function. *Ann Biomed Eng*. 42: 1224–1237.

Erdemir, A., Hamel, A.J., Fauth, A.R., Piazza, S.J. & Sharkey, N.A. (2004) Dynamic loading of the plantar aponeurosis in walking. *J Bone Joirn Surg Am*. 86: 546–552.

Fasuyi, F.O., Fabunmi, A.A. & Adegoke, B.O.A. (2017) Hamstring muscle length and pelvic tilt range among individuals with and without low back pain. *J Bodyw Mov Ther*. 21: 246–250.

Feldman, D.E., Shrier, I., Rossignol, M. & Abenhaim, L. (2001) Risk factors for the development of low back pain in adolescence. *Am J Epidemiol*. 154: 30–36.

Findley, T., Chaudry, H. & Dhar, S. (2015) Transmission of muscle force to fascia during exercise. *J Bodyw Mov Ther*. 19(1): 119–123.

Franca, F.R., Burke, T.N., Caffaro, R.R., Ramos, L.A. & Marques, A.P. (2012) Effects of muscular stretching and segmental stabilization on functional disability and pain in patients with

chronic low back pain: a randomized, controlled trial. *J Manipulative Physiol Ther*. 35: 279–285.

Garrett, T.R. & Neibert, P.J. (2013) The effectiveness of a gastrocnemius–soleus stretching program as a therapeutic treatment of plantar fasciitis. *J Sport Rehabil*. 22: 308–312.

Grieve, R., Goodwin, F., Alfaki, M., Bourton, A.J., Jeffries, B. & Scott, H., (2012) The immediate effect of bilateral self myofascial release on the plantar surface of the feet on hamstring and lumbar spine flexibility: A pilot randomised controlled trial. *J Bodyw Mov Ther*. 19: 544–552.

Halbertsma, J.P., Göeken, L.N., Hof, A.L., Groothoff, J.W. & Eisma, W.H. (2001) Extensibility and stiffness of the hamstrings in patients with nonspecific low back pain. *Arch Phys Med Rehabil*. 82: 232–238.

Harty, J., Soffe, K., O'Toole, G. & Stephens, M.M. (2005) The role of hamstring tightness in plantar fasciitis. *Foot Ankle Int*. 26: 1089–1092.

Joseph, L., Hussain, R.I., Naicker, A.S., Htwe, O., Pirunsan, U. & Paungmali, A. (2014) Myofascial force transmission in sacroiliac joint dysfunction increases anterior translation of humeral head in contralateral glenohumeral joint. *Polish Ann Med*. 21.

Kim, J.W., Kang, M.H. & Oh, J.S. (2014) Patients with low back pain demonstrate increased activity of the posterior oblique sling muscle during prone hip extension. *PM&R*. 6: 400–405.

Kirilova, M., Stoytchev, S., Pashkouleva, D. & Kavardzhikov, V. (2011) Experimental study of the mechanical properties of human abdominal fascia. *Med Eng Phys.* 33: 1–6.

Labowitz, J.M., Yu, J. & Kim, C. (2011) The role of hamstring tightness in plantar fasciitis. *Foot Ankle Int.* 4: 141–144.

Lin, W., Shuster, S., Maibach, H.I. & Stern, R. (1997) Patterns of hyaluronan staining are modified by fication techniques. *J Histochem Cytochem.* 45: 1157–1163.

Martin, D.C., Medri, M.K., Chow, R.S. & Oxorn, V. (2001) Comparing human skeletal muscle architectural parameters of cadavers with in vivo ultrasonographic measurements. *J Anat.* 199: 429–434.

Monteagudo, M., Maceira, E., García-Virto, V. & Canosa, R. (2013) Chronic plantar fasciitis: plantar fasciotomy versus gastrocnemius recession. *Int Orthop.* 37: 1845–1850.

Mooney, V., Pozos, R., Vleeming, A., Gulick, J. & Swenski, D. (2001) Exercise treatment for sacroiliac pain. *Orthopedics.* 24: 29–32.

Norton-Old, K.J., Schache, A.G., Barker, P.J., Clark, R.A., Harrison, S.M. & Briggs, C.A. (2013) Anatomical and mechanical relationship between the proximal attachment of adductor longus and the distal rectus sheath. *Clin Anat.* 26: 522–530.

Otsuka, S., Shan, X. & Kawakami, Y. (2019) Dependence of muscle and deep fascia stiffness on the contraction levels of the quadriceps: an in vivo supersonic shear-imaging study. *J Electromyogr Kinesiol.* 45: 33–40.

Otsuka, S., Yakura, T., Ohmichi, Y., Ohmichi, M., Naito, M., Nakano, T. & Kawakami, Y. (2018) Site specificity of

mechanical and structural properties of human fascia lata and their gender differences: A cadaveric study. *J Biomech.* 77: 69–75.

Puentedura, E.J., March, J., Anders, J., Perez, A., Landers, M.R., Wallmann, H.W. & Cleland, J.A. (2012) Safety of cervical spine manipulation: are adverse events preventable and are manipulations being performed appropriately? A review of 134 case reports. *J Man Manip Ther.* 20: 66–74.

Schleip, R., Duerselen, L., Vleeming, A., Naylor, Lehmann-Horn, F., Zorn, A., Jäger, H. & Klingler, W. (2012) Strain hardening of fascia: static stretching of dense fibrous connective tissues can induce a temporary stiffness increase accompanied by enhanced matrix hydration. *J Bodyw Mov Ther.* 16: 94–100.

Schleip, R., Gabbiani, G., Wilke, J., Naylor, I., Hinz, B., Zorn, A., Jäger, H., Schreiner, S. & Klingler, W. (2019) Fascia is able to actively contract and thereby influence musculoskeletal dynamics: a histochemical and mechanographic investigation. *Front Physiol.* 10: 336.

Stecco, A., Machhi, V., Stecco,C., Porzionato, A., Day, J.A., Delmas, V. & De Caro, R. (2009) Anatomical study of the myofascial continuity in the anterior region of the upper limb. *J Bodyw Mov Ther.* 13: 53–62.

Stecco, C., Pavan, P., Pachera, P., De Caro, R. & Natali, A. (2014) Investigation of the mechanical properties of the human crural fascia and their possible clinical implications. *Surg Radiol Anat.* 36: 25–32.

Stecco, C., Porzionato, A., Machhi, V., Stecco, A., Vigato, E., Parenti, A., Delmas, V., Aldegheri, R. & De Caro, R.

(2008) The expansions of the pectoral girdle muscles onto the brachial fascia: morphological aspects and spatial disposition. *Cells Tissues Organs.* 188: 320–329.

Tafazzoli, F. & Lamontagne, M. (1996) Mechanical behavior of hamstring muscles in low-back pain patients and control subjects. *Clin Biomech.* 11: 16–24.

Valent, A., Frizziero, A., Bressan, S., Zanella, E., Gianotti, E. & Masiero, S. (2012) Insertional tendinopathy of the adductors and rectus abdominis in athletes: a review. *Muscles Ligaments Tendons J.* 2: 142–148.

van Wingerden, J.P., Vleeming, A., Snijders, C.J. & Stoeckart, R. (1993) A functional-anatomical approach to the spine-pelvis mechanism: interaction between the biceps femoris muscle and the sacrotuberous ligament. *Eur Spine J.* 2: 140–144.

Vleeming, A., Pool-Goudzwaard, A.L., Stoeckart, R., van Wingerden, J.P. & Snijders, C.J. (1995) The posterior layer of the thoracolumbar fascia. Its function in load transfer from spine to legs. *Spine* 20: 753–758.

Vleeming, A., van Wingerden, J.P., Snijders, C.J., Stoeckart, R. & Stijnen, T. (1989) Load application to the sacrotuberous ligament; influences on sacroiliac joint mechanics. *Clin Biomech.* 4: 204–209.

Wilke, J., Debelle, H., Tenberg, S., Dilley, A., Maganaris, C. (2020) Ankle motion is associated with soft tissue displacement in the dorsal thigh: an in vivo investigation suggesting myofascial force transmission across the knee joint. *Front Physiol.*

Chapter 13

doi: 10.3389/fphys.2020.0018010.3389/fphys.2020.00180

Wilke, J., Kalo, K., Niederer, D. & Vogt, L. (2019) Gathering hints for myofascial force transmission under in vivo conditions: are remote exercise effects age-dependent? *J Sport Rehabil.* 28(7): 758–763.

Wilke, J., Niederer, D., Vogt, L. & Banzer, W. (2016) Remote effects of lower limb stretching: preliminary evidence for myofascial continuity? *J Sport Sci.* 34: 2145–2148.

Wilke, J., Niederer, D., Vogt, L. & Banzer, W. (2017) Is remote stretching as effective as no-local exercise? A randomized-controlled trial. *J Sport Sci.* 35: 2021–2027.

Myofascial force transmission to synergistic and antagonistic muscles

Can A. Yucesoy

Muscular force transmission

Muscular force transmission is central to bodily movement. Clearly, the tendon is the dedicated organ for the forces produced in the skeletal muscle to be transmitted to the bone to produce joint motion. Therefore, myotendinous force transmission is the key to muscular force transmission. However, force production in the muscle and transmission of the force to the joint are not independent processes. The muscle-tendon complex with its two mechanical elements arranged in series is exposed to forces coming from the joint, sharing them based on their relative stiffness. Consequently, for each muscle-tendon complex length, the muscle and the tendon attain certain lengths, and the length the muscle attains is a central determinant of muscular force production. This is because the global length of the muscle will affect the lengths of sarcomeres locally, which in turn is the key determinant for force production. Nevertheless, when it comes to local sarcomere lengths and particularly to what determines it mechanically, the picture is much more complex than just the question of how the muscle-tendon complex length is shared by the muscle and the tendon. In recent years, it has been shown in many studies that muscular force transmission is not limited to the tendon, but also involves muscle related connective tissues, that is, intramuscular fasciae (endo-, peri- and epimysium) as well as collagen-reinforced connective tissues connecting the muscle belly from its epimysium to its surroundings, for example, the neurovascular tracts (Huijing, 2009; Wilke et al., 2018; Yucesoy, 2010). The important issue here is that the tendon is still the main component that will transmit the force to the joint to cause motion. However, the effect of considering those connective tissues as well is that the tendon's mechanical interaction with the muscle is not the only mechanism that will determine sarcomere lengths locally. Therefore, overall, muscular force transmission is a misnomer or represents an insufficient terminology. This is because, as argued above, myotendinous force transmission involves aspects of force production as well, but myofascial force transmission is more about force production than sole force transmission. This chapter will elaborate on these new viewpoints, aiming to provide movement practitioners with related background knowledge for their daily work with clients and patients.

Among other works by our research groups, an animal study published back in 2003 showed remarkable new scopes of muscle mechanics (Yucesoy et al., 2003). In that experiment, the isometric forces at both the proximal and distal tendons of the extensor digitorum longus (EDL) were measured simultaneously (Figure 14.1A) in two different conditions. In the first, the entire anterior crural compartment was kept intact. After lengthening the EDL distally, its distal forces, measured at different muscle lengths, were substantially higher (maximally by 46%)

Chapter 14

than the proximal forces. This proximo-distal force difference implies that part of the muscle's force may have been transmitted to other structures. This was supported by the second condition, in which the muscle's synergistic muscles, the tibialis anterior (TA) and the extensor hallucis longus (EHL), were removed. As a result, the EDL forces measured were different to those in the first condition although the testing protocol was identical (Figure 14.1B). At first sight, and considered together, these changes hence indicate the presence of force transmission between these synergistic muscles. Recall that, in general, the central mechanism of muscular force transmission to the joint involves the tendon. However, as the three muscles tested do not share a common tendon, the reported force transmission must be via the muscle-related connective tissue system. This mechanism has been referred to as myofascial force transmission (Yucesoy, 2010).

Note that the proximal forces of the EDL were lower in both conditions with such proximodistal force differences being more pronounced in the intact condition. This means that the amplitude of muscle force produced at different lengths of the target muscle can change depending on the activity and positions of the surrounding muscles. Nevertheless, that was not the only remarkable effect shown. The EDL muscle's length range of force exertion was greater in the intact condition (Figure 14.1C). This means that the muscle length range between the muscle's active slack length (i.e. the shortest muscle length of non-zero muscle force production) and optimum length (i.e. the muscle length at which the peak force is measured) was manipulated. Therefore, the effect of inter-synergistic myofascial force transmission was not limited to integration of the force of one muscle into the force exerted at the tendon of another. Instead, the effect of inter-synergistic myofascial force

transmission is its capability to manipulate the mechanics of the target muscle substantially.

Muscle fiber-extracellular matrix integrity and mechanical interactions between these two domains

A condition-dependent varying output of a muscle as described above indicates altered force production, which can best be characterized with the mechanical interaction concept, that is, inter-synergistic myofascial force transmission is mechanical interaction between synergistic muscles. As lengths of sarcomeres of the muscle will determine the force the muscle can produce in every condition within which it functions, condition-dependent varying output of a muscle suggests that, despite being at an identical muscle length globally, the muscle's sarcomeres should attain differing lengths in different conditions. Note that sarcomere length is the result of a mechanical equilibrium between the forces acting on the sarcomere to change its length and the force the sarcomere produces to resist those. Sarcomeres with differing lengths within the muscle and even along the same muscle fibers will have differing force production. For this to take place, there must be forces acting on the sarcomere ends with varying amplitudes and directions. Such variable forces cannot be coming from the sarcomeres arranged in series within the same muscle fibers. However, in the level of a single muscle, they can come from the extracellular matrix (ECM) in the first place, and also from sarcomeres in adjacent muscle fibers, and act on the z-disks. Moreover, beyond the muscle level (compartment or even limb level, i.e. the muscle within the context of its intact connective tissue surroundings, which is the *in vivo* condition), these forces can also come from other myofascial structures outside the muscle, which are

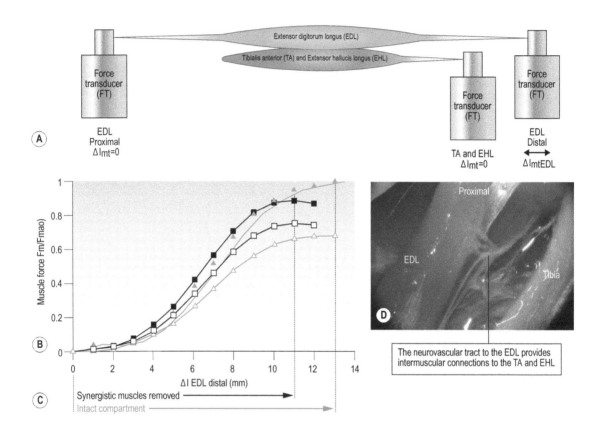

Figure 14.1 Assessment of the functional effects of intermuscular mechanical interactions

(A) In experiments performed for such a specific purpose, (1) the muscle belly was not dissected free from the surrounding structures, and instead of measurement of the muscle force only in one end and assuming identical force at the other end, (2) the forces exerted at both proximal and distal tendons of the target muscle were measured simultaneously using separate force transducers (FTs). The experiment discussed in the text involves anterior crural muscles. The forces of the EDL as the targeted muscle and the TA and the EHL were measured after activating these muscles maximally. Length changes of the EDL were imposed by changing the position of its distal force transducer (Δl_{mt} EDL), whereas the positions of the other FTs were kept constant ($\Delta l_{mt} = 0$). Further detailed illustrations and pictures of the experimental set-ups are available (Ateş and Yucesoy, 2014; Yucesoy and Ateş, 2018; Yucesoy et al., 2010a; 2012; 2015). **(B)** This approach was repeated under two conditions: (1) intact compartment and (2) after the synergistic muscles TA and EHL were removed. The results showed the characteristic effect: proximo-distal force differences (Yucesoy et al., 2003) quantified as a function of muscle length, in which changes indicate condition-dependent variable muscular force production. **(C)** Another remarkable effect is that the muscle's length range of force exertion is also condition-dependent instead of being a unique property. **(D)** The more proximal and stiffer part of the collagen neurovascular tract of the anterior crural compartment interconnects the EDL to the TA and EHL at their muscle belly and is continuous with compartmental connective tissues. These muscle-related connective tissues facilitate intermuscular mechanical interactions, which causes the changes in muscular mechanics, as illustrated in **(B)** and **(C)**.

Chapter 14

in continuity with the muscle's ECM. Therefore, if this is a tenable mechanism, inter-synergistic myofascial force transmission is not as simple as forces of other muscles being integrated to the tendon force of other muscles. Instead, it needs to be considered as mechanical interaction between synergistic muscles, which is characterized by a myofascial load concept (Yucesoy, 2010) with local sarcomere level effects translating into condition-dependent variable global output of the muscle to influence the joint moment and movement.

Tenability of that mechanism first requires presence of mechanical connections between the muscle fibers and the ECM. Although a certain general knowledge has existed for a long time that myofibers are connected to the ECM (Pond, 1982), this knowledge has not been implemented in physiological experiments. However, these two domains are connected mechanically along the full periphery of muscle fibers with complex structures. Inside the muscle fiber, internal myofibrils are interconnected via the protein desmin. On the other hand, the peripheral myofibrils are connected by trans-sarcolemmal molecules to the basal lamina (Berthier and Blaineau, 1997), which is connected to the endomysium. The endomysium forms a 3D structure of tunnels (Trotter and Purslow, 1992) within which the muscle fibers are operating (see, for an example illustration, Figure 1 in Yucesoy, 2010). A common simplistic consideration involves ascribing the mechanical connections between the muscle fibers and the endomysial tunnels only to the ends of the muscle fiber, where the myotendinous junctions are present. Mechanically, this is equivalent to considering muscle fiber as an uni-axially loaded member, which means that the only forces acting on the muscle fiber are located at the ends, and have identical amplitudes. Consequently, the length changes

along that member, that is, the lengths of sarcomeres arranged in series have been considered as identical. Another consequence of that has been to consider muscle fibers as units functioning independently of each other.

However, because of the trans-sarcolemmal connections, these viewpoints are not accurate hence tenable. Mechanical interactions between a muscle fiber and its epimysium as well as between several muscle fibers in a bundle (Street, 1983; Street and Ramsey, 1965), and the importance of the continuity of the ECM in intramuscular force transmission (Huijing, 1999) were shown in passive and active states. Therefore, muscle fibers cannot be considered as units functioning independently of each other. Additionally, the length of a sarcomere cannot be determined exclusively by its interaction with the sarcomeres arranged in series with it in the same muscle fiber. Instead, a more complex mechanical equilibrium, involving that and the forces exerted on the sarcomere by the fiber-reinforced ECM as well as the forces of the sarcomeres located in the neighboring muscle fibers, should be considered. Therefore, theoretically, a muscle fiber is a mechanical member with various loads acting on it along its length. Consequently, it is plausible that the forces acting at both ends of the muscle fiber are unequal and different parts of the muscle fiber may undergo unequal length changes. However, even this is unlikely to be the exhaustive consideration of muscle fiber-myofascial structure continuity and hence mechanical interactions.

Myofascial continuity between muscle and its surroundings

Intramuscular fasciae, including endomysium, perimysium and epimysium, are continuous within the muscle, but the epimysium also has connections to structures beyond the muscle. Within the same compartment, collagenous linkages between epimysia of adjacent muscles provide direct intermuscular connections, which can be considered as shared epimysia of those muscles. Additionally, with collagen-reinforced structures such as neurovascular tracts (Figure 14.1D), muscles within the same compartment and distant ones in other compartments, that is, antagonistic muscles, are interconnected. On the other hand, those myofascial structures are also continuous with intermuscular septa, compartmental fasciae, interosseous membranes, the periosteum and even ligaments. In certain locations, direct insertions of skeletal muscles into the myofascia are present. For example, the deltoideus, latissimus dorsi and pectoralis muscles have fibrous expansions connecting to the brachial fascia (Stecco et al., 2008). In other locations, muscles originate from such fascial structures. The extensor hallucis longus muscle in the anterior crural compartment and the two muscles of the peroneal compartment originate from the anterior intermuscular septum. Note that these are antagonistic muscles. Structural continuity is not limited to the linkages between the fascia and the muscle. The connective tissue enveloping the adjacent compartmental muscles of the lower limb has been shown to fuse tightly with each other. In addition, myofascial continuity in an in-series arrangement is also present (Chapter 12). Therefore, via several different forms of structural continuity, synergistic and antagonistic muscles are mechanically integrated with each other. Taking into account such close morphological relationships between muscles and muscle-related fascial tissues, the effects of local stiffness changes and altered local muscular forces might affect both the tissue of origin and the surroundings. Conceivably, the insertions and origins of certain muscles onto and from myofascial structures allow for selective tensioning of the fascia,

which, in turn, supports and facilitates muscle activity via muscle and fascia mechanical interactions. Continuity of the lateral collateral ligament with fasciae suggests that muscle forces acting directly on the fascial system via muscle fiber attachments or indirectly via the continuity described above can manipulate not only muscle function, but also proprioception.

Effects of intermuscular mechanical interactions: Burden or fact with major functional implications?

Note that, using the terminology of muscular force transmission, the proximo-distal force differences addressed above comprise a solid example for the myofascial structures' force-transmitting capability. Yet this has sometimes been considered as unusual, even as a threat, in, for example, skeletal muscle physiology and musculoskeletal biomechanics communities. One common reason for this is because the proximo-distal force difference has been considered as a loss of some of the muscle's produced force being distracted away from the joint. However, due to the following reasons, alternative viewpoints can enable improvement of our understanding of skeletal muscle mechanics considerably.

First, this is not a realistic concern because all the connective tissues described above and, in particular, the neurovascular tracts, are vital elements of the machinery. They serve the absolutely necessary functions of accommodating or anchoring the force-producing motors and keeping them in physiological state. Additionally, they house the mechanoreceptors, so also serve the sensory aspect of the functioning of the motor. Therefore, those structures must be there, and intermuscular mechanical interactions attributable to them represent a fact to recognize rather than to ignore or fear.

Chapter 14

Second, the proximo-distal force difference needs to be considered as a mechanical mechanism determining the muscle's force production. This difference is the result of myofascial loads of possibly different amplitudes and directions acting on different locations of the epimysium. These loads arise from relative position changes of the muscle with respect to its surroundings, which occur due to: (1) differential length changes among muscles of the limb, for example, among mono- and bi-articular muscles, or among agonist and antagonistic muscles, (2) moment arm differences, also imposing differences in the length changes of several muscles. Such relative position changes cause the epimuscular myofascial connections of the muscles to become stretched and, in return, those structures exert myofascial loads on the muscle belly at the locations where they insert into the muscle, based on their non-linear mechanical properties and possible pre-strain (Yucesoy et al., 2005). Numerous finite element modeling studies have shown that such loads cause changes in sarcomere lengths and corresponding stress distributions along the muscle fibers, which is a metric for the muscle's force production (Yucesoy and Huijing, 2012; Turkoglu et al., 2014, Turkoglu; Yucesoy, 2016). Such stress values were shown to be in concert with the proximo-distal force differences, for example, lower values of stresses are calculated in the proximal segments of muscle fibers than in the distal segments in a muscle, which shows a smaller proximal force. This indicates that the proximo-distal force difference does not necessarily represent forces of other muscles to be integrated with the target muscle's force at the tendon, or otherwise some of the target muscle's forces leaking out to elsewhere. Instead, they represent myofascial loads acting on the target muscle, which affects the internal mechanics and modifies the muscle's force production.

However, another remarkable effect is that such mechanical interaction of the target muscle with its surroundings can yield changes to the shape of the muscle's length-force characteristics, including a change in the muscle's length range of force exertion, that is, its excursion (Yucesoy et al., 2003). This is determined by the heterogeneity of sarcomere lengths along, but more importantly, across different muscle fibers. A good metric for that is the mean sarcomere length of muscle fibers, the elevated heterogeneity of which across different muscle fibers was shown to shift the muscle's optimum length to a longer muscle length (Willems and Huijing, 1994), which means that the muscle's contribution to joint movement will be effective for a wider range of joint angles.

Muscle's effect at the joint moment and movement modified by its interaction with other structures in the compartment opens up new perspectives in musculoskeletal biomechanics as well as rehabilitation and sports science. That is why its extent beyond the compartment has become an issue of interest. In animal experiments involving multiple compartments, Huijing (2007) studied the interaction between the various lower leg muscles. For example, distal lengthening of the peronei muscles caused the active force of the TA to decrease by 25%. Such inter-antagonistic mechanical interaction was shown to affect the entire lower leg of the rat (Yucesoy et al., 2010b). Therefore, with a large body of evidence derived from animal studies and matching finite element modeling, the effects and mechanism of intermuscular mechanical interactions within the level of a whole limb has been revealed yielding epimuscular myofascial force transmission as a novel muscle mechanics paradigm. Note that the central component of this mechanism, that is, the heterogeneity of sarcomere lengths, has been shown by other groups as well (Moo et al., 2017), however, without addressing the cause of the heterogeneity or mentioning either intermuscular mechanical interactions or epimuscular myofascial force transmission.

Intermuscular mechanical interactions and sarcomere length inhomogeneity in human muscles *in vivo*

Effects of intermuscular mechanical interactions in terms of muscle belly displacements, stiffness or sarcomere length changes have been studied. Electrical percutaneous stimulation of the gastrocnemius was shown to cause displacement of the soleus suggesting presence of force transmission between these muscles (Bojsen-Møller et al., 2010). Also, Tian et al. (2012) studied those muscles' mechanical interaction and showed that knee flexion imposed at a constant ankle position affected soleus length. Although the source of such an effect could be myofascial force transmission, it could also be ascribed to the two muscles' mechanical interaction via their common Achilles tendon. Ultrasound shear wave elastography was used to assess the muscle shear modulus of the lower (Ateş et al., 2018a) and upper (Yoshitake et al., 2018) muscles. The former study showed mechanical interaction effects of the gastrocnemius lateral (GL) with the soleus, TA and peronei muscles in terms of altered shear modulus (an index of changes in muscle force) due to manipulated knee angle, despite the fact that the muscles do not cross the knee. The latter showed altered shear modulus effects between the biceps brachii and the brachialis, which was considered to isolate the myofascial channel as, in contrast to the gastrocnemius and the soleus, those muscles do not share a common tendon.

Magnetic resonance imaging (MRI) allows quantifying of local length changes of muscle tissue in human limb. Huijing et al. (2011) combined MRI analyses with a cadaver experiment for the assessment of global length changes of the GM. This showed that local length changes caused by passively imposed knee motion at constant ankle angle are heterogeneous and the amplitudes of the global muscle length changes are much smaller. Note that Yaman et al. (2013) studied the remaining lower leg muscles, which do not cross the knee joint. Despite undergoing no global length changes, the local length changes shown, for example, for the TA, indicates effects of intermuscular mechanical interaction.

In particular, (Pamuk et al., 2016) and (Karakuzu et al., 2017) quantified length changes along GM muscle fibers as an indicator of sarcomere length changes. They used another MRI technique, that is, diffusion tensor imaging (DTI) to determine muscle fiber directions for that purpose. The former study showed that knee extension imposed in the passive state yielded strain heterogeneity along medial gastrocnemius (GM) fascicles. The latter study, conducted in the active state (15% of sustained maximal voluntary contraction), confirmed previous anticipations based on modeling that different parts of GM fascicles showed varying amplitudes and directions of length changes. Notably, Karakuzu et al. (2017) also specifically studied the neurovascular tracts and showed that the altered muscle position and activation yields local length changes within those structures. This was interesting in two ways: (1) straining of these collagen-reinforced tissues, interconnecting GM to other muscles implies their exposure to myofascial loads; (2) the locations where they insert into the muscle are the locations of high strain along muscle fiber length changes.

Therefore, MRI-DTI studies indicate that intermuscular mechanical interactions can lead to inhomogeneous length changes of sarcomeres along muscle fibers of human muscles *in vivo*. As addressed in the preceding sections, because

Chapter 14

this means that the muscle's contribution to joint moment and range of movement is not independent of other muscles' actions and positions, these techniques provide an important asset for our understanding of muscular mechanics. Note that evidence of variable sarcomere lengths across different regions of human muscle has been shown using other techniques such as microendoscopy (Lichtwark et al., 2018) with laser scanning microscopy (Llewellyn et al., 2008). This elegantly confirms the described mechanism of condition-dependent variable sarcomere lengths in general. However, again the resolution is very low, as only a few locations along selected fascicles can be studied. Note that some authors have questioned the relevance of epimuscular myofascial force transmission for physiologically representative or *in vivo* conditions (Maas, 2019). Although these are mostly animal studies, limited or trivial effects of such force transmission have also been reported, for example, altered knee angles imposing no effects on the soleus ankle moment in the rat (Tijs et al., 2015). It is important to consider the possibility of test conditions, joint position combinations or individuals showing marginal effects of intermuscular mechanical interactions. Nevertheless, even in the absence of such effects on the gross metrics, it may be hard to conclude that there are no local effects. After all, myofascial loads are supposed to impose no local effects only if the muscle is a rigid body, which is not true.

Implications for joint movement in health and disease

Pathological conditions involving impeded joint movement are highly conceivable implications for this mechanism. Cerebral palsy (CP) is one remarkable pathology, the etiology and treatment of which has been studied in the context of epimuscular myofascial force transmission.

This will be elaborated on here as an example of how this mechanism can affect muscle's contribution to joint moment and range of movement, and not specifically for the purpose of addressing pathological conditions. Instead, this can be considered as an overall phenomenon, which can be reflected to joint function in health and also to sport and other movement. In CP, limited joint mobility is ascribed to higher force production of spastic muscles typically in flexed joint positions and a narrow joint range of force production. Accordingly, it is considered that the muscle's peak force is encountered at shorter muscle lengths and it is incapable of producing active force at longer muscle lengths. However, intra-operative experiments showed that spastic gracilis (Ateş et al., 2013), semitendinosus (Ateş et al., 2016) and semi-membranosus (Yucesoy et al., 2017) show no profound force production in flexed knee positions and a narrow joint range of force exertion, if they are stimulated alone. This indicates the following: (1) spastic muscles do not necessarily have the assumed mechanics, and (2) the mechanical interactions between the target-activated spastic muscle and lower leg muscles in the passive state do not affect its mechanics. However, the simultaneous co-activation of knee flexor (Kaya et al., 2018) and extensor (Ateş et al., 2018b) muscles considerably elevated spastic semitendinosus forces. In gait relevant joint positions, such increases are highly relevant for the clinically observed limited knee extension (Kaya et al., 2019; 2020). Spastic gracilis also showed a shift of its peak force due to intermuscular mechanical interactions in the active state. Epimuscular myofascial force transmission should therefore be considered as a determinant of the pathological knee joint condition in CP, suggesting that tissue adaptations occur in the fascial structures rather than in spastic muscle's contractile apparatus. This also has major implications for surgical treatments and spasticity management using botulinum toxin. Muscle-lengthening surgery on a target muscle was shown to also affect other muscles, which were not interfered with because of their mutual mechanical interactions (Ateş et al., 2013). Botulinum toxin leads to stiffening of the exposed muscle's ECM. Via muscle fiber-ECM mechanical interactions, this leads to unintended contraindicated outcome of the treatment, including increased passive resistance and narrowed range of force production (Ateş and Yucesoy, 2014). Based on these studies, and leaving aside the abnormal neurological control in CP, the pathological condition may be formulated as mechanically abnormally linked muscles, which may not necessarily be abnormal themselves. Accordingly, the movement therapy is advised to focus on muscle-related connective tissues. On the other hand, overall, considering epimuscular myofascial force transmission as a determinant for muscle's force and movement production, suggests that this mechanism is also quite relevant for sports. This can, for example, be a determinant for the sportsman's talent for the particular branch of sports they are enrolled in. Co-activating an antagonistic muscle may lead to an extra force exerted at the joint to perform the particular task, or mechanical interactions between different muscles may be reflected as a widened joint range of movement. Such properties may help the athlete to reach the ball with appropriate joint positioning, and afterwards to exert sufficient force to either shoot it (e.g. in football after dribbling past a defender or after controlling a passed ball) or block it (e.g. in defense in basketball or volleyball, taking the necessary hand position and resisting the offensive action by avoiding a wrist joint extension or even applying a flexor moment) at the right moment. This is also likely to fine-tune the muscle's output for precision tasks such as playing a musical instrument. Additionally, the possible influence of epimuscular myofascial force transmission on the mechanoreceptor function can be relevant. Proximo-distally exerted unequal forces as a central effect implies that Golgi tendon organs may sense force differences instead of just muscle force. Along muscle fiber length heterogeneity suggests that muscle spindles may sense local length changes rather than simply the muscle's length. Therefore, proprioception may be influenced by muscle-related connective tissues. A recent kinesio taping study indicated that the tape as a source of externally applied mechanical loading could have local effects within the entire limb (Pamuk and Yucesoy, 2015). This suggests that myofascial loads can affect other mechanoreceptors as well. Therefore, the sensory aspects of epimuscular myofascial force transmission may also be relevant both for improved movement performance as well as pain management. However, more involved investigations need to be conducted to achieve specific and clinically applicable knowledge.

In conclusion, data made available over the last 2 decades suggest that mechanical interactions between muscles and between muscle fibers and the ECM open new perspectives for understanding previously unknown aspects of muscular mechanics. This is paramount in identifying mechanisms of the etiology and treatment techniques of pathological conditions. Effects on local muscle tissue lengths are central to those. This may have a direct effect on the muscle's contribution to joint moment and movement, but even for joint positions in which muscle force is not directly affected, there may be effects on mechanoreceptors, sensory organs and sarcomeres. Therefore, the potential effects of such mechanical interactions on, for example, pain, joint position sense, proprioception, joint range of motion and precision tasks, which require dosing of the muscle's output, are highly plausible.

Chapter 14

References

Ateş, F., Andrade, R.J., Freitas, S.R., Hug, F., Lacourpaille, L., Gross, R., Yucesoy, C.A. & Nordez, A. (2018a) Passive stiffness of monoarticular lower leg muscles is influenced by knee joint angle. *Eur J Appl Physiol.* 118: 585–593.

Ateş, F., Özdeşlik, R.N., Huijing, P.A. & Yucesoy, C.A. (2013) Muscle lengthening surgery causes differential acute mechanical effects in both targeted and non-targeted synergistic muscles. *J Electromyogr Kinesiol.* 23: 1199–1205.

Ateş, F., Temelli, Y. & Yucesoy, C.A. (2013) Human spastic gracilis muscle isometric forces measured intraoperatively as a function of knee angle show no abnormal muscular mechanics. *Clin Biomech.* 28: 48–54.

Ateş, F., Temelli, Y. & Yucesoy, C.A. (2016) The mechanics of activated semitendinosus are not representative of the pathological knee joint condition of children with cerebral palsy. *J Electromyogr Kinesiol.* 28: 130–136.

Ateş, F., Temelli, Y. & Yucesoy, C.A. (2018b) Effects of antagonistic and synergistic muscles' co-activation on mechanics of activated spastic semitendinosus in children with cerebral palsy. *Hum Movement Sci.* 57: 103–110.

Ateş, F. & Yucesoy, C.A. (2014) Effects of botulinum toxin type A on non-injected bi-articular muscle include a narrower length range of force exertion and increased passive force. *Muscle Nerve.* 49: 866–878.

Berthier, C. & Blaineau, S. (1997) Supramolecular organization of the subsarcolemmal cytoskeleton of adult skeletal muscle fibers. A review. *Biol Cell.* 89: 413–434.

Bojsen-Møller, J., Schwartz, S., Kalliokoski, K.K., Finni, T. & Magnusson, S.P. (2010) Intermuscular force transmission between human plantarflexor muscles in vivo. *J Appl Physiol.* 109: 1608–1618.

Huijing, P.A. (1999) Muscle as a collagen fiber reinforced composite material: Force transmission in muscle and whole limbs. *J Biomech.* 32: 329–345.

Huijing, P.A. (2007) Epimuscular myofascial force transmission between antagonistic and synergistic muscles can explain movement limitation in spastic paresis. *J Electromyogr Kinesiol.* 17: 708–724.

Huijing, P.A. (2009) Epimuscular myofascial force transmission: a historical review and implications for new research. International Society of Biomechanics Muybridge Award Lecture, Taipei, 2007. *J Biomech.* 42: 9–21.

Huijing, P.A., Yaman, A., Ozturk, C. & Yucesoy, C.A. (2011) Effects of knee joint angle on global and local strains within human triceps surae muscle: MRI analysis indicating in vivo myofascial force transmission between synergistic muscles. *Surg Radiol Anat.* 33: 869–879.

Karakuzu, A., Pamuk, U., Ozturk, C., Acar, B. & Yucesoy, C.A. (2017) Magnetic resonance and diffusion tensor imaging analyses indicate heterogeneous strains along human medial gastrocnemius fascicles caused by submaximal plantarflexion activity. *J Biomech.* 57: 69–78.

Kaya, C.S., Temelli, Y., Ates, F. & Yucesoy, C.A. (2018) Effects of inter-synergistic mechanical interactions on the mechanical behaviour of activated spastic semitendinosus muscle of patients with cerebral palsy. *J Mech Behav Biomed.* 77: 78–84.

Kaya, C.S., Bilgili, F., Akalan, N.E., Temelli, Y., Ates, F. & Yucesoy, C.A. (2019) Intraoperative experiments combined with gait analyses indicate that active state rather than passive dominates the spastic gracilis muscle's joint movement limiting effect in cerebral palsy. *Clinical Biomechanics.* 68: 151–157.

Kaya, C.S., Bilgili, F., Akalan, N.E., & Yucesoy, C.A. (2020) Intraoperative testing of passive and active state mechanics of spastic semitendinosus in conditions involving intermuscular mechanical interactions and gait relevant joint positions. *Journal of Biomechanics.* 103: 109755.

Lichtwark, G.A., Farris, D.J., Chen, X.F., Hodges, P.W. & Delp, S.L. (2018) Microendoscopy reveals positive correlation in multiscale length changes and variable sarcomere lengths across different regions of human muscle. *J Appl Physiol.* 125: 1812–1820.

Llewellyn, M.E., Barretto, R.P.J., Delp, S.L. & Schnitzer, M.J. (2008) Minimally invasive high-speed imaging of sarcomere contractile dynamics in mice and humans. *Nature.* 454: 784–788.

Maas, H. (2019) Significance of epimuscular myofascial force transmission under passive muscle conditions. *J Appl Physiol.* 126: 1465–1473.

Moo, E.K., Leonard, T.R. & Herzog, W. (2017) In vivo sarcomere lengths become more non-uniform upon activation in intact whole muscle. *Front Physiol.* 8: 1015.

Pamuk, U., Karakuzu, A., Ozturk, C., Acar, B. & Yucesoy, C.A. (2016) Combined magnetic resonance and diffusion tensor imaging analyses provide a powerful tool for in vivo assessment of deformation along human muscle fibers. *J Mech Behav Biomed Mater.* 63: 207–219.

Pamuk, U. & Yucesoy, C.A. (2015) MRI analyses show that kinesio taping affects much more than just the targeted superficial tissues and causes heterogeneous deformations within the whole limb. *J Biomech.* 48: 4262–4270.

Pond, C.M. (1982) The importance of connective tissue within and in between muscles. *Behav Brain Sci.* 5: 562.

Stecco, C., Porzionato, A., Macchi, V., Stecco, A., Vigato, E., Parenti, A., Delmas, V., Aldegheri, R. & De Caro, R. (2008) The expansions of the pectoral girdle muscles onto the brachial fascia: morphological aspects and spatial disposition. *Cells Tissues Organs.* 188: 320–329.

Street, S.F. (1983) Lateral transmission of tension in frog myofibers: a myofibrillar network and transverse cytoskeletal connections are possible transmitters. *J Cell Physiol.* 114: 346–364.

Street, S.F. & Ramsey, R.W. (1965) Sarcolemma: transmitter of active tension in frog skeletal muscle. *Science.* 149: 1379–1380.

Tian, M.Y., Herbert, R.D., Hoang, P., Gandevia, S.C. & Bilston, L.E. (2012) Myofascial force transmission between the human soleus and gastrocnemius muscles during passive knee motion. *J Appl Physiol.* 113: 517–523.

Tijs, C., van Dieen, J.H. & Maas, H. (2015) No functionally relevant mechanical effects of epimuscular myofascial connections between rat ankle plantar flexors. *J Exp Biol.* 218: 2935–2941.

Trotter, J.A. & Purslow P.P. (1992) Functional morphology of the endomysium in series fibered muscles. *J Morphol.* 212: 109–122.

Turkoglu, A.N., Huijing, P.A. & Yucesoy, C.A. (2014) Mechanical principles of effects of botulinum toxin on muscle length-force characteristics: an assessment by finite element modeling. *J Biomech.* 47: 1565–1571.

Turkoglu, A.N. & Yucesoy, C.A., (2016) Simulation of effects of botulinum toxin on muscular mechanics in time course of treatment based on adverse extracellular matrix adaptations. *J Biomech.* 49: 1192–1198.

Wilke, J., Schleip, R., Yucesoy, C.A. & Banzer, W. (2018) Not merely a protective packing organ? A review of fascia and its force transmission capacity. *J Appl Physiol.* 124: 234–244.

Willems, M.E. & Huijing, P.A. (1994) Heterogeneity of mean sarcomere length in different fibres: effects on length range of active force production in rat muscle. *Eur J Appl Physiol Occup Physiol.* 68: 489–496.

Yaman, A., Ozturk, C., Huijing, P.A. & Yucesoy, C.A. (2013) Magnetic resonance imaging assessment of mechanical interactions between human lower leg muscles in vivo. *J Biomech Eng.* 135: 091003.

Yoshitake, Y., Uchida, D., Hirata, K., Mayfield, D.L. & Kanehisa, H. (2018) Mechanical interaction between neighboring muscles in human upper limb: evidence for epimuscular myofascial force transmission in humans. *J Biomech.* 74: 150–155.

Yucesoy, C.A. (2010) Epimuscular myofascial force transmission implies novel principles for muscular mechanics. *Exercise Sport Sci Rev.* 38: 128–134.

Yucesoy, C. A. & Huijing, P. A. (2012) Specifically tailored use of the finite element method to study muscular mechanics within the context of fascial integrity: the linked fiber-matrix mesh model. *Int J Multiscale Comput Eng.* 10: 155–170.

Yucesoy, C.A., Arıkan, E. & Ates, F. (2012) BTX-A administration to the target muscle affects forces of all muscles within an intact compartment and epimuscular myofascial force transmission. *J Biomech Eng.* 134: 111002.

Yucesoy, C.A. & Ates, F. (2018) BTX-A has notable effects contradicting some treatment aims in the rat triceps surae compartment, which are not confined to the muscles injected. *J Biomech.* 66: 78–85.

Yucesoy, C.A., Baan, G. & Huijing, P.A. (2010a) Epimuscular myofascial force transmission occurs in the rat between the deep flexor muscles and their antagonistic muscles. *J Electromyogr Kinesiol.* 20: 118–126.

Yucesoy, C.A., Baan, G.C. & Huijing, P.A. (2010b) Epimuscular myofascial force transmission occurs in the rat between the deep flexor muscles and their antagonistic muscles. *J Electromyogr Kinesiol.* 20: 118–126.

Yucesoy, C.A., Baan, G.C., Koopman, H.J.F.M., Grootenboer, H.J. & Huijing, P.A. (2005) Pre-strained epimuscular connections cause muscular myofascial force transmission to affect properties of synergistic EHL and EDL muscles of the rat. *J Biomech Eng.* 127: 819–828.

Yucesoy, C.A., Koopman, H.J.F.M., Baan, G.C., Grootenboer, H.J. & Huijing, P.A. (2003) Effects of inter- and extramuscular myofascial force transmission on adjacent synergistic muscles: assessment by experiments and finite element modeling. *J Biomech.* 36: 1797–1811.

Yucesoy, C.A., Temelli, Y. & Ates, F. (2017) Intra-operatively measured spas-tic semimembranosus forces of children with cerebral palsy. *J Electromyogr Kinesiol.* 36: 49–55.

Yucesoy, C.A., Turkoglu, A.N., Umur, S. & Ates, F. (2015) Intact muscle compartment exposed to botulinum toxin type a shows compromised intermuscular mechanical interaction. *Muscle Nerve.* 51: 106–116.

Fascia as sensory organ

Robert Schleip and Carla Stecco

No longer an inert wrapping tissue

For most anatomical researchers, fascia was mainly considered an inert wrapping organ, giving mechanical support to our muscles and most other organs. Yes, there were some early histological reports about the presence of sensory nerves in fascia (Sakada, 1974; Stillwell, 1957), but these were largely disregarded and did not affect the common understanding of musculoskeletal dynamics. While both Moshe Feldenkrais and Ida Rolf, the founders of the related somatic therapies, were apparently not aware of the importance of fascia as a sensory organ, Andrew Taylor Still, the founder of osteopathy, proclaimed that, "No doubt nerves exist in the fascia…" and suggested that all fascial tissues should be treated with the same degree of respect as if dealing with "the branch offices of the brain" (Still, 1902).

Van der Wal reported, with painstaking detail, the substantial presence of sensory nerve endings in the fascia of rats, yet this finding was ignored for several decades (van der Wal, 1988). As far as ligaments were concerned, their proprioceptive innervation was recognized during the 1990s, which subsequently influenced the guidelines for joint injury surgeries (Johansson et al., 1991). Similarly, the plantar fascia was found to contribute to the sensorimotor regulation of postural control in standing (Erdemir and Piazza, 2004). However, what really changed the "view" in a more powerful manner was the first international Fascia Research Congress, held at Harvard

Medical School in Boston in 2007. During the Congress, three teams from different countries reported, independently, their findings of a rich presence of sensory nerves in fascial tissues (Findley and Schleip, 2007). Following that event, several papers were published about fascial innervation, suggesting that the fasciae can be seen as our largest sensory organ in terms of overall surface area, but also that they can play an active role in proprioception and in the perception of pain.

Thanks to recent research insights, it is becoming evident that the fasciae are more complicated than anyone had thought. Indeed, the different fasciae have different type of innervation: the superficial fascia is more related with the exteroception and shares with the skin many nerve elements, the deep fasciae have above all free nerve endings including Pacini, Ruffini and spindle cell corpuscles for proprioception, the visceral fasciae have more an autonomic innervation (Stecco et al., 2017). Besides, spatial analysis indicates that in different areas there is a different density and types of nerve endings (Stecco et al., 2007) and, also in the same area, the various sublayers forming the aponeurotic fascia are innervated in a different way (Tesarz et al., 2011).

A detailed calculation by Martin Grunwald estimated the quantity of nerve endings in the body-wide fascial net as 100 million (Grunwald, 2017). This calculation related to the total mass of dense fibrous connective tissues only, which,

Chapter 15

based on Tanaka and Kawamura (2013) was estimated at 5 kg for an average male body. However, there are good reasons for also including the loose connective tissues in the calculation, not only because these tissues are part of the modern functional definition of the "fascial net" (see Chapter 1), but also because, based on Tesarz et al. (2011), we know that the loose subcutaneous connective tissue tends to express an even higher innervation density compared with the denser fascial layers underneath. Based on the data from Tanaka and Kawamura (2013), the mass of fibrous connective tissues in the human then increases to 12.5 kg (thus representing 17% of the total body weight). Taking this reasoning into account, the total quantity of nerve endings in the fascial net can then be estimated as ~2.5 times larger than the 100 million endings suggested by Grunwald, therefore arriving at the impressive number of 250 million nerve endings in the fascial net. Compared with an estimated quantity of 200 million nerve endings in the skin (Grunwald, 2017) or with the estimated 126 million endings for vision in our eyes, this new calculation suggests that the body-wide fascial network may possibly constitute our richest sensory organ.

Why sensory receptors?

Those of us who deal with the muscles and tissues of the human body often forget the importance of the sensory receptors. The brain, which is part of the central nervous system (CNS), is a very busy organ that requires its own army to continuously inform itself so that it can create movements that are accurate, opportunely timed, with proper force. Kendal et al. (2013) state that the brain relies on input from receptors in muscles, tendons, joints and skin to provide it with the information it needs to direct smooth and coordinated muscle movements. It therefore becomes extremely important for individuals who deal with any method of movement therapy to have an understanding of our potential influence on these sensory receptors. The CNS is directly responsible for all global movement directions such as raising our arms overhead, but must depend on sensory receptors for information about the movements of specific muscles.

Our bodies contain a somatosensory system containing sensory (afferent) neurons that respond to changes at the surface or inside our body. The somatosensory system regulates three major functions: proprioception, exteroception and interoception. Because this chapter is concerned with the sensory receptors of the fascial system, we will mainly be concerned with proprioceptive function. Proprioception refers to our ability to determine muscle activity and joint position. It is based on the stimulation of particular mechanoreceptors such as muscle spindle cells, Golgi tendon organs, joint capsule receptors and stretch-sensitive free nerve endings. Mechanoreceptors react when they are deformed by movement such as pressure, muscle stretch or contraction. These receptors produce and send sensory information to the brain, enabling it to detect the position and posture of the body and its parts. The sensory receptors that are classified as proprioceptors are the muscle spindles, Golgi tendon organs and joint receptors. Sometimes, Pacini and Ruffini corpuscles have a proprioceptive function, as they also report to the CNS regarding position. The CNS integrates information from proprioceptors and other sensory systems, such as vision and the vestibular system, to create an overall representation of body position, movement and acceleration. The sense of proprioception is essential for the motor coordination of the body. Proprioceptors can form reflex circuits with motoneurons to provide rapid feedback about body and limb position. These mechanosensory circuits are important for flexibly maintaining posture and balance, especially during locomotion.

Different types of sensory receptors in the fascial net

Free nerve endings

In the fasciae, we can recognize different types of sensory receptors, each one with a specific characteristic (Figure 15.1). Surely the most represented nerve receptors are the free nerve endings (Figure 15.2). They form a net, strongly connected with the extracellular matrix (viscous tissue providing support, segregating tissues from one another, and regulating intercellular communication) of the fasciae, and consequently they are particularly responsive to either stretch or shear loading. This is not surprising, since from a morphological and embryological perspective, the fascial net consists of those connective tissues that have adapted their architecture in response to a local dominance of tensional, rather than compressive loading (Schleip et al., 2012). The free nerve endings are very thin and delicate threads, sensitive to mechanical stimuli. Besides, if the extracellular matrix is altered or if

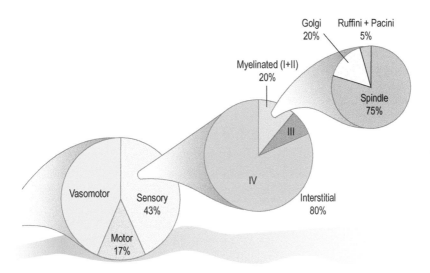

Figure 15.1 Composition of neurons in musculoskeletal connective tissues

The quantities of respective axons shown were derived from detailed analysis of the combined nerve supplying the lateral gastrocnemius and soleus muscle of a cat. While a small portion of the interstitial neurons may terminate inside bone, the remaining neurons can all be considered to terminate in fascia! tissues. Even the sensory devices called muscle spindles are nestled within fibrous collagenous intramuscular tissues. Interstitial neurons terminate in free nerve endings. Some of these clearly have a proprioceptive, interoceptive or nociceptive function. Recent investigations, however, suggest that the majority of the interstitial neurons in fascia serve a polymodal function, meaning that they are open for stimulation from more than one of these mentioned sensorial categories.

(Illustration courtesy offascialnet.com)

Chapter 15

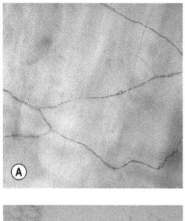

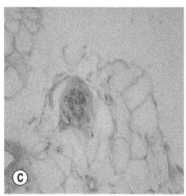

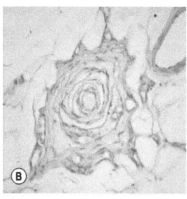

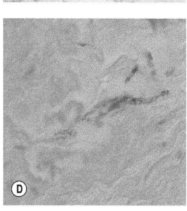

Figure 15.2

(A) Immunostaining of the thora-columbar fascia in rat with S100 antibody reveals the rich network of visible nerves (20×).

(B) Pacinian corpuscles and **(C)** Ruffini corpuscles on the surface of the human crural inter-osseous membrane, as stained for S100 (40x)

(D) Free nerve endings in the human capsule of the hip joint as stained for PGP9.5 (40 ×).

Images from Department of Neurosciences, Institute of Human Anatomy, University of Padova.

the stimuli is too strong, these free nerve endings could also become nociceptors (pain receptors). Taguchi et al. (2013) have demonstrated that the mechanical activation threshold of the fascial free nerve endings is 2-fold greater than the skin and muscle. Schilder et al. (2014) demonstrated that the free nerve endings in the thoracolumbar fascia are more sensitive to chemical irritation compared with the underlying muscles, and that they can maintain a long-lasting hypersensitiv-ity. Finally, Deising et al. (2012) have shown that the free nerve endings of the fascia are stimu-lated in the most effective way when the fascia is "pre-stretched" before muscle contraction. For health-oriented practitioners, it is important to realize that not all the free nerve endings can be classified as nociceptive. Some of them are sen-sory devices for thermoception, and others moni-tor muscular activity to the sympathetic nervous system to allow for a locally specific fine-tuning of the blood flow to respective muscle portions, which is then called ergoreception. Interestingly, in fascial tissues, the majority of the interstitial (between fibrous tissue) neurons are so-called polymodal receptors, meaning that they are responsive to more than one kind of stimulation. While their respective synapses in the posterior horn of the spinal cord are hungry and eager for any kind of stimulation, they seem to be easily satisfied if sufficient proprioceptive information is supplied to them via these polymodal recep-tors. However, in cases of alterations in the con-nective tissue matrix surrounding the respective nerve endings, these free nerve endings tend to actively lower their threshold for nociceptive stimulation, that is, expressing increased pain. In addition, they may actively give off cytokines that sensitize polymodal neurons in their neighborhood and predispose them towards a nociceptive function. A seemingly miniscule mechanical stimulation, such as a leg length difference of only 1 mm, can then lead to a nociceptive response within the intricate network of these intrafascial polymodal receptors.

In the fasciae there are four types of specialized mechanoreceptors (Stecco, 2015): Pacini, Ruffini and Golgi corpuscles, as well as the muscle spindles. Each type serves different functions accommodated by their different structures and activating stimuli. The Pacini corpuscles are rapidly adapting mechanoreceptors, so they decrease their discharge rate to extinction within milliseconds of the onset of a continuous stimulus. They are very sensitive to changes in stimulation and are therefore considered to mediate the sensation of joint motion, and may be more important in sports characterized by sudden directional changes, such as pivoting, shifting and tackling (Ergen et al., 2007).

Ruffini corpuscles are slowly adapting mechanoreceptors, so they remain discharging in response to a continuous stimulus. Ruffini are maximally stimulated at certain fascial tensions, and thus they can mediate the sensation of body position, but they are also highly sensitive to shear loading, so they can perceive a directional difference in tensional loading between one tissue layer and an adjacent one.

The muscle spindle receptor is a complex, fusiform receptor composed of several intrafusal muscular fibers, innervated by nerve fibers and surrounded by a strong capsule of connective tissue (Stecco et al., 2014). This capsule is in continuity with the perimysium of the surrounding muscle bundles, so the muscle spindles can perceive the tension developing inside the perimysium. We need to remember that it only takes a tension of 3 g to trigger a muscle spindle.

This means that small alteration of the perimysium, as often happens after immobilization, can alter the threshold of these receptors, and this causes alteration in proprioception and muscle activation. Indeed, the muscle spindles play a key role in proprioception because they inform the CNS of the continually changing status of muscle tone, movement and position of body parts. Mense (2011) affirms that "structural disorders of the fascia can surely distort the information sent by the spindles to the central nervous system and thus can interfere with proper coordinated movement. Particularly the primary spindle afferents are so sensitive that even slight distortions of the perimysium will change their discharge frequency."

Golgi endings are slowly adapting receptors that respond to tension. Stimulation of Golgi receptors tends to trigger a relaxation response in skeletal muscle fibers that are directly linked with the respectively tensioned collagen fibers. However, if tendinous extramuscular tissues are stretched in a condition in which they are arranged in series with muscle fibers that are in a relaxed condition, then most of the respective elongation will be "swallowed" by the more compliant myofibers. In this way, the respective stretching impulse may not provide sufficient stimulation for eliciting any muscular tonus change (Jami, 1992). A practical conclusion of this may be that a stretching impulse, aimed at reaching the tendinous tissues, may profit from including some moments in which the lengthened muscle fibers are actively contracting or are temporarily resisting their overall elongation.

While the Golgi receptors were previously considered to only exist in tendinous tissues, their presence in other fascial tissues has been confirmed by two independent studies (Stecco et al., 2007; Yahia et al., 1992). The Golgi corpuscles are located in the myotendineous junctions close to

Chapter 15

the intermuscular septa, and play a role in the coordination between agonist and antagonist muscles. So the Golgi endings can also contribute to the proprioceptive sense of force and heaviness of muscles.

The presence of the mechanoreceptors inside the fasciae is not homogeneous, for example, the Ruffini and Pacini corpuscles are located in the superficial fascia, while in the deep fascia they are present only where the proprioceptive inputs are stronger, as in the joint retinacula, and in the palmar and plantar fasciae. The muscle spindles are present only in the perimysium of the muscles and not in the thicker fasciae such as the thoracolumbar fascia and fascia lata.

Not all fasciae share the same innervation

Does it make a difference, which locations of the body-wide fascial network are stimulated in order to supply the spinal cord with new proprioceptive input? Two new insights regarding the density of sensory receptors in fascia provide valuable insight into this issue. First, the recent studies from the group around Mense at the University of Heidelberg have shown that in human and rat lumbar fascia, the density of sensory neurons is significantly higher in the superficial tissue layers between the dermis and fascia profunda compared with the respective density within the deeper tissue layer called lumbodorsal fascia, just underneath these superficial layers (Tesarz et al., 2011). In our own experimental examinations at Ulm University, we also observed an increased density of visible nerves in the transitional shearing zone between fascia profunda and fascia superficialis. In healthy body regions, this zone is where a lateral "skin sliding" movement, in relation to the underlying tissues, can easily be induced. It is also the zone whose architecture

determines whether a skin fold can be pulled away from the body or not. It makes sense to assume that the lateral gliding movements given by everyday movements provide an important source of fascial proprioception. It is also an intriguing thought that the often profound reported therapeutic effects of various skin-taping techniques in sports medicine may partially be explained by their local amplification of respective skin movements in normal joint functioning.

The second recent insight regarding areas of increased density of sensory nerves in the fascial net comes from the Stecco group at Padua University in Italy (Stecco et al., 2007). Their histological examinations of upper and lower limb fasciae in human cadavers revealed huge differences in the density of proprioceptive nerve endings, such as Golgi, Pacini and Ruffini corpuscles. These recent data indicated that fascial tissues, which clearly serve an important force-transmitting function (such as the lacertus fibrosus on the upper forearm as an extension of the biceps femoris), hardly contain the same proprioceptive endings as the biceps fascia. On the other hand, they observed that some fascial structures seem to have very little role in force transmission, as witnessed when cutting them away, as is the case of the retinacula around the ankle and wrist regions. Interestingly, these more obliquely running fascial bands seem to be located at specific approximations to major joints and they contain a very high density of proprioceptive nerve endings (Figure 15.3). Some researchers suggest that the prime function of these fascial bands may not be their biomechanical but their sensorial function in providing detailed proprioception to the CNS. If verified, this could suggest that proprioception-enhancing approaches, whether in skin taping, yoga, stretching, foam roller self-treatment, or continuum movement-like micro movements, could each possibly be augmented

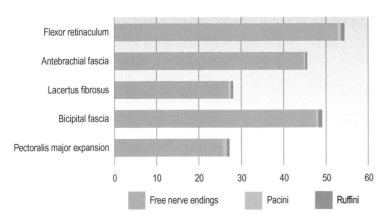

Figure 15.3

The mean number of the types of mechanoreceptors found in different areas of the upper limb (data from Stecco et al., 2007).

in their respective therapeutic effectiveness by stimulating fascial tissue movements in regions with an increased proprioceptive innervation.

The superficial fascia is also richly innervated, presenting both free nerve endings and corpuscular receptors such as Pacini and Ruffini. The corpuscular receptors are located inside the superficial adipose tissue and the superficial fascia, suggesting that these receptors are in this way able to perceive the mechanical stimuli applied to the superficial fascia. However, very few nerve receptors are present in the deep adipose tissue (DAT), which may be considered the watershed between the exteroceptive system (formed by skin, superficial adipose tissue and superficial fascia) and the proprioceptive system (placed in the muscles and deep fasciae). Where the DAT disappears and the superficial and deep fasciae fuse (as in the palm of the hand and in the plantar part of the foot), the exteroceptive and proprioceptive systems are combined (Stecco et al., 2017).

A surprising new finding is the discovery of the so-called tactile C-fibers in the superficial fascia of humans and other primates. These interstitial neurons are present in body areas where our ancestors had furry skin (e.g. not on the palms of the hands or the soles of the feet) and they are associated with grooming behavior as a social health function in primates. When stimulated,

these intrafascial neurons do not signal any proprioceptive information (and the brain cannot apparently locate the regional origin of the stimulation); however, they trigger activation in the insular cortex, which is expressed as a sense of peaceful well-being and social belonging (McGlone et al., 2014).

In the visceral fasciae the innervation is very different according to the type of fascia under consideration. Indeed, the fasciae closely related to the individual organ, such as the visceral peritoneum, the liver capsule and the esophagus adventitia, are very well innerved, but only with autonomic nerve elements. On the contrary, the parietal peritoneum, the pericardial sac, the renal fascia, and all the insertional fasciae, have a somatic innervation, exactly the same as the overlying muscles (Stecco et al., 2017).

Fasciae and pain

One of the most studied fasciae is the thoracolumbar fascia (TLF), because many studies have suggested that it can play a role in non-specific low back pain (Langevin et al., 2011; Schleip et al., 2007; Yahia et al., 1992). Indeed, the TLF is a densely innervated tissue and its free nerve endings can send nociceptive input to lumbar dorsal horn neurons (Taguchi et al., 2008). The work of Schilder et al. (2014) clearly demonstrated that

Chapter 15

the deep fascia, if altered, can be a prime candidate for pain, more so than muscles and subcutis. Injections of hypertonic saline into the deep fascia resulted in longer pain duration and higher peak pain ratings than injections into subcutaneous tissue or muscle. Also, pain radiation and pain affect evoked by fascia injection significantly exceeded those of the muscle and the subcutaneous tissue. The pain descriptors after fascia injection were burning, throbbing and stinging. After induction of delayed onset muscle soreness, pain thresholds of the fascia decrease significantly more than those of the underlying muscle tissue (Lau et al., 2015). Moreover, chronic irritation of the TLF can induce sensitization phenomena at the spinal level (Hoheisel et al., 2011). After experimentally induced chronic inflammation of the TLF, the density of nociceptive fibers was significantly increased from 4% to 15%. Also, the metamers affected by the nociceptive afference increased (Hoheisel et al., 2015). Similar results were reported in another fascia, the knee retinaculum, by Sanchis-Alfonso and Rosello-Sastre (2000), who highlighted the growth of nociceptive, substance P immunoreactive fibers in patients with patellofemoral syndrome. Pedersen et al. (1956) mechanically pinched the TLF of decerebrated cats and were able to elicit spastic contractions of the back muscles (mostly ipsilateral), as well as the hamstring and gluteal muscles (ipsilateral leg). Compared with pinching the underlying muscle tissues, the observed responses were much stronger in response to pinching the fascia. A similar result was obtained in the tibial anterior fascia of the lower leg. Taguchi et al. (2013) pinched the rat crural fascia and found an increased neural activation in the spinal dorsal horn.

The increased density of nociceptive fibers under chronic painful circumstances may suggest that the fasciae can play a role in peripheral sensitization. This is an increased sensitivity to inputs that usually are not painful, and could be due to increased numbers of free nerve endings in the fascial tissue or to a decreased threshold to the stimulus. For example, a fascial tension before injury is not painful and is useful to provide proprioceptive information, but after trauma is interpreted as pain. Hypersensitivity following an injury could be an important self-preservation mechanism to avoid further injury to this area, but if this hypersensitivity becomes prolonged, it provides the body with no benefit. It is important to identify patients with peripheral sensitization because if we restore the correct fascial tissue elasticity, the sensitivity of the free nerve endings can decrease, and consequently the pain intensity.

Interoception and the insular cortex

An often overlooked aspect of fascial stimulation is the presence of interstitial nerves in fascia that serve an interoceptive, rather than proprioceptive or nociceptive, function. Stimulation of those free nerve endings provides the brain with information about the condition of the body in its constant search for homeostasis in relation to its physiological needs. Many of the respective free nerve endings are located in visceral connective tissues and constitute an important part of what is frequently referred to as the enteric brain. However, other interoceptive interstitial neurons are located within endomysial and perimysial intramuscular connective tissues. Interoceptive signaling is associated with feelings like warmth, nausea, hunger, soreness, effort, heaviness and lightness, as well as a sense of belonging or alienation regarding specific body regions (Craig, 2002).

The neural stimulation from the respective nerve endings does not follow the usual afferent pathways towards the somatomotor cortex of the brain, rather these neurons project to the so-called insular cortex, an internally folded area of cortical gray matter located inside the forebrain.

Fascia as sensory organ

In this walnut-sized cortical area, perceptions about internal somatic sensations are associated with emotional preferences and feelings. People with disturbed functioning of the insula may still have full biomechanical functioning and achieve high IQ levels in respective tests; however, they are usually socially dysfunctional and unable to make reasonable decisions in complex situations (Damasio, 1999).

Whereas some health-related conditions, such as low back pain, scoliosis or complex regional pain syndrome, are associated with diminished proprioceptive acuity, other conditions seem to be more clearly related to dysfunctional interoceptive processing. These latter conditions include anorexia, anxiety, depression, irritable bowel syndrome, alexithymia (inability in recognizing and expressing one's own emotional states) and possibly fibromyalgia. It therefore makes sense that movement instructors, whether in yoga, pilates or martial arts, carefully examine their habitual preferences in fostering the direction of the suggested somatic curiosity of their clients. A rigid reliance on proprioceptive perception—"Where exactly is your lower back touching the ground?"—may provide limited long-term effects if applied to clients for whom a more interoceptive perceptual refinement approach may be required. In these cases, a skillful fostering of visceral fascial sensations, via specific yoga postures, for example, may sometimes provide more profound effects than the often habitual focus on musculoskeletal sensations (Table 15.1).

Table 15.1 Health conditions associated with dysfunctions in proprioceptive or interoceptive processing

Several pathologies have been shown to be associated with dysfunctions in proprioception. Other conditions are associated with an altered interoceptive processing. In the pathways of interoception, the insular cortex plays a leading role, in which all sensory input is combined with affective associations. In prioprioception, the somatomotor cortex and its representational mapping of the body (body schema) are of central importance. Depending on the involved pathway of dysfunction, a different emphasis in fascia-oriented therapies may be indicated

Proprioceptive impairment	Interoceptive dysregulation
Low back pain	Eating disorders
	Irritable bowel syndrome
Whiplash	Post-traumatic stress disorder
Complex regional pain syndrome (CRPS)	Substance use disorders
Attention deficit hyperactivity disorder (ADHS)	Depression
	Panic disorder
	Generalized anxiety disorder
Scoliosis diagonal chain	Autism spectrum disorders
	Depersonalization/derealization disorder
Systemic hypermobility	Somatic symptom disorders
	Functional disorders
Other myofascial pain syndromes	Fibromyalgia
	Chronic fatigue syndrom

Chapter 15

Conclusions

- Fascia constitutes a body-wide tensional network, which serves as our richest and most important sensory organ for perceiving changes in our own bodies.

- Related sensory nerves include receptors that clearly signal proprioceptive information.

- Visceral fasciae tend to primarily have an autonomic innervation, rather than a somatosensory one.

- Proprioceptive signaling tends to inhibit potential myofascial nociception, particularly if accompanied by a state of mindfulness and if the proprioceptive stimulation occurs in a body region, which is innervated by the same (or nearby) level of the spinal cord.

- The mutually inhibiting influences between myofascial nociception and proprioception seem to be particularly relevant in working with low back pain.

- Other smaller receptor neurons in fascia are focused on interoceptive or nociceptive sensations.

- Therapeutic enhancement of proprioceptive stimulation can be beneficial in many myofascial pain conditions.

- A skillful facilitation of interoceptive perceptions, on the other hand, may work equally well in several complex somatic dysfunctions by fostering an improved insular processing.

References

Bednar, D.A.1., Orr, F.W. & Simon, G.T. (1995) Observations on the pathomorphology of the thoracolumbar fascia in chronic mechanical back pain. A microscopic study. *Spine.* 20: 1161–1164.

Craig, A.D. (2002) How do you feel? Interoception: the sense of the physiological condition of the body. *Nat Rev Neurosci.* 3: 655–666.

Damasio, A. (1999) *The feeling of what happens: body and emotion in the making of consciousness.* New York, NY: Harcourt-Brace.

Erdemir, A. & Piazza, S.J. (2004) Changes in foot loading following plantar fasciotomy: a computer modeling study. *J Biomech Eng.* 126: 237–243.

Ergen, E. (2007) Proprioception and Coordination, Bülent Ulkar, in *Clinical Sports Medicine.*

Findley T. & Schleip R. (eds) (2007) *Fascia research. Basic science and implications for conventional and complementary health care.* Munich, Germany: Elsevier Urban & Fischer.

Gibson, W., Arendt-Nielsen, L., Taguchi, T., Mizumura, K. & Graven-Nielsen, T. (2009) Increased pain from muscle fascia following eccentric exercise: animal and human findings. *Exp Brain Res.* 194: 299–308.

Grunwald, M. (2017) *Homo hapticus.* Munich, Germany: Droemer Verlag.

Jami, A. (1992) Golgi tendon organs in mammalian skeletal muscles: functional properties and central actions. *Physiol Rev.* 72: 623–666.

Johansson, H., Sjölander, P. & Sojka, P. (1991) A sensory role for the cruciate ligaments. *Clin Orthop Relat Res.* 268: 161–178.

Koike, S., Mukudai, S. & Hisa, Y. (2016) *Muscle Spindles and Intramuscular Ganglia/Neuroanatomy and Neurophysiology of the Larynx.* Tokyo, Japan: Springer, 11–20.

Liptan, G.L. (2010) Fascia: A missing link in our understanding of the pathology of fibromyalgia. *J Bodyw Mov Ther.* 14: 3–12.

McGlone, F., Wessberg, J. & Olausson, H. (2014) Discriminative and affective touch: sensing and feeling. *Neuron.* 82: 737–755.

Mense, S. & Hoheisel, U. (2016) Evidence for the existence of nociceptors in rat thoracolumbar fascia. *J Bodyw Mov Ther.* 20: 623–628.

Mitchell, J.H. & Schmidt, R.F. (1977) Cardiovascular reflex control by afferent fibers from skeletal muscle receptors. In: Shepherd JT et al. (eds) *Handbook of physiology.* Section 2, Vol. III, Part 2: 623–658.

Moseley, G.L.1., Zalucki, N.M. & Wiech, K. (2007) Tactile discrimination, but not tactile stimulation alone, reduces chronic limb pain. *Pain.* 137: 600–608.

Sakada, S. (1974) Mechanoreceptors in fascia, periosteum and periodontal ligament. *Bull Tokyo Med Dent Univ.* 21(Suppl 0): 11–13.

Sandkühler, J. (2009) Models and mechanisms of hyper-algesia and allodynia. *Physiol Rev.* 89: 707–758.

Schilder, A., Hoheisel, U., Magerl, W., Benrath, J., Klein, S. & Treede, R.D. (2014) Sensory findings after stimulation of the thoracolumbar fascia with hypertonic saline suggest its contribution to low back pain. *Pain.* 155: 222–231.

Schleip, R., Jäger, H. & Klingler, W. (2012) What is 'fascia'? A review of different nomenclatures. *J Bodyw Mov Ther.* 16: 496–502.

Schleip, R., Naylor, I.L., Ursu, D., Melzer, W., Zorn, A., Wilke, H.J., Lehmann-Horn, F. & Klingler, W. (2006) *Med Hypotheses.* 66: 66–71.

Standring, S., et al. (2009) *Gray's Anatomy: the Anatomical Basis of Clinical Practice*, 40th edn. Edinburgh, UK: Churchill Livingstone, 1101.

Stecco, C. (2014) *Functional atlas of the human fascial system.* Elsevier Health Sciences.

Stecco, C., Gagey, O., Belloni, A., Pozzuoli, A., Porzionato, A., Macchi, V., Aldegheri, R., De Caro, R. & Delmas, V. (2007) Anatomy of the deep fascia of the upper limb. Second part: study of innervation. *Morphologie.* 91: 38–43.

Stecco, C., Sfriso, M.M., Porzionato, A., et al. (2017) Microscopic anatomy of the visceral fasciae. *J Anat.* 231: 121–128.

Stecco, A., Stecco, C. & Raghavan, P. (2014) Peripheral mechanisms contributing to spasticity and implications for treatment. *Curr Phys Med Rehabil Rep.* 2: 121–127.

Still, A.T. (1902) *The philosophy and mechanical principles of osteopathy.* Kansas City: Hudson-Kimberly, 62.

Stillwell, D.L. (1957) Regional variations in the innervation of deep fasciae and aponeuroses. *Anat Rec.* 127: 635–648.

Tanaka, G. & Kawamura, H. (1992) Reference Man Models Based on Normal Data from Human Populations. Report of the Task Group on Reference Man, The International Commission on Radiological Protection, Nr. 23. http://www.irpa.net/irpa10/cdrom/00602.pdf.

Tesarz, J., Hoheisel, U., Wiedenhöfer, B. & Mense, S. (2011) Sensory innervation of the thoracolumbar fascia in rats and humans. *Neuroscience.* 194: 302–308.

van der Wal, J.C. (1988) The organization of the substrate of proprioception in the elbow region of the rat. PhD thesis. Maastricht, the Netherlands: Maastricht University, Faculty of Medicine.

Yahia, L., Rhalmi, S., Newman, N. & Isler, M. (1992) Sensory innervation of human thoracolumbar fascia. An immunohistochemical study. *Acta Orthop Scand.* 63: 195–197.

Fascia and musculoskeletal injury: An underestimated association?

Jan Wilke

Introduction

The prevention and treatment of musculoskeletal disorders represent superordinate goals of training in sports. Extensive research efforts have therefore been made to identify and describe the most frequent injuries occurring during athletic activity. However, while numerous studies meticulously report the incidence and prevalence of muscle, bone, tendon, ligament or capsular injuries, the deep fascia remains a Cinderella tissue in this regard: it is largely unknown to what extent it can be damaged although its vulnerability is highly plausible. This chapter gives two examples of the involvement of fascia in the genesis and symptomatology of musculoskeletal disorders, highlighting its potential role in soft tissue strain injury and delayed onset muscle soreness.

Soft tissue strain injuries

Muscle injuries are one of the most frequent health problems in sports. According to epidemiological data, 10–55% of all acute injuries sustained during athletic activity are muscle strains (Chan et al., 2012). The pathology is particularly prevalent in sports such as football (soccer), basketball, rugby and running (Maffulli et al., 2015). Its typical location is in the lower limb as the quadriceps femoris, gastrocnemius, as well as the adductor and hamstring muscles (the latter particularly in football), represent the most commonly damaged structures (Barroso and Thiele,

2011; Ekstrand et al., 2011). The susceptibility of the listed muscles can be ascribed to a variety of features: among others, a high percentage of glycolytic fast twitch muscle fibers, pennate fiber arrangement and bi-articularity have been suggested to be predisposing factors (Maffulli et al., 2015).

Pathophysiology of soft tissue strains

Powerful decelerations requiring eccentric contraction (see Chapter 26) represent the main pathomechanism of injury (Maffulli et al., 2015). This implies that the affected tissue has to counteract high elongating forces in the presence of active muscle work. While a certain amount of stress is tolerated by a resilient muscle-tendon complex, its load-bearing capacity can be exceeded by repetitive and cumulative stimuli, finally leading to rupture. In particular, end game situations in sports represent a dangerous period for athletes. In football, the number of injuries rises almost proportionally until the end of the two halves (Ekstrand et al., 2011), which seems to be explained by accumulating exhaustion. Results from animal experiments revealed that the force necessary to provoke muscle failure is reduced by ~3–7% in the fatigued state (Mair et al., 1996). This, in turn, is of relevance because biomechanical studies in human athletes demonstrated that eccentric strength, probably representing a crucial protective factor, decreases with increasing playing time (Grieg and Siegler, 2009).

Chapter 16

The role of fascia in soft tissue strains

Although clinical diagnostics and associated therapies traditionally focus on the skeletal muscle and the tendon, it is not the only actuator that may be strained during injury. The collagenous connective tissue forms a functional and structural unit with the active component of the locomotor system. This can be observed on both a micro and a macro level. The micro level includes the connectivity of the individual fibers with the endomysium as well as another surprising architectural feature: in some muscles, as few as one fifth of the fibers extend over the entire distance between origin and insertion, whereas the rest of the fibers terminate within the muscle belly, being linked through their endomysium (Figure 16.1; Hijikata and Ishikawa, 1997). Hence, the connective tissue appears to represent a relevant mechanical hub transmitting and distributing forces within the muscle and can be stretched during eccentric contraction. The macro level, in addition to the micro-arrangement, includes the tight linkages of muscles with their deep fascia as well as the tissue fusion with adjacent (e.g. synergists and antagonists) and serially connected (e.g. gastrocnemius and hamstrings) structures (for a more detailed summary on myofascial continuity, see Chapter 12). Taken together, the intimate micro- as well as macro-level fusions of the connective tissue with the skeletal muscles suggest that the former assists the latter mechanically by helping to absorb and damp peak stresses produced during explosive movements such as accelerations, stops, or changes of direction. The hypothesis that the deep fascia may be injured in athletic movements, thus appears tenable and merits further contemplation.

The findings of a recent systematic review with meta-analysis (Wilke et al., 2019) corroborate the assumed vulnerability of fascial tissues during sports. Analyzing a total of 1433 muscle strain injuries registered in 15 observation studies (diagnosis verified by magnet resonance imaging and/or ultrasound), it found 9 out of 10 lesions included structural damage to the fascia or the tendon. While the deep fascia exhibited tears in 32% of the cases, an even higher share was detected for the myotendinous junction (68%), which seems highly plausible in view of the force transmitting function of the tendon. In contrast to these surprisingly high values, isolated damage to the muscle occurred only in 1 out of 10 injuries (11%). The term muscle injury, therefore, ignores the morphological substrate of the disorder and may better be replaced by "myofascial injury" or "myocollagenous injury".

Fascia-specific therapy of muscle injuries and new approaches for prevention

From a theoretical point of view, both sports performance and the duration of the rehabilitation

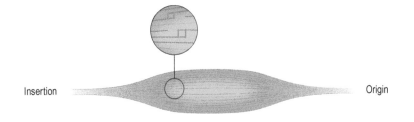

Insertion   Origin

Figure 16.1 Schematic illustration of a skeletal muscle

While spanning muscle fibers bridge the entire distance between insertion and origin, non-spanning fibers (circle) are linked only by means of connective tissue (red vertical lines).

Fascia and musculoskeletal injury: An underestimated association?

process may be adversely affected by connective tissue damage detected in soft tissue injuries. In fact, after fasciotomy (a longitudinal incision of the fascia), Garfin et al. (1986) found force decreases of up to 16% in the leg muscles of dogs. The authors suggested that the force loss was related to substantial (~50%) reductions in intra-compartmental pressure. A recent study made similar observations: removal of the deep fascia surrounding the wing muscles of wild turkeys decreased the maximal force output by 28% compared with the pre-surgery state (Ruttiman et al., 2018). It therefore remains to be elucidated if the typical size of fascial ruptures in myocollagenous injury is sufficiently large to have similar consequences in athletes. In addition to force production, fascial lesions could also affect joint range of motion. Bishop et al. (2018) examined the effect of a 2 cm-long injury on tissue thickness and shear strain mobility of the porcine lumbar fascia. The incision led to a slightly higher thickness and a decrease of ~15% in fascial layer sliding. Both factors may impair range of motion (Wilke et al., 2018). Interestingly, the magnitude of the changes was markedly more pronounced if the animals were subjected to an 8-week immobilization period. Although the downtimes following soft tissue strains are not as long, the reciprocal aggravation of injury and lack of movement could also be of relevance in humans.

With regard to the potential impact of fascial injury on the duration of the rehabilitation process, the available data is hitherto insufficient. Some observation studies registered a higher return to play time in case of greater fascial damage (Prakash et al., 2018; Werner et al., 2017). Other studies (Connell et al., 2004; Ekstrand et al., 2016; Pedret et al., 2015; Pollock et al., 2016) compared return to play after myofascial and myotendinous injuries. Mostly, they revealed similar

durations for both types, which seems expected as both are characterized by collagen failure. Although not distinguishing tendinous and fascial lesions, one study investigated the potential difference between myocollagenous and purely muscular soft tissue strain injuries. In a sample of 70 elite athletes, Renoux et al. (2018) demonstrated that myocollagenous lesions required a 3-week longer rehabilitation process than isolated muscle lesions (7.6 vs. 3.9 weeks). While this finding needs to be solidified by further studies, it is congruent with the fact that the connective tissue has a substantially higher turnover rate than the skeletal muscle (Heinemeier et al., 2013).

Despite the lack of data clearly delineating the impact of fascial tissue on return to play time, a focused treatment providing specific stimuli to the connective tissue could still speed up recovery when assuming it had not been optimal to date. Basically, two factors determine the resilience of the connective tissue to strain forces: the relative amount of type I collagen and the arrangement of the fibers. To stimulate the production of type I collagen and to elicit an optimal fiber orientation (in tendons parallel, lattice-like in fascia), the application of mechanical forces lengthening the targeted tissue is required. As an example, this can be achieved by means of eccentric training and stretching. Eccentric exercise is already widely used in current rehabilitation paradigms. Both acutely and in the long term, it leads to a substantial shift of the optimal force production angle towards longer muscle lengths (Brockett et al., 2001). The enhanced mechanical output in stretched positions may represent a protective mechanism against strain injury. When designing preventive interventions, clinicians should particularly consider the eccentric-concentric strength ratio. Croisier et al. (2002) examined this outcome in a sample of athletes with injury history and recurrent strains.

Chapter 16

Most of the study participants had substantial bilateral deficits in eccentric strength. After a focused eccentric training program, the imbalance was restored and none of the athletes suffered from a recurrence during the observation period of 12 months. In general, three meta-analyses have examined the effectiveness of eccentric training in the prevention of hamstring strains. All conformably conclude that the exercises, if performed with high compliance, have a prophylactic impact (Al Attar et al., 2017; Goode et al., 2015; Schache, 2012).

With regard to the effectiveness of stretching, there is a paucity of evidence. Findings from fundamental research basically support its application, suggesting a crucial role in regulating the inflammatory response and tissue remodeling. Corey et al. (2012) stretched previously inflamed lumbar mice fasciae twice daily for 10 minutes. After 12 days, they observed a normalization of the step length, less macrophage expression, and a reduced mechanical sensitivity. In a follow-up trial by the same research group, a similar treatment protocol was applied to examine the acute impact of stretching (Berrueta et al., 2016). Forty-eight hours after induction of connective tissue inflammation, rats which had performed flexibility exercises displayed a decreased thickness of the inflammatory lesion and had a smaller neutrophil count. While increased collagen production following the inflammatory phase is an essential part of functional healing, an overshooting synthesis can lead to fibrosis and excessive scarring. Interestingly, a 20–30% subcutaneous connective tissue stretch in mice has been shown to decrease the injury-induced expression of the transforming growth factor beta 1 (TGF-ß1) and procollagen type-1. The production of both substances can lead to fibrosis and, with this, to adhesions reducing tissue functionality and flexibility. It has to be

reiterated that a large elongation, like the one applied in the experiment, may be difficult to achieve in humans under *in vivo* conditions: according to biomechanical testing, the normal deep fascia ruptures at strains of 12–15% (Wang et al., 2009; Yahia et al., 1993). However, with a continuous lengthening protocol, progressively performed over several consecutive days, the failure threshold can increase by up to 27–37% (Wang et al., 2009). Another issue relates to the optimal timing of when to apply a stretching intervention within the rehabilitation period as it cannot be extrapolated from the experimental data.

Despite its potentially beneficial impact on tissue regeneration, stretching should be used cautiously. If the exercise stimulus is too strong, the positive effect may vanish or even reverse. Comparing two stretch intensities, Wang et al. (2007) found that rabbit leg lengthening at a rate of 2 mm per day caused collagen fibril necrosis whereas 1 mm per day induced regenerative changes. Furthermore, the higher stretching rate was shown to foster collagen type III production (Wang et al., 2008). This collagen type is typically synthesized after trauma and provides provisional, but less stable, tissue healing. Under normal circumstances, the deep fascia consists almost exclusively of type I collagen, which is directly related to the tensile strength of a tissue. The shift towards a higher type III share may therefore be the result of an excessive strain rate.

Only one study has investigated the value of an explicit stretching exercise program on the success of the return-to-play process. Malliaropoulos et al. (2004) examined the recovery of 80 elite athletes with hamstring strain injuries. The study participants were randomly allocated to two groups: while the first group stretched once a day, the second group performed four stretching sessions. The intensified protocol led to a 2-day faster restoration of the normal range of motion and a significantly shorter return-to-play process (13.3 vs. 15.1 days) compared with the controls, who were stretching less. Although more trials are needed to solidify the evidence for the effectiveness of stretching as a treatment of soft tissue strain injuries, it may at least be used as an adjunct element of a multifaceted rehabilitation program.

Similar to its application with therapeutic purposes, stretching is also often used as a prophylactic measure. Several systematic reviews clearly showed that it does not reduce the overall occurrence of injuries (Thacker et al., 2004; McHugh & Cosgrave, 2010; for a complete review see Chapter 10). However, there appears to be a small beneficial effect if only muscle injuries are considered (McHugh & Cosgrave, 2010). More importantly, the available studies mostly used static stretching, which may not provide sufficient repeated lengthening stimuli.

In summary, specific cyclic stretching interventions with higher volumes tailored to mainly load the extramuscular fascia (see Chapter 10) could open new frontiers in the prevention of myocollagenous injuries. Myocollagenous healing may also be improved using nutritional supplementation. Orally ingested vitamin C-enriched gelatin and rope-skipping exercises have been shown to enhance collagen synthesis *in vivo* (Shaw et al., 2016). Interestingly, there seems to be a linear dose response relationship because the intake of 15 g elicited a stronger response than the use of 5 g. Although no effects on mechanical stability were found, it was further demonstrated in a placebo-controlled trial that supplementation with collagen peptides (5 g) can improve self-perceived functional stability of the foot in participants with chronic ankle instability (Dressler et al., 2018).

Delayed onset muscle soreness

Delayed onset muscle soreness (DOMS) is a well-known phenomenon for both couch potatoes as well as high-level athletes getting back to action after the off-season: when training loads are rapidly increased or new, previously unfamiliar exercise stimuli are applied, motion-related muscle pain can develop on the days after activity. It has long been thought that DOMS primarily originates from the muscle. In fact, compelling evidence suggests that eccentric exercise in particular results in increased levels of creatine kinase, an enzymatic marker of muscle damage. Findings from biopsy studies, furthermore, revealed structural changes such as damage of z-disks and disruption of myofibers (Stauber et al., 1990). Taken together, these processes are suggested to lead to tissue inflammation, swelling and pain, representing the characteristic hallmarks of DOMS (Cleak and Eston, 1992; Kanda et al., 2013).

Despite the proven existence of muscle damage following severe or unaccustomed exercise, recent research has challenged the classical theory about the pathogenesis of DOMS, showing that the delayed discomfort felt after exercise does not seem to stem from the muscle. Gibson et al. (2009) required their participants to perform eccentric contractions of the tibialis anterior muscle. One day later, hypertonic saline (a solution eliciting pain) was injected into the muscle as well as into the surrounding fascia. Interestingly, the pain ratings of the participants were substantially higher upon fascial injection, while the nociceptive response to muscle irritation was not even different to the non-exercised control leg. A similar study by Lau

Chapter 16

et al. (2015) confirmed these surprising findings. After inducing DOMS in the elbow flexors, the pain reaction of different tissues was assessed by means of the electrical pain threshold, which identifies the current intensity corresponding to the first pain sensation. Again, the stimulation of the surrounding fascia was demonstrated to be more painful than the irritation of the muscle. From the data of Gibson et al. (2009) and Lau et al. (2015), it can be inferred that the deep fascia (and not the muscle itself) appears to represent the source of nociception in DOMS. This hypothesis fits with the data of Barry et al. (2015), who found the lumbar fascia to exhibit a 3-fold higher nerve density than the back muscles.

With regard to the pathophysiology of DOMS, the evidence pointing towards the existence of structural damage in the skeletal muscle and pain perception stemming from the fascia enables two slightly different explanation models (Langevin & Sherman, 2006; Wilke et al., 2017). First, when assuming structural muscle damage as a cause, the nociceptors of the connective tissue surrounding it may be stimulated by the inflammation-induced muscular swelling. Connected to this, it is also conceivable that the lesion of the muscle would trigger an increased sensitivity of the fascia due to its innervation by the same spinal segment. Then even light stimuli such as touch or moderate muscle contractions could evoke pain. Another theory completely negates the pathogenic value of the muscle damage, which may then rather be considered an essential part of the remodeling/adaptation process following training. In this case, both origin and manifestation of pain could be in the connective tissue. As the fascia is intimately connected to the skeletal muscle and needs to adapt to its volume and length changes, it may be damaged particularly during heavy-load eccentric contractions (see above). To date, the presence of micro-ruptures within the deep fascia has not been investigated explicitly. However, after 50 maximal eccentric contractions leading to DOMS, increased excretion of urinary hydroxyproline and hydroxylysine have been reported (Brown et al., 1997). Both amino acids are suggested to reflect collagen breakdown and, with this, possibly also lesions of the intra- or extramuscular connective tissue. In another study (Crameri et al., 2004), biopsies were taken from the human vastus lateralis muscle. Unaccustomed high-intensity eccentric exercise led to tenascin C staining and the detection of reactive macrophages in the perimysium and epimysium. Tenascin C is a surrogate of high loading and/or failure of a tissue, whereas the presence of macrophages is indicative of inflammatory processes. Finally, in a recent experiment, ultrasound imaging was used to quantify the thickness of the biceps brachii fascia in response to fatiguing eccentric exercise (Nosaka & Lau, 2018). On the day after the induction of DOMS, thickness was described to be ~30% higher. During subsequent days, further increases were registered, reaching the maximum (+104%) on the fifth day. Although there are multiple potential causes for the observed fascial thickening, it may be the result of injury-provoked edema. Taken together, the experimental findings appear to reveal that exercise causing DOMS does not only provoke structural muscle damage but also micro-lesions within the fascia. It is, hence, tenable to assume that the mechanisms underlying the two hypotheses presented above act in concert when muscle soreness occurs following physical activity.

Summary

Musculoskeletal traumas can substantially affect the deep fascia of the skeletal muscle. This becomes highly evident in soft tissue strain injuries, which mainly manifest in the extramuscular and tendinous connective tissue. By contrast, isolated morphological damage to the muscle occurs only in a very few cases. Although the effectiveness of specific preventive and therapeutic approaches has yet to be fully established, the development and application of interventions targeting fascia offer interesting opportunities for coaches and therapists. Based on the available evidence, eccentric training and dynamic stretching exercises seem to be capable of providing adequate stimuli. In DOMS, the connective tissue surrounding the muscle also seems to plays an important role as the pain experienced by the individual is likely to originate from the fascia. While further research is still warranted definitively confirming the presence of fascial micro-ruptures, treatments aiming to ease the post-exercise phenomenon should be tailored according to the new findings.

References

Al Attar, W.S.A., Soomro, N., Sinclair, P.J., Pappas, E. & Sanders, R.H. (2017) Effect of injury prevention programs that include the Nordic hamstring exercise on hamstring injury rates in soccer players: a systematic review and meta-analysis. *Sports Med.* 47: 907–916.

Barroso, C.G. & Thiele, E.S. (2011) Muscle injuries in athletes. *Rev Bras Ortop.* 46: 354–358.

Barry, C.M., Kestell, G., Gillan, M., Haberberger, R.V. & Gibbins, I.L. (2015) Sensory nerve fibers containing calcitonin gene-related peptide in gastrocnemius, latissimus dorsi and erector spinae muscles and thoracolumbar fascia in mice. *Neuroscience* 291: 106–117.

Berrueta, L., Muskaj, I., Olenich, S., Butler, T., Badger, G.J., Colas, R.A., Spite, M., Serhan, C.N., Langevin, H.M. (2016) Stretching impacts inflammation resolution in connective tissue. *J Cell Physiol.* 231(7): 1621–1627

Bishop, J.H., Fox, J.R., Maple, R., Loretan, C., Badger, G.J., Henry, S.M., Vizzard, M.A. & Langevin, H.M. (2016) Ultrasound evaluation of combined effects of thoracolumbar fascia injury and movement restriction in a porcine model. *PLoS One.* 11: e0147393.

Brockett, C.L., Morgan, D.L. & Proske, U. (2001) Human hamstring muscles adapt to eccentric exercise by changing optimum length. *Med Sci Sports Exerc.* 33: 783–790.

Brown, S.J., Child, R.B., Day, S.H. & Donnelly, A.E. (1997) Indices of skeletal muscle damage and connective tissue breakdown following eccentric muscle contractions. *Eur J Appl Physiol Occup Physiol.* 75: 369–374.

Chan, O., Del Buono, A., Best, T.M. & Maffulli, N. (2012) Acute muscle strain injuries: a proposed new classification system. *Knee Surg Sports Traumatol Arthrosc.* 20: 2356–2362.

Cleak, M.J. & Eston, R.G. (1992) Delayed onset muscle soreness: mechanisms and management. *J Sports Sci.* 10: 325–341.

Connell, D.A., Schneider-Kolsky, M.E., Hoving, J.L., Malara, F., Buchbinder, R., Koulouris, G., Burke, F. & Bass, C. (2004) Longitudinal study comparing sonographic and MRI assessments of acute and healing hamstring injuries. *Am J Roentgenol.* 183: 975–984.

Crameri, R.M., Langberg, H., Teisner, H., Magnusson, P., Schroder H.D., Olsesen, J.L., Jensen, C.H., Koskinen, S., Suetta, C. & Kjaer, M. (2004) Enhanced procollagen processing in skeletal muscle after a single bout of eccentric loading in humans. *Matrix Biol.* 23: 259–264.

Croisier, J.L., Forthomme, B. & Namurois, M.H. (2002) Hamstring muscle strain recurrence and strength performance disorders. *Am J Sports Med.* 30: 199–203.

Dressler, P., Gehring, D., Zdieblik, D., Oesser, S., Gollhofer, A. & König, D. (2018) Improvement of functional ankle properties following supplementation with specific collagen peptides in athletes with chronic ankle instability. *J Sports Sci Med.* 17: 298–304.

Ekstrand, J., Hägglund M. & Waldén, M. (2011) Epidemiology of muscle injuries in professional football (soccer). *Am J Sports Med.* 39:1226–1232.

Garfin, S.R., Tipton, C.M., Mubarak, S.J., Savio, L.Y., Hargens, A.R. & Akeson, W.H. (1981) Role of fascia in maintenance of muscle tension and pressure. *J Appl Physiol Respir Environ Exerc Physiol.* 51: 317–320.

Gibson, W., Arendt-Nielsen, L., Taguchi, T., Mizumura, K. & Graven-Nielsen, T.

(2009) Increased pain from muscle fascia following eccentric exercise: animal and human findings. *Exp Brain Res.* 194: 299–308.

Goode, A.P., Reiman, M.P., Harris, L., DeLisa, L., Kauffman, A., Beltramo, D., Poole, C., Ledbetter, L. & Taylor, A.B. (2015) Eccentric training for prevention of hamstring injuries may depend on intervention compliance: a systematic review and meta-analysis. *Br J Sports Med.* 49: 349–356.

Grieg, M. & Siegler, J.C. (2009) Soccer-specific fatigue and eccentric hamstrings muscle strength. *J Athl Train.* 44: 180–188.

Heinemeier, K.M., Schjerling, P., Heinemeier, J., Magnusson, S.P. & Kjaer, M. (2013) Lack of tissue renewal in human adult Achilles tendon is revealed by atomic nuclear bomb 14C. *FASEB J.* 27: 2074–2079.

Hijikata, T. & Ishikawa, H. (1997) Functional morphology of serially linked skeletal muscle fibers. *Acta Anat.* 159: 99–107.

Kanda, K., Sugama, K., Hayashida, H., Sakuma, J., Kawakami, Y., Miura, S., Yoshioka, H., Mori, Y. & Suzuki, K. (2013) Eccentric exercise-induced delayed-onset muscle soreness and changes in markers of muscle damage and inflammation. *Exerc Immunol Rev.* 19: 72–85.

Langevin, H.M. & Sherman, K.J. (2007) Pathophysiological model for chronic low back pain integrating connective tissue and nervous system mechanisms. *Med Hypotheses.* 68: 84–80.

Lau, W.Y., Blazevich, A.J., Newton, M.J., Wu, S.S. & Nosaka, K. (2015) Changes in electrical pain threshold of fascia and muscle after initial and secondary bouts of elbow flexor eccentric exercise. *Eur J Appl Physiol.* 115: 959–968.

Maffulli, N., Del Buono, A., Oliva, F., Giai Via, A., Frizziero, A., Barazzuol, M., Brancaccio, P., Freschi, M., Galletti, S., Lisitano, G., Melegati, G., Nanni, G., Pasta, G., Ramponi, C., Rizzo, D., Testa, V. & Valent, A. (2015) Muscle injuries: a brief guide to classification and management. *Transl Med UniSa.* 12: 14–18.

Mair, S.D., Seaber, A.V., Glisson, R.R. & Garrett, W.E. (1996) The role of fatigue in susceptibility to acute muscle strain injury. *Am J Sports Med.* 24: 137–143.

Malliaropoulos, N., Papalexandris, S., Papalada, A. & Papacostas, E. (2004) The role of stretching in rehabilitation of hamstring injuries: 80 athletes follow-up. *Med Sci Sports Exerc.* 36: 756–759.

McHugh, M.P. & Cosgrave, C.H. (2010) To stretch or not to stretch: the role of stretching in injury prevention and performance. *Scand J Med Sci Sports* 20: 169–181.

Nosaka, K. & Lau, W.Y. (2018) Increases in biceps brachii fascia thickness after eccentric exercise of the elbow flexors. *J Bodyw Mov Ther.* 22: 858.

Pedret, C., Rodas, G., Balius, R., Capdevil, L., Bossy, M., Vernooij, R.W. & Alomar, X. (2015) Return to play after soleus injuries. *Orthop J Sports Med.* 3: doi: 10.1177/2325967115595802

Prakash, A., Entwisle, T., Schneider, M., Brukner, P. & Connell, D. (2018) Connective tissue injury in calf muscle tears and return to play: MRI correlation. *Br J Sports Med.* 52: 929–933.

Renoux, J., Brasseur, J.L., Wagner, M., Frey, A., Folinais, D., Dibie, C., Maiza, D. & Crema, M.D. (2018) Ultrasound-detected connective tissue involvement in elite athletes and return to play: the French National Institute of Sports (INSEP) study. *J Sci Med Sport.* 22: 641–646.

Ruttiman, R.J., Sleboda, D.A. & Roberts, T.J. (2018) Release of fascial compartment boundaries reduces muscle force output. *J Appl Physiol.* 126: 593–598.

Schache, A. (2012) Eccentric hamstring muscle training can prevent hamstring injuries in soccer players. *J Physiother.* 58: 58.

Shaw, G., Lee-Barthel, A., Ross, M.L., Wang, B. & Baar, K. (2017) Vitamin C-enriched gelatin supplementation before intermittent activity augments collagen synthesis. *Am J Clin Nutr.* 105: 136–143.

Stauber, W.T., Clarkson, P.M., Fritz, V.K. & Evans W.J. (1990) Extracellular matrix disruption and pain after eccentric muscle action. *J Appl Physiol.* 69: 868–874.

Thacker, S.B., Gilchrist, J., Stroup, D.F. & Kimsey, C.D. (2004) The impact of stretching on sports injury risk: a systematic review of the literature. *Med Sci Sports Exerc.* 36: 371–378.

Wang, H.Q., Li, X.K., Wu, Z.X., Wei, Y.Y. & Luo, Z.J. (2008) The effect of the extracellular matrix of the deep fascia in response to leg lengthening. *BMC Musculoskelet Disord.* 9: 101.

Wang, H.Q., Li, M.Q., Wu, Z.X. & Zhao, L. (2007) The deep fascia in response to leg lengthening with particular reference to the tension-stress principle. *J Pediatr Orthop.* 27: 41–45.

Wang, H.Q., Wei, Y.Y., Wu, Z.X., Luo, Z.J. (2009) Impact of leg lengthening on viscoelastic properties of the deep fascia. *BMC Musculoskelet Disord.* 10: 105.

Wilke, J., Hespanhol, L. & Behrens, M. (2019) Is it all about the fascia? A systematic review and meta-analysis of the prevalence of connective tissue lesions in muscle strain injury, Volume 7. doi: 10.1177/2325967119888500.

Wilke, J., Macchi, V., De Caro, R. & Stecco, C. (2018) Fascia thickness, aging and flexibility: is there an association? *J Anat.* 234: 43–49.

Wilke, J., Schleip, R., Klingler, W. & Stecco, C. (2017) The lumbodorsal fascia as a potential source of low back pain: a narrative review. *Biomed Res Int.* ePaper, doi: 10.1155/2017/5349620

Yahia, L.H., Pigeon, P., DesRosiers, E.A. (1993) Viscoelastic properties of the human lumbodorsal fascia. *J Biomed Eng.* 15(5): 425–429.

Classification of athletic injuries to muscular tissues

Hans-Wilhelm Müller-Wohlfahrt

Athletic muscle injuries

Muscle injuries in sports are very common. For instance, they represent about 30% of all injuries in elite soccer (Ekstrand et al., 2011). The term muscle injury is used here to describe a lesion to the whole muscular tissue complex, including muscle fibers, intramuscular connective tissues (such as the endo- and perimysium), the fascial envelope around the muscle (epimysium), as well the tendinous extensions. Most athletic muscle injuries affect the lower limb. Even in sports such as tennis and those which are throwing disciplines, injuries of the upper extremity are rare. Age also seems to constitute an important factor. Muscle injuries significantly increase from the age of 25 years upwards. An involvement of connective tissue disruptions in such injuries tends to be associated with longer times needed before returning to play (Renoux et al., 2019). Muscle injuries can have severe consequences for athletic performance, returning to play as well as motivation, and can even lead to financial losses in the case of elite athletes.

Muscles frequently involved in muscle injuries:

- Bi-articular muscles (crossing two joints)
- Muscles with a more complex architecture (e.g., adductor longus)
- Muscles that undergo eccentric contraction
- Muscles that contain primarily fast-twitch type 2 muscle fibers.

The first treatment step in an athletic muscle injury is the establishment of a precise diagnosis, which is crucial for a reliable prognosis. Even although muscle injuries are among the most frequent of all sports injuries (see Chapter 16), they are often evaluated incorrectly and treated inadequately. At the heart of questionable treatment recommendations lies uncertainty, not least because current clinical and imaging diagnosis are inconsistent and not yet sufficiently classified. Consequently, it is frequently difficult to achieve proper assessment of muscle injury and clear communication between practitioners, and the rResulting miscommunication can affect rehabilitation progress, recurrence and complication rates.

To facilitate diagnostic, therapeutic and scientific communication, a precise definition of the English muscle injury terminology is needed.

Classification of athletic muscle injuries

Defining and categorizing athletic muscle disorders has traditionally been difficult because they present a heterogeneous group of muscle disorders. Muscles exist in many different shapes and sizes, and their functional and anatomical organization is complex (Armfield et al., 2006). It is therefore challenging to develop a generally applicable terminology and classification of muscle injuries.

While a number of different classification systems have been published in the literature, little

Chapter 17

consistency exists. The limitations of previous grading systems (e.g. by O'Donoghue, Ryan, Takebayashi, Peetrons, Stoller) include the lack of a differentiated spectrum of muscle injuries in athletes. Furthermore, prior grading systems do not include terminology for muscle injuries without macroscopic evidence of structural damage, even although they have high clinical relevance in professional athletes (Ekstrand et al., 2012).

To better reflect the differentiated spectrum of muscle injuries observed in athletes, and to foster discourse centering on the topic of athletic muscle injuries, a new classification system is proposed and introduced in Table 17.1.

The core aspects of the classification system consist of distinguishing between indirect muscle disorders/injuries and direct muscle injuries, and also explicitly recognizing that functional muscle disorders "without macroscopic" evidence (e.g. in MRI or ultrasound) are a category of athletic muscle injury.

Functional muscle disorder

Functional muscle disorders can be described as acute indirect muscle disorders without macroscopic evidence in MRI or ultrasound. They are often associated with an increase of muscle tone in varying dimensions.

Functional muscle disorders are indirect injuries. They cause more than 50% of the absence of players in professional soccer clubs (Ekstrand et al., 2012). They can also lead to functional limitations. For instance, painful increase of muscle tone can constitute a risk factor for structural injury. However, functional muscle disorders do not show evidence of structural damage in imaging methods such as MRI and are therefore not readily diagnosed with standard diagnostic methods.

Functional muscle disorders can be further distinguished according to the clinical origin of the disorder. There are "overexertion-related" and "neuromuscular" muscle disorders. This distinction is important as it influences the chosen treatment pathway.

Fatigue-induced muscle disorder (type 1A) and delayed onset muscle soreness (type 1B)

Muscle fatigue has been shown to predispose to injury (Opar et al., 2012), for instance, through

Table 17.1 Classification of acute muscle disorders and injuries (adapted from Mueller-Wohlfahrt et al., 2013. Reproduced with permission.)					
A) Indirect muscle disorder/injury				**B) Direct muscle disorder**	
Functional muscle disorder		Structural muscle injury		Contusion	Laceration
Type 1: Overexertion related muscle disorder	Type 2: Neuromuscular muscle disorder	Type 3: Partial muscle tear	Type 4: (Sub)total tear		
Type 1A: Fatigue-induced muscle disorder	Type 2A: Spine-related	Type 3A: Minor partial muscle tear	Subtotal or complete muscle tear		
Type 1B; Delayed-onset muscle soreness (DOMS)	Type 2B: Muscle-related	Type 3B: Moderate partial muscle tear	Tendinous avulsion		

increased stiffness. As warming up prior to activity and maintaining flexibility has been shown to decrease muscle stiffness, it is recommended to include these systematically into each training regimen.

Delayed onset muscle soreness (DOMS) is different to fatigue-induced muscle injury. While it occurs several hours after unaccustomed deceleration movements, fatigue-induced muscle disorders can also manifest during athletic activity. As another distinguishing feature, DOMS causes acute inflammatory pain, stiff and weak muscles, as well as pain at rest. It usually resolves spontaneously within a week. By contrast, fatigue-induced muscle disorders lead to aching muscle firmness that increases with continued activity. If it is unrecognized and untreated, it can persist for a longer time, and consequently may cause structural injuries such as partial tears.

Spine-related (type 2A) and muscle-related (type 2B) neuromuscular muscle disorders

Two different types of neuromuscular disorders can be differentiated, (1) a spinal or spinal nerve-related and (2) a neuromuscular endplate-related type.

In the spine-related neuromuscular muscle disorder, functional or structural spinal or lumbopelvic disorders may lead to an irritation of a spinal nerve root and consequently cause an increase of muscle tone.

Back injuries, particularly at the L4/5 and L5/S1 level, are common among elite athletes. It is also well established that pathologies relating to the lumbar spine, such as disc prolapses at L5/S1 level, may present with hamstring and/or calf pain as well as limitations in flexibility. This, in turn, may result in or mimic a muscle injury (Orchard et al., 2004). Such "lumbar spine-related" hamstring injuries are supported by various studies, although this is a controversial paradigm to researchers.

Against the background sketched above, in the case where a hamstring injury was related to the lumbar spine region, mere treatment of the muscle-tendon unit would not be sufficient. Thus it is important that an assessment of hamstring injury should include a thorough biomechanical evaluation, especially of the lumbar spine, pelvis and sacrum (Woods et al., 2004).

A diagnosis of spine-related neuromuscular disorder is established through clinical functional examination. MRI imaging is usually negative or only shows muscle edema.

The second type of neuromuscular disorder is related to dysfunctions of neuromuscular control mechanisms such as reciprocal inhibition (Figure 17.1).

The neurologic reflex called reciprocal inhibition causes an antagonist muscle to relax when the agonist of a muscle action is contracting. On a neurological level, when sensory information from the agonist muscle is transmitted to the brain, some signals enter the spinal cord, exciting the motoneurons of the associated muscle. Simultaneously, motoneurons of the antagonistic muscles are stimulated via interneurons in the spinal cord, which act via inhibitory synapses.

When the inhibition of the antagonistic muscle is disturbed and agonistic muscles over-contract to compensate for this, normal muscle tone can be significantly impaired, resulting in painful muscle firmness. This may prevent the athlete from participating in sporting activities.

Structural muscle injury

A structural muscle injury is any acute indirect muscle injury "with macroscopic" evidence of muscle damage in MRI or ultrasound.

Chapter 17

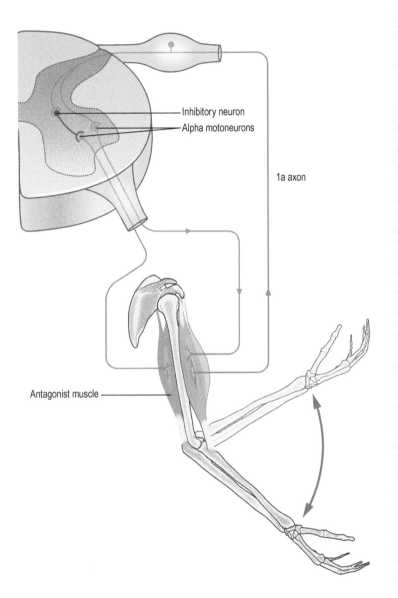

Inhibitory neuron
Alpha motoneurons

1a axon

Antagonist muscle

Figure 17.1 Reciprocal inhibition

When sensory information from the agonist muscle (here: M. biceps brachii) is carried to the brain, afferent signals enter the spinal cord on the alpha motoneuron of the agonist muscle. At the same time, interneurons in the spinal cord act via inhibitory synapses on the alpha motoneurons of antagonistic muscles (here: M. triceps brachii).

The most relevant structural athletic muscle injuries are indirect injuries, that is, stretch-induced injuries caused by a sudden forced lengthening over the viscoelastic limits of muscles occurring during a powerful contraction (internal force) (Figure 17.2).

While a tear can theoretically occur anywhere along the muscle-tendon-bone chain, these injuries are usually located at the muscle-tendon junction because these areas present biomechanically weak points. Due to their large

Classification of athletic injuries to muscular tissues

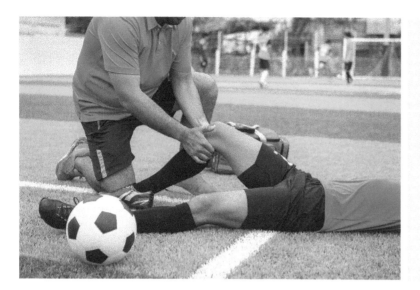

Figure 17.2

In football/soccer, most muscle injuries affect the four major muscle groups of the lower limbs: hamstrings, adductors, quadriceps and calf muscles; 96% of all muscle injuries in football/soccer occur in non-contact situations (Ekstrand et al., 2011).

© iStock.com/nirat.

tendinous structures, the quadriceps muscle and the hamstrings are often affected.

Partial muscle tears (type 3)

The majority of indirect structural injuries are partial muscle tears. We distinguish between minor and moderate partial tears. To differentiate between the two can have consequences for therapy, and consequent return to sports. Minor partial tears present a maximum diameter of less and moderate partial tears a diameter of greater than a muscle fascicle/bundle (Figure 17.3).

In addition to the size, it is the participation of the connective tissue that can distinguish a minor from a moderate partial muscle tear. The fascial structures of endomysium, the perimysium, and the epimysium can be affected. Simultaneous injury of the external perimysium seems to play a special role: the external perimysium has a barrier function within the muscle in case of bleeding. It may be the injury to this connective tissue structure that discerns a moderate from a minor partial muscle tear. While minor partial muscle tears may be accompanied with intramuscular edema, intermuscular edema are more frequently found in moderate partial muscle tears.

Differentiating between partial muscle tears seems difficult because muscles can be structured very differently. Moreover, today's technical capabilities (MRI and ultrasound) are not accurate enough to assess such differences. MRI can be oversensitive and may lead to an overestimation of the actual damage. Further research is needed to be able differentiate minor from moderate partial muscle tears in the future.

Most muscle injuries heal without forming scar tissue. Greater muscle tears can result in a defective healing with scar formation. Minor partial tears usually heal completely while moderate partial tears can result in a fibrous scar.

(Sub)total muscle tears and tendinous avulsions (type 4)

While complete muscle tears are very rare, subtotal muscle tears and tendinous avulsions are more frequent. Subtotal tears involving more than 50% of the muscle diameter usually heal within the same timeframe as complete tears.

Chapter 17

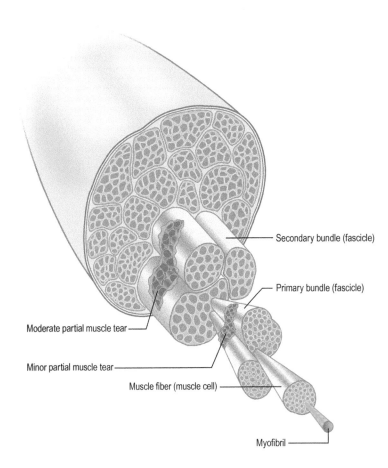

Secondary bundle (fascicle)

Primary bundle (fascicle)

Moderate partial muscle tear

Minor partial muscle tear

Muscle fiber (muscle cell)

Myofibril

Figure 17.3 Illustration of minor and moderate partial muscle tears in relation to the anatomical structures

Understanding the macro- and microanatomy of musculature is important to correctly classify indirect structural injuries. An individual muscle fiber has an average diameter of 60 μm. Usually, an isolated tear of an individual muscle fiber remains without clinical relevance. Secondary muscle bundles are 2 to 5 mm in diameter, are visible to the human eye, and can be palpated by experienced practitioners when they are torn.

(Adapted from Mueller-Wohlfahrt et al., 2013, with permission).

Biomechanically, tendinous avulsions equal a total tear of the origin or insertion of the muscle. The most often involved sites are the proximal parts of rectus femoris, hamstrings and adductor longus, as well as the distal semitendinosus.

Muscle contusions

Indirect injuries, lacerations or contusions are caused by external forces; these are frequently observed in athletes and present a complex injury that includes defined blunt trauma of the muscular tissue and hematoma (Beiner and Jokl, 2001; Kary, 2010). In clinical practice, it is often observed that such contusions do not go along with any recognizable tearing injuries to muscular tissues.

Factors affecting the severity of the injury include the contact force and the contraction state of the affected muscle at the moment of injury. Contusion injuries can be classified as mild, moderate or severe. The muscles that are most frequently affected are the rectus femoris and the intermediate vastus. As they lie next to the bone, they have limited space for movement when exposed to a direct blunt blow and are thus prone to contusion injuries. Interestingly, the

Classification of athletic injuries to muscular tissues

intermediate vastus has been observed to have a very strong tendency towards a degenerative ossification if treated improperly (e.g. with premature loading during a hematoma phase).

Direct injuries such as contusions do not necessarily present with structural damage of muscle tissue. Without such structural damage, athletes may be able to continue competing for a long time, even with more severe contusions. By contrast, an athlete may need to stop immediately when they suffer a fairly small indirect structural injury. However, contusion injuries should not be underestimated. Acute compartment syndrome, active bleeding or large hematomas can be serious and severe complications of contusions.

Diagnosis of muscle injuries

In order to diagnose an athletic muscle injury, we recommend including a precise history of the occurrence. The circumstances and symptoms of the injury as well as previous problems should also be noted. The clinical examination should include inspection, palpation of the injured area, comparison with the unaffected side and functional muscle testing.

Palpation requires experience, sensitivity and intuitive aptitude. The skillful clinical examiner can gather substantial information from palpating the affected area. More superficial and larger tears, particularly of secondary muscle fiber bundles (diameter ~5 mm), as well as perimuscular edema and increased muscle tone, can be detected with seasoned hands.

Practical tip
The physiologic muscle tone varies greatly in athletes. It differs greatly between individuals and depends on training load, type of sport and other factors. It can also vary from side to side.

An ultrasound taken early after the muscle trauma (between 2 and 48 h after injury; Peetrons, 2002) can provide helpful information about any disturbances of the muscle structure. An ultrasound examination is particularly recommended if the clinical examination points towards a functional disorder without the evidence of structural evidence, or if there is any hematoma.

For every injury which is suspicious for structural muscle injury, an MRI examination is recommended. This helps to determine whether and in what pattern edema is present. Furthermore, an MRI can show structural lesions, including approximate size and site of injury. A possible tendon involvement can also be detected via MRI imaging (Askling et al., 2008). However, MRI alone is not sufficiently sensitive to measure the extent of muscle tissue damage accurately. For instance, it cannot be obtained from MRI imaging where edema/hemorrhage is obscuring muscle tissue that has not been structurally damaged.

Practical tip
Changing surfaces, for example, from turf to hall floor or hard courts, leads to an altered demand profile for the musculoskeletal system through, for instance, a receptor-mediated change of muscle tone. The resulting increase in proprioception by the internal structure of the joints inevitably leads to an increase in muscle tone and premature fatigue. This reaction would impede the recovery process after an athletic muscle injury (Figure 17.4). During regenerative training, frequent changes of training surfaces should be avoided.

Typical examples of unnecessary and unfavorable changes of training surface for soccer players include warming up on artificial turf, as well as sprints on all-weather synthetic tracks instead of natural turf.

Chapter 17

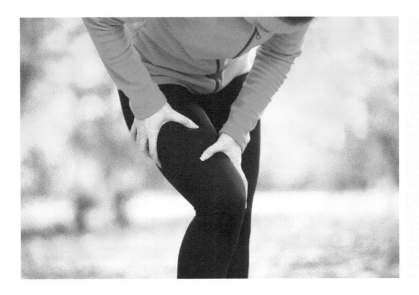

Figure 17.4

Injuries are sometimes under-estimated or not recognized. A consequent premature return to full training constitutes one possible cause for recurrent athletic muscle injury. Muscle and other connective tissue heal gradually. The immature connective tissue scar is the weakest point of the injured muscle (while mature scars are stiffer or stronger than healthy muscle tissue). Regaining full strength of the injured tissue takes time. Size and localization of the injury also plays a significant role on the healing process.

© iStock.com/fizkes

References

Armfield, D.R., Kim, D.H., Towers, J.D., et al. (2006) Sports-related muscle injury in the lower extremity. *Clin Sports Med.* 25: 803–842.

Askling, C.M., Tengvar, M., Saartok, T., et al. (2007) Acute first-time hamstring strains during high-speed running: a longitudinal study including clinical and magnetic resonance imaging findings. *Am J Sports Med.* 35: 197–206.

Beiner, J.M. & Jokl, P. (2001) Muscle contusion injuries: current treatment options. *J Am Acad Orthop Surg.* 9: 227–237.

Ekstrand, J., Hagglund, M. & Walden, M. (2011) Epidemiology of muscle injuries in professional football (soccer). *Am J Sports Med.* 39: 1226–1232.

Ekstrand, J., Healy, J.C., Walden, M., et al. (2012) Hamstring muscle injuries in professional football: the correlation of MRI findings with return to play. *Br J Sports Med.* 46: 112–117.

Kary, J.M. (2010) Diagnosis and management of quadriceps strains and contusions. *Curr Rev Musculoskelet Med.* 3: 26–31.

Mueller-Wohlfahrt, H.W., Haensel, L., Mithoefer, K., et al. (2013) Terminology and classification of muscle injuries in sport: the Munich consensus statement. *Br J Sports Med.* 47: 342–350.

Opar, D.A., Williams, M.D. & Shield, A.J. (2012) Hamstring strain injuries: factors that lead to injury and re-injury. *Sports Med.* 42: 209–226.

Orchard, J.W., Farhart, P. & Leopold, C. (2004) Lumbar spine region pathology and hamstring and calf injuries in athletes: is there a connection? *Br J Sports Med.* 38: 502–504.

Peetrons P. (2002) Ultrasound of muscles. *Eur Radiol.* 12: 35–43.

Renoux, J., Brasseur, J.L., Wagner, M., Frey, A., Folinais, D., Dibie, C., Maiza, D. & Crema, M.D. (2019) Ultrasound-detected connective tissue involvement in acute muscle injuries in elite athletes and return to play: the French National Institute of Sports (INSEP) study. *J Sci Med Sport.* 22: 641–646.

Woods, C., Hawkins, R.D., Maltby, S., et al. (2004) The Football Association Medical Research Programme: an audit of injuries in professional football—analysis of hamstring injuries. *Br J Sports Med.* 38: 36–41.

Fascia, exercise and oncology

Susan Shockett and Thomas Findley

Exercise and cancer

Fascia plays an integral role in physical exercise, contributing to the powerful protective effects that exercise provides against many diseases, including cancer, cardiovascular disease and diabetes (Zügel et al., 2018). Exercise induces a cascade of biological, metabolic and epigenetic changes, with immediate health benefits, and benefits that amplify over time (Hojman et al., 2018). It is one of several lifestyle factors that have been shown to reduce the risk of developing cancer, the second leading cause of death, following cardiovascular disease (Thomas et al., 2017). Globally, one in six deaths is due to cancer. According to the World Health Organization (2018), physical inactivity, dietary factors, tobacco smoking and alcohol consumption are the biggest behavioral risk factors for disease, including cancer.

In addition to helping to prevent cancer, exercise can slow cancer progression (Hofmann, 2018), and can even improve the efficacy of anti-cancer treatments (Hojman et al., 2018). Aerobic exercise has been associated with lower relapse and better survival rates among those living with cancer, as well as improved quality of life (Thomas et al., 2017). Globally, chronic diseases were responsible for 71% of deaths in 2015, and diseases other than cancer were identified as substantial independent risk factors for cancer development. Among people with signs of chronic disease other than cancer, physical activity is associated with a 40% reduced risk of cancer incidence and death. With the global burden of cancer expected to rise by 70% in the next 20 years, leveraging the potential of exercise to prevent cancer incidence and to manage progression and symptoms seems essential (Tu et al., 2018).

Fascia, exercise and adaptation

When evaluating the importance of exercise in disease prevention, it is impossible to assess the effects of our musculoskeletal and cardiovascular systems without considering the contributions of fascia (Zügel et al., 2018). Fascial tissues interpenetrate and surround muscles, and connect muscles (tendons) and bones (ligaments) to bones. The high collagen content of dense fascial tissues allows for the distribution of tensional forces throughout the body. Through secretion of lubricating hyaluronan (e.g., in synovial fluid within joints), the different layers of fascia can slide against each other and other structures, facilitating functional movement (Cowman et al., 2015). Fascia also houses our blood and lymphatic vasculature, and surrounds every organ (Langevin et al., 2016). Fascia is integral in most aspects of physiological function, and it is involved in many avenues of functional improvement as we increase demand.

Our bodies adapt to increased intensity and duration of exercise over time, making it feel easier and less effortful. Our heart and lung functions

Chapter 18

improve, and our muscles become stronger. Within muscle, the numbers of mitochondria (the "powerhouses" of our cells) increase, facilitating greater energy production. Our nervous system extends and strengthens neural connections, providing efficient patterned movements (Kenney et al., 2012). In turn, our multilayered fascial connective tissue system adapts to support the new demands (Langevin et al., 2016).

In response to sufficient aerobic and resistance exercise, our capillary beds expand, allowing for quicker delivery of oxygenated blood, nutrients

and immune cells to key organs and peripheral tissues, as well as removal of waste. Our vascular network, which decreases in both span and range with age, can increase with exercise (Kwak et al., 2018). These are just some of the ways in which our bodies' adaptations to exercise can improve cancer prevention and treatment outcomes, via our intraconnected fascial nets.

Exercise prescription

People who exercise regularly live longer and enjoy a greater quality of life than those who are sedentary (Powell et al., 2019). However, it is estimated that only 20% of adults and adolescents are meeting the minimum recommendations for exercise in the USA (Piercy et al., 2018), with varying rates globally (World Health Organization, 2018). Aerobic capacity decreases by 5–10% per decade in people who are sedentary, with the decline accelerating rapidly with age (Gremeaux et al., 2012). Fortunately, it is never too late in life to start exercising to reap the rewards (Leirós-Rodríguez et al., 2018).

According to the Physical Activity Guidelines for Americans (Piercy et al., 2018), the minimum amount of aerobic exercise recommended per week for adults is 150 min (2.5 h) to 300 min (5 h) at moderate intensity, or 75 min to 150 min (2.5 h) at vigorous intensity, or a combination of both, ideally spread throughout the week. Note that higher intensity exercise is associated with a lower mortality rate than moderate intensity exercise (Samitz et al., 2011). Note also that additional health benefits can be gained by participating in greater amounts of aerobic exercise per week that those levels recommended by the guidelines (Piercy et al., 2018). Children and adolescents aged 6–17 years are advised to participate in ≥60 min of moderate-to-vigorous physical activity each day (Piercy et al., 2018).

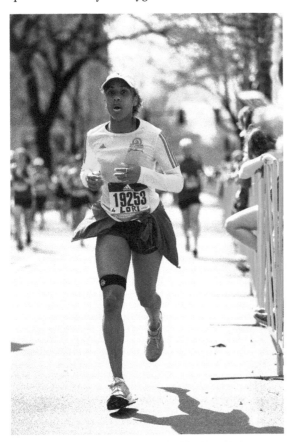

Figure 18.1

It's not so much that I love running but I love how it makes me feel: confident, fit and healthy.

Fascia, exercise and oncology

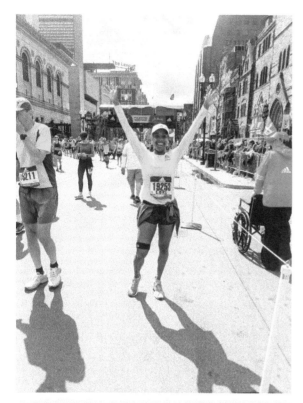

Figure 18.2
Lori Caldon finishing her 16th Marathon; Boston, 2019.

Aerobic exercise (also called endurance or cardio-exercise) is characterized by use of the large muscles of the body in a rhythmic manner over a sustained time period, causing an elevated heart rate and labored breathing. As a benchmark for what defines "moderate" versus "vigorous" aerobic exercise, someone doing moderate-intensity aerobic activity can talk but not sing, and someone doing vigorous-intensity activity typically cannot speak more than a few words without pausing for breath (Samitz et al., 2011).

Light-intensity physical activity such as slow walking may provide some benefit, depending on baseline fitness. And the greatest health benefits have been shown to result from moderate to vigorous intensity exercise, for those who can tolerate this (Aslan et al., 2020). Short increments of aerobic exercise count and are additive (even 1–2 min), particularly at high intensities. And longer durations of sustained aerobic exercise can provide additional benefits. Long duration and high intensity exercise will also more effectively burn fat (Kenney et al., 2012). Remember that while ≥5 h per week at a gym may sound like a lot, time passes quickly on a hiking trail, bike path, dance floor, soccer field, basketball court or ski slope.

In addition to aerobic exercise, adults are recommended to participate in strength training activities of moderate or greater intensity ≥2 days per week, and involving all major muscle groups. Strength training helps to build and maintain muscle, connective tissue and bone, which is particularly important as we age (Leirós-Rodríguez et al., 2018). Older adults should also include balance training in their exercise routines to reduce the risk of falls (Gremeaux et al., 2012). For anyone with acute or chronic conditions or a disability, prior consultation with their medical doctor and exercise physiologist is advisable, to optimize exercise protocol and progression (Piercy et al., 2018).

Exercise has a myriad of health benefits, including increased energy, strength, stamina, weight management, better mood, lower anxiety and depression, and improved sleep. Exercise can reduce resting blood pressure and heart rate (Kenney et al., 2012), decrease "bad" cholesterol and improve insulin sensitivity, with incremental benefits over the long term (Thomas et al., 2017). It also offers powerful cognitive benefits, including improved attention and memory, and may also reduce the risk of and slow progression of Alzheimer's disease (Cass, 2017).

With sufficient intensity and duration, aerobic and resistance exercise have also been

Chapter 18

shown to reduce pain. Exercise can decrease pain both during and after the activity, benefiting people suffering from low back pain, neuropathy, osteoarthritis, fibromyalgia, as well as other painful conditions (Da Silva Santos et al., 2018). While pain reduction is, unfortunately, relevant to us all, it is especially important to those suffering from pain due to disease and its treatment, including cancer. Given the high level of innervation within fascial tissue (Chapter 15) and the recent discovery of endocannabinoid receptors within fascia (Fede et al., 2016), fascia is likely to play a key role in the analgesic (pain reduction) benefits of exercise, among many others (Zügel et al., 2018).

Fascia, exercise and immune function

Fascia is involved in the body's physiological response to exercise, which stimulates immune function (Figure 18.3). Fight or flight hormones (catecholamines), triggered by sufficiently vigorous exercise, induce a rapid increase in immune cells, in particular the Natural Killer (NK) cells (Idorn and Hojman, 2016). Blood vessels, wrapped in part by delicate, adhesive, fascial sheaths called "basement membranes", widen to allow faster flow, based on demand (Pozzi et al., 2017). Then, as blood rushes to supply working muscles with oxygen and nutrients during exercise, immune cells are quickly distributed throughout the body, through fascia-enclosed channels (Thomas et al., 2017).

Some fluid is osmotically pulled out of blood vessels and filtered through the fascial membranes within capillary walls into the surrounding loose fascial connective tissue matrix (termed "the interstitium", i.e., the space in between). In addition to collagen and elastin fibers, the extracellular matrix contains a bed of large, negatively charged, highly absorbant molecules called glycosaminoglycans (GAGs). Hyaluronan (i.e., hyaluronic acid) is one type of GAG common in connective tissue and skin, contributing to the gooey quality of interstitial spaces, and more broadly to tissue hydration. The watery fluid filtered from capillaries forms rivulets, flowing through the denser gel of the interstitial matrix (Scallan et al., 2010).

Most interstitial fluid is absorbed back into the blood. Some interstitial fluid is also picked up from the extracellular matrix by adjacent lymphatic capillaries, to be filtered and recycled. Like blood vessels, lymph vessels are lined in part by adhesive fascial membranes, which serve as filters (Pozzi et al., 2017). Once inside lymph vessels, interstitial fluid is termed "lymph" (Scallan et al., 2010). While the passage of fluid from blood to interstitium to lymph happens continuously, the rate increases dramatically during exercise due to increased blood flow (McFarlane-Parrott, 2018).

Lymph, rich in infection-fighting white blood cells, travels through lymphatic channels to lymph nodes, where pathogens are neutralized, including pre-cancer and cancer cells. Unlike blood, which is pumped by the heart, lymph relies primarily on contractions and movement of skeletal muscle and its associated fascia to accelerate flow. Aerobic exercise, therefore, can rapidly accelerate the rate of lymphatic system filtration, ridding the body of toxins and waste, and helping to prevent disease (McFarlane-Parrott, 2018). It may be that the paucity of metastases found in skeletal muscle (Langevin et al., 2016) is due to the steady cycling of immune cells from our circulatory system, as oxygen and nutrients are fed into working muscles, and waste is filtered out and removed, via fascial enclosures and conduits, and lymphatics.

Fascia, exercise and oncology

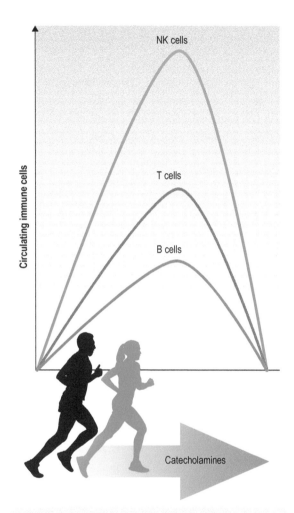

Figure 18.3 Exercise stimulates immune system

During exercise of sufficient intensity and duration, catecholamine (fight/flight hormones) levels in blood rise, including adrenaline. This triggers an increased concentration of circulating immune cells, especially Natural Killer (NK) cells.

Adapted from: Idorn & Hojman. (2016). Exercise-Dependent Regulation of NK Cells in Cancer Protection. Trends in Molecular Medicine, 22(7), 565–577, with permission from Elsevier Science & Technology Journals.

Inflammation, fibrosis and cancer

Fascia is much more than a passive actor in immune function. The extracellular fascial matrix is responsive to the local microenvironment, adapting both biochemically and structurally to demand (Langevin et al., 2016). Fascia houses many bioactive cells, including macrophages, scavenger immune cells which are resident in all tissues. Macrophages identify, engulf and kill bacteria, debris and anything else that the body does not recognize as healthy cells, including cancer cells. Macrophages also play an important role in our adaptive immunity, recruiting additional immune cells to point out unwanted intruders for destruction by "Killer T" cells (Idorn and Hojman, 2016).

Acute inflammation in response to injury facilitates healing, as white blood cells are rushed to injury sites to neutralize invaders and promote wound resolution. Chronic inflammation, however, can become pathological. With the continued release of pro-inflammatory signaling molecules such as Tumor Necrosis Factor, inflammation can damage tissue over the long term and contribute to cancer development (Koelwyn et al., 2015). Chronic inflammation has been linked to tumor formation in several types of cancer (Pedersen et al., 2016).

In response to injury and inflammation, the extracellular fascial matrix will protectively reinforce itself. Excess formation of connective tissue, however, can be damaging, creating stiffness and potentially fibrosis. If not checked, fibrosis can lead to functional limitations. Fascial matrix stiffness has also been identified as a determinant of tumor invasion and progression (Multhaupt et al., 2016). Fortunately, chronic inflammation and associated connective tissue fibrosis can be mitigated to some extent by exercise, which can reduce cancer proliferation, and may help to prevent or slow metastasis (Langevin et al., 2016).

Oncogenesis

Oncogenesis is the process by which healthy cells are transformed into cancer cells. It is characterized by a series of genetic and cellular changes

Chapter 18

that leads to cells dividing in an uncontrolled manner. Cancer is not one single disease; different types of cancer have different risk factors, trajectories and treatment options (World Health Organization, 2018). New research studies are investigating the roles of fascia in both oncogenesis and tumorigenesis.

In general, cancer initiation seems to be due to a combination of environmental and genetic factors, in addition to random DNA replication errors. In support of the role of random duplication errors, tissues with the highest rates of cell division have the greatest risk of developing cancer. Approximately three mutations (replication errors) occur every time that a normal human stem cell divides (Tomasetti et al., 2017).

There are two broad categories of genes affected by replication errors that are most relevant to cancer: oncogenes and tumor suppressor genes. Oncogenes promote the malignant properties of cancer cells and tumor suppressor genes inhibit cancer cell division and survival. Tumor suppressor genes are often disabled by cancer-promoting genetic changes, while oncogenes are turned on. Mutations of the oncogenes can provide the signals for cancer cells to start dividing uncontrollably (López-Lázaro, 2009). These genes have normal, productive functions in healthy cells, but become cancer-promoting when they are mutated or altered in some way.

Certain viruses are considered oncogenic because they incite cancer formation and growth (López-Lázaro, 2009). Globally, it is estimated that 12% of human cancers may be attributable to viruses, including human immunodeficiency virus type 1 (HIV-1), Epstein-Barr virus, hepatitis B and C, and human papilloma viruses (HPVs). Note that while HPV is common, it does not often lead to cancer (National Toxicology Program, 2016).

Environmental and behavioral factors combine with genetic risk and random errors to cause cancer cells to grow and proliferate, and eventually form tumors. DNA damage is frequent and DNA repair processes can eventually become overwhelmed. Multiple genetic changes can accumulate, potentially over many years, to form cancer. Factors that promote oncogenesis include smoking, being overweight or obese, inadequate consumption of fruit and vegetables (resulting in lower levels of antioxidants and potential vitamin and mineral deficiencies), consumption of carcinogenic foods (e.g., red meat), consumption of alcohol, exposure to pollution and physical inactivity (Brown et al., 2012). Fascial connective tissue plays a vital role in preventing tumors from uncontrolled growth and metastasis, and spreading to new sites.

Tumorigenesis and metastases

In order for tumors to grow, they need a steady supply of energy. Tumors eventually need to develop their own vasculature (angiogenesis) as a route for nutrients to be brought in and for waste to be sent out (Kwak et al., 2018). Fascial basement membranes act as mechanical barriers, restricting tumors from forming new blood vessels (Pozzi et al., 2017).

If tumors do develop their own vasculature, they eventually adopt, in effect, a "sweet tooth". All cancer cells seem to have a unique metabolic adaptation that allows them to continuously use glucose for fuel, with or without oxygen (the Warburg effect). This adaptation, common to all cancer types, is the focus of great attention among cancer researchers (Hofmann, 2018).

When oxygen is available, healthy cells typically switch from relying on glucose (glycolysis) to a different metabolic pathway, which can use additional fuel sources such as fat, and generate more ATP (energy). Lactate, a regular by-product of glycolytic metabolism in all cells, is usually recycled efficiently by the liver into glucose, preventing build-up. Only with sufficient duration of high-intensity exercise does lactate production exceed the rate at which it can be recycled, increasing blood lactate concentration. With regular endurance exercise, skeletal muscle can adapt, thus preventing or reducing lactic acid build-up (Kenney et al., 2012).

Lactate is regularly produced in great abundance in cancer cell metabolism. Excess lactate production by cancer cells is shuttled out to the surrounding interstitial spaces and can lead to acidosis and cachexia (wasting) of adjacent tissue. Breakdown of skeletal muscle is a characteristic symptom of cachexia, which can be caused by a number of disease conditions, including cancer (Alves et al., 2015) as well as cancer treatment (Hojman et al., 2018). Cachexia in cancer patients can be due to other factors as well, including increased levels of Tumor Necrosis Factor (involved in inflammation), and is associated with physical inactivity (Hofmann, 2018).

The flexibility that tumor cells have in common, including alterations in fuel utilization and bioenergetics, and resilience to oxidative stress, allows for survival in the face of adverse conditions such as starvation, and during cancer treatments such as chemotherapy. The degree to which cancer cells actively develop these traits does not yet seem to be fully known, versus those cells that have these traits surviving, in a nefarious natural selection process.

Fascial connective tissue serves as a final frontier, preventing metastasis. Fascial membranes surrounding adjacent tissues act as mechanical barriers, preventing tumors from invading and spreading. To infiltrate the vascular or lymphatic systems, tumors must again surpass their protective fascial coverings (Pozzi et al., 2017). A healthy and resilient fascial connective tissue system plays a key role in our defense against tumorigenesis and metastasis.

Efforts to prevent and intercept the complex and potentially deadly progression of cancer development to tumor formation and metastasis are essential. Regular cancer screenings, allowing for early detection and intervention, can be life-saving.

Exercise oncology

Exercise reduces the risk of developing cancer, and of cancer progression and recurrence (Figure 18.4), in concert with an adaptive and responsive fascial network. Immune system stimulation and dissemination through the pores and tunnels of our fascial system is one way that exercise can suppress oncogenesis, tumor formation and growth. Exercise has a variety of effects on immune function, which are accelerated by fight or flight hormones produced during vigorous exercise, such as adrenaline (Pedersen et al., 2016). During intense exercise, our tissues are bathed in blood rich with immune cells. As our vascular network expands and the strength of our heart increases with repeated aerobic exercise, the potential force of this army of immune cells increases over time (Kwak et al., 2018).

As previously discussed, exercise stimulates production and circulation of NK and Killer T cells, among other immune cells (Idorn and Hojman, 2016). These potent protectors against bacteria and viruses are activated and mobilized by intense exercise, reducing systemic inflammation. Since inflammation occurs in a variety of diseases including cardiovascular disease, diabetes and obesity, this anti-inflammatory effect of exercise is key to reducing the risk of cancer for

Chapter 18

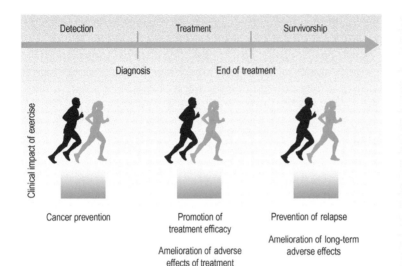

Detection | Diagnosis | Treatment | End of treatment | Survivorship

Clinical impact of exercise

Cancer prevention

Promotion of treatment efficacy

Amelioration of adverse effects of treatment

Prevention of relapse

Amelioration of long-term adverse effects

Figure 18.4 Protective effects of exercise

Aerobic exercise reduces cancer risk, and improves prognosis and quality of life among cancer survivors. Adapted from: Hojman, Gehl, Christensen, & Pedersen. (2018). Molecular Mechanisms Linking Exercise to Cancer Prevention and Treatment.

Adapted from Hojman, J., Gehl, J., Christensen, J.F., et al. (2018). Molecular mechanisms linking exercise to cancer preventions and treatment. *Cell Metabolism*, 27(1): 10–21, with permission from Elsevier Science & Technology Journals.

much of the population. The anti-inflammatory effect of exercise is particularly important for the elderly, who are prone to systemic inflammation, and bear most of the burden of this disease (Thomas et al., 2017).

Exercise has been shown to have epigenetic effects, influencing gene expression and stimulating DNA repair processes. It exerts protective effects against cellular aging over the long term. Telomeres, the protective caps at the end of our chromosomes, indicate biological aging by their length. While telomeres typically shorten as we age, telomeres of people who exercise regularly are longer than those who do not. Decreased oxidative stress is one mechanism by which exercise reduces cellular aging. Oxidative stress can also lead to cancer, particularly when combined with vitamin and mineral deficiencies and other risk factors (Thomas et al., 2017). Exercise can literally keep us "young", and, in turn, decreases the risk of cancer development (Gremeaux et al., 2012).

Exercise also reduces cancer development and progression through effects on metabolism, most notably by helping people to maintain a healthy weight (World Health Organization, 2018). High body fat is linked to an increased risk of developing cancer, due in part to chronic low-grade inflammation (Hojman et al., 2018). In addition, fat cells secrete estrogen and leptin (our satiety hormone), both of which are linked to cell proliferation and cancer growth in high quantities, and both of which are reduced by exercise, independent of weight loss (Thomas et al., 2017). Overweight/obese people also have higher levels of insulin, as well as insulin-like growth factor (IGF-1), linked to cancer proliferation, which can also be reduced by exercise. Decreased levels of IGF-1 are associated with improved survival rates in physically active cancer patients (Thomas et al., 2017). Exercise increases insulin sensitivity (Mctiernan, 2008), allowing healthy cells better access to available glucose for use as fuel. It also plays an important role in helping to reduce visceral fat, which is linked to cancer as well as cardiovascular disease (Koelwyn et al., 2015).

Exercise has a number of additional metabolic and hormonal effects relevant to cancer

Fascia, exercise and oncology

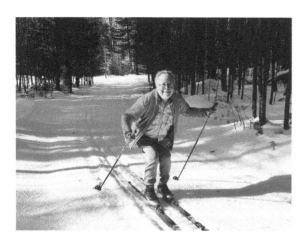

Figure 18.5 Exercise is good medicine.
Tom skiing with Susan, 2018.

prevention and reduction, some of which are not yet fully understood. When muscles contract, hundreds of small proteins are released, some of which have endocrine (hormonal) effects. In response to aerobic exercise, one protein produced by muscle cells is irisin, which has anti-tumor benefits. Irisin has been demonstrated to reduce cancer cell proliferation, and was shown in one study to enhance the effects of chemotherapy without affecting healthy cells (Thomas et al., 2017).

Exercise of sufficient intensity and duration may also play a role in essentially poisoning tumor cells with high lactic acid build-up in the blood, reducing glycolysis and the fuel available for tumor growth. As new blood vessels are formed both in and around tumors in response to repeated exercise, the potency of this effect and others may increase as tumors are dosed with more immune cell- and lactate-rich blood (Hofmann, 2018). This effect is one of many by which exercise can fight tumor growth, delay metastasis and improve treatment outcomes, in addition to preventing cancer development.

Exercise for cancer survivors

Based on recent guidelines, exercise is safe for people diagnosed with cancer, both during and after treatment (Campbell et al., 2019). Very few, if any, negative effects of exercise have been seen in studies of people living with cancer. It is recommended that exercise protocols be adapted for any disease- or treatment-related adverse effects, which can be done in consultation with a medical professional and exercise physiologist (Segal et al., 2017). Depending on the stage of illness and the type of treatment, physical activity may initially need to be light for some people, and increased gradually.

Exercise can improve fitness and strength among people living with cancer, which is important before, during and after treatment. Exercise intensity of moderate and higher levels has been found to most effective in improving fitness (as expected), and has been linked to greater quality of life improvements among cancer survivors, as well as health outcomes. Higher intensity aerobic exercise is suggested for the greatest protective effects against cancer and reduced recurrence, if tolerable (Hofmann, 2018). However, moderate intensity aerobic exercise might be preferred by some people, and thus be more sustainable over their lifetimes, which is the goal (Segal et al., 2017).

In addition to aerobic exercise, resistance training can improve strength and the quality of life for cancer survivors, and it is recommended as part of a regular exercise routine. Patients undergoing androgen deprivation therapy have made substantial increases in strength and endurance with resistance training. Strength training can also improve treatment outcomes (Segal et al., 2017).

Exercise during chemotherapy has been shown to benefit patients with early-stage breast cancer,

Chapter 18

improving the quality of life, chemotherapy completion rates, and possibly contributing to cancer-free survival rates. In a randomized study that compared standard exercise guidelines of 75 min of vigorous aerobic exercise spread over 3 days per week with high-exercise volumes which doubled those durations (50–60 min per session), higher dose exercise was more effective in improving physical functioning and fitness, reducing pain and depression, and improving sleep quality. Among women without significant medical issues (i.e., incomplete axillary or reconstructive surgery), who were approved by their oncologists to participate, higher dose exercise was also enjoyed much more than had been anticipated. Note that study participants with higher initial fitness levels benefited the most from higher dose exercise; those who did not already exercise and were unfit did not show any improvement in sleep quality and neuropathy (Courneya et al., 2016). Unquestionably there are benefits to starting an exercise routine sooner rather than later, and to starting cancer treatment feeling as strong and resilient as possible.

For cancer patients at 4–6 weeks post-chemotherapy treatment without contraindications for high intensity exercise, both low-to-moderate and high-intensity exercise programs combining aerobic and resistance training have been shown to improve physical functioning and reduce fatigue. Higher intensity exercise can yield additional benefits, increasing quality of life and reducing anxiety (Kampshoff et al., 2015). For people unaccustomed to rigorous physical activity, it is not yet known whether it is safe to recommend higher intensity exercise right before or immediately after chemotherapy (Thomas et al., 2017). Therefore it is important to exercise discretion, and to seek medical guidance should there be any question regarding the appropriateness of a new exercise routine.

People are encouraged to decide for themselves what type of exercise program they prefer, incorporating both aerobic exercise and resistance training (if possible). It is important to schedule sufficient recovery time from exercise, particularly for those undergoing cancer treatment. During and immediately after treatment, lighter intensity physical activity might be the most manageable, including slower walking, yoga and other restorative wellness activities. It is good, however, to build fitness and strength to the greatest extent possible, and not to underestimate individual potential. Participation in a group physical activity program can have added social and psychological benefits, and increase motivation and fun (Kenney et al., 2012).

The psychological benefits of exercise are not insignificant for people dealing with cancer, or for anyone else for that matter. Fatigue is a major symptom of cancer treatment and can be debilitating. Fatigue may initially be an obstacle to exercise, but can improve if physical activity is built up gradually. Any amount of physical activity can be beneficial, and some is much better than none. Feeling physically capable and independent is empowering. By reducing pain and improving mood, confidence and cognitive function, exercise can increase quality of life, and indirectly boost immune function, health and longevity (Segal et al., 2017).

Exercise is clearly of significant therapeutic value for people diagnosed with cancer at various stages, as well as for cancer prevention. Our fascial system is integral to the protective benefits of exercise against cancer development and progression, and to overall health. While the extensive roles that fascia plays in exercise oncology have not yet been fully investigated, this is a potent avenue for future research.

References

Alves, C.R.R., Da Cuna, T.F., Da Paixão, N.A., et al. (2015) Aerobic exercise training as therapy for cardiac and cancer cachexia. *Life Sciences*. 125: 9–14.

Aslan, D.H., Collette, J.M., & Ortega, J.D. (2020) Bicycling exercise helps maintain a youthful metabolic cost of walking in older adults. *J Aging Phys Act* [published online ahead of print, 2020 Jul 28]:1–7.

Brown, J., Winters-Stone, K., Lee, A., et al. (2012) Cancer, physical activity, and exercise. *Compr Physiol*. 2: 2775–2809.

Campbell, K.L., Winters-Stone, K.M., & Wiskemann, J., et al. (2019) Exercise Guidelines for Cancer Survivors: Consensus Statement from International Multidisciplinary Roundtable. *Med Sci Sports Exerc*. 51(11): 2375–2390.

Cass, S.P. (2017) Alzheimer's disease and exercise: a literature review. *Curr Sports Med Rep*. 16: 19–22.

Courneya, K., Segal, S., Vallerand, R., et al. (2016) Motivation for different types and doses of exercise during breast cancer chemotherapy: a randomized controlled trial. *Ann Behav Med*. 50: 554–563.

Cowman, M.K., Schmidt, T.A., Raghavan, P., et al. (2015) Viscoelastic properties of hyaluronan in physiological conditions. *F1000 Research*. 4: 622.

Da Silva Santos, R., & Galdino, G. (2018) Endogenous systems involved in exercise-induced analgesia. *J Physiol Pharmacol*. 69: 3–13.

Fede, C., Albertin, G., Petrelli, L., et al. (2016) Expression of the endocannabinoid receptors in human fascial tissue. *Eur J Histochem*. 60: 2643.

Gremeaux, V., Gayda, M., Lepers, R., et al. (2012) Exercise and longevity. *Maturitas*. 73: 312–317.

Hofmann, P. (2018) Cancer and exercise: Warburg hypothesis, tumour metabolism and high-intensity anaerobic exercise. *Sports*. 6: 10.

Hojman, J., Gehl, J., Christensen, J.F., et al. (2018) Molecular mechanisms linking exercise to cancer prevention and treatment. *Cell Metab*. 27(1): 10–21.

Idorn, M. & Hojman, P. (2016) Exercise-dependent regulation of NK cells in cancer protection. *Trends Mole Med*. 22: 565–577.

Kampshoff, C., Chinapaw, M., Brug, J., et al. (2015) Randomized controlled trial of the effects of high intensity and low-to-moderate intensity exercise on physical fitness and fatigue in cancer survivors: results of the Resistance and Endurance exercise After ChemoTherapy (REACT) study. *BMC Med*. 13: 275.

Kenney, W.L., Wilmore, J.H., Costill, D.L., et al. (2012) *Physiology of Sport and Exercise*. Champaign, IL: Human Kinetics.

Koelwyn, G.J., Wennerberg, E., Demaria, S., et al. (2015) Exercise in regulation of inflammation-immune axis function in cancer initiation and progression. *Oncology*. 29: 908–922.

Kwak, S., Lee, J., Zhang, D., et al. (2018) Angiogenesis: focusing on the effects of exercise in aging and cancer. *J Exerc Nutrition Biochem*. 22: 21–26.

Langevin, H., Keely, P., Mao, J., et al. (2016) Connecting (T)issues: how research in fascia biology can impact integrative oncology. *Cancer Res*. 76: 6159–6162.

Leirós-Rodríguez, R., Soto-Rodríguez, A., Pérez-Ribao, I., & García-Soidán, J. (2018) Comparisons of the health benefits of strength training, aqua-fitness, and aerobic exercise for the elderly. *Rehabil Res and Pract*. 8: 5230971–5230978.

López-Lázaro, M. (2009) A new view of carcinogenesis and an alternative approach to cancer therapy. *Mole Med*. 16: 144–153.

McFarlane-Parrott, S.C. (2018) Lymphatic System. *The Gale Encyclopedia of Nursing and Allied Health*, 4th ed. Editor: Jacqueline L. Longe. Volume 4, 2124–2128.

Mctiernan, A. (2008) Mechanisms linking physical activity with cancer. *Nat Rev Cancer*. 8: 205–211.

Multhaupt, H., Leitinger, B., Gullberg, D., & Couchman, J. (2016) Extracellular matrix component signaling in cancer. *Adv. Drug Deliv Rev*. 97: 28–40.

National Toxicology Program (2016) *Report on Carcinogens*, 14th edition. Research Triangle Park, NC: U.S. Department of Health and Human Services, Public Health Service. https://ntp.niehs.nih.gov/go/roc14

Pedersen, L., Idorn, M., Olofsson, G., et al. (2016) Voluntary running suppresses tumor growth through epinephrine- and IL-6-dependent NK cell mobilization and redistribution. *Cell Metab*. 23: 554–562.

Piercy, K.L., Troiano, R.P., Ballard, R.M., et al. (2018) The physical activity guidelines for Americans. *JAMA*. 320: 2020–2028.

Powell, K., King, A., Buchner, D. et. al. (2019) The Scientific Foundation for the Physical Activity Guidelines for Americans, 2nd Edition. *J Phys Act Health.* 16(1): 1–11.

Pozzi, A., Yurchenco, P.D., & Iozzo, R.V. (2017) The nature and biology of basement membranes. *Matrix Biol.* 57–58: 1–11.

Samitz, G., Egger, M., & Zwahlen, M. (2011) Domains of physical activity and all-cause mortality: systematic review and dose–response meta-analysis of cohort studies. *Int J Epidemiol.* 40: 1382–1400.

Scallan, J., Huxley, V.H. & Korthuis, R.J. (2010) *Capillary Fluid Exchange: Regulation, Functions, and Pathology.* San Rafael, CA: Morgan & Claypool Life Sciences. Chapter 2, The Interstitium.

Segal, R., Zwaal, C., Green, E., et al. (2017) Exercise for people with cancer: a systematic review. *Curr Oncol.* 24: E290–E315.

Thomas, R.J., Kenfield, S.A. & Jimenez, A. (2017) Exercise-induced biochemical changes and their potential influence on cancer: a scientific review. *Br J Sports Med.* 51: 640–644.

Tomasetti, C., Li, L., & Vogelstein, B. (2017) Stem cell divisions, somatic mutations, cancer etiology, and cancer prevention. *Science* 355(6331): 1330–1334.

Tu, H., Wen, C.P., Tsai, S.P., et al. (2018) Cancer risk associated with chronic diseases and disease markers: prospective cohort study. *BMJ.* 360: K134.

World Health Organization (2018, September 12) Cancer [Fact sheet]. Retrieved from https://www.who.int/news-room/fact-sheets/detail/cancer

Zügel, M., Maganaris, C.N., Wilke, J. et al. (2018) Fascial tissue research in sports medicine: from molecules to tissue adaptation, injury and diagnostics: consensus statement. *Br J Sports Med.* 52: 1497.

Further reading

American Cancer Society: ACS Guidelines on Nutrition and Physical Activity for Cancer Prevention. https://www.cancer.org/healthy/eat-healthy-get-active/acs-guidelines-nutrition-physical-activity-cancer-prevention.html

National Cancer Institute: Physical Activity and Cancer. https://www.cancer.gov/about-cancer/causes-prevention/risk/obesity/physical-activity-fact-sheet

National Comprehensive Cancer Network: Exercise During Cancer Treatment. https://www.nccn.org/patients/resources/life_with_cancer/exercise.aspx

American College of Sports Medicine: ACM Guidelines for Exercise and Cancer. https://www.acsm.org/blog-detail/acsm-certified-blog/2019/11/25/acsm-guidelines-exercise-cancer-download

U.S. Department of Health & Human Services: Physical Activity Guidelines for Americans, 2nd Edition. https://health.gov/sites/default/files/2019-09/Physical_Activity_Guidelines_2nd_edition.pdf

2
Assessment methods

Assessment of joint mobility

Robert Schleip

Hypermobility and hypomobility: two ends of a phenotypic spectrum

Masi et al. (2007) suggest that myofascial tonicity is regulated as a polymorphic human trait and might contribute to clinical disorders, if the degree is either excessive or insufficient. They propose that evolutionary selection among some of our human ancestors living in artic climates may have favored the increased expression of specific myofascial traits that go along with an increase in tonicity and a concomitant decrease in joint mobility. By contrast, the evolutionary conditions of living in a tropical climate may have fostered myofascial traits associated with increased laxity of the joints. In support of that hypothesis, the authors state the increased prevalence of ankylosing spondylitis (a stiffening of spinal structures) and the relative immunity towards scoliosis among descendants of Scandinavian ancestors and, in addition, the increased occurrence of scoliosis and relative immunity towards ankylosing spondylitis in persons with general hypermobility.

Indeed, population studies indicate that interindividual variation in generalized joint mobility tends to follow a Gaussian distribution. Increasing age and being male are associated with reduced laxity, and a strong effect of family was observed in respective sibling studies. Interestingly, general joint mobility in Asians was shown to be similar to that of non-Asians, although the female/male difference—with women expressing a more "lax" condition—is greater within the Asian group (Silman et al., 1987).

General joint hypermobility can therefore be seen as a natural phenotypical expression of traits observed at the looser end of the continuous spectrum. This condition has been examined as a separate medical entity for several decades (Graham, 1990). Many people with loose joints experience no ill effects and enjoy a symptom-free life. In some professional fields, such as gymnastics and dancing, it is even considered an advantage (Engelbert et al., 2004). When the condition is associated with an increase in chronic musculoskeletal pain, a diagnosis of benign joint hypermobility is applied, provided the individual does not show any signs of neurological, rheumatic, metabolic or skeletal pathologies. The term "benign joint hypermobility syndrome" is used because of the relatively favorable prognosis when comparing this condition with more serious connective tissue disorders associated with hypermobility, such as Marfan syndrome or Ehlers-Danlos syndrome (see Chapter 7).

The prevalence of generalized joint hypermobility in adults as well as children has been reported to vary between 10% and 25% and it appears to be associated with gender, age and race (Engelbert et al., 2004). While general joint hypermobility tends to be associated with an

Chapter 19

increased inclination towards a vast variety of medical disorders, its frequent distribution among chronic myofascial pain patients has been increasingly recognized (Kumar and Lenert, 2017).

The other end of the phenotypic spectrum, generalized hypomobility, has only recently been proposed as a new clinical entity, with specific clinical characteristics that tend to be associated with an increased stiffness of connective tissue as a result of higher amounts of collagen with increased cross-linking (Engelbert et al., 2014). It is believed to be primarily caused by an altered collagen metabolism, which is associated with increased stiffness of dense fascial tissues around the joints, leading to decreases in range of motion of nearly all joints. Interestingly, in children, it tends to be associated with an increased prevalence of habitual toe-walking, an occurrence of hypertrophic scars and an increase in exercise-induced pain in calf, knee and/or hip muscles. Biopsy probes indicated higher amounts of collagen with increased cross-linking. Based on these findings, Engelbert et al. (2004) suggested that similar modifications in collagen metabolism may also be present in other collagenous connective tissues in the body, such as bones and ligaments.

A comparison of children with generalized joint hypomobility and musculoskeletal complaints with healthy children of normal mobility of joints revealed that the following parameters showed a significant difference in joint mobility between the two groups: elbow extension, wrist palmar flexion, wrist dorsal flexion, hip flexion, hip extension, knee flexion, knee extension, ankle dorsal flexion, hip extension and ankle plantar flexion. By contrast, no clear difference was found between the groups for shoulder flexion (i.e. arm elevation in a forward direction),

elbow flexion and hip flexion (Engelbert et al., 2004). It is also of interest that other studies suggest that joint mobility tends to decrease with aging in children (Al-Rawi et al., 1985).

How to measure joint range of motion?

Several assessment methods have been developed. For example, to measure active and passive cervical range of motion, "good" reliability and validity have been confirmed for the CROM device, the Spin-T goniometer and the single inclinometer (Williams et al., 2010). A more recent review concluded that the use of expensive devices (>$500) to measure ACROM in adults with non-specific neck pain did not appear to improve the reliability of the assessment, and that side bending had a lower level of intra-examiner reliability (Rondoni et al., 2017), meaning that repeated assessments by the same examiner in this movement direction lead to more incongruent measurement results. To measure range of motion in lumbar flexion, the fingertip-to-floor distance test and the modified Schober test showed excellent inter-examiner reliability. However, they were not particularly sensitive in detecting the smallest possible changes. The medium correlation between these two assessments suggested that they do not assess precisely the same phenomenon and hence should be used in combination (Robinson and Mengshoel, 2014). A more recent study documented good-to-excellent reliability and validity for measuring lumbar spine flexion and extension range of motion with either a gravity-based goniometer or an iPhone® application (Pourahmadi et al., 2016).

Assessment tools for hypermobility

Several questionnaires have been developed for assessing general joint hypermobility (Meyer et al., 2017; Nicholson and Chan, 2018). However,

Assessment of joint mobility

in clinical practice, the use of an *in vivo* examination of joint mobility is more common, such as the Beighton scale (see Chapter 6) or the Hospital del Mar criteria (Bulbena et al., 1990). A method comparison investigation confirmed that the inter- and intra-rater reliability for total scores was good-to-excellent for the Beighton scale as well as the Hospital del Mare criteria when following a structured protocol. However, the reliability was poor-to-moderate in some single joint measurements of the latter protocol, indicating difficulties in the performance of these tests (Schlager et al., 2018). No wonder that the Beighton scale, straightforward as it is, continues to enjoy a very wide application among therapists working with hypermobility.

Measuring hypomobility

In contrast to hypermobility, the assessment for limited joint range of motion (hypomobility) is less well developed. Engelbert et al. (2004) developed a procedure of measuring active joint range of motion by use of a standard goniometer applied to specific anatomical landmarks. The examination was conducted bilaterally to the nearest 5 degrees. The investigation included shoulder flexion, elbow motion (flexion/extension), wrist motion (palmar/dorsal flexion), hip joint (flexion/extension), knee motion (flexion/extension) and ankle mobility (plantar/dorsal flexion). The index of total range of motion consisted of a summing up of all measurements. The authors propose a scoring system, in which local hypomobility is present when the range of joint motion in that joint is lower than -1 standard deviation of a healthy control group. In addition, the authors suggest that if local joint hypomobility is present in several joints of the lower and of upper extremities then the term "generalized hypomobility syndrome" may be applicable.

Their mean values and standard deviations from 284 healthy children are available from Engelbert et al. (2004). Unfortunately, no comparable data pool exists concerning the data distribution from healthy adults.

Schleip and Buschman (2016) introduced a "Viking Test" as well as a separate "Cross Over Test" for the self-assessment of joint mobility restrictions. Similar to the well-established Beighton test (described in Chapter 7), these free-of-charge tests do not require any professional measurement equipment and aim for a relatively quick preliminary indication as to whether an individual may be prone to general hypomobility and/or to a more selective expression of only a few typical joint restrictions.

While both of these tests have been frequently used by athletes as well as lay persons and each has demonstrated good applicability in almost all practiced administrations, to date no statistical data have been published regarding the normative distribution of measurement results in different gender and age groups in a healthy population. This lack of scientific exploration is partially comparable with the previously described hypomobility assessment from Engelbert et al. (2004) in its application to adult individuals.

The Viking Test for general hypomobility

The name Viking Test is inspired by the reportedly increased prevalence of fascial contractures, such as Morbus Dupuytren (a shortening and stiffening of the palmar fascia of the hand; also called Viking's disease) and other fibrotic pathologies among descendants of northern European ancestors (Masi et al., 2007).

In this test the person collects points for movement restrictions. The more points you get, the more Viking-like, or more hypomobile, you are.

Chapter 19

VIKING TEST

Your Viking points:

Having less than 3 points in the Beighton test (see Figure 7.1)

If so then start this test by giving yourself 3 Viking points.

By contrast, a Beighton score of ≥3 will result in zero Viking points at this time.

(Note: if you have between 0 and 2 points in the Beighton test, you need to award yourself 3 Viking points. And if you have between 3 and 9 points in the Beighton test then you will need to give yourself 0 Viking points.)

Hands reaching behind back

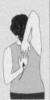

If you cannot touch your hands behind your back and the minimal distance between them is more than 1½ hand-length (no matter on which side):

1 Viking point

Trunk rotation

Sitting on a stool or chair (without leaning against a backrest), try to rotate your head and upper torso as far as possible to the right and to the left while keeping your legs and pelvis fixated.

If you cannot turn at least 90 degrees to the easier side:

1 Viking point

Trunk extension

Sitting on a stool or chair as before, place one hand on your lower belly with your thumb touching the navel and the other hand in front of your sternum (or chest bone).

Now try to move your hands as far as possible away from each other by extending your whole torso, including your head, thorax and pelvis.

If you cannot increase the distance between your hands by at least one handwidth:

1 Viking point

Knee to forehead

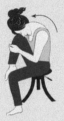

While sitting, try to touch your forehead with one knee at a time.

If you cannot touch your forehand with either of your knees:

1 Viking point

Forward bending

Repeat the forward bending test (from the previous Beighton test). Make sure not to bend your knees.

If you cannot get closer with your fingertips to the floor than one hand-length distance:

1 Viking point

Total points
(up to a maximum of 9)

Continued

Continued

Additional age and gender bonus

Choose one option only:

Male aged >35 years: minus 2 points	
Male aged ≤35 years: minus 1 point	
Female aged >35 years: minus 1 point	
Female aged ≤35 years: no minus points	
Corrected final point total:	

Evaluation:

5–9 points:
   You are most likely genetically equipped with a Viking (i.e. hypomobile) body constitution, which partly sacrifices mobility in favor of stability.

3–4 points:
   Your genetic constitution is not conclusive. Your life history and training may shape your tissue constitution as much as your genetic constitution.

1–2 points:
   No clear constitutional tendency towards hypomobility.

The Crossover Test for assessment of "lifestyle-associated" local movement restrictions

This test examines to what degree your body expresses movement restrictions, which were described by the Czech rehabilitation expert Vladimir Janda (1928–2002). He observed that many people in Western society express particular postural and movement patterns, which are characterized by chronic contractures of certain muscles as well as muscular weakness in other areas (Janda, 1989, 1993). While his publications mainly emphasized the neuromuscular components, several of his followers extended this concept to also include the tonicity of myofascial connective tissues (Liebenson, 2001; Page et al., 2009).

According to this concept, a common pattern of muscular (or myofascial) imbalance is described as "upper-crossed syndrome" and includes an increased tonicity and stiffness in the region of the upper posterior neck and pectoral region. This is accompanied by a decreased tonicity in the anterior neck and of the inferior shoulder blade stabilizers, while the posture is characterized by rounded shoulders and a head-forward position.

The "lower-crossed syndrome" is characterized by an increased tonicity and stiffness in the lower back, hip flexors and posterior leg muscles. This is accompanied by weakness and flaccidity in the abdominal muscles and the gluteus maximus, while the habitual posture expresses a lumbar lordosis and forward tilted pelvis (Figure 19.1).

While the more detailed assessment of Janda required more time than many therapists were willing to invest for quick client evaluation, the following short test was developed with the aim of providing an initial orientation to what degree (if at all) the myofascial system of a given client matches the typical imbalances described by this model. Note that proponents of Janda's model tend to attribute these imbalances to lifestyle features, such as habitual over-usage and under-usage of specific muscles, which tends to change their

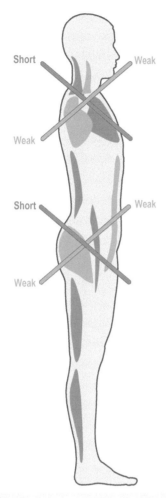

Figure 19.1

Typical patterns of hypomobility (described as "short") versus areas of muscular weakness described by Vladimir Janda's mode of "upper-crossed syndrome" and "lower-crossed syndrome". These patterns describe frequent expressions of muscular imbalance, most often caused by habitual over- and under-usage of specific motor patterns in everyday life.

© fascialnet.com.

chronic tonicity. The test, therefore, relates less to genetic than to acquired musculoskeletal patterns. It also emphasizes primarily the related mobility restrictions in the assessment, while considering associated muscular weaknesses as secondary and supportive parameters.

CROSSOVER TEST

In this test, the client also collects points for movement restrictions. The more points you get, the more of these specific restrictions you have, and the more likely it is that you may fit into this typology. Each single test describes a specific movement exploration as well as a typical "pattern description" that characterizes a respective movement restriction.

If a described pattern description fits
clearly for you: 2 points
If it could possibly fit: 1 point
If it clearly does not fit: 0 points

	Points:
Chin-to-chest test With your mouth closed, tilt your forehead downwards while trying to touch your chest bone with your chin. Pattern description: you cannot bring the chin and the chest bone to touch each other, and the minimal distance between them is more than the width of two fingers.	
Knee-to-wall test 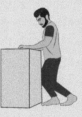 Stand in front of a wall, solid furniture, or similar, while touching the wall or furniture with both hands at an easy height. Place one foot so far forward on the ground that it touches the wall in front slightly, while you allow the same knee to be bent. Now slide this foot very slowly backwards on the ground while maintaining the contact between that knee and the wall.	

Continued

Find out how far you can slide the foot backwards until the knee loses the contact with the wall in front.

Pattern description: the maximal distance between the front of the sliding foot and the wall is one handwidth or more, no matter on which leg you perform this test.

Resting angel test

Lying on your back place your arms (if possible) into a position with 90 degree angles at the shoulder and elbow joints. In this position, slowly slide your upper arms towards the head while keeping your elbows and lower arms in contact with the ground.

Find out how far you can slide in this manner until the elbow and/or lower arms start to detach from the floor.

Pattern description: you cannot abduct the arms further than 45 degrees from the starting position (without detaching from the ground), no matter which arm you examine.

Hip-extension test

Lying prone on the ground, lift one lower leg towards the ceiling and then try to lift that knee slowly off the ground, while checking with one of your hands how far you can lift that knee without tilting your pelvis into a lordosis.

Pattern description: you are unable to lift the knee further than one hand-length away from the floor (without any pelvic tilt motion), no matter on which leg you conduct this examination.

Total (up to a maximum of 8 points)	

Evaluation:

6–8 total points:	clear Crossover type.
3–5 total points:	partially a Crossover type.
0–2 total points:	you are not a typical Crossover type.

Clinical summary

- While assessment of hypermobility is supported with evidence-based examinations, this is less the case with the respective assessments of either general or localized movement restrictions.

- While general hypermobility and general hypomobility tend to express two opposite ends of a phenotypic spectrum (and therefore usually exclude each other), the described cross-over pattern expresses myofascial features that are primarily shaped by habitual lifestyle factors and can therefore sometimes be found to coexist with either a general hypermobile or hypomobile constitutional tendency.

- If the Beighton test (described in detail in Chapter 7) indicates a clear hypermobility pattern, it is advisable to seek additional input and advice from a qualified health professional, particularly if this situation is accompanied with chronic myofascial pain.

Continued

Chapter 19

- A similar recommendation can be given if a clear Viking pattern or cross-over pattern is indicated with the respective mobility assessments, and if it is accompanied with chronic myofascial pain.

- It is also not uncommon for many people to function happily and healthily in their biopsychosocial environment while expressing a clear hypermobility or Viking pattern. Nevertheless, the described examinations may support these people in better understanding the relative strength and weaknesses of their specific musculoskeletal system.

References

Al-Rawi, Z.S., Al-Aszawi, A.J. & Al-Chalabi, T. (1985) Joint mobility among university students in Iraq. *Br J Rheumatol.* 24: 326–331.

Bulbena, A., Duro, J.C., Porta, M., Faus, S., Vallescar, R. & Martin-Santos, R. (1992) Clinical assessment of hypermobility of joints: assembling criteria. *J Rheumatol.* 19: 115–122.

Engelbert, R.H., Uiterwaal, C.S., van de Putte, E., Helders, P.J., Sakkers, R.J., van Tintelen, P. & Bank, R.A. (2004) Pediatric generalized joint hypomobility and musculoskeletal complaints: a new entity? Clinical, biochemical, and osseal characteristics. *Pediatrics.* 113: 714–719.

Graham, R. (1990) The hypermobility syndrome. *Ann Rheum Dis.* 49: 199–200.

Grahame R. (2009) Joint hypermobility syndrome pain. *Curr Pain Headache Rep.* 13: 427–433.

Janda, V. (1989) Impaired muscle function in children and adolescents. *J Man Med.* 6: 157–160.

Janda V. (1993) *Muscle Function Testing.* London, UK: Butterworths.

Kumar, B. & Lenert, P. (2017) Joint hypermobility syndrome: recognizing a commonly overlooked cause of chronic pain. *Am J Med.* 130: 640–647.

Liebenson, C. (2001) Sensory-motor training. *J Bodyw Movem Ther.* 5: 264–268.

Masi, A.T., Benjamin, M. & Vleeming, A. (2007) Anatomical, biomechanical, and clinical perspectives on sacroiliac joints: an integrative synthesis of biodynamic mechanisms related to ankylosing spondylitis. In: *Movement, Stability and Lumbopelvic Pain,* 2nd edn (eds Vleeming, A., Mooney, V. & Stoeckart, R.), pp. 205–227. Edinburgh, UK: Churchill Livingstone Elsevier.

Meyer, K., Chan, C., Hopper, L. & Nicholson, L. L. (2017) Identifying lower limb specific and generalised joint hypermobility in adults: validation of the Lower Limb Assessment Score. *BMC Musculoskelet Dis.* 18: 1–9.

Nicholson, L.L. & Chan, C. (2018) The Upper Limb Hypermobility Assessment Tool: A novel validated measure of adult joint mobility. *Musculoskelet Sci Pratt.* 35: 38–45.

Page, P., Frank, C.C. & Lardner, R. (2009) *Assessment and Treatment of Muscle Imbalance: The Janda Approach.* Champaign, IL: Human Kinetics.

Pourahmadi, M.R., Taghipour, M., Jannati, E., Mohseni-Bandpei, M.A., Ebrahimi Takamjani, I. & Rajabzadeh, F. (2016) Reliability and validity of an iPhone® application for the measurement of lumbar spine flexion and extension range of motion. *Peer J.* 4: e2355.

Robinson, H.S. & Mengshoel, A.M. (2014) Assessments of lumbar flexion range of motion: intertester reliability and concurrent validity of 2 commonly used clinical tests. *Spine.* 39: E270–E275.

Rondoni, A., Rossettini, G., Ristori, D., Gallo, F., Strobe, M., Giaretta, F., Battistin, A. & Testa, M. (2017) Intrarater and inter-rater reliability of active cervical range of motion in patients with nonspecific neck pain measured with technological and common use devices: a systematic review with meta-regression. *J Manipulative Physiol Ther.* 40: 597–608.

Schlager, A., Ahlqvist, K., Rasmussen-Barr, E., Bjelland, E.K., Pingel, R., Olsson, C., Nilsson-Wikmar, L. & Kristiansson, P. (2018) Inter- and intra-rater reliability for measurement of range of motion in joints included in three hypermobility assessment methods. *BMC Musculoskelet Disord.* 19: 376.

Schleip, R. & Buschmann, B. (2016) *Faszien Krafttraining.* Munich, Germany: Riva Verlag.

Silman, A.J., Day, S.J. & Haskard, D.O. (1987) Factors associated with joint mobility in an adolescent population. *Ann Rheum Dis.* 46: 209–212.

Williams, M.A., McCarthy, C.J., Chorti, A., Cooke, M.W. & Gates, S. (2010) A systematic review of reliability and validity studies of methods for measuring active and passive cervical range of motion. *J Manipulative Physiol Ther.* 33: 138–155.

Imaging techniques (ultrasound)

Wolfgang Bauermeister and Frieder Krause

Introduction

The health status of soft tissue can be estimated by measuring its elasticity, which has an impact on tissue motion. The examination of soft tissue with conventional ultrasound helps to detect lesions in the fascia, muscles and organs, but without gaining information about its elastic properties. The measurement of elastic properties can be achieved by tracking the deformation of soft tissue in B-Mode images using speckle tracking or by using cross-correlation techniques, either as direct motion measurement or elastography for strain assessment. Finding the areas of altered elasticity and reinstating normal elasticity through appropriate treatment makes tissue movement analysis and elastography an important diagnostic feature for treatment decisions and for monitoring the reaction to different treatment modalities.

In vivo evaluation of connective tissue movement

Sonography is the only method that allows the clinician a radiation-free evaluation of tissue movement with the necessary temporal and graphical resolution *in vivo*. When recording high-definition ultrasound videos, these can be used to track the movement of connective tissue. One possibility is the cross-correlation method developed in MATLAB (MathWorks, Natick, MA) by Dilley et al. (2001). It is basically a speckle- or pixel-tracking algorithm that uses the digital information of video data to track the movement of selected regions. The method is described and discussed in the following section.

Cross-correlation analysis

As previously mentioned, the cross-correlation analysis uses videos recorded with a high-definition ultrasound device to track the movement of selected areas or tissues. In the first step, the video is loaded into the software and converted into individual gray level frames. In the next step, you can select as many rectangle-shaped regions of interest (ROIs) as you wish to track from the first frame of the video. In the actual analysis, the correlation coefficient between the pixel gray levels for all selected ROIs in two adjacent images is calculated. The pixel shift providing the maximum correlation coefficient corresponds to the relative movement between two frames (Dilley et al., 2001). This is repeated for all adjacent frames to calculate the movement off the ROIs during the recorded period. To control background movement, an additional ROI can be placed on the skin or a bony structure, which remain static during the movement that is being tracked. The background movement is then subtracted from the original results.

The method was originally developed for and has been extensively used to quantify nerve movement *in vivo*. Studies on reliability show promising results, so it has been described as a reliable method with an ICC ranging from 0.70–0.99 (Boyd et al., 2012; Carroll et al., 2012; Dilley et al., 2001, 2007; Ellis et al., 2008, 2012).

Chapter 20

It has also been used in research to quantify the movement of connective tissue during passive movement. Langevin et al. (2011) were the first to show changes in fascial shear strain in the thoracolumbar fascia in patients with unspecific low back. More recently, Griefahn et al. (2017) used a similar approach to quantify the fascial mobility of the thoracolumbar fascia after foam rolling at the dorsal body. Unfortunately, no measures for reliability were calculated in these studies.

In our laboratory, we used the cross-correlation method to quantify the movement of different layers of the fascia lata at the anterior thigh. Here, movement of the superficial ($ICC_{(3,1)} = 0.88$ (0.75–0.95), $P < 0.0001$) and deep layer ($ICC_{(3,1)} = 0.77$ (0.55–0.91), $P < 0.0001$) showed good reliability (Krause, 2018). To provide a better understanding of the methodology of the cross-correlation, our research approach is described below.

To evaluate the movement of different fascial layers at the anterior thigh, six equidistant ROIs per fascial layer were chosen to steadily evaluate movement of the layers. Figure 20.1 shows the original US signal at the beginning of the video (Figure 20.1A) and the six ROIs per fascial layer

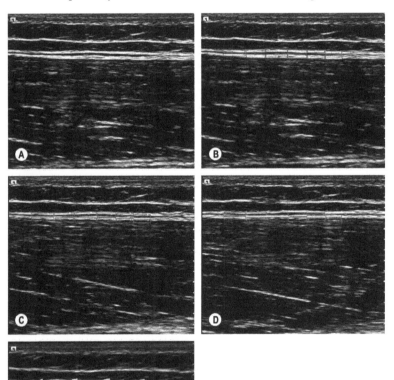

Figure 20.1

20.1A Raw ultrasound video signal at the beginning of the recorded video.

Structures (top to bottom): skin, subcutaneous fat, subcutaneous connective tissue, superficial layer of deep fascia, loose connective tissue (enriched with hyaluronic acid), deep layer of the deep fascia and rectus femoris muscle.

20.1B Selection of six equidistant ROIs in each fascial layer in the first video frame.

20.1C Graphical results of the cross-correlation analysis after 5 s of the recorded video.

20.1D Graphical results of the cross-correlation analysis after 10 s of the recorded video.

20.1E Resulting line graph of the movement of all selected ROIs.

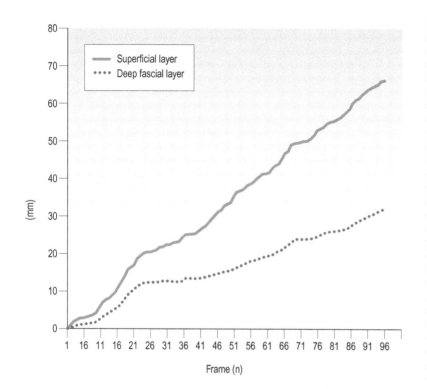

Figure 20.2

Movement of the superficial and the deep fascial layer during the recorded video sequence.

(Figure 20.1B). The movement of each individual ROI in the middle (5 s) and at the end (10 s) of the recorded video is shown in Figures 20.1C and 20.1D, respectively. Figure 20.1E shows the resulting line graph of the movement of all selected ROIs.

The blue boxes are the selected ROIs in each fascial layer, the small white squares represent the mean movement of all twelve ROIs, while the slightly bigger yellow squares represent the movement of individual ROIs. To quantify the movement of each layer, the mean movement of the six ROIs per fascial layer was calculated (Figure 20.2).

Traditionally, ultrasound has extensively been used in internal medicine, cardiology and gynecology. However, new improvements in temporal and graphical resolution have led to increased use in orthopedics as well as in exercise and sport science research in recent years. The cross-correlation analysis is a useful method to extract quantitative information on tissue movement from high-frequency ultrasound data.

Ultrasound elastography

Introduction

Manual palpation is an important assessment tool for estimating the pathological state of soft tissue. The goal is to identify myofascial areas that are structurally or functionally compromised. Surface pressure application gives feedback about the tissue strain, and skin drag provides information about shear strain. Communication about these findings is difficult

Chapter 20

because of a lack of numerical values that would accurately quantify them. Palpation is often limited to larger superficial structures with a high stiffness contrast compared to the surrounding areas. Smaller, areas with lower stiffness contrast or deep lying changes can often be overlooked even though they can play an important role in pain and dysfunction.

Conditions causing myofascial stiffness

Soft tissue health can be reflected by the degree of stiffness changes caused by various conditions and in sports often through neurogenic inflammation (NI) as a reaction to trauma of any kind (Toumi and Best, 2003); conversely tendons can react with a softening (Aubry et al., 2015). With micro-analytical techniques *in vivo*, it is possible to identify those biochemicals which are associated with NI of the myofascia in active myofascial trigger points (Shah et al., 2008). Under experimental conditions increase of fascia stiffness can be related to isometric strain and changes in tissue hydration (Schleip et al., 2012). Clinically myofascial trigger points, fibrosis and or densification are possible causes of increased fascial stiffness.

Myofascial stiffness can affect the joint range of motion, fascial glide, strength, posture and motor unit recruitment measured with electromyography. Conventional X-ray, MRI, CT-scan or ultrasound cannot identify stiffness, but magnetic resonance elastography (MRE) and forms of ultrasound elastography (UE) can.

Ultrasound elastography methods

Besides MRE which is exclusively available for research, strain elastography (SE) and shear wave elastography (SWE) are in clinical use for tumor detection, staging of liver fibrosis and musculoskeletal applications. Both methods differ by the way of stress application to create tissue-motion, by their results—quantitative vs. qualitative—operator dependency, depth of penetration and the size of the region of interest (ROI) .

Strain elastography

SE (synonym: compression-, or static-elastography) was first introduced by Ophir at al. (1991). It requires rhythmic manual pressure on the surface of the tissue with the ultrasound transducer producing a compressive strain. Compressive strain is the ratio of an objects change in thickness Δl to its initial thickness l (Compressive strain = $\Delta l/l$) which is dimensionless (Figure 20.3).

An elastogram is an image with color-coded strain representation. In stiff tissue the strain is small; in softer tissue high (Garra, 2007). SE produces qualitative images and requires areas of different strain within the region of interest (ROI). The consequence is that equally stiff tissue within the ROI does not give a result because of a lack of strain differences. From the qualitative elastogram numeric values can be obtained by counting the pixels which represent hard or soft with the software Image J (Abramoff et al., 2004). SE allows semi-quantitative measurements by calculating a strain ratio (SR) of two different areas. It is calculated by dividing the strain of a reference area by the strain of a target area. SR = Strain of reference (B)/Strain of a target (A). When the target area has a higher strain (softer) the SR is >1, when the target area has a lower strain (stiffer) the SR is <1. A Strain elastogram (Figure 20.4) shows a strain ratio of 2.59 between the fascia (Target 1A) with a strain of 0.19% and the muscle (Reference 2B) 0.50%. The fascia has a lower strain value, which means it is 2.59 times stiffer compared to the muscle with higher strain.

Imaging techniques (ultrasound)

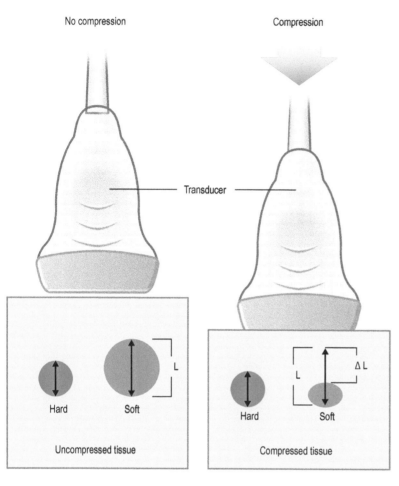

No compression

Compression

Transducer

L

Hard   Soft

Uncompressed tissue

Hard   Soft

L   ΔL

Compressed tissue

Figure 20.3

Through a rhythmic compression of the tissue a time shift occurs in the echo signal which is proportional to the strain of the tissue.

The quality of the elastogram can be strongly operator dependent when the compression/decompression cycle requires and amplitude of several millimeters. Newer technologies need minimal transducer motion for excitation or even use internal motion generated through pulse or breathing to obtain the elastogram. Interrater reliability studies show a relatively good agreement provided the tissue is not too soft (Boettner 2018). When the transducer is driven by a computer-controlled shaker, all operator induced artefacts can be eliminated resulting in a stable reproducible elastogram (Bauermeister 2017).

Shear wave elastography

Shear wave elastography was first mentioned 1995 (Sarvazyan et al. 1995) as a quantitative measure of tissue stiffness versus the qualitative assessment with SE. Instead of manual compression in SE with a tissue displacement up to 3 mm like, tissue peak displacement in the order of i.e. 10 μm or more is achieved through a push beam generated with an acoustic radiation force impulse (ARFI) emitted from the ultrasound probe (Nightingale et.al., 2002). The resulting shear waves are perpendicular to the direction of excitation force in a transverse

Chapter 20

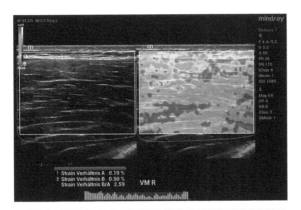

Figure 20.4

Mindray Resona 7 Strain elastography. The fascia (Target 1A) with a strain of 0.19 and the muscle (Reference 2B) 0.50%. The fascia has a lower strain value, which means it is 2.59 times stiffer compared to the muscle with higher strain.

direction (Figure 20.5). The resulting shear waves detected through the tracking beam of the ultrasound probe which generates the push beam. In Figure 20.6 the shear waves are shown as they travel through the ROI. Parallel lines indicate reliable, distorted lines unreliable measurements.

The push beam has a duration of less than a microsecond, the resulting shear waves persist for several milliseconds (Sarvazyan et. al. 1998). By measuring the peak to peak duration, the speed of the shear wave v (nu) propagation expressed in m/sec can be derived. The propagation speed v is higher in stiff and lower in soft tissue. From the propagation speed v the Shear Modulus G in kPa or Young's Modulus E in kPa can be estimated with the formula: $E = 3G = 3\rho v^2$. In this formula ρ (rho) is the mass density of the tissue, assumed to be ≈ 1. Figure 20.7 shows a shear wave elastogram of the thoraco lumbar fascia TLF (Trace 1) with a mean Young's

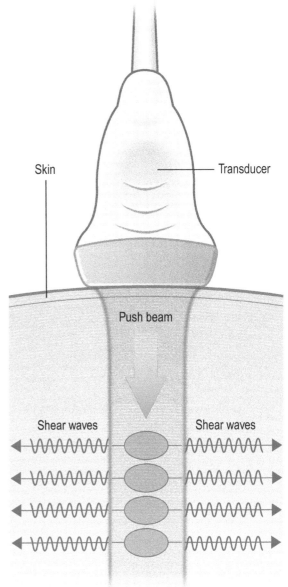

Figure 20.5

The resulting shear waves are perpendicular to the direction of the push beam in a transverse direction.

Imaging techniques (ultrasound)

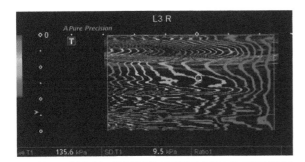

Figure 20.6

Canon Aplio 500. Shear wave pattern. Parallel lines indicate reliable—distorted lines unreliable—measurements.

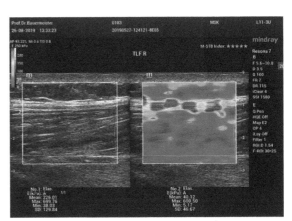

Figure 20.7

Mindray Resona 7. Shear wave elastogram of the thoraco lumbar fascia TLF (Trace 1) with a mean Young's modulus of 226.01 kPa and muscle (Trace 2) with a mean Young's modulus of 40.12 kPa

modulus of 226.01 kPa and muscle (Trace 2) with a mean Young's modulus of 40.12 kPa.

Other shear wave forms are supersonic shear wave imaging (SSI) (Bercoff et.al., 2004) which has been used widely in muscle research and acoustic radiation force impulse imaging (ARFI) (Sarvazyan et.al., 2011).

Ultrasound elastography research of the myofascial and clinical application

The focus of myofascial research with ultrasound-elastography is to establish normative values for muscle, fascia and tendons. In sports medicine injury prevention is a major concern where early recognition of increased myofascial stiffness could play an important role. A pilot study on 20 juvenile soccer players, mean age 15 years, showed a statistical difference for the rectus femoris muscle/fascia and the fascia of the vastus medialis and adductor magnus (highlighted yellow). (Table 20.1) (K. Bauermeister, 2021). Table 20.2 shows measurements of muscles, the thoraco lumbar and the plantar fascia of 45 males, mean age 35 years, with a high physical work load with statistically significant left/right differences of the

rectus femoris and the plantar fascia (highlighted yellow). Table 20.3 is an example of how to translate SWE measurements into a treatment strategy. Here the patient is its own control by comparing the left to the right side. Significant discrepancies between the left and the right side are marked in red. The effect of a therapeutic intervention can be monitored by reevaluating at the same measurement points after the intervention.

Comparing SWE results obtained with equipment from different manufacturers can produce different results. There are no agreed standards about the generation and frequency of the push beam. The size of the area where measurements within the ROI can be made varies widely.

They range from some square millimeters to several square centimeters. Comparing study results is difficult because researches arbitrarily chose regions of the fascia or within the muscles which appear homogeneous to them. Areas with very high kPa-values are usually omitted

Chapter 20

Table 20.1 Medians and means of Young's moduli in left/right comparison. Significant differences are highlighted yellow (see text page 231)

Region	Fascia left	Fascia right	Muscle left	Muscle right
Tensor fasciae latae	43.33 (17.75)	43.85 (20.06)	30.82 (13.65)	32.03 (9.63)
Rectus femoris middle	24.19 (8.91)	20.46 (9.02)	20.62 ± 8.34	17.36 ± 3.56
Distal rectus femoris	22.46 (20.35)	22.91 (14.12)	26.46 (38.98)	29.51 (22.73)
Vastus medialis	13.73 (4.70)	11.53 (5.60)	13.67 (3.04)	13.43 (3.60)
Vastus lateralis	111.52 ± 37.12	115.84 ± 37.04	28.65 (11.03)	30.34 (9.52)
Tibialis anterior	91.28 (34.2)	34.63 (6.41)	34.86 ± 5.21	34.63 ± 6.41
Peroneus longus	82.64 ± 27.23	78.56 ± 21.83	27.12 (8.57)	27.94 (8.57)
Gluteus medius	23.10 (38.73)	17.46 (27.66)	21.75 ± 7.81	19.95 ± 7.54
Gluteus maximus	9.38 (2.33)	10.28 (2.88)	20.33 ± 4.75	20.31 ± 5.60
Adductor magnus	13.98 (4.73)	15.86 (5.73)	15.79 (3.21)	17.24 (4.12)
Biceps femoris	31.99(14.39)	32.57 (19.35)	18.41 (4.59)	19.35 (4.44)
Gastrocnemius medial head	33.70 (16.04)	38.27 (22.14)	20.42 ± 6.24	19.52 ± 4.11
Gastrocnemius lateral head	42.22 ± 17.55	43.91 ± 14.85	18.92 ± 4.34	19.31 ± 4.91

Table 20.2 Medians and means of Young's moduli in left/right comparison. Significant differences are highlighted yellow (see text page 231)

Region	Left	Right
Adductor magnus	13.91 (6.59)	15.1 (7.63)
Biceps femoris middle	12.26 (3.95)	12.64 (4.95)
Erector spinae L4	25.57 ± 4.75	25.8 ± 6.12
Gastrocnemius lateral head	14.00 (4.50)	13.00 (5.25)
Gluteus maximus	9.17 (5.62)	9.17 (3.09)
Gluteus medius	9.00 (3.00)	8.00 (3.00)
Plantar fascia	27.51 ± 8.67	23.99 ± 6.65
Rectus femoris middle	15.50 (6.00)	14.00 (5.00)
Tibialis anterior	36.00 (7.50)	36.00 (9.00)
Thoraco lumbar fascia TLF L4	58.86 ± 30.18	55.57 ± 29.54
Upper trapezius	25.00 (17.00)	26.00 (11.00)

because most researchers don't know how to interpret these "red and brown dots" within them. Especially these areas can provide valuable information for practitioners in sports- and pain medicine. They can represent "disease" state like MTrPs with increased neurogenic inflammation which develop through overuse or trauma.

SE has its place in research and clinical use as well even though it does not produce quantitative data like SWE. It can provide valuable information when the elastograms are analyzed for the number of hard pixels comparing the myofascia of the left and the right side. The validity of these findings has been shown in several preliminary studies. The stiffness patterns are correlated to pain location, range of motion (Bauermeister, 2012), pressure pain threshold and tissue indentometry (Bauermeister, 2015; Farasyn and Lassat, 2015).

Conclusion

Soft tissue pain and dysfunction is a problem of altered tissue stiffness not just in one myofascial location but along myofascial chains requiring an assessment of the entire myofascia from head to toe. SE is a qualitative and semi quantitative method which is integrated even into small portable ultrasound devices. It is useful in clinical practice for identifying the stiffest myofascial areas in all tissue layers. It serves as an objective enhancement of manual palpation.

Imaging techniques (ultrasound)

Table 20.3 Young's moduli in left right comparison in one pain patient with mean, maximum and minimum values. Significant differences between both sides are highlighted in red (see text page 231).

Region	E Mean L	E Mean R	E Max L	E Max R	E Min L	E Min R
Upper trapezius upright	42.71	54.93	172.08	228.04	4.84	4.17
Upper trapezius supine	53.30	32.06	189.80	204.63	5.16	0.17
Thoracic 1	31.99	37.62	267.38	340.05	4.01	5.45
Thoracic 2	37.55	33.07	467.69	357.50	3.36	3.60
Thoracic 3	25.97	24.48	74.89	174.48	0.13	1.34
Thoracic 4	25.73	17.72	126.78	83.55	6.15	0.02
Thoracic 5	24.88	19.36	113.96	226.67	4.12	4.48
Lumbar 1	22.29	16.96	76.42	83.90	4.43	2.35
Lumbar 2	28.59	16.74	125.96	73.93	4.31	3.86
Lumbar 3	25.39	20.35	141.70	89.65	0.99	1.31
Lumbar 4	27.27	20.09	154.60	167.16	3.64	2.96
Sacrum	24.24	25.92	208.97	168.89	0.48	0.00
Gluteus medius	25.46	12.68	210.19	110.74	3.01	0.00
Biceps femoris middle	14.53	15.47	94.39	67.77	1.74	3.17
Biceps femoris distal	27.61	17.66	185.55	99.97	2.70	0.28
Biceps femoris proximal	11.17	14.85	63.13	66.91	2.84	3.02
Gastrocnemius lateral	32.25	17.94	201.88	105.12	1.48	0.01
Gastrocnemius medial	22.90	19.25	161.15	234.21	1.74	0.99
Adductor magnus	17.53	11.01	84.88	55.56	3.68	2.91
Soleus	20.84	28.57	295.90	232.92	3.22	4.53
Plantar fascia	25.30	26.79	75.70	59.00	2.15	6.56
Rectus femoris middle	34.76	22.77	323.70	77.14	4.39	6.72
Tibialis anterior	38.41	39.04	230.84	147.17	14.94	14.48
Tensor fasciae latae	37.55	25.56	124.16	127.69	5.66	2.96

SWE is a quantitative method which measures the shear wave speed. To obtain individual values of shear wave speed, one or several areas within the ROI must be chosen for analysis. Some devices offer immediate results of shear wave speed or Young's modulus over the entire ROI with mean, maximum, minimum and standard deviation values. More research is needed to obtain representative standard values for all relevant areas of the myofascia. As long as we do not have normative values we need to use the patient as their own control. This is at present the best approach to decide on a target area for treatment.

Chapter 20

References

Abramoff, M.D., Magelhaes, P., Ram, S.J. (2004) Image processing with image. *J Bio-photonics Int.*11: 36–42.

Aubry, S., Nueffer, J.P., Tanter, M.,Becce, F., Vidal, C. & Michel, F. (2015) Viscoelasticity in Achilles tendonopathy: quantitative assessment by using real-time shear-wave elastography. *Radiology.* 274: 821–829.

Bauermeister, W. (2012) Ultraschall-Elastographie zur Diagnose myofaszialer Schmerzsyndrome. Der Deutsche Schmerz- und Palliativtag 2012. Frankfurt, Germany.

Bauermeister, W. (2015) Ultrasound elastography for the evaluation of the elastic properties of fascia and muscle. Fourth International Fascia Research Congress, 2015. Reston, VA, USA.

Bauermeister, W. (2017) Optimierung des Strain-Elastografie durch Computer assistierte Steuerung der Ultraschallsonde. *Ultraschall in Med.* 38: P2.011.

Bauermeister, K. (2021) The role of elastography in sports injury prevention. School of Medicine, Technical University Munich, unpublished.

Böttner, C. (2018) Interrater reliability of ultrasound elastography to examine the stiffness and elasticity of muscles and fascia of the lower extremity in healthy adults. *J Bodyw Mov Ther.* 22(4): 849–850. doi:10.1016/j.jbmt.2018.09.015

Boyd, B.S., Gray, A.T., Dilley, A., et al. (2012) The pattern of tibial nerve excursion with active ankle dorsiflexion is different in older people with diabetes mellitus. *Clin Biomech.* 27: 967–971.

Carroll, M., Yau, J., Rome, K., et al. (2012) Measurement of tibial nerve excursion during ankle joint dorsiflexion in a weight-bearing position with ultrasound imaging. *J Foot Ankle Res.* 5: 1.

Dilley, A., Greening, J., Lynn, B., et al. (2001) The use of cross-correlation analysis between high-frequency ultrasound images to measure longitudinal median nerve movement. *Ultrasound Med Biol.* 27: 1211–1218.

Dilley, A., Summerhayes, C. & Lynn, B. (2007) An in vivo investigation of ulnar nerve sliding during upper limb movements. *Clin Biomech (Bristol, Avon).* 22(7): 774–779.

Ellis, R., Hing, W., Dilley, A., et al. (2008) Reliability of measuring sciatic and tibial nerve movement with diagnostic ultrasound during a neural mobilisation technique. *Ultrasound Med Biol.* 34: 1209–1216.

Ellis, R.F., Hing, W.A. & McNair, P.J. (2012) Comparison of longitudinal sciatic nerve movement with different mobilization exercises: an in vivo study utilizing ultrasound imaging. *J Orthop Sports Phys Ther.* 42: 667–675.

Farasyn, A. & Lassat, B. (2015) Cross friction algometry (CFA): comparison of pressure pain thresholds between patients with chronic non-specific low back pain and healthy subjects. *J Bodyw Mov Ther.* 20: 224–234.

Garra, B.S. (2007) Imaging and estimation of tissue elasticity by ultrasound. *Ultrasound Q.* 23: 255–268.

Griefahn, A., Oehlmann, J., Zalpour, C., et al. (2017) Do exercises with the foam roller have a short-term impact on the thoracolumbar fascia? A randomized controlled trial. *J Bodyw Mov Ther.* 21: 186–193.

Krause, F. (2018) *Akuteffekte von Self-Myofascial-Release auf Beweglichkeit, passive Gewebesteifigkeit, Dehnwahrnehmung und fasziale Gleitbewegung—Eine randomisierte & kontrollierte Cross-Over Studie.* Inaugural dissertation. Frankfurt am Main, Germany.

Langevin, H.M., Fox, J.R., Koptiuch, C., et al. (2011) Reduced thoracolumbar fascia shear strain in human chronic low back pain. *BMC Musculoskelet Disord.* 12: 203.

Ophir, J., Cespedes, I., Ponnekanti, H., Yazdi, Y. & Li, X. (1991) Elastography: a quantitative method for imaging the elasticity of biological tissues. *Ultrason Imaging.* 13: 111–134.

Sarvazyan, A., Skovoroda, A., Emelianov, S., Fowlkes, J., Pipe, J., Adler, R., Buxton, R., and Carson, P. (1995) Biophysical bases of elasticity imaging. *In: Acoustical imaging.* Springer, pp. 223–240.

Sarvazyan, A., Hall, T.J., Urban, M.W., Fatemi, M., Aglyamov, S.R. & Garra, B.S. (2011) An overview of elastography – an emerging branch of medical imaging. *Curr Med Imaging Rev.* 7: 255–282.

Sarvazyan, A.P., Rudenko, O.V., Swanson, S.D., Fowlkes, J.B. & Emelianov, S.Y. (1998) Shear wave elasticity imaging: a new ultrasonic technology of medical diagnostics. *Ultrasound Med Biol.* 24: 1419–1435.

Shah, J.P., Danoff, J.V., Desai, M.J., Parikh, S., Nakamura, L.Y., Phillips, T.M. & Gerber, L.H. (2008) Biochemicals associated with pain and inflammation are elevated in sites near to and remote from active myofascial trigger points. *Arch Phys Med Rehabil.* 89: 16–23.

Schleip R, Duerselen L, Vleeming A, et al. (2012) Strain hardening of fascia: static stretching of dense fibrous connective tissues can induce a temporary stiffness increase accompanied by enhanced matrix hydration. *J Bodyw Mov Ther.* 16(1): 94–100. doi:10.1016/j.jbmt.2011.09.003

Toumi, H. & T. M. Best (2003) The inflammatory response: friend or enemy for muscle injury? Brit *J Sports Med.* 37: 284–286.

Mechanical assessment

Robert Schleip and Katja Bartsch

Introduction

Changes in the mechanical properties of fascial tissues are of interest to researchers and clinicians. In order to assess such changes, invasive as well as non-invasive methods can be used. Invasive examination methods on a cellular and molecular level, in essence, include needle biopsy and immunohistochemistry. Non-invasive methods of assessing biomechanical tissue properties are employed in research as well. They have become increasingly relevant in clinical practice.

Rapid developments in technology are offering useful diagnostic and assessment tools that can be used to examine different physical and physiological features of fascial tissues. As considerable demand for diagnostic methods related to fascial tissue function has arisen, overviews of such methods have helped to gain better understanding and evaluation of the different methodologies (Wilke and Banzer, 2014; Zugel et al., 2018). This chapter draws from these current literature overviews and describes and evaluates various techniques, ranging from traditional and cost-neutral practices such as palpation to relatively new and costly methods such as ultrasound elastography (Table 21.1).

Assessment methods

Palpation

Examining tissue through touch traditionally plays an important role in clinical practice.

Assessments of properties such as tissue stiffness represent a frequent (although not always precise) tool in the detection of cancer, injuries and other diseases (Fowlkes et al., 1995). Palpation is cost-neutral and widely used by physicians and physiotherapists. However, many palpation methods, particularly when targeting soft tissue structures, appear to be subjective and lack reliability. For instance, investigations into the reproducibility of palpation in myofascial trigger point identification yielded conflicting results (Myburgh et al., 2008). To render the art of manual palpation more reliable, standardized assessment and training methodologies are necessary

> **Palpation insight: assessing palpation skills**
> - Various methods and materials for assessing and teaching palpatory skills can be found in the literature. They range from simple self-built tools to more costly and technically engineered variants.
> - Examples include the palpation of a coin under different layers of copy paper (Kamp et al., 2019), the use of grating domes (Mueller et al., 2014) as well as virtual reality simulations of mechanical properties of human tissue designed as an aid to teaching palpatory diagnosis (Howell et al., 2008).

Questionnaires/scales

In order to evaluate the effects of fascia-related interventions, questionnaires and scales related to the client's pain level are often used. Such

Chapter 21

Table 21.1 Overview of diagnostic methods to examine fascial tissues

Method	Assessment target	Advantages	Disadvantages
Palpation	Stiffness, elasticity, shearing mobility, as well as other tissue parameters	Cost-effectiveness Differentiation between structures partly possible Psychosocial factors	Subjective/depends on patient's and examiner's experience Differentiation between structures limited Palpation of deeper structures difficult
Questionnaires/scales	Perception of pain	Cost-effectiveness Generally reliable	Differentiation between structures limited Subjective results
Algometry	Perception of pain	Semi-quantifiable results Reliable	Differentiation between structures only limited Good applicability only with superficial structures
Indentometry	Stiffness and elasticity	Quantification of results possible Reliable	Limited depth Differentiation between structures only limited
Myometry	Stiffness	Quantification of results possible Reliable	Limited depth Differentiation between structures not possible
Electrical bioimpedance	Hydration changes	High sensitivity	Reliability data are lacking Validity for smaller body regions are lacking
Ultrasound	Thickness of layers, tendon elongation, relative shearing motion of adjacent layers	Differentiation between structures possible Reliable Relatively cost-efficient	Lack of standardization regarding selection of exact viewing angles
Ultrasound-elastography	Stiffness	Differentiation between structures possible Quantification of results possible Reliable	Lack of standardization Frequent appearance of artefacts High acquisition cost

scales reflect the client's perception of the therapeutic effect of an intervention. While easy to use, they are an inherently subjective measurement tool and do not allow for conclusions related to a specific anatomical structure. Widely used scales include the Visual Analogue Scale (VAS), the Numerical Rating Scale (NRS) as well as the Verbal Rating Scale (VRS) (Figure 21.1; Williamson and Hoggart, 2005)

Algometry

The use of the Pressure Algometer (Park et al., 2011) allows the clinician/trainer not only to test tissue sensitivity, but also to evaluate the client's pain threshold in a specific body location. With the tip of the algometer, the clinician applies increasing amounts of pressure to a particular area, for example, a trigger point (Myburgh et al., 2008), and asks the client to signal when the pain is uncomfortable. By doing this, the client gets an impression of the scale of pain, from 0 to 10, with 10 representing unbearable pain. The clinician then repeats the procedure at several points around the problem area, before and after treatment, and records the results. Tenderness pressure is measured in pounds (lbs) and tissue penetration is measured in millimeters (mm).

Mechanical assessment

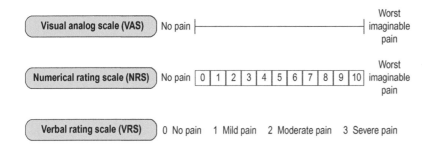

Figure 21.1

Common pain rating scales (Williamson and Hoggart, 2005).

Indentometry

Indentometry is an affordable and easy to handle technology to assess soft tissue stiffness. Hand-held devices such as the semi-electronic tissue compliance meter (STCM) or the IndentoPro consist of a modified algometer with a probe tip that is pressed into the tissue until a predefined penetration depth or force is reached. Stiffness is then specified as force per indentation depth (e.g. N/mm). While simple in handling, the STCM was reported to deliver reliable and valid measurements. As with other modes of assessment, reference values (e.g. for different body regions or musculoskeletal disorders) are still to be elucidated by future research (Wilke et al., 2018). The IndentoPro (Chemnitz, University of Technology; Figure 21.2) can provide measurements for both algometry and indentometry. It is easy to handle and has the advantage of providing a digital measurement.

Myometry

Hand-held myotonometer devices such as the Myotonometer or the MyotonPro aim to quantify the mechanical muscle properties. A testing probe is placed on the tissue so that short impulses generate oscillations in the tissue. The oscillation wave form reflects the viso-elastic properties of the tissue.

The MyotonPro is a myometer that gives numerical feedback on biomechanical tissue properties such as dynamic stiffness and

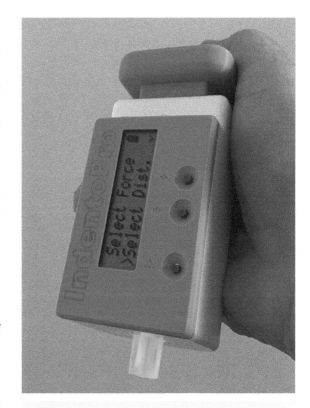

Figure 21.2

The IndentoPRO tool which can be used as an algometer (for the assessment of pressure pain sensitivity) and as indentometer (for stiffness assessment at different tissue depths).

Photo: fascialnet.com

elasticity. This method for measuring tissues close to the skin (up to depths of 1.5–2 cm) works by creating an external mechanical impulse. The

Chapter 21

muscle response is then recorded, in the form of an acceleration graph, and subsequently, the tone, elasticity and stiffness are computed. Reliability studies related to various body regions such as paraspinal muscles, gastrocnemius or Achilles tendon have reported that the MyotonPro can be used to reliably assess the mechanical properties of these tissues (Feng et al., 2018; Hu et al., 2018).

While the MyotonPro (Figure 21.3) has been used in various studies to assess the biomechanical properties of muscle tissue, the device generally does not only measure muscle tissue itself, but assesses various tissue layers. It is therefore important to note that the parameters quantified with this type of diagnostic, similar to those of the indentometer, relate to different tissue layers.

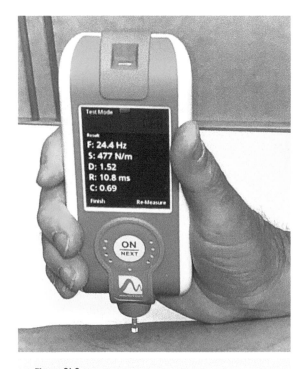

Figure 21.3

Myometry with MyotonPRO.

Research highlight: MyotonPro in space

In April 2018, a MyotonPro device was successfully launched to the International Space Station (ISS) for monitoring astronauts' muscle health and physical condition. The study funded by the European Space Agency, German Aerospace Center and UK Space Agency is called "Myotones–Muscle Tone in Space". It is the first time muscle tone assessment became technically possible in space. Staying fit through the space mission allows astronauts to return to normal life on earth as smoothly as possible. Measuring muscle tone with the MyotonPro is a crucial device to test muscle adaptation in space as part of the astronauts' daily routine. Scientists at the Charité University Berlin analyze the data on how muscles change during and after time on the ISS.

Electrical bioimpedance

Tissue hydration is frequently used as a hypothetical explanation for the benefits of many different types of bodywork. Schleip et al. (2012) showed that an increase in tissue stiffness may, at least, be partially caused by a temporarily altered matrix hydration.

Electrical bioimpedance is a fast, safe and inexpensive method using portable devices. The method has been used to assess nutritional status, cellular health and integrity as well as body composition (Martins et al., 2020). In sports, bioelectrical impedance analysis is used to determine the body composition and related hydration changes. It has been shown that athletic performance is influenced by and dependent on the distribution and total amount of fat-free mass and body fat. Bioimpedance has also been used to detect hydration changes before and after treatment and to help to determine influences that might change fluid distribution such as positioning. Lower impedance was shown along collagenous bands. Along these bands, some of the Traditional Chinese Medicine

Mechanical assessment

meridians could be represented. It is, therefore, of great interest to have a measurement tool that detects fluid distribution within the body.

The measured bioimpedance is the sum of the ohmic resistance of all fluids in the body, which is called resistance, and the capacitive resistance due to body cells, which is called reactance. Compared with muscle and blood, bone and fat are poorly conductive in the body. Therefore, if there is more bone and fat, the body is less conductive.

In electrical bioimpedance, several measurement methods can be performed using different frequencies and mathematical models. The use of different frequencies is necessary as they are required to estimate the various parameters such as fat-free mass or changes in the extra cellular water.

Whole-body impedance measurement is typically performed in supine position with four surface electrodes placed on one side of the body. Two current source electrodes are placed on the backside of the foot and hand and two detecting electrodes are positioned on the backs of the wrist and ankle (Foster and Lukaski, 1996; Kyle et al., 2004). A minimum distance of 3 cm should be kept between the current and the detecting electrode (Figure 21.4). While segmental measurements of body regions are possible and have advanced substantially in recent years, data on the reliability and validity of measurements in smaller body regions are still a matter of controversy. For instance, segmental impedance analysis tends to underestimate fat-free mass and overestimate fat mass (Jaffrin and Morel, 2008; Ward, 2012).

Ultrasound

Except for medical doctors, up until very recently, clinicians and coaches within the fields of sports and movement therapy rarely used any ultrasound equipment for their assessments.

However, technological advances have made portable ultrasound equipment an increasingly useful diagnostic tool within this field (Figure 21.5). Ultrasound technology has, for instance, been used to assess muscle activation, thickness of fascial tissues and "shear strain" between tissue layers.

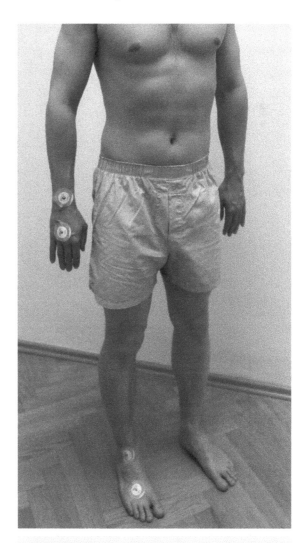

Figure 21.4

Standard electrode position for whole-body impedance measurement.

Chapter 21

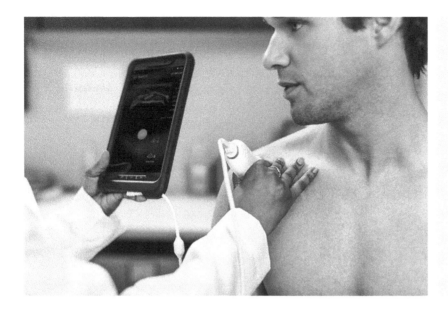

Figure 21.5

Use of ultrasound to visualize and assess fascial properties. Use of portable ultrasound allows for the measurement of thickness of various fascial membranes positioned close to the surface.

Photo: Philips Health System

Practitioners focusing on segmental stabilization, via muscular activation training, have successfully used ultrasound in their daily practices to assess proper (or lacking) activation of muscle layers related to "core stability", such as the transversus abdominis or the multifidus muscle (Hodges et al., 2003).

Ultrasound may also be used effectively to measure the thickness of fascial tissues (Figure 21.5).

Research highlights: tissue thickness from head to heel

- An impressive clinical study by Stecco et al. (2014) showed that in patients with chronic neck pain, the thickness of the sternocleidomastoid fascia corresponded to the amount of pain and disability, and also to the degree of therapeutic improvement after a myofascial manipulation treatment. Furthermore, a fascial thickness of 1.5 mm was found to be a reliable cut-off point in this study for the diagnosis of fascia-generated neck pain.

- Langevin et al. (2009) reported assessed connective tissue structures in the lumbar region with ultrasound. Connective tissue structure was altered in a group of subjects with chronic or recurrent low back pain. The perimuscular tissue layer was ~25% thicker in the low back pain group compared with controls without low back pain. Differences in age, sex, body mass index or activity level did not influence the results. The differences found may have their cause in genetic factors, abnormal movement patterns or chronic inflammation.

- Holowka et al. (2019) used portable ultrasound technology in Kenya and the USA to assess foot callus thickness. They found that people who frequently walk barefoot have thicker calluses than those who usually use footwear. However, callus thickness did not trade-off protection for the ability to perceive tactile stimuli. Furthermore, callus thickness did not affect how hard the feet strike the ground during walking.

A prominent study by Langevin et al. (2011) showed, via ultrasound assessment, that patients

Mechanical assessment

with chronic low back pain tend to express significantly less shear strain (corresponding to the ability to slide in relation to one another) between different layers of their lumbar fasciae compared with a pain-free control group. This type of assessment has also been used to research the effect of foam rolling on the low back region in healthy young adults (Frieder et al., 2019). Foam rolling significantly increased the mobility of the thoracolumbar fascia in the studied population.

Some studies use ultrasound to visualize myofascial trigger points. While the value of an ultrasound diagnostic for trigger point detection is still a matter of debate (Wilke and Banzer, 2014), most of the available studies found it to be a suitable method of diagnosis, and novel methods to measure myofascial trigger points using ultrasound imaging are still being developed (Jafari et al., 2018).

Ultrasound-elastography

A fairly new development with increasing application in musculoskeletal research is ultrasound elastography. This technology was created in the 1990s but has only recently been applied to soft tissue imaging of muscles. This cutting-edge technology provides images reflecting the hardness of the analyzed region (Zugel et al., 2018).

A mechanical vibration of the respective tissue is induced, for which the detected resonance frequency allows an assessment of the tissue stiffness. The softer a fascial tissue is, the slower its induced vibratory frequency. This non-invasive technology is already used to assist in the detection of liver fibrosis, breast cancer and prostate cancer as well as plantar fibrosis (Sconfienza et al., 2013). Furthermore, its real-time measurement of muscle stiffness can aid the diagnosis and rehabilitation of musculoskeletal injuries and chronic myofascial pain and also help to monitor intervention outcomes (Brandenburg et al., 2014).

Ultrasound elastography insight: strain versus shear wave elastography

- Strain elastography: the examiner compresses the ultrasound transducer against the body surface (e.g. muscle) manually. Softer tissue shows more deformation (and therefore experiences larger strain) than stiffer tissue. This is shown in an elastogram and represents a qualitative assessment. Translating this into a quantitative measure is challenging. One semi-quantitative method is the strain ratio. The elastography software first calculates the average strain in the normal area and then divides it by the average strain in the diseased area (e.g. a myofascial trigger point). However, these techniques are not in reality quantitative, but rather a relative assessment of tissue stiffness.

- Shear wave elastography: this technique uses shear waves to assess tissue stiffness. The shear waves travel perpendicularly through tissue to the direction of the particle motion. As the stiffness of underlying tissue increases, the shear wave speed increases. When looking at shear wave elastography studies, it is important to note that both the Young and shear modulus have been used in reporting outcomes, with the latter being the more accurate measure. The two measures differ slightly in their theoretical assumptions, but display good agreement with one other. The Young modulus can be converted to the shear modulus by dividing by 3 (Brandenburg et al., 2014).

Unfortunately, the prices of new equipment are still comparatively high. However, the respective technological industry has started to target physiotherapists, and others, as a new customer group. This has created the necessity to develop more affordable versions, with impressive imaging quality incorporated into smaller therapeutic practices.

Apart from the acquisition cost, the technology has a couple of other limitations. The amount of

Chapter 21

pressure to be applied to the tissue, the distance between the probe and the tissue, as well as the size of the region of interest, need to be carefully selected and standardized, as these factors can influence the results and their interpretation. Artefacts such as fluctuant changes at the edges of the elastogram and at the borders of thin structures can occur. Familiarity with such artefacts is important for the interpretation of results. Furthermore, there are currently many different techniques and processing algorithms in use. Accordingly, the findings and artefacts may be highly dependent on the technique used (Drakonaki et al., 2012).

Application and benefits

Measuring biomechanical tissue qualities before and after treatment or training has many benefits. The most obvious advantage is being able to track client progress. The practitioner or trainer has a better tool for communication with the client by being able to demonstrate objective evidence of treatment progress. This means less reliance is placed on the patient's subjective accounts of improvement (or lack thereof), and more on objective assessment tools, which measure an array of parameters.

Objective assessment allows for monitoring the quality and effectiveness of treatments. Clinicians can improve techniques through self-assessment, which leads to better methodologies and advancements in this field of health.

As in any field characterized by rapid technological advancements, evidence-based recommendations for clinical application will develop and then be refined within the next few years. Meanwhile, the enthusiastic clinician should combine methods and interpret findings with care, bearing in mind that factors such as the operator's experience or measuring technique may influence the results.

References

Brandenburg, J.E., et al. (2014) Ultrasound elastography: the new frontier in direct measurement of muscle stiffness. *Arch Phys Med Rehabil*. 95: 2207–2219.

Drakonaki, E.E., Allen, G.M. & Wilson, D.J. (2012) Ultrasound elastography for musculoskeletal applications. *Brit J Radiol*. 85: 1435–1445.

Feng, Y.N., et al. (2018) Assessing the elastic properties of skeletal muscle and tendon using shearwave ultrasound elastography and MyotonPRO. *Sci Rep*. 8: 17064.

Foster, K.R. & Lukaski, H.C. (1996) Whole-body impedance—What does it measure? *Am J Clin Nutr*. 64: S388–S396.

Fowlkes, J.B., et al. (1995) Magnetic-resonance imaging techniques for detection of elasticity variation. *Med Phys*. 22: 1771–1778.

Griefahn, A. et al. (2017) Do exercises with the Foam Roller have a short-term impact on the thoracolumbar fascia? - A randomized controlled trial. *J Bodyw Mov Ther*. 21(1): 186–193.

Hodges, P.W., et al. (2003) Measurement of muscle contraction with ultrasound imaging. *Muscle Nerve*. 27: 682–692.

Holowka, N.B., et al. (2019) Foot callus thickness does not trade off protection for tactile sensitivity during walking. *Nature*. 571: 261–264.

Howell, J.N., et al. (2008) The virtual haptic back: a simulation for training in palpatory diagnosis. *BMC Med Educ*. 8: 14.

Hu, X., et al. (2018) Quantifying paraspinal muscle tone and stiffness in young adults with chronic low back pain: a reliability study. *Sci Rep*. 8: 14343.

Jafari, M., et al. (2018) Novel method to measure active myofascial trigger point stiffness using ultrasound imaging. *J Bodyw Mov Ther*. 22: 374–378.

Jaffrin, M.Y. & Morel, H. (2008) Body fluid volumes measurements by impedance: A review of bioimpedance spectroscopy (BIS) and bioimpedance analysis (BIA) methods. *Med Eng Phys.* 30: 1257–1269.

Kamp, R., Moltner, A. & Harendza, S. (2019) "Princess and the pea" – an assessment tool for palpation skills in postgraduate education. *BMC Med Educ.* 19: 177.

Krause, F., et al. (2019). Acute effects of foam rolling on passive stiffness, stretch sensation and fascial sliding: a randomized controlled trial. *Hum Mov Sci.* 67: 102514.

Kyle, U.G., et al. (2004) Bioelectrical impedance analysis—Part I: Review of principles and methods. *Clin Nutr.* 23: 1226–1243.

Langevin, H.M., et al. (2009) Ultrasound evidence of altered lumbar connective tissue structure in human subjects with chronic low back pain. *BMC Musculoskelet Disord.* 10: 151.

Langevin, H.M., et al. (2011) Reduced thoracolumbar fascia shear strain in human chronic low back pain. *BMC Musculoskelet Disord.* 12: 203.

Martins, P.C., Moraes, M.S. & Silva, D.A.S. (2020) Cell integrity indicators assessed by bioelectrical impedance: a systematic review of studies involving athletes. *J Bodyw Mov Ther.* 24(1): 154–164.

Mueller, S., et al. (2014) Occupation-related long-term sensory training enhances roughness discrimination but not tactile acuity. *Exp Brain Res.* 232: 1905–1914.

Myburgh, C., Larsen, A.H. & Hartvigsen, J. (2008) A systematic, critical review of manual palpation for identifying myofascial trigger points: evidence and clinical significance. *Arch Phys Med Rehabil.* 89: 1169–1176.

Park, G., et al. (2011) Reliability and usefulness of the pressure pain threshold measurement in patients with myofascial pain. *Ann Rehab Med.* 35: 412–417.

Schleip, R., et al. (2012) Strain hardening of fascia: static stretching of dense fibrous connective tissues can induce a temporary stiffness increase accompanied by enhanced matrix hydration. *J Bodyw Mov Ther.* 16: 94–100.

Sconfienza, L.M., et al. (2013) Real-time sonoelastography of the plantar fascia: comparison between patients with plantar fasciitis and healthy control subjects. *Radiology.* 267: 195–200.

Stecco, A., et al. (2014) Ultrasonography in myofascial neck pain: randomized clinical trial for diagnosis and follow-up. *Surg Radiol Anat.* 36: 243–253.

Ward, L.C. (2012) Segmental bioelectrical impedance analysis: an update. *Curr Opin Clin Nutr Metab Care.* 15: 424–429.

Wilke, J., et al. (2018) Reliability and validity of a semi-electronic tissue compliance meter to assess muscle stiffness. *J Back Musculoskelet Rehabil.* 31: 991–997.

Wilke, J. & Banzer, W. (2014) Non-invasive screening of fascial tissues—a narrative review. *Physikalische Medizin Rehabilitationsmedizin Kurortmedizin.* 24: 117–124.

Williamson, A. & Hoggart, B. (2005) Pain: a review of three commonly used pain rating scales. *J Clin Nursing.* 14: 798–804.

Zugel, M., et al. (2018) Fascial tissue research in sports medicine: from molecules to tissue adaptation, injury and diagnostics: consensus statement. *Brit J Sports Med.* 52: 1497.

Further reading

Huang, Y.-P. & Yong-Ping, Z. (2019) *Measurement of Soft Tissue Elasticity in Vivo: Techniques and Applications.* Boca Raton, FL: CRC Press Taylor & Francis Group.

Palpation and functional assessment methods for fascia-related dysfunction

Leon Chaitow

Introduction

Fascia provides structural and functional continuity between the body's hard and soft-tissues. It is a ubiquitous elastic–plastic, sensory component that invests, supports, separates, connects, divides, wraps and gives both both shape and functionality to the rest of the body, while allowing gliding, sliding motions, as well as playing an important role in transmitting mechanical forces between structures (Chapter 1). At least, that is how fascia behaves when it is healthy and fully functional. In reality, due to age, trauma or inflammation, for example, fascia may shorten, becoming painful and restricted and fail to painlessly allow coherent transmission of forces, or smooth sliding interactions, between different layers of body-tissues (Langevin, 2009).

Adaptation

One way of viewing fascia-related dysfunction, that occurs gradually over time, happens suddenly following trauma or inflammation or which may be part of inevitable age-related changes, is as physiological or biomechanical adaptation or as compensation. Neuromyofascial tissue contraction may result in varying degrees of pain-inducing binding, or "adhesions", between layers that should be able to stretch and glide on each other, potentially impairing motor function (Grinnel, 2009; Fourie & Robb, 2009) (Chapter 2).

A process evolves that can be neatly summarized as "densification" of, previously, more pliable tissues including fascia. This involves interference with complex myofascial relationships, altering muscle balance, motor control and proprioception (Stecco and Stecco, 2009). These slowly evolving adaptive processes may become both habitual and built-in. For example, in an individual with a chronically altered postural pattern involving a forward head position, protracted shoulders, a degree of dorsal kyphosis and lumbar lordosis, there will be both a range of soft-tissue changes, fibrosis, etc., as well as the evolution of ingrained, habitual, postural patterns that are usually difficult to modify unless the chronic tissue features are altered via exercise and/or therapeutic interventions. Myers (2009) has expressed this progressive adaptive phenomenon as involving a process in which chronic tissue loading leads to "global soft tissue holding patterns", where clear postural and functional imbalance and distress are both visible, as well as being palpable.

A shorthand summary of such processes may describe them as being the result of:

- Overuse, for example, repetitive actions
- Misuse, for example, postural or ergonomic insults

Chapter 22

- Disuse, for example, lack of exercise
- Abuse, for example, trauma
- Or any combination of these.

Whatever the single or multiple contributing features may be, the end result is of structural and functional modifications that prevent normal activity, result in discomfort or pain, and which, themselves, make further adaptive demands as the individual attempts to compensate for restrictions and altered use patterns.

Assessment objectives

When evaluating possible interventions, whether therapeutic or exercise related, it is important to ascertain which tissues, structures, patterns and mechanisms may be involved? For example, is there any evidence of soft-tissue change, involving hypertonicity or fibrosis? Is there joint or neurological involvement? Are the tissues inflamed? In other words: Why is this happening? What causative or maintaining features are identifiable? What actions might usefully be taken to modify, improve, and correct the situation?

As a starting point, in order to encourage rehabilitation, areas of restriction need to be identified and assessed so that they can be encouraged towards normality. The question as to how best to identify such pathophysiological changes is, therefore, one of the key challenges that face practitioners, before manual and/or movement therapies or modalities can be safely applied. Fortunately, a range of palpation and assessment tools is available to help achieve the identification and localization of dysfunction, as will be described later in this chapter.

Gathering evidence

Clinical decision-making needs to be based on a combination of the unique history and characteristics of the individual combined with objective and subjective information, gathered from assessment, observation, palpation and examination. The findings of such information gathering endeavours need to be correlated with whatever evidence exists, research studies, experience, etc. that offers guidance, regarding different therapeutic choices. The objectives of palpation and assessment are, therefore, the gathering of evidence regarding function and dysfunction, so that informed clinical decisions can be made, rather than being based on guesswork. What's too tight? What's too loose? What functions are impaired? Which kinetic and structural chains are involved? What are the causes? What can be done to remedy or improve the situation?

There are many functional assessment methods and protocols, as well as a variety of palpation methods that can assist in this search for information, and answers. Some of these have been tested for reliability, others are used extensively, without any clear evidence that they are reliable.

This leads to a key recommendation: that no single piece of "evidence" gained from observation, or from the results of functional tests and assessment, or from palpation, should be used alone as evidence to guide clinical choices. It is far safer to rely on combinations of evidence that support each other and which point towards rehabilitation and/or treatment options.

Therapeutic options

When the sliding/gliding motion potential of fascia is reduced, is painful or has been lost, restoration of normal function requires attention to the causative, as well as the maintaining, factors associated with the dysfunctional fascial layers. This chapter focuses on evaluation, palpation and assessment of fascial changes that may be contributing to functional or pain-related symptoms. The intent of using such findings is to decide on the best ways of encouraging more normal function. There are, of course, multiple strategies that aim to improve, correct or rehabilitate such dysfunction but their underlying ambitions can briefly be summarized as follows:

- To reduce adaptive load: for example, to modify overuse, or misuse, or other features that are contributing to the problem

- To enhance functionality: for example, to improve posture, breathing function, nutrition, sleep, exercise patterns, as well as the local mobility and stability of tissues

- To focus on symptom reduction: which might be a poor, potentially short-term, choice unless and until adaptive demands are reduced and/or function improved.

Postural assessment

A general evaluation of posture and movement patterns offers initial clues as to areas that are either underactive or overactive in their ranges of motion or functionality.

Information gathering

1. A general evaluation of postural and movement patterns offers an overview of what is functional and which tissues, structures and areas require further investigation (see Therapeutic options).

2. Testing particular key muscles for relative shortness, as well as for functional efficiency, allows a more focused evaluation as to where restrictions exist.

3. Within identified areas, such as shortened muscles, local areas of dysfunction may be isolated by means of direct palpation (see notes on ARTT later in this chapter).

Crossed syndromes (Figure 22.1)

Patterns of imbalance, such as the upper and the lower crossed syndrome patterns, have classically been interpreted as demonstrating hypertonic extensor muscles overwhelming inhibited abdominal flexors (Janda, 1996).

Greenman (1996) explained this perspective as follows: "Muscle imbalance consists of shortening and tightening of muscle groups (usually the tonic 'postural' muscles), and weakness of other muscle groups (usually the phasic muscles), and consequent loss of control on integrated muscle function. The lower crossed syndrome involves hypertonic, and therefore shortened, iliopsoas, rectus femoris, TFL, the short adductors of the thigh and the erector spinae group with inhibited abdominal and gluteal muscles.

Chapter 22

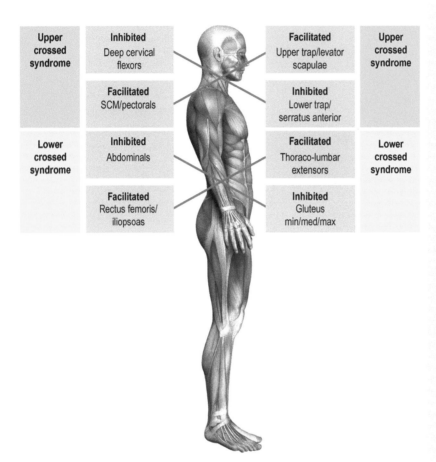

Upper crossed syndrome	Inhibited Deep cervical flexors	Facilitated Upper trap/levator scapulae	Upper crossed syndrome
Facilitated SCM/pectorals	Inhibited Lower trap/serratus anterior
Lower crossed syndrome	Inhibited Abdominals	Facilitated Thoraco-lumbar extensors	Lower crossed syndrome
Facilitated Rectus femoris/iliopsoas	Inhibited Gluteus min/med/max

Figure 22.1

The so-called "crossed syndrome" postural pattern, as described by Janda (1983).

This tilts the pelvis forward on the frontal plane, while flexing the hip joints and exaggerating lumbar lordosis." In addition, it is not uncommon for quadratus lumborum to shorten and tighten, while gluteus maximus and medius weaken.

The upper crossed syndrome involves, among other muscles, hypertonic cervical extensors, upper trapezius, pectorals, thoracic erector spinae, with inhibited deep neck flexors and lower fixators of the shoulders.

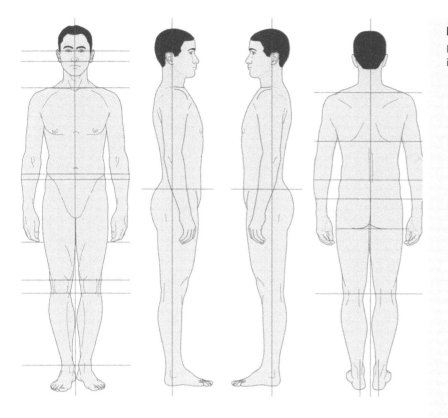

Figure 22.2
Postural evaluation recording form

Key et al. (2010) note that this pattern may involve "a posterior (pelvic) shift with increased anterior sagittal rotation or tilt", together with an anterior shunt/translation of the thorax, and the head. In such instances diaphragmatic control and altered pelvic floor function would result.

Chapter 22

Visual assessment for overall postural impression (i.e. not diagnostic)

The individual being assessed is standing (Figure 22.2).

Static assessment

1. Posterior view
   Note: symmetry and levels of shoulders and scapulae and any evidence of winging, head position, any spinal curvature as well as relative fullness of paraspinal msucles, position of pelvis, fat folds (creases) at waist and gluteals, symmetry and position of knees, feet, malleoli, Achilles tendons, arms and any obvious morphological asymmetry such as scars or bruises.

2. Lateral view
   Note: status of knees: relaxed or locked in extension, spinal curves: exaggerated or reversed, head position: forward or balanced, evidence of abdominal ptosis ("sagging") or any obvious morphological asymmetry such as scars or bruises.

3. Anterior view
   Note: shoulder levels: symmetrical at the midsternal line, head tilt, deviation of clavicles, asymmetry of pelvis: are crests level, patella symmetry and any obvious morphological asymmetry such as scars or bruises.

Do the imbalances you observe suggest a pattern where there may be restrictions, structures involving 'crossed-syndrome' patterns, rotations, side-shifts, or particular fascial chain involvement? If so, investigate further using palpation as well as functional assessments (see below).

Active assessment

Now observe the individual walking away from and back towards you, as well as from the side. Do this slowly and more rapidly, as you evaluate stride, balance/symmetry, weight transfer, unusual patterns of movement. Record the findings of your impressions. Observe a variety of potentially significant normal movements, particularly those that the individual complains of as painful or limited, and, in addition, look closely at any abnormal patterns when the individual is "long-sitting" (Figure 22.5) or bends forward, backwards and reaching upwards, as well as the breathing pattern.

Ask yourself:

- What needs to change to help improve/normalize this person's posture?

- What is tight, loose, rotated, off-center, unbalanced, folded, crowded and/or compressed and where might restrictions exist that relate to such observations?

- What fascial structures might be involved in such restrictions that, if released, would allow for a postural lengthening, opening out or unfolding to occur?

The soft tissue palpation puzzle: Problems are not necessarily where they appear to be!

In the descriptions of crossed syndromes, individual muscles are named. However, it has become obvious in recent years that the concept of individual muscles is flawed. The multiple fascial connections between "named" muscles and other muscles means that their action is not independent. Force is transmitted in many directions offering muscles additional leverage and functionality, as well as adding load to sometimes-distant muscles. Individually named muscles can, no longer, be considered to be discrete and separate, operating individually. Huijing (1999) has pointed out that agonists and antagonists are coupled structurally and mechanically via the fascia that connects them, so that when force is generated by a prime mover it can be measured in the tendons of antagonist muscles.

Franklyn-Miller and colleagues (2009) have shown that, for example, a hamstring stretch produces 240% of the resulting strain in the iliotibial tract and 145% in the ipsilateral lumbar fascia compared with the hamstrings. Strain (load) transmission, during contraction or stretching, therefore affects many other tissues beyond the muscle being targeted, largely due to fascial connections. Importantly, this suggests that apparent muscular restrictions, such as "tight hamstrings", might not originate in the affected muscle but elsewhere. In the case of hamstring restriction, there may be fascial dysfunction in the tensor fasciae latae, or the ipsilateral thoracolumbar, creating, encouraging or maintaining hamstring symptoms. This sort of fascial

interconnectedness exists throughout the body so, as knowledge accumulates as to what structures are linked to others via fascia and at which orientation, understanding sources of dysfunction should become more predictable.

Palpation and assessment and load-transfer: The thoracolumbar fascia

Palpation and assessment strategies need to take account of this load-sharing phenomenon. The scale of the palpation puzzle can be seen in the illustration of the huge number of potential links available from just one massive fascial structure, the thoracolumbar fascia. This ties together the erector spinae, latissimus dorsi, quadratus lumborum, psoas, transversus abdominis, and diaphragm muscles, as well as countless other minor muscle structures (Figures 22.3 and 39.4).

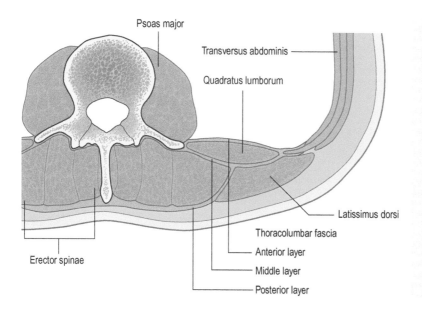

Figure 22.3

A transverse view of the fascial wrapping that binds together key muscles including quadratus lumborum, psoas, erector spinae, latissimus dorsi and transversus abdominis. (Gray's Anatomy)

Psoas major

Transversus abdominis

Quadratus lumborum

Latissimus dorsi

Thoracolumbar fascia

Anterior layer

Middle layer

Posterior layer

Erector spinae

Chapter 22

Unraveling the puzzle

As we focus attention on the assessment of relative shortness in named muscles, we need to maintain awareness that multiple fascial connections exist that bind together muscles with different names into a virtual interconnecting tensegrity structure (Chapter 6). An important distinction needs to be made in our search for culprit areas of restriction. There is a need to identify both the *location* of restriction, for example shortened hamstrings, as well as the *source* of the restriction that, as has been explained, could be in the hamstrings but also possibly in the thoracolumbar fascia, or elsewhere.

Testing particular, key, muscles for relative restriction/loss of full range of motion, as well as for functional efficiency, allows a more focused evaluation as to where restrictions exist. There are strategies that can help to identify areas that may be responsible for dysfunction:

1. General observation: for example of normal posture and movement, such as standing and walking as described above (page 250).

2. Observation of functional movements or postures: for example walking (Chapter 17), long-sitting (see Figure 22.4), bending, as well as Janda's (1996) Hip Abduction and Hip Extension tests.

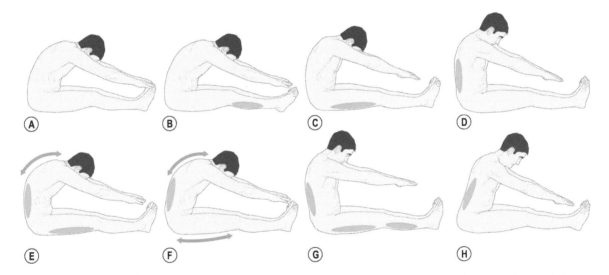

Figure 22.4

Tests for shortness of the erector spinae and associated postural muscles.

(A) Normal length of erector spinae msucles and posterior thigh muscles.

(B) Tight gastrocnemius and soleus; the inablilty to dorsiflex the feet indicates tightness of the plantar-flexor group.

(C) Tight hamstring muscles, which cause the pelvis to tlit posteriorly.

(D) Tight low-back erector spinae muscles.

(E) Tight hamstrings; slightly tight low-back muscles and overstreteched upper back muscles.

(F) Slightly shortened lower back muscles, stretched upper back muscles and slightly stretched hamstrings.

(G) Tight low-back muscles, hamstrings and gastrocnemius/soleus.

(H) Very tight low-back muscles, with lordosis maintained even in flexion.

3. Specific tests for muscle shortness: (see Table 22.1, Postural Muscle Assessment Sequence)

4. Direct manual palpation: see palpation exercises described later in the chapter.

Functional assessment: Hip abduction test, hip extension test

There are hundreds of functional assessment methods that offer evidence of overuse, inhibition, restriction and other aspects of dysfunction, as well as, potentially, discomfort or pain, when being demonstrated, due to space constraints, just two examples are described below.

Hip abduction test

This assessment can be performed by including palpation; however, it is possible that adding digital touch to the muscles being evaluated would add sensory motor stimulation that might reduce the reliability of any findings. Observation alone is encouraged initially, with direct palpation being added subsequently (Figure 22.5A).

The aim of this test is to screen for stability of the lumbopelvic region. The patient should be side lying with the superior leg resting on the lower leg, which is flexed at the hip and knee. The upper-most leg should be in line with the torso. The patient is requested to slowly lift

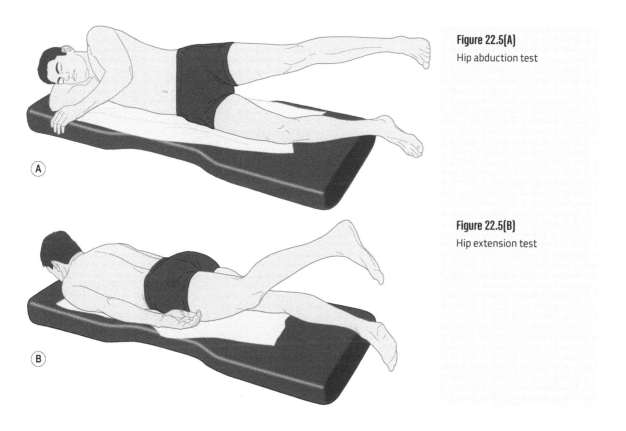

Figure 22.5(A)
Hip abduction test

Figure 22.5(B)
Hip extension test

Chapter 22

the leg toward the ceiling. If normal, the leg should abduct to 20° with no internal or external rotation, or hip flexion, and without any ipsilateral "hip-hike" (pelvic cephalad elevation). There should be an initial moderate contraction of the lumbar erector spinae and/or quadratus lumborum, in order to stabilize the pelvis. However, this should not involve any obvious contraction, merely an indication of toning.

The test is regarded as positive if any of the following are observed:

1. Ipsilateral external hip/leg rotation which suggests overactivity and probable shortening of piriformis.

2. Ipsilateral external pelvic rotation, which suggests piriformis and other external hip rotator overactivity and probable shortness.

3. Ipsilateral hip flexion, which suggests overactivity and probable shortening of the hip flexors, including psoas and/or tensor fasciae latae.

4. Cephalad elevation of the ipsilateral pelvis before 20º of hip abduction, which suggests overactivity and shortening of quadratus lumborum.

5. An obvious hingeing should be noted at the hip, rather than in the waist area if gluteus medius and tensor fasciae latae are working optimally, and quadratus lumborum is not overactive.

6. Any pain reported in performance of the abduction movement. For example, discomfort noted on the inner thigh may represent adductor shortness.

7. Any combination of the above.

Hip extension test

The aim of this test is to evaluate coordination of a number of muscles (Figure 22.5B) during prone hip extension. The patient should lie prone with the arms at the side and feet extending beyond the table end. The patient is then requested to lift a specific leg toward the ceiling. An initial toning contraction of the thoracolumbar erector spinae, to stabilize the torso before the limb extends, is considered normal, if the action is achieved by coordinated activity of the ipsilateral hamstrings and gluteus maximus.

The test is considered positive if any of the following are observed:

1. Knee flexion of the leg being extended suggests overactivity and probable hamstring shortness.

2. Delayed or absent ipsilateral gluteus maximus. Absence of a meaningful contraction of gluteus maximus at the outset of the extension movement is considered significant, as this should be a prime mover. Inhibition may indicate overactivity of the erector spinae group and/or of the ipsilateral hamstrings.

3. False hip extension occurs, where the hinging/pivot point of the leg, during the first 10° extension, occurs in the low back rather than at the hip itself, suggesting overactivity of the erector spinae and inhibition of gluteus maximus.

4. Early contraction of the contralateral periscapular musculature suggests a functional low back instability, involving recruitment of the upper torso as compensation for inhibition of the intended prime movers.

Palpation and functional assessment methods for fascia-related dysfunction

Table 22.1 Postural muscle assessment sequence

The table lists the main muscles of the body that are prone to shortening when overused, misused (for example, poor posture), or abused (traumatized)(Janda 1996).

The letters E L R represent: E = equally-bilaterally-short, L = left short, R = right short.

The other abbreviations relate to lack of flexibility of: LL= low lumbar, LDJ = lumbodorsal junction, LT = lower thoracic, MT-mid-thoracic, UT = upper thoracic. Details for assessment of these muscles can be found in *Palpation & Assessment Skills,* Chaitow (2010).

Name: _____

E + Equal (circle both if both are short)

L or R are circled if left or right are short

Spinal abbreviations indicate low-lumbar, lumbo dorsal junction, low-thoracic, mid-thoracic and upper thoracic areas (of flatness and therefore reduced ability to flex – short erector spinae)

1. Gastrocnemius E L R	12. Latissimus dorsi E L R
2. Soleus E L R	13. Upper trapezius E L R
3. Medial hamstrings E L R	14. Scalenes E L R
4. Short adductors E L R	15. Sternocleidomastoid E L R
5. Rectus femoris ELR	16. Levator scapulae E L R
6. Psoas E L R	17. Infraspinatus E L R
7. Hamstrings	18. Subscapularis E L R
a) upper fibers E L R	19. Supraspinatus E L R
b) lower fibers E L R	20. Flexors of the arms E L R
8. Tensor fasciae latae E L R	21. Spinal flattening:
9. Piriformis E L R	a) seated legs straight LL LDJ LT MT UT
10. Quadratus lumborum E L R	b) seated legs flexed LL LDJ LT MT UT
11. Pectoralis major E L R	22. Cervical spine flexors short? Yes No

Observed posture, together with observation of movement patterns, as well as in long-sitting, hip abduction and hip extension tests, offers clues as to which muscles/groups of muscles may be overactive and potentially shortened, and which may be inhibited. This information can be refined by testing specific muscles for shortness, as indicated in Table 22.1.

Having identified muscles with reduced range of motion, local areas, or areas distant from them, may be sought that could be affecting them. These may then be usefully assessed (see discussion of thoracolumbar fascia above).

ARTT palpation features of local dysfunction

Fascial, or general musculoskeletal dysfunction, involving pain and/or restriction for example, is commonly associated with a number of predictable features that can be summarized using the acronym ARTT.

Chapter 22

- **A** stands for **A**symmetry, since one-sided fascial dysfunction is more usual than bilateral.

- **R** stands for **R**ange of motion restriction. In almost all cases of fascial or general musculoskeletal dysfunction, there will be a reduction in the range of movement available to the tissues involved.

- **T** stands for **T**enderness or sensitivity/pain, which is common but not universal. Fryer et al. (2004) have confirmed that sites in the thoracic paravertebral muscles, identified by deep palpation as displaying "abnormal tissue texture", also showed greater tenderness than adjacent tissues characteristic of dysfunction. Fascial dysfunction frequently involves a particular quality of sharp, cutting or "burning" sensation, when moved, compressed or stretched.

- **T** stands for **T**extural or **T**issue changes. Dysfunctional tissues are commonly associated with hypertonicity, fibrosis, induration/hardening, oedema or other palpable modifications from the norm. Fryer et al. (2005) examined the possibility that tissue texture irregularity of paravertebral sites might be due to greater cross-sectional thickness of the paraspinal muscle bulk. Diagnostic ultrasound (Chapter 24) showed that this was not the case. Changes in the "feel" of fascia, when dysfunctional, have been described as "densification": a word that neatly summarizes what is commonly palpated. Fryer et al. (2007) examined the EMG activity of deep paraspinal muscles, lying below paravertebral thoracic muscles with "altered texture", that were also more tender than surrounding ones. This demonstrated increased EMG activity in these dysfunctional muscles, i.e. they were hypertonic.

All four elements of ARTT are not always apparent when dysfunctional tissues are assessed/palpated. However, it would be unusual for there to not be at least two, and ideally three, of these characteristics in evidence when fascia is functioning other than optimally.

ARTT Exercise

Have the patient stand flexing from the waist, as you stand in front, viewing the paraspinal musculature from the head. One side of the paraspinals will commonly be more "mounded" than the other. Note the level at which this occurs and have the individual lie prone.

In this example let's assume it is the lower thoracic/upper lumbar area on the left. At this stage you will have established that the "A" (asymmetry) in ARTT is identifiable. Now palpate both left and right sides of this area of the back in order to evaluate the relative tone on each side. The more mounded side, left in this example, will inevitably be felt to be "tighter", more hypertonic.

Testing for the "R" element of ARTT is easily achieved by gently attempting to lengthen the paraspinal tissues, either via simply pressing into them, or by trying to flex the tissues laterally with thumb, finger or hand. There will be reduced range of motion on the hypertonic, shortened, side.

Once you have sensed the difference in tone, one side to the other, palpate a little deeper into the musculature, possibly from a slightly lateral angle rather than vertically, and sense any differences you can identify in the texture of the tissues. It should usually be possible to sense greater rigidity and possibly, depending on chronicity, some fibrotic elements on the hypertonic side. If so, you will have established one of the "T" (texture, or tissue) elements of ARTT.

Palpation and functional assessment methods for fascia-related dysfunction

Pressure applied into the tissues, on each side should establish that, in most instances, the hypertonic side will be tender (producing the second "T") in ARTT.

Translating ARTT into fascial assessment is less obvious than when applying it to muscles or joints, since many fascial restrictions may be deep and not directly palpable. However, superficial fascia and loose areolar tissues are easily evaluated, as described below.

Exercises: Skin and fascia palpation

Ideally the exercises below should be practiced on "normal" tissue as well as on areas where dysfunction is apparent or suspected. In addition, practice on tissues that are overlying large muscle masses and also where there is minimal muscle between the palpating contact and underlying bone. The more variety of tissues, and individuals of different ages and physical condition, that are involved in palpation exercises the more rapidly palpatory literacy will be achieved (Chaitow, 2010).

Exercise 1

Skin drag

- Before starting the exercise itself remove any watches or jewellery.
- With no pressure at all, only the very lightest of touch of one or two finger pads, stroke the skin of the area where the watch had been, so that you move from skin that was not covered by the strap, to cross over that area and back again several times.
- Do you notice an obvious difference, as you cross this more "moist" area, compared with the dryer areas?
- Increased skin hydrosis (sweat) changes should be palpable. What you are feeling is

known as "drag" and you are using drag palpation to identify increased hydrosis, which is often associated with hypertonicity, tissue dysfunction and fascial resistance to sliding.

- When you are comfortable that you can recognize the feeling of drag and using no pressure at all, only the very lightest of touch of one or two finger pads, stroke the skin of your anterior thigh (for the purpose of this exercise), in various directions.
- Then do the same on the lateral thigh, overlying the densest aspects of the iliotibial band.
- Try to sense and identify areas of drag. These will be far less obvious than the area under a watchstrap but should make themselves known when smooth finger-movement, over the skin, becomes slightly "rough".

Exercise 2

Sliding and rolling superficial fascia

- Place two or three finger pads on the skin of the anterior thigh with minimal compressive force (grams only) and slide it (the skin together with superficial fascia, to which it is bound) towards the knee, until you feel resistance. Then return to where you started and slide the skin towards the hip.
- Compare the ease of movement in one direction with the other.
- Was there greater resistance in one direction or the other?
- Perform the action over areas that displayed "drag" sensations, as well as those that did not.
- Now perform the same actions on the lateral surface of that leg, overlying the iliotibial band. Compare ease of movement with the anterior surface, or areas free of, as well as displaying "drag".

Chapter 22

- After exploring one leg, perform the same evaluations on the other leg, as well as in other easily accessible areas of the body, such as the anterior and the lateral calf area, comparing and remembering the different feel of these tissues as you lift, slide and roll them.

- Compare your findings. Was there greater resistance to sliding skin/superficial fascia in some locations compared to others and did this correlate with drag?

- Was there greater resistance on one surface of the leg, or aspect of the leg, compared with the other?

- What differences did you notice when trying to perform the same exercises on areas with little muscle cover or where there were dense fascial layers (iliotibial band)?

Exercise 3

Testing skin elasticity

- Now gently hold a pinch of skin between your index and middle finger pads, and your thumb in an area already tested for skin "slideability", as in Exercise 2.

- Lift this to sense its degree of elasticity, which will differ greatly in different areas of the body.

- What you are holding is skin and superficial fascia, together with some of the adipose/areolar/loose connective tissue that lie between those layers and the underlying dense connective tissue. This "loose" material includes a variety of cells and substances, such as proteoaminoglycans, which facilitate the "slideability" of

the various layers of tissue, on each other (Chapter 3).

- When this facility is reduced or lost, dysfunction, restriction and pain are almost inevitable consequences.

Repeat this light pinch-and lift in various parts of the thigh, both where there is a thick layer of muscle and also where there is minimal muscle and more fascial tissue.

- Now see if you can "roll the skin" and superficial fascia between fingers and thumbs, in the different areas you are testing, in various directions.

- Did you notice that where reduced sliding (Exercise 2) was observed, skin is less easy to lift/stretch and roll?

- In general, the greater the degree of underlying hypertonicity and shortening, the greater will be the resistance to free sliding on underlying structures of the skin/superficial fascia.

- In many instances, there will be a correlation between drag, and lack of easy sliding capacity, and loss of elastic quality (Chapter 8).

Note that several elements of ARTT are being demonstrated via this exercise. A degree of increased tenderness is also likely in areas where drag is noted, where there is reduced ability to slide and to roll. Sometimes rolling the tissue will be more uncomfortable, adding the final element of ARTT (tenderness).

Exercise 4

Apply tests 1, 2, 3 to somebody else's sacrum and/or lower back and, as you do so, try evaluate directions of relative restriction in the ability of superficial tissues to slide. You are now on your way towards palpatory literacy.

Clinical summary

- Global evaluation via observation: static and during movement offers indications of areas that are restricted or dysfunctional

- Functional assessments allow you to identify specific structures that deserve further investigation

- Direct palpation isolates local areas of tissue change

Your only remaining concern is what to do about what you have identified. This book offers solutions to those concerns.

References

Barker, P.J., Briggs, C.A. & Bogeski, G. (2004) Tensile transmission across the lumbar fasciae in unembalmed cadavers: effects of tension to various muscular attachments. *Spine*. 29(2): 129–138.

Chaitow, L. (2010) *Palpation and assessment skills*. Edinburgh: Churchill Livingstone.

Fourie, W. & Robb, K. (2009) Physiotherapy management of axillary web syndrome following breast cancer treatment: Discussing the use of soft tissue techniques. *Physiotherapy*. 95: 314–320.

Franklyn-Miller, A. et al. (2009) IN: *Fascial Research II: Basic Science and Implications for Conventional and Complementary Health Care Munich:* Elsevier GmbH.

Fryer, G., Morris, T., Gibbons, P. et al. (2007) The activity of thoracic paraspinal muscles identified as abnormal with palpation. *JMPT*. 29(6): 437–447.

Fryer, G., Morris, T. & Gibbons, P. (2004) The relationship between palpation of thoracic paraspinal tissues and pressure sensitivity measured by a digital algometer. *J Ost Med*. 7: 64–69.

Fryer, G., Morris, T. & Gibbons, P. (2005) The relationship between palpation of thoracic tissues and deep paraspinal muscle thickness. *Int J Ost Med*. 8: 22–28.

Greenman, P.E. (1996) *Principles of manual medicine*. 2nd Edition. Maryland: Williams and Wilkins.

Grinnel, F. (2009) *Fibroblast mechanics in three-dimensional collagen Matrices. Fascia Research II: Basic Science Implications for Conventional and Complementary Health Care*. Munich: Elsevier GmbH.

Hammer, W. (1999) Thoracolumbar Fascia and Back Pain. *Dynamic Chiro Canada*. 31(10): 1.

Huijing, P. (1999) Muscular force transmission: a unified, dual or multiple system. *Arch Physiol Biochem*. 107: 292–311.

Janda, V. (1983) Muscle function testing. London: Butterworths.

Janda, V. (1996) Evaluation of muscular balance. In: Liebenson, C. (ed.) *Rehabilitation of the spine*. Baltimore: Williams and Wilkins.

Langevin, H. et al. (2009) Ultrasound evidence of altered lumbar connective tissue structure in human subjects with chronic low back pain. Presentation 2nd Fascia Research Congress.

Myers, T. (2009) *Anatomy Trains*. 2nd edition. Edinburgh: Churchill Livingstone.

Stecco, L. & Stecco, C. (2009) *Fascial Manipulation: Practical Part*. Italy: Piccini.

Willard, F.H., Vleeming, A., Schuenke, M.D. et al. (2012) The thoracolumbar fascia: anatomy, function and clinical considerations. *Jnl Anatomy*. 221(6): 507–536.

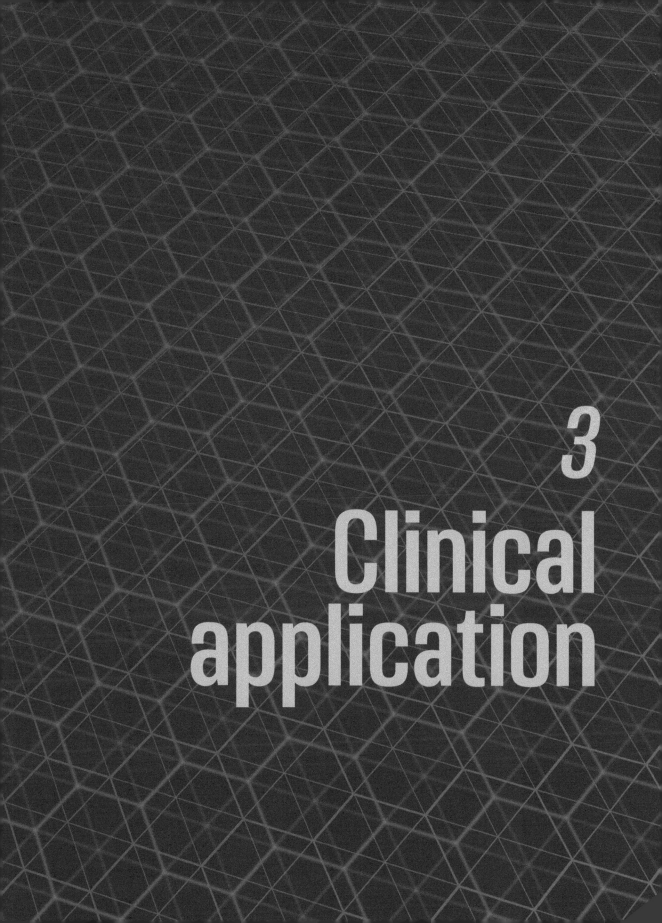

3
Clinical application

Integrating clinical experience and scientific evidence: Roadmap for a healthy dialog between health practitioners and academic researchers

Robert Schleip and Jan Wilke

Imagine you are back at school and eagerly waiting for your teacher to appear. When the teacher does not show up, you start inspecting the other classrooms, spying through each door's keyhole. Two rooms attract your interest: in the first stands no other than the great Albert Einstein, one of the most famous physicists in the history of humankind. His profession reflects objectivity and precision. In the second classroom, you see Yoda, a 900-year-old, very wise fictional character from the fantasy film saga, *Star Wars*. In the galactic movies, Yoda, a so-called Jedi master, is the go-to-guy for the main protagonists fighting against a dark empire. Using his mental superpowers, Yoda can move spaceships and create illusions: pure magic, although it is not exactly known how this works. Upon which door would you knock? (Figure 23.1). Think wisely, we will further delineate the role of Einstein and Yoda later.

The following chapters are devoted to clinical applications. Because many of these are written by clinicians rather than professional scientists, it is helpful to add a reflection on the different types of language frequently used by these two groups. A more sceptical language is used among scientists, which only makes careful suggestions without any absolute predictions, is usually regarded as the more respectable. It serves the purpose of scientific publication and scientific debates but often frustrates outsiders, who require something more concrete than the response of "We don't know. Further research is needed" from scientists answering their questions.

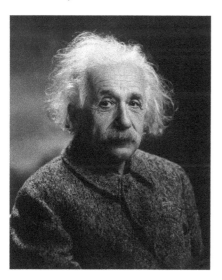
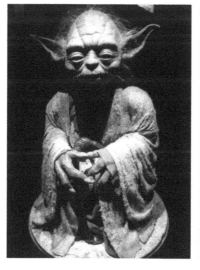

Figure 23.1

Physicist Albert Einstein (left) and master Yoda (right), the supposedly 900-year-old Jedi master from the *Star Wars* trilogy, represent two seemingly opposite orientation contexts, which are frequently used in complementary and integrative movement therapies. The editors of this book recommend a strong scientific reasoning orientation while being open to inspiration by intuitive concepts originating from clinical experience.

Chapter 23

On the other side, it is common practice, particularly among personal trainers, fitness coaches and manual therapists, to describe the effectiveness of their treatments with absolute and very positive predictions. These practitioners tend to be very enthusiastic about their preferred explanation of the physiological mechanism behind the respective treatment modality. This is often the case, even if a careful evidence-based literature analysis only supports a less fulminant prediction and explanation. However, since the majority of experts agree that motivation of the client is an essential contributor to therapeutic success, and because the therapeutic effectiveness tends to matter more for a good therapist than the academic correctness of their statements, it is easy to understand their overzealous descriptions. While this kind of enthusiastic language tends to work well for communication with the public and with most clients, it does hamper a constructive interaction and mutual learning process among enthusiastic practitioners of different treatment concepts, and, also, scientists and clinicians.

Despite having a strong clinical focus, as book editors we are primarily scientists and therefore tend to prefer the more careful language, as it is common practice in academic publications. However, we are also strongly impressed by the rich experience and reflections of the leading practitioners in the fields covered in the following chapters. While not wanting to downsize their valuable and impressive experience and motivation, we, therefore, suggested adding some careful distinctions between the different levels of evidence behind their statements, even if this was their previous practice and approach. We truly thank those authors who have inserted critical reflections congruently into their chapters, and also understand if this was not always possible. We also want to encourage the reader to treat these chapters with a healthy mixture of open-minded curiosity, critical scepticism and eagerness for learning.

The common slogan "Who heals is right" deserves special support in the field of complementary and integrative therapies. This slogan certainly makes sense in terms of clinical effectiveness, meaning that whoever achieves long-lasting therapeutic improvements is doing something right. We would, however, question that this necessarily applies to the personal interpretation of the therapist regarding the physiological mechanisms involved. Basically, when the effect of a treatment has to be explained, there are three possible avenues: first, a practitioner may be simply right with their theoretical rationale. Second, they may be wrong, and what is induced is a placebo response. Third, they may be wrong because the true mechanism is different to the one initially proposed.

The placebo response represents an area of discord in discussions among researchers and practitioners. It is believed that the word placebo first occurred due to a mistranslation of the Hebrew bible. Around the 1300s, the phrase "I will walk before the Lord in the land of the living" was expressed in Latin as "I shall please the lord in the land of the living" ("Placebo Domino in regione vivorum"; Aronson, 1999). While controversy exists as to how the word entered medical literature, its original use could not be closer to what placebo represents today: it is centered around the patient or athlete, pleasing them with the aim to make them feel better or stronger. Having said this, it is clear that satisfying a patient can have multiple contributors: as well as the actual effect of a treatment (which indicates the non-placebo part), this also includes the behavior of the therapist or coach, the atmosphere and setting, the attitudes, beliefs and expectations of the client as well as the

Integrating clinical experience and scientific evidence: Roadmap for a healthy dialog between health practitioners and academic researchers

credibility of the disposed intervention (Finniss et al., 2010). The named placebo factors can be strongly interrelated. For instance, the credibility of acupuncture will also depend on a patient's interest in alternative treatment methods.

Enemies of the placebo effect frequently disqualify it by commentating that it is imagined. This position, however, is both simultaneously right and wrong. While it certainly needs some imagination/expectation from the client, the effects observed are not unreal: research has shown that credible treatments without an actual effect, among others, can trigger the production of opioids or dopamine, induce changes in brain activation, and affect the secretion of hormones and immune mediators (e.g., interleukin; Finniss et al., 2010). The common remark that "this is just placebo" is thus hiding a useful aspect of a treatment method. However, why should practitioners still seek to treat according to the best evidence? First, they should be aware that a placebo can also be harmful, which is called nocebo. Here, a treatment thought to have no direct effect induces a worsening because of the possibility of triggering psycho-physical adaptations can also have harmful consequences (e.g., increased nervousness, fear). Second, albeit to a varying degree, the placebo is always specific: because it depends on the practitioner, client and the specifics of the situation, it is quite obvious that it cannot always be reproduced reliably. An effective method, however, should be available for multiple therapists, coaches, clients and situations. Finally, while the positive effects of the placebo are deeply welcome, they still compete with the true effects of an effective treatment, which can be considerably higher. As a consequence, the discussion as to whether the placebo is the good, the bad or the ugly is meaningless. The actual treatment effects and the placebo are not false but best friends: each treatment has an inert effect, whose size can be trivial or large. High credibility may enhance the effect. Treatment effectivity is hence determined by the true effect of the intervention (research shows it is the most important part) plus the placebo effect. Our recommendation can hence be broken down to one simple imperative: find the best available evidence and apply it in the best possible setting, which depends on the client.

Besides the placebo, a second reason why practitioners may be wrong with their proposal for a treatment's mechanism is that the intervention has an effect, but that the assumed explanation is incorrect. A good example for the difference between the effectiveness of a treatment and its explanatory mechanism is the history of aspirin. While natural origins of the substance—for example, in the form of willow's extract—had already been successfully used by Hippocrates, and even before in ancient Egypt, the modern pharmacological substance acetylsalicylic acid was originally invented in 1898. It was subsequently used as one of the most successful analgesic medicines for many decades, and yet without any proper understanding of its physiological mechanism (Miner and Hoffhines, 2007). In fact, during the early decades of its usage, the most accepted theory for its physiological mechanism was that aspirin relieves pain by working on the central nervous system. However, later research revealed that this assumption was wrong, as the drug mainly works locally by combatting pain and inflammation. It was not until 1970 that the basic mechanism—its inhibition of prostaglandin synthesis—was finally discovered, and this important insight was even honored with a Nobel award. Further clarifications about the exact pathways of its inhibitory effect led to the development of other powerful analgesic substances, but also to important additional applications of aspirin, which is currently not

Chapter 23

only used as an analgesic and anti-inflammatory medicine, but also as a heart drug.

Similarly, it is quite possible that some of the therapeutic approaches described in the following chapters may have proven their clinical effectiveness long before their physiological working mechanism will be properly understood. For many powerful fascia therapies, the first explanations of their founders may subsequently prove to be considered "noble guessing attempts" by practitioners and scientists once new scientific insights become available. Some clinicians therefore take the standpoint: "Why bother about the mechanism? If a treatment works, that is enough to know." However, we suggest that, as witnessed in the case of aspirin, a scientific explanatory model can indeed lead to a refinement of and additional applications of the original therapy. If acupuncture works equally strongly on points several centimeters apart from the official acupuncture point location then that is indeed helpful to know, and may lead to therapeutic advances in the next few decades. And if a positive relationship context between patient and practitioner is required as an essential ingredient for a given therapeutic modality, that insight should also be included in the respective explanatory model.

A good orientating principle to follow when looking for improved explanatory mechanisms among scientists is known as Occam's razor. Attributed to the 14th century philosopher, William of Ockham, this principle suggests that among competing hypotheses, the one with the fewest number of wild assumptions is preferable. For example, if a patient has influenza-like symptoms during an epidemic, it is more likely that the patient suffers from influenza, rather than from a new type of intergalactic brain infection. Or, as medical interns are often advised, "When you hear hoofbeats, think horses, not zebras."

We suggest that this principle could also be applied—not as an absolute rule but rather as a first orientation—when examining different explanatory models in these chapters on clinical applications. One good example of this could be how to account for what is often called "tissue memory" (Tozzi, 2014). Some patients are not able to remember the details of a past injury until a practitioner works on the affected tissue, at which point the patient sometimes suddenly sees, hears or smells an incident that happened decades before. For some practitioners these incidences have been used as proof that fascial tissue can store and process memory via some yet-to-be-discovered electromagnetic (or quantum-based) signaling system, independent of the nervous system.

While it would be unwise to completely rule out the possibility that such additional and exotic signaling systems will be discovered in the future, and may then also correctly apply to this phenomenon, we suggest that the much simpler models of context-dependent or state-dependent memory in conventional psychology are probably sufficient. According to these well-established principles, it is not unusual that during memory retrieval by the brain that a specific sensory stimulus pattern works as a cue for accessing previously forgotten episodic events. This could be a specific smell, sound or tissue sensation in the body. Similarly, a specific state of the nervous system—such as the influence of alcohol or the experience of a particular pain—can access memories associated with that physiological condition, but which were considered to be forgotten before. In other words, a Nobel award is not very likely if a future study proves that this simple and rather unspectacular psychological explanation is valid in the described tissue memory phenomenon. By contrast, a future study revealing support for the exotic

267

Integrating clinical experience and scientific evidence: Roadmap for a healthy dialog between health practitioners and academic researchers

alternative hypothesis of fascia as a quantum dynamics-based signaling system—enabling much faster and more complex communications compared with the nervous system—would certainly cause more excitement and attention. However, Occam's razor suggests placing our bets on the former rather than the latter outome.

It is not known whether Albert Einstein and Yoda would have agreed upon most of their standpoints. In this chapter, the physicist represents the researchers, while Yoda stands for the practitioners. Both have their place in the world—and they probably would have enjoyed talking to each other.

References

Aronson, J. (1999) Please, please me. *BMJ*. 318: 716.

Finniss, D.G., Kaptchuk, T.J., Benedetti, F., et al. (2010) Placebo effects: biological, clinical and ethical advances. *Lancet*. 375: 686–695.

Miner, J., & Hoffhines, A. (2007) The discovery of aspirin's antithrombotic effects. *Tex Heart Inst J*. 34: 179–186.

Tozzi, P. (2014) Does fascia hold memories? *J Bodyw Mov Ther*. 18: 259–265.

Fascial Fitness

Robert Schleip, Divo G. Müller and Bill Parisi

How to build a youthful, resilient fascial body

The elegant movements of a dancer, the impressive performance of a circus artist, the powerful throw of an Olympic javelin thrower, are not only a matter of muscular strength, good cardiovascular condition, neuromuscular coordination (Jenkins, 2005) and good luck in genetics. According to current findings in the international field of fascia research, the muscular connective tissues, called myofasciae, have more meaning for a body in motion than had been generally considered several decades ago. Recent research findings prove that the body-wide fascial network plays a significant role in force transmission, hydration (fluid dynamic) and proprioception (Chapters 9, 12, 13 and 15).

Specific training, focusing on the question of how to build a strong and flexible fascial body, could be of great value to athletes, dancers, martial arts students and somatic oriented movement advocates. It could also contribute to better prevention of the wide distribution of fascial injuries in athletes (Wilke et al., 2019). The optimal fascial body is both elastic and resilient, and can, therefore, be relied upon to respond effectively to a variety of challenges and circumstances, thereby providing a high degree of injury prevention (Kjaer et al., 2009) (Chapters 4–6).

This chapter mainly focuses on one specific aspect of Fascial Fitness, the elastic storage capacity of kinetic energy by the collagenous tissues. How to stimulate the fibroblasts to lay down new collagenous fibers in a healthy and youthful network architecture is explored. The physiological and biomechanical foundations that underlie the training principles which follow are described in Chapters 1–6.

The basic principles of a fascia-focused movement training approach, called Fascial Fitness, were first developed by an international group of scientists and clinicians (including Thomas Myers, James Earls, Wilbour Kelsick, Stephen Mutch, Markus Rossmann, Stefan Dennenmoser, Carina Trippelsdorf and Simone Lindner, in addition to the authors of this chapter as well as other contributors). This happened subsequent to the 2009 Fascia Research Congress, at which the surprising changes in length of aponeurotic fasciae versus muscular sarcomeres during hopping movements were impressively demonstrated by Kawakami and Fukunaga (2006). The training principles of Fascial Fitness, as developed by its founders, were first described by Müller and Schleip (2011) and have continued to evolve since then.

Three modes of fascia-muscle interaction

Previous descriptions of Fascial Fitness, including the corresponding chapter on this topic in the first edition of this book, mainly emphasized the energy conservation mode, in which the

Chapter 24

strain and subsequent recoil of fascial elements are maximally utilized, as typified by the hopping of a kangaroo (Figure 24.1A). This important mode of fascia-muscle interaction is described in greater detail in Chapter 8.

However, there are two additional modes of functional interaction between fascial elements and muscle fibers that should also be implemented in training routines. Figure 24.1B illustrates the alternative mode of power amplification as used in a single frog jump or in squat jump exercises in plyometrics. Here, a rapid concentric muscular contraction induces a lengthening strain of fascial fibers,

whose subsequent recoil motion then leads to the rapid body dislocation. Regular practice of that modality not only enhances an increase in fascial stiffness, but also in fast-twitch muscle fibers.

Figure 24.1C describes a third mode of fascia-muscle interaction, in which kinetic energy is dampened by lengthening of collagenous fibers as well as by eccentric muscular contraction. Examples of this mode of 'power attenuation' include the soft and quiet landing of a gymnast or of a jumping cat on the ground as well as the smooth catching of a flying medicine ball.

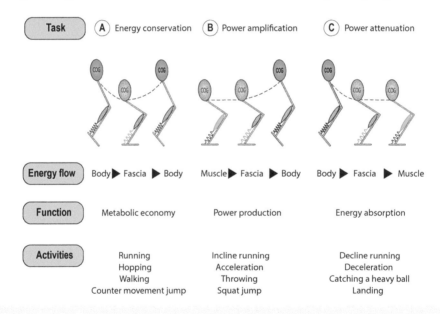

Figure 24.1

Three modes of functional interaction between parallel fibered fascial tissues (here, mainly tendon and aponeuroses) and muscle. In **(A)**, the energy conservation mode, the center of gravity (COG) shifts down and up, mainly changing the length and tonus of the fascial elements, while the muscle fibers are less strongly involved. In **(B)**, the power amplification mode, a rapid concentric muscular contraction leads the process, which then strains the fascial elements, whose subsequent recoil action then increases the upwards momentum of the COG. In **(C)**, the power amplification mode, the kinetic energy generated by a drop of COG is absorbed in a dampening fascial elongation, as well as in an orchestrated eccentric muscular contraction. Red color: current storage location of kinetic energy (in terms of an increase in the relative height of COG, or as temporary strain of fascial fibers, or as an active muscular contraction). Illustration modified after Roberts and Azizi (2011) with permission.

Fascial Fitness

The rapid lengthening of both fascial as well as muscular fibers in this application mode tends to go along with more frequent tissue micro-ruptures (or irritations) in both tissues than the other two interaction modes, as seen in a higher incidence of delayed onset muscle soreness (DOMS), which has been shown to include a high sensitization of intrafascial nerve endings (The clinical observation of us authors of the respective fascial length changes during loading suggest that an increase in tendon crimp seems to be particularly expressed in athletes emphasizing mode A, such as runners, whereas an additional increase in epimysial thickness has been observed in athletes emphasizing mode B, such as javelin throwers. In addition, an increase in endomysial thickness has been observed after regular downhill running (mode C) based on yet unpublished work of Prof. Wilhelm Bloch (Univ. of Cologne, Germany). Further research is necessary to clarify the complex architectural tissue adaptations to the three different modes of fascia loading.

Practical application to enhance power conservation (elastic recoil)

Preparatory counter-movement

To increase the dynamics of elastic recoil (type A in Figure 24.1), the movement is first initiated with a pre-tensioning in the opposite direction, followed by the actual movement. A suitable metaphor would be an archer who pre-stretches the tendon of their bow in the opposite direction before shooting the arrow in the desired direction. Applying muscular effort in pushing the arrow forward would not be of a comparable effectiveness (Chapter 8).

Frontal leg

Standing with feet hip-width apart, shift the weight onto one leg (Figure 24.2). At the beginning, to aid balance, hold on to the back of a chair. To progress, you may later remove the balancing aid, once the movement is familiar and fluent.

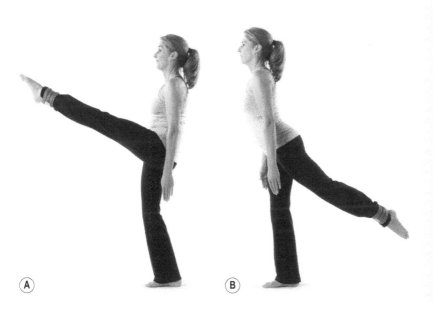

(A) (B)

Figure 24.2 Leg swing

(A) The leg is first extended backwards in such a way that a pre-stretch is created in the front.

(B) The stored tension is then suddenly released and the leg is accelerated forward like a swinging pendulum. Alternating between a dorsiflexed foot position (as shown here) and a plantarflexed position will add variation of the loading focus to different portions of the swinging leg.

Chapter 24

- Start with easy swings of the free leg, swinging backwards and forwards like a pendulum. In such a swinging motion, kinetic energy is rhythmically stored and released; however, the storage of kinetic energy occurs in the spatial relationship of the swinging weight towards gravity, whereas the fascial tissues are not—or not yet—stretch-loaded.

- Increase the loading by deliberately pre-stretching in the opposite direction (backwards), followed by releasing the stored energy through the frontal swing. Here, the kinetic energy is also stored and released, although this time the storage involves an elastic elongation (stretch) of collagenous tissues within the body.

- To further enhance the elastic recoil effect, initiate the frontal leg swing proximally, from your pubic bone or sternum, immediately followed by the distal end, via the pre-stretched leg and foot.

- To load the tissues even more effectively and enhance proprioceptive refinement, use ankle weights.

Fascial effects

The frontal leg swings are optimal to increase elasticity in short hip flexors and to lengthen hamstrings.

Fascial Fitness: Basic elastic recoil exercise – Flying Sword

The Fascial Fitness exercise called the Flying Sword is one of the core exercises to train elastic recoil, especially in the lumbodorsal fascia. Beginners start with steps 1 to 3, subsequently adopting the more refined aspects presented in steps 4 and 5 once the earlier steps have been mastered. Most important is the orchestration of the movement, without muscular effort or strain, and optimally performed as fast, fluid and powerful.

Three basic steps

1. Preparatory counter-movement
2. Proximal initiation of the power motion
3. Sequential delay of more distal body parts in following this movement.

Equipment

Weight, dumbbell, kettle bell, swing dumbbell.

Stand with feet a little wider than hip-width apart so that the weight can easily be moved between your knees.

Step 1: Preparatory counter-movement

Hold the weight with both hands and lift your arms up above your head. Pre-tensioning is achieved, while bending the body's axis slightly backward and extending it in an upward direction, lengthening at the same time (Figure 24.3A). This quick backward bounce initiates the movement and increases the elastic tension in the front fascial "body suit".

Bring the weight down, by releasing the pre-tension through the upper body and arms. This allows them to spring forward and down like a dynamic catapult, allowing the weight to "fly" like a sword between your knees (Figures 24.3B and 24.3C).

Next, reverse this process. Here, the recoil capacity of the fascia is activated by an active pre-tensioning of the posterior fascia by directing the weight further backwards. Before moving from the forward bending position, the flexor muscles on the front of the body are first, briefly, activated. This momentarily pulls the body even further back and down and at the same time the fascia

Fascial Fitness

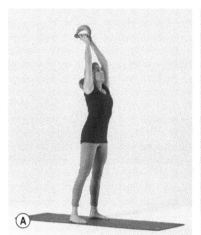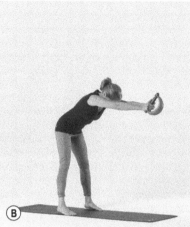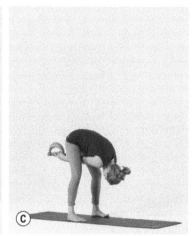

Figure 24.3 Flying Sword

(A) The principle of preparatory counter-movement is an effective way to load the fascial tissues, before performing the actual movement in the desired direction. For example, in this exercise we start the movement with a pre-stretch into the opposite direction, slightly bending backwards.

(B) Releasing down: the stored energy in the connective tissues allow a dynamic and efficient movement performance. In this phase we "fly" down, with hardly any muscular effort, but relying instead on the capacity of fascia to store kinetic energy and release it.

(C) At the turning point: pull the weight and the upper body slightly more backwards into the preparatory counter-movement. To increase the recoil effect and loading of the fascia of the back, briefly activate the flexor muscles on the front of the body first, before releasing the stored energy in flying up into the starting position.

Photograph reprints with permission from www.blackroll.com.

on the back of the body is loaded with greater tension. The kinetic energy, which is stored on the posterior side of the fascial net, is dynamically released via a passive recoil effect as the upper body flies back to the original upright position.

Rhythm is it

A feeling of rhythm is required to ensure that the individual is not relying on the muscle work of their back muscles, but rather on the dynamic recoil activity of the fascia, in addition to the preparatory counter-movement. This is similar to the timing necessary when playing with a yo-yo. If the inherent rhythm is met, it swings with almost effortless ease and flow (Chapter 8).

Step 2: Proximal initiation to perform the actual motion

From the pre-tensed backward bending position, the forward movement is initiated by a proximal pull of the sternum followed by the distal parts of the body (Figure 24.4). In this exercise, the sternum or pubic bone initiates the release forwards and downwards.

Step 3: Sequential delay of more distal body parts following this movement

The proximal initiation of Step 2 is immediately followed by a sequential delay of the more distal body parts. In this exercise, the arms and

Chapter 24

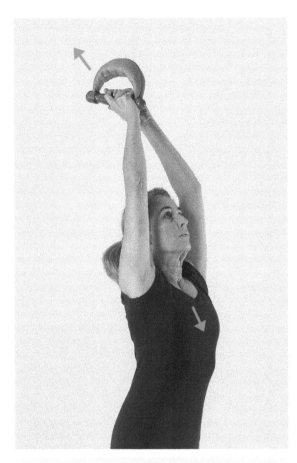

Figure 24.4 Proximal initiation and distal delay

To increase the elastic recoil effect and its power in action, we initiate the movement by the proximal pull of the sternum, followed by a distal delay of the upper body, in this example by the arms and the hands, creating a flowing whip-like movement and thereby increasing the energy storage and release.

hands holding the weight follow behind, creating a wave-like movement. By using the proximal initiation and sequential delay of the distal parts, the pre-tension of the body is further increased, and dynamic power and acceleration are enhanced.

Two advanced steps to enhance elastic recoil

Having mastered these basic steps in a recoil movement exercise, add these two more advanced steps to refine the orchestration of the movement.

The following two steps are practiced immediately prior to the three basic steps described above.

Advanced step 1: Increase of sensory awareness – proprioceptive refinement

One of the big surprises resulting from fascial research was the discovery that fascia contains a rich supply of sensory nerves, including proprioceptive receptors, multimodal receptors and nociceptive nerve endings. This means that fascia is alive (Chapter 15)!

Histologial findings indicate that the superficial fascial layers of the body are, in fact, much more densely populated with sensory nerve endings than the connective tissues situated internally (Benetazzo et al., 2011; Tesarz et al., 2011). In particular, the transition zone between the fascia profunda and the subdermal loose connective tissue seems to have the highest sensorial innervation (Tesarz et al., 2011). The body-wide connective tissue network is certainly our most important organ for proprioception (Schleip, 2003).

For a long time, proprioception shared a similar history to fascia, and, at the start of the 21st century, was rediscovered as our main movement sense. In a movement training routine, there are a variety of ways to train and stimulate sensory or proprioceptive refinement. Common and effective ways before the actual movement include rubbing, tapping, rolling, brushing or kinesiotaping specific bodyparts to stimulate the receptors of the superficial fascial layers.

In a more refined preparation, mindfulness and the benefits of conscious attention focus may be used (Moseley et al., 2008). For example, by focusing on the natural expansive wave of inhalation to expand from within into the surrounding space or by sensing the slightest touch of the air on the skin (Chapter 47).

Advanced step 2: Tensegral expansion

Tensegrity (Chapter 11), and the essential role that fascial membranes play in the structural well-being of the body, are utilized in the principle of tensegral expansion. However, before we move into action, we must first engage a 360-degree body-wide spacious expansion. This can be achieved by an all-over pre-tensioning of the superficial fascia, which envelopes the body as a whole. In Fascial Fitness training, we describe this as "tensing the tiger body suit". Research findings show that this kind of tensegral pretension is a substitute for a "power pose" that is known from the animal kingdom. This has instant positive effects by changing our psychological condition (Carney et al., 2010).

In the Flying Sword exercise, this would be created by bringing attention to the body's "poles", engaging a slight bi-directional movement apart, from top to toe; or in fascial terms, from the plantar fascia to the galea aponeurotica, as well as a widening from front to back. The same kind of attention is added while bending backwards, to load the fascial chain of the front. Here, the tensegral expansion between the vertebrae is enhanced, to avoid any buckling and, therefore, straining in the cervicals or the lumbars.

Practical application to enhance power amplification

In the principle of power amplification (Figure 24.1B), the motion is started with a rapid concentric muscular contraction. This is partially transmitted into a lengthening strain of tendons, aponeuroses and other fascial tissues, whose subsequent elastic recoil action then adds additional momentum to the overall joint motion. It is ideal if the tonicity (pre-stress) of the fascial tissues fits exactly to the expected magnitude of the muscular contraction, that is, for a moderate muscular contraction, a moderate fascial pre-stress may be best suited, while a very powerful overall motion may require a much stronger fascial pre-stress.

Contrary to the previously described elastic recoil motions, such power amplification motions are not initiated with a quick preparatory counter-movement. In the athletic field of plyometrics, many forms of "squat jump" training variations exist, which are well suited to this method of muscle-fascia interaction. Similarly, many athletic throwing techniques, such as javelin throwing, fit well into this basic principle.

Frog jump

Start in a squatted position, with your knees directly over your front feet. Keep your arms extended backwards and raise your chest slightly in an upward/forward direction. Experiment with finding the ideal bending position for your ankles, knees and hip joints, as well as the best position for your arms, to give you maximum momentum. Do not initiate the jump with a preparatory downwards bounce, but rather start the jumping with an explosive upwards motion.

Chapter 24

Figure 24.5 shows the more joyous motion variation, in which the arms are allowed to contribute additional momentum. An alternative version can also be conducted without the upwards arm swing. In this version, the power amplification of the legs is more strongly emphasized.

Practical applications to enhance power attenuation

Daily fascial training: Stair dancing

Walking up and down stairs can become an instant fascial recoil training when the Ninja principle (see below) is applied. A variation of easy bounces in stepping is suggested with the focus of making as little noise as possible. The "no sound parameter" provides useful feedback to engage the fascial springiness: the quieter and gentler the better. Dancing fascially up and down the stairs would be of additional benefit using a barefoot-like plantar-foot contact with the ground (Chapter 32).

The Ninja principle

The Ninja principle uses the metaphor of the legendary Japanese warriors, who reputedly moved as silently as cats leaving no trace. When engaging fascial elements in bouncy movements, such as jumping, running or dancing, the quality of motion should be as smooth and quiet as possible. A change in direction is preceded by a gradual deceleration of the movement before the turning point and a gradual acceleration afterwards. Any harsh, jerky or noisy movement would be counter-productive. The sensed benefits could be a perception of fluid, elegant and effective movement, like a cat in a dynamic leap or stalking while hunting (Figure 24.6).

Fascial stretching

In Fascial Fitness, both dynamic and slow stretching applications are used. Instead of stretching isolated muscle groups, the aim is finding body movements that engage the longest possible myofascial chains (Chapter 13). In the slower

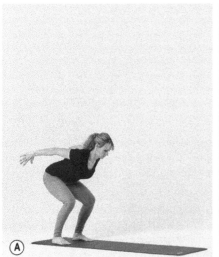
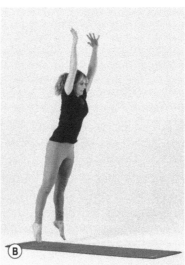

Figure 24.5 The exercise frog jump demonstrates one of several options for the principle of power amplification

(A) In a squatted position, proper pre-tension is tensegrally distributed throughout the whole body, including the arms.

(B) The release of this pre-tension is then immediately followed by an explosive upwards jumping motion.

Fascial Fitness

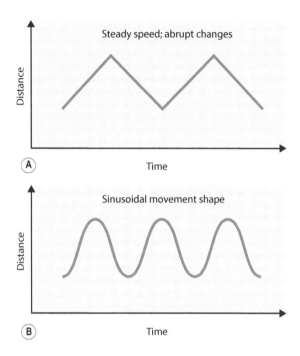

Steady speed; abrupt changes

(A) Time

Sinusoidal movement shape

(B) Time

Figure 24.6 Movement quality in change of direction: jerky versus elegant turns

When a dynamic arm movement (e.g. forward and back), is performed with lack of proprioceptive refinement, the tendency is to use sudden turns and provoke **(A)** abrupt loading patterns. By contrast, when the same movements are conducted with an internal search for elegance, then **(B)** a more sinusoidal movement directional change can be observed. This is characterized by a gradual deceleration before the turning point, which is followed by a subsequent gradual acceleration. In this pattern, the loaded tissues are less prone to injuries, and the movements appear fluid and graceful.

stretches, this is not done by passively waiting, as in a lengthening classical Hatha yoga pose, or in a conventional isolated muscle stretch. Because the majority of the human fascial net is composed of membranous sheets, rather than long narrow stripes, multidirectional angular variations are frequently explored during stretching. This might include sideways or diagonal movement variations as well as spiraling rotations. With this method, large areas of the fascial network are simultaneously involved.

The dynamic stretching variation may be familiar to many readers, as it was part of the physical education in the first half of the 20th century. In recent decades, such bouncing stretches were considered to be generally harmful to the tissue, but contemporary research has confirmed the method's merits. While stretching immediately before athletic performance (e.g. 30 s before a competitive run) may induce minor attenuations in the performance of world-class athletes, long-term and regular use of dynamic stretching, when correctly performed, can positively influence the architecture of the connective tissue, in that it becomes more elastic and injury resistant (Decoster et al., 2005; Chaabene et al., 2019). For dynamic stretching, the muscles and tissue should be warmed up first, and any jerking or abrupt movements should be avoided. The aforementioned principles of elastic recoil can often be applied, including the proprioceptive refinement, using a sinusoidal deceleration and the preparatory counter-movement.

When the elongated myofibers are in a relaxed condition then a slow stretching approach is sufficient to reach many intramuscular fascial tissues. However, this approach does not reach the tendinous tissues as they are arranged in

Chapter 24

series with the relaxed and soft myofibers (Figure 24.7C). In order to stimulate these tendinous and aponeurotic tissues, more dynamically swinging stretch movements are recommended, similar to the elegant and fluid extensional movements of rhythmic gymnasts. The same tissues can also be targeted by muscular activation (e.g. against resistance) in a lengthened position, similar to how a cat sometimes enjoys pulling their front claws towards the trunk when stretching (Figure 24.7D). Finally, so-called "mini-bounces" can also be employed as soft and playful explorations in the lengthened stretch position.

Fascial training guidelines

One main intention of a connective tissue-oriented training routine is to influence the matrix remodeling via specific training activities, which may, after 3–12 months, result in a more resilient "silk-like body suit". This creates a strong and elastic fibrous network that is at the same time flexible, allowing smooth gliding joint mobility over wide angular ranges. A few Fascial Fitness training guidelines to support optimal results are listed below.

Low loading

Inclusion of fascial rebound and long myofascial chains often triggers an exhilarating sense of playfulness, fun and adventure orientation. However, if untamed, this can also lead to more frequent injuries than standard muscle training, which features monotonous repetitions. Start with much lower loads and repetitions than usual. Increase load only if a sense of elegance can be maintained, particularly during the elastic rebound phase.

Low frequency

The examination of collagen turnover in a tendon after exercise has shown that collagen synthesis is, indeed, increased after exercise.

Yet the fibroblasts also break collagen down at the same time. Furthermore, 24–48 h after exercise, collagen degradation is greater than collagen synthesis. After 48 h and thereafter this situation is reversed. Therefore, it is suggested that this appropriate tissue stimulation only occurs 1–2 times per week (Magnusson et al., 2010) (Chapter 1).

Long-lasting effect

In contrast to muscular strength training, in which big gains occur rapidly in only a few weeks, fascia renewal is much slower (Chapter 1). Therefore, the improvements during the first few weeks may be small and less obvious on the outside. It usually takes 3–9 months to see tissue remodeling effects from the outside as well as "to feel" them in palpation. In muscular training, a plateau is reached relatively quickly, with further increases difficult to achieve. However, fascial improvements have a cumulative effect and will not be lost as quickly (e.g. when training is stopped because of health- or work-related reasons), and are, therefore, of a more sustainable quality (Kjaer et al., 2009) (Chapter 5). Regular application over 2–3 years will definitely be expected to yield long-lasting tissue improvements in the form of improved strength and elasticity of the global fascial network.

Clinical summary

Fascial Fitness training does not seek to compete with neuromuscular or cardiovascular training, both of which can have very important health effects that are not possible with fascial training on its own. On the contrary, fascial training is suggested as either a sporadic or more regular addition to comprehensive movement training. It promises to lead towards remodeling of the body-wide fascial network in such a way that it works with increased effectiveness and refinement

Fascial Fitness

in terms of its kinetic storage capacity, as well as a sensory organ for proprioception. Further research is required to validate whether it does, indeed, fulfill its basic promise of increased protection against repetitive strain injuries in sports medicine.

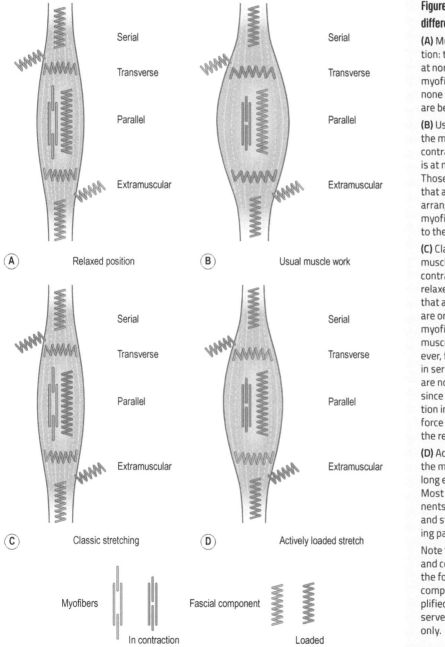

Figure 24.7 Loading of different fascial components

(A) Muscle in relaxed position: the tissue muscle is at normal length and the myofibers are relaxed. Here, none of the fascial elements are being stretched.

(B) Usual muscle work: the myofibers are actively contracted while the muscle is at normal length range. Those fascial tissues that are loaded are either arranged in series with the myofibers or run transverse to them.

(C) Classic stretching: the muscle is elongated and its contractile myofibers are relaxed. Here, fascial tissues that are being stretched are oriented parallel to the myofibers, as well as extramuscular connections. However, fascial tissues oriented in series with the myofibers are not sufficiently loaded, since most of the elongation in that serially arranged force chain is taken up by the relaxed myofibers.

(D) Actively loaded stretch: the muscle is activated in long end range positions. Most of the fascial components are being stretched and stimulated in that loading pattern.

Note that various mixtures and combinations between the four different fascial components exist. This simplified abstraction therefore serves as a basic orientation only.

Chapter 24

References

Benetazzo, L., Bizzego, A., De Caro, R., Frigo, G., Guidolin, D. & Stecco, C. (2011) 3D reconstruction of the crural and thoracolumbarfasciae. *Surg Radio Anat*. 33: 855–862.

Carney, D.R., Cuddy, A.J. & Yap, A. (2010) Power posing: brief nonverbal displays affect neuroendocrine levels and risk tolerance. *J Psychol Sci*. 21: 1363–1368.

Chaabene, H., Behm, D.G., Negra, Y. & Granacher, U. (2019) Acute effects of static stretching on muscle strength and power: An attempt to clarify previous caveats. *Front Physiol*. 10: 1468.

Decoster, L.C., Cleland, J., Altieri, C. & Russell, P. (2005) The effects of hamstring stretching on range of motion: a systematic literature review. *J Orthopedi Sports Phy Ther*. 35: 377–387.

Jenkins, S. (2005) Sports Science Handbook. In: *The Essential Guide to Kinesiology, Sport & Exercise Science*, volume 1. Essex, UK: Multi-science Publishing.

Kawakami, Y., & Fukunaga, T. (2006) New insights into in vivo human skeletal muscle function. *Exerc Sport Sci Rev*. 34: 16–21.

Kjaer, M., Langberg, H., Heinemeier, K., Bayer, M.L., Hansen, M., Holm, L., Doessing, S., Kongsgaard, M., Krogsgaard, M.R. & Magnusson, S.P. (2009) From mechanical loading to collagen synthesis, structural changes and function in human tendon. *Scand J Med Sci Sports*. 19: 500–510.

Lau, W.Y., Blazevich, A.J, Newton, M.J., Wu, S.S.X. & Nosaka, K. (2015) Changes in electrical pain threshold of fascia and muscle after initial and secondary bouts of elbow flexor eccentric exercise. *Eur J Appl Physiol*. 115: 959–968.

Magnusson, S.P., Langberg, H. & Kjaer, M. (2010) The pathogenesis of tendinopathy: balancing the response to loading. *Nat Rev Rheumatol*. 6: 262–268.

Moseley, G.L., Zalucki, N.M. & Wiech, K. (2008) Tactile discrimination, but not tactile stimulation alone, reduces chronic limb pain. *Pain*. 137: 600–608.

Müller, D.G. & Schleip, R. (2011) Fascial Fitness – Fascia oriented training for bodywork and movement therapies. *Terra Rosa E-Magazine*. 7: 2–11.

Roberts, T.J. & Azizi, E. (2011) Flexible mechanisms: the diverse roles of biological springs in vertebrate movement. *J Experim Biol*. 214: 353–361.

Schleip, R. (2003) Fascial plasticity – a new neurobiological explanation. Part 1. *J Bodyw Mov Ther*. 7: 11–19.

Tesarz, J., Hoheisel, U., Wiedenhofer, B. & Mense, S. (2011) Sensory innervation of the thoracolumbar fascia in rats and humans. *Neuroscience*. 194: 302–308.

Wilke, J., Hespanhol, L. & Behrens, M. (2019) Is it all about the fascia? *Orthop J Sports Med*. 7: 2325967119888500.

Basic principles of plyometric training

Robert Heiduk

Introduction

Plyometric training is commonly performed with the aim of improving power, movement, speed and/or economy of movement. The aim of this chapter is to provide information about its origins and to review potential physiological mechanisms. In addition, this chapter provides some guidelines and recent developments for application and training program design to optimize performance associated with plyometric training.

Origin of plyometric training

The term plyometric is composed of two Greek words: plio, meaning "more", and metric, meaning "to measure". Measurable increase might be the most accurate definition (Chu, 1998). Commonly known as plyometrics, this category of exercise is mostly referred to as jump training. The earliest references have been found in a publication by Zanon (1989). In the early 1960s, Soviet Union track and field coach Yuri Verkhoshansky experimented with maximal jumps and hops to increase power in his high level athletes. He found that "depth" jumping, with landing and take-off on both feet, was particularly effective for improving jump performance. He termed his new training the "Shock Method". The name referred to the mechanical shock stimulation used to force the muscle to produce as much tension as possible (Verkhoshansky and Siff, 2009). Verkhoshansky's strange new system of jumps

and bounds quickly became very popular in the world of sport. In Germany it was popularized by Peter Tschiene, in South Africa by Mel Siff, and in Italy by Carmello Bosco (Verkhoshansky and Siff, 2009). It has been suggested that the dominance of the Eastern European countries in track and field, weightlifting and gymnastics during the 1970s can be partially attributed to the Shock Method (Chu, 1998). In the USA, the term "plyometrics" was coined in 1975 by Verkhoshansky's colleague, the track and field coach Fred Wilt (Chu, 1998).

The stretch-shortening cycle

Walking, running, throwing, jumping, hopping, swinging, hitting and kicking are examples of activities that allow muscle-tendon units (MTUs) to be stretched before shortening rapidly, without delay, between the eccentric and concentric phases. This is known as the stretch-shortening cycle (SSC) (Komi, 2000). There are variations in time characteristics in different types of SSC movement patterns. Güllich and Schmidtbleicher (2000) classify SSC movements into a short (<200 ms) and long (>200 ms) SSC. Examples of a short SSC are sprinting with a ground contact time of ~100–110 ms, the long jump with 120 ms and the high jump with 170–180 ms (Bührle, 1989). The long SSC can be observed in the jump of a volleyball smash with ground contact times of 300–360 ms.

Compared with the pure concentric rate of force development, without a preceding

Chapter 25

eccentric movement phase, use of the SSC creates a significant performance enhancement (Komi, 2000). For example, Cavagna (1964) demonstrated an increase in running economy of ~50%, thus maximizing energy efficiency and improving aerobic performance (Spurrs et al., 2003). In plyometric patterns like bouncing, Dean and Kuo (2011) observed how the properties of the elastic tissues reduce the work needed from active muscle fibers, which leads to a decrease in energy expenditure. In maximum performance, Markovic (2004) found an 8% gain in vertical jump height by utilizing the SSC.

Physiological mechanisms

Currently, elastic and contractile mechanisms are considered to be responsible for performance-enhancing effects in the SSC (Blazevich, 2011). The relative contribution of each mechanism seems to be dependent on the force and time characteristics of the movements. In addition, individual anthropometrics and genetics come into play (Sano et al., 2015). The energy storage and spring-like release of potential energy in elastic tissues, like tendons, mean that MTUs shorten at speeds exceeding those using muscle contraction on its own (Blazevich, 2011).

Zatsiorsky and Kraemer (2008) point out that the amount of elastic energy storage in tendons is largely dependent on the stiffness of the muscles. If we consider muscle and tendon as two springs connected in series, more energy is stored on the compliant spring. Muscle stiffness is dependent on the level of contractile force a muscle can produce, which depends on factors such as muscle size and neural activation.

An additional factor for the importance of muscle force during a countermovement is the ability to decelerate in the eccentric or yielding phase. This specific contractile ability seems to be a supporting factor for the recoil mechanisms in elastic tissues.

Kawakami et al. (2002) showed that, during the eccentric phase of a countermovement plantar flexion, the gastrocnemius only works in a near-isometric manner, which means that only very few length changes in the muscle fibers are observable in this phase. Because, by contrast, the tendon elongates significantly, the SSC cannot be considered as a muscle-related phenomenon. Kangaroos are a perfect example of an efficient use of the SSC (Morgan et al., 1978). Despite comparably small muscles, their long and compliant hind limb tendons allow the storage of large amounts of kinetic energy, which can be used to achieve tremendously long jumping distances. While the role of the tendon in the SSC has been extensively researched, to date there are no data for the deep fascia. However, a similar contribution is conceivable, albeit probably to a smaller degree. In summary, the higher power output observed during the SSC can, at least partially, be attributed to the recoil properties of the connective tissue. A second key factor in the SSC is the amount of coupling time between the eccentric and concentric phase, which is described as the "amortization phase" (Chu, 1998). If the amortization phase lasts too long, the energy being absorbed is lost as heat (Radcliffe and Farentinos, 1999). Schmidtbleicher and Gollhofer (1985) found that in trained athletes the amortization phase was ~100 ms, significantly shorter than in untrained subjects. Other research suggests that the ideal coupling time lasts 15–25 ms (Bosco et al., 1981). Chu (1998) characterizes the amortization phase as quasi-isometric muscle action, which means that muscle length does not significantly change during this period.

Besides elastic recoil and eccentric-concentric contraction coupling, another mechanism for enhanced performance in SSC movements suggests that the rapid pre-stretch of the muscle during the eccentric phase leads to a stretch reflex, which is initiated in the muscle spindle receptor. Consequently, a more powerful muscle contraction is produced, due to the activation of more motor units (Komi, 1992). Rassier and Herzog (2005) propose that the magnitude of force enhancement may come from three different factors: (1) the magnitude of stretch, (2) the rate of stretch and (3) the duration of stretch. The faster the eccentric loading phase then the stronger the concentric muscle contraction (Böhm et al., 2006). Bubeck (2002) adds, that under different loading conditions, the neuromuscular activation patterns change. This would indicate that adaptations in a SSC are highly context-specific. Some authors suggest that the stretch reflex may be not be initiated in all muscles (Nardone et al., 1990): monoarticular muscles, which cross one joint only, may benefit more strongly from the stretch reflex than biarticular muscles (Nicol and Komi, 1998).

The spring-like properties of the elastic tissues vary for subjects of different genders, injury state and athletic background. This would be one explanation for the differences in the effects of plyometric training. It seems that there are movement- and age-specific differences in the behavior of elastic tissues in plyometric training (Arampatzis et al., 2007; Hoffrén et al., 2007).

Preconditions for plyometric training

The implementation of proper plyometric training requires some preliminary considerations. The success of training programs for optimal individual adaptations strongly relies on personalization. At the beginning a specific goal should be defined. Like every other kind of exercise, the training effects are highly movement-specific.

A plyometric training program for golfers is different to one for sprinters, jumpers, gymnasts, strength athletes, or for rehabilitation. Moreover, the current performance level of the athlete has to be considered. A beginner needs a different training stimulus to an intermediate or a top-level athlete. Age, body weight, skill and previous injury play an important role (Holocomb et al., 1998). Starting with plyometric training, the development of a proper exercise technique under qualified instruction and supervision is paramount. The goal is to increase efficiency and avoid injury.

Injury prevention is a critical factor in plyometric training. High impulsive peak forces produce serious injury risks for the joints. Coaches should be aware that plyometric exercises can lead to muscle damage and collagen breakdown of the connective tissues without decreases in skeletal muscle capacity (Tofas et al., 2008). Therefore, risks may result from inappropriate or excessive use, rather than from plyometric training itself (Verkhoshanky and Siff, 2009). Being technically proficient and creating appropriate progression seem to be the most important factors in injury prevention. In addition, the coach has to ensure a proper warm-up and the use of an adequate landing surface (Borkowski, 1990). Wathen (1994) highlights that the quality of the landing surfaces plays a major role in performing plyometric drills. Allerheiligen and Rogers (1996) suggest spring-loaded floors or rubber mats and caution against practicing on concrete or asphalt. Firm natural grass may also be a sufficient training surface. However, overly soft surfaces diminish the effectiveness of plyometrics, as the mechanical stimulus on the body is lowered.

It is suggested that a carefully designed plyometric training regime, over the course of a season, may reduce the incidence of knee injury

Chapter 25

in athletes involved in sports with large jumping and cutting components (Hewett et al., 1999). In addition to the enhancement of the athlete's movement skills, the increased musculotendinous stiffness may be another possible factor for injury prevention (Spurrs et al., 2003).

Depth jumps are the most advertized form of plyometric training, but they also exert the highest loads on body structures (Allerheiligen and Rogers, 1996). Thus, these should only be used by a small percentage of athletes. The jump height is the most critical factor. People weighing more than 98 kg should not perform depth jumps from platforms higher than 45 cm (Chu, 1992). Ishikawa et al. (2005) reported that different drop heights in depth jumps have a specific impact on connective tissues. It seems that overly high eccentric loads limit the effectiveness of the catapult mechanism (Figure 25.1).

Strength and conditioning practitioners should never design a plyometric training routine as a stand-alone program. Every athlete needs an adequate strength base prior to

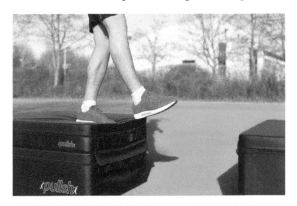

Figure 25.1

Incorporating depth jumps require a well-founded strength base and precise technique. These should only be used by athletes who have advanced to levels that are appropriate for them.

With permission from Pullsh, Germany.

starting plyometric drills. When strength is not adequate, it results in a loss of stability and forces are excessively absorbed by the joints. This leads to an increased risk of injury. For high-intensity drills, like depth jumps, the literature suggests a strength ratio of 1.5–2.5 times body weight in the One Repetition Maximum (1-RM) barbell-squat (Allerheiligen and Rogers, 1996; Chu, 1992; Gambetta, 1992).

These recommendations may not be appropriate for female athletes and, to date, no specific research has addressed this topic. Experience in daily sport practice suggests that for female athletes 1–1.5 times body weight in the 1-RM barbell-squat would be a suitable value. There is also a lack of research on recommendations for strength values in upper body plyometrics and for application in recreational athletes.

In addition, a sufficient amount of specific flexibility is needed to perform plyometric training safely (Chu, 1992). Davies and Matheson (2001) report the following contraindications to plyometrics: pain, inflammation, ligament and capsular sprains, muscle and tendon strains, joint instability, connective tissue limitations based on postoperative conditions, and a lack of strength base.

Basic principles for training program design

First and foremost, there is no general design that can be applied consistently to all competitive athletes. Hence, at this juncture, it would make no sense to lay out a specific training regime because the requirements in each area of training are highly individualized. However, there are some basic rules that apply.

Two different kinds of guidelines are useful when creating a training program. The first approach uses coaching principles, which describe instructions in a deeper context, such as educational aspects to ensure optimal training progression. The four coaching principles in this approach are:

1. Move from simple to complex

2. Move from light to heavy

3. Technique first – quality over quantity

4. Avoid fatigue.

These principles suggest systematically increasing loads and the complexity of movements. Moreover, the principles promote the importance of movement quality instead of quantity—the coach has to ensure the perfect execution of the movement and must avoid fatigue. In the SSC, fatigue is absolutely counterproductive. It causes a decrease in neuromuscular activity and a loss of elastic energy potential (Komi, 2000). This leads to reduced muscle and joint stiffness, which can cause injury. Thus, turning plyometrics into a conditioning program, which is usually designed to develop energy systems, is not advisable. One key to avoid fatigue is to keep a specific work:rest ratio between sets. For rehabilitation, Chu and Cordier (2001) suggest a ratio of 1:5–1:10. When the exercise takes 10 s, 50–100 s rest would be appropriate. True Shock Training, for example, depth jumps, demands considerably longer rest periods. Depending on the intensity, 3–10 min rest is advised (Bubeck, 2001; Sialis, 2004).

The second approach determines the specific load. In plyometric training, intensity is determined by the jumping height or effort, the usage of additional weight, or the style of exercise, like single- or double-leg exercises. Volume and frequency describe more quantitative variables, such as the amount of work within a training session, the total number of jumps, the number of

sets and repetitions, the work:rest ratio between exercise and break within a training session, and the number of sessions per week. According to the literature, a sufficient recovery time of 48–72 h is required. This means a training frequency of approximately twice a week (Chu and Cordier, 2001).

Fluid periodisation

From a biological point of view, general training frequency suggestions can be far removed from the individual's needs, because time courses of adaptation are never linear but instead are based on instability. Therefore, recovery times are not always equal, not even in the same athlete. This is due to environmental changes, as well as asynchronous reactions, of different biological systems in the body.

As previously stated, true plyometric training is very taxing on the nervous system, therefore, for optimal trainability, the timing of a plyometric training session has to be scheduled when the central nervous system (CNS) is in a state of optimal readiness without fatigue. Measurements of the brain's electrical direct current (DC) potential have been proven to be a valid and reliable method for assessment of the functional state of the CNS (Morris, 2015). DC potential is an ultraslow (<0.5 Hz) brainwave that is sensitive to short- and long term adaptational changes in the organism (Iliukhina, 2011).

Practically spoken, measuring DC potential is valuable for detecting CNS fatigue as a result of the effects of different training sessions and interventions. With this additional information it is possible to make adjustments to individual adaptation, because the coach has more information to work with and, via long-term monitoring trends, it can be deduced how an individual responds to certain forms of training. In summary, gaining

Chapter 25

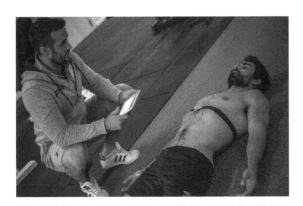

Figure 25.2

Measurement of the brain's electrical direct current (DC) potential with a mobile computer device to detect adaptational changes in the organism and determine the current trainability of the athlete. The setup consists of one electrode on the forehead, a reference electrode on the palm for the central nervous system (CNS), and a chest unit for measuring the heart's electrical activity at the same time.

With permission from Omegawave, Finland

a more objective insight enables optimization of training beyond just guessing or general recommendations (Figure 25.2).

Eccentric overload training

The modality of eccentric overload training has a reasonable value as part of a comprehensive training program, particularly in regard to the importance of specific strength ability in the deceleration phase of the SSC and related MTU stiffness. An eccentric muscle contraction occurs when the external force exceeds the force developed by the muscle.

In a systematic approach to eccentric training, there has to be distinguishment between training with eccentric emphasis and eccentric overload. The first can be employed with almost all resistance training exercises, because this modality is simply a conventional strength training with a slower execution in the yielding phase, that is, 1 s concentric and 3 s eccentric contraction.

This eccentric training modality has different effects that are not specific to the physiological changes seen in the SSC or eccentric overload. Eccentric emphasis training can lead to significant hormonal reactions and elevations in resting metabolic rate, immediately after a training session (Hackney et al., 2008; Preuß, 2010). Nevertheless, in a long-term approach, this modality has value for the body's preparation before progressing to higher loads, as well as providing a means to support recovery during de-load periods.

A true eccentric overload is achieved when the external force is on a level where an isometric contraction is almost impossible. With regard to the SSC a specific eccentric overload has to go beyond submaximal slow eccentrics. This is because, in the eccentric phase, higher loads than the voluntary concentric maximum are possible (Güllich and Schmidtbleicher, 2000), and in the braking phase movement speeds are quite high. In traditional strength training, which is based on gravity, respectively, mass, this is called supramaximal load, (i.e. 105% of the 1-RM).

For a safe and effective eccentric overload, gravity-based equipment, like barbells, dumbbells or kettlebells, are less convenient, because these tools expose the body to an unnecessarily high risk of injury. Spotters are also always needed to keep the weight moving and to overcome the weaker concentric phase.

Therefore, the implementation of eccentric overload strength training has been lacking in traditional strength and conditioning program designs. In addition, traditional weight training using gravity-dependent equipment is limited to vertical action in the frontal plane, leaving out most horizontal and lateral actions in the mode of eccentric overload.

Flywheel training has been proven to close the gap where traditional gravity-based weights and machines have their limits. Instead of working against gravity, in flywheel training the resistance is created through the inertia of a flywheel, which is accelerated or decelerated with muscle force. The level of inertia of the flywheel rather than the weight determines the force needed. The principle is equivalent to that of a traditional yoyo device. Thanks to technological progress and growing research on eccentric training, flywheel training is enjoying a remarkable comeback (Figure 25.3).

The principle of the flywheel became popular in the late 1980s when researchers began to focus on how to maintain lean muscle mass and bone density during extended space travel (Dudley et al., 1991). The effectiveness of flywheel training for developing strength, hypertrophy, power, injury prevention and rehabilitation has been confirmed by extensive research (Alfredson, 2003; Gonzalo-Skok et al., 2016). For improvements in plyometric performance, it is noteworthy that recent research indicates that using eccentric overload training leads to a significantly greater braking and propulsive contact time (de Hoyo et al., 2016). From a practical point of view, the simplicity of training and infinite amount of exercise variation within an eccentrically overloaded environment is the biggest advantage of flywheel training. Last but not least, rehabilitation training with flywheel devices has proven to be an effective means for tendinopathy (Murtaugh and Ihm, 2013), and for the elderly (Onambélé et al., 2008).

Wearable resistance

With increasing performance levels of athletes, specificity of training is paramount to ensure a transfer to performance, because neuromuscular and functional changes induced by exercise are specific to the mode of exercise performed. Thus, plyometric training must exactly match the movement kinetics, kinematics, and metabolic demands of the sport. Therefore, the sport itself would be the most specific way to improve

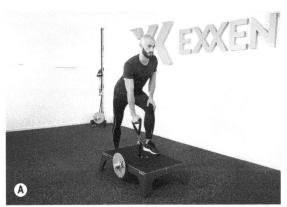
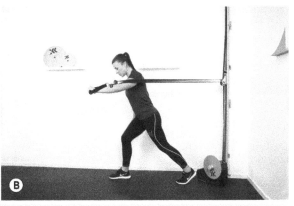

Figure 25.3

A flywheel device is a safe and effective way to apply an eccentric overload at high movement speeds in any movement pattern.

With permission from Exxentric, Sweden.

Chapter 25

performance. (The most specific plyometric training for a sprinter is sprinting.)

Unfortunately, in traditional resistance training, the equipment defines the movement, not the user. This means that the user is attached to a piece of equipment and the characteristics of the equipment determine what he or she can do with it.

The approach of wearable resistance is exactly the opposite by matching resistance equipment to movement. This is achieved by new garment technology, where flexible drop-shaped weights of 50, 100 or 200 g can be stuck to increase the weight of a particular body part. The protocols and loading conditions are different to traditional resistance training. Applied loads are generally measured and progressed in grams not in kilograms and total loading generally does not exceed 10% of body weight in order to maintain movement speeds within 10% of competition speed. Furthermore, the loads should not disrupt the athlete's skill-based range of motion. Here, there is greater focus on maintaining the body-mind connection in a proprioceptively enriched resistance training because in these protocols there is less emphasis on traditional resistance parameters, like repetitions or weight (Figure 25.4).

Conclusions

Reviewing the development of plyometric training from its origins to the present, few significant changes are observable since the 1980s. However, decisive progress has been made in complementary and overarching methods, mainly based on the further development of new technologies. These technological advances open up new opportunities to increase efficiency of training, gaining results with less cost of adaptation and providing a more specific, demand-oriented approach.

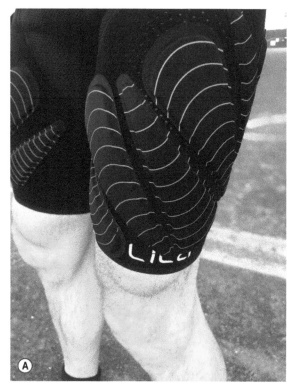

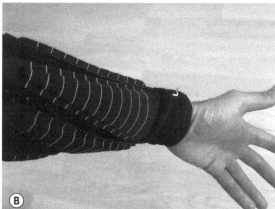

Figure 25.4

Wearable resistance on different body parts. The flexible drop-shaped weights (50, 100 and 200 g) can be placed at any body part in any direction. This methodology allows a proprioceptively enriched resistance training, since the flexible weights are not perceived as foreign bodies, as in conventional weight vests.

With permission from Robert Heiduk, Germany.

References

Alfredson, H. (2003) Chronic midportion achilles tendinopathy: An update on research and treatment. *Clin Sports Med.* 22: 727–741.

Allerheiligen, B. & Rogers, R. (1996) Plyometrics program design. National Strength and Conditioning Association (Eds), *Plyometric and Medicine Ball Training*. Colorado Springs: National Strength and Conditioning Association, 3–8.

Arampatzis, A., Karamanidis, K., Morey-Klapsing, G., De Monte, G. & Stafilidis, S. (2007) Mechanical properties of the triceps surae tendon and aponeurosis in relation to intensity of sport activity. *J Biomech.* 40: 1946–1952.

Blazevich, A. (2011) The stretch-shortening cycle (SSC). In: Cardinale, M., Newton, R. & Nosaka, K. (Eds), *Strength and conditioning: Biological principles and practical applications*. Chichester, UK: Wiley-Blackwell, 209–222.

Böhm, H., Cole, G., Brüggemann, G. & Cole, H. (2006) Contribution of muscle series elasticity to maximum performance in drop jumping. *J Appl Biomech.* 22: 3–13.

Borkowski, J. (1990) Prevention of preseason muscle soreness: plyometric exercise. Abstract. *Athletic Training.* 25: 122.

Bosco, C., Komi, P.V. & Ito A. (1981) Prestretch potentiation of human skeletal muscle during ballistic movement. *Acta Physiologica Scandinavica.* 111: 135–140.

Bubeck, D. (2002) Belastungsvariation und funktionelle Anpassungen im Dehnungs-Verkürzungs-Zyklus. PhD Thesis. Fakultät für Geschichts-, Sozial- und Wirtschaftswissenschaften der Universität Stuttgart.

Bührle M. (1989) Maximalkraft-Schnellkraft-Reaktivkraft. *Sportwissenschaft.* 3: 311–325.

Chu, D. (1992) *Jumping into Plyometrics*. Champaign, IL: Human Kinetics.

Chu, D. & Cordier D. (2000) Plyometrics in Rehabilitation. In: Ellenbecker T.S. (Ed), *Knee Ligament Rehabilitation*. New York, NY: Churchill Livingstone, 321–344.

Davies, G.J. & Matheson, J.W. (2001) Shoulder plyometrics. *Sports Med Arthrosc.* 9: 1–18.

Dean, J.C. & Kuo, A.D. (2011) Energetic costs of producing muscle work and force in a cyclical human bouncing task. *J Appl Physiol.* 110: 873–880.

de Hoyo, M., Sanudo, B., Carrasco, L., Mateo-Cortes, J., Dominguez-Cobo, S., Fernandes, O. & Gonzalo-Skok, O. (2016) Effects of 10-week eccentric overload training on kinetic parameters during change of direction in football players. *J Sports Sci.* 34: 1380–1387.

Dudley, G.A., Tesch, P.A., Miller, B.J. & Buchanan, P. (1991) Importance of eccentric actions in performance adaptations to resistance training. *Aviat Space Environ Med.* 62: 543–550.

Gambetta, V. (1992) New plyometric training techniques: designing a more effective plyometric training program. *Coaching Volleyball*. April/May: 26–28.

Gonzalo-Skok, O., Tous-Fajardo, J., Valero-Campo, C., Berzosa, C., Bataller, A.V., Arjol-Serrano, J.L., Mendez-Villanueva, A. (2016) Eccentric overload training in team-sports functional performance: constant bilateral vertical vs. variable unilateral multidirectional movements. *Int J Sports Physiol Perform.* 1–23.

Güllich, A. & Schmidtbleicher, D. (2000) Struktur der Kraftfähigkeiten und ihrer Trainingsmethoden. In: Siewers, M. (Ed.), *Muskelkrafttraining. Band 1: Ausgewählte Themen – Alter, Dehnung, Ernährung, Methodik*. Kiel: Siewers Eigenverlag, 17–71.

Hackney, K.J., Engels, H.J. & Gretebeck, R.J. (2008) Resting energy expenditure and delayed-onset muscle soreness after full-body resistance training with an eccentric concentration. *J Strength Cond Res.* 22: 1602–1609.

Hewett, T.E., Lindenfeld, T.N., Riccobene, J.V. & Noyes, F.R. (1999) The effect of neuromuscular training on the incidence of knee injury in female athletes. *Am J Sports Med.* 27: 699–705.

Hoffrén, M., Ishikawa, M. & Komi, P.V. (2007) Age-related neuromuscular function during drop jumps. *J Appl Physiol.* 103: 276–283.

Iliukhina, V.A. (2011) Continuity and prospects of development of researches in area system-integrativity of psychophysiology of functional state and cognitive activity. *Human Physiol.* 37: 105–123.

Ishikawa, M., Niemalä, E. & Komi, P.V. (2005) Interaction between fascicle and tendinous tissues in short-contact stretch-shortening cycle exercise with varying eccentric intensities. *J Appl Physiol.* 99: 217–223.

Komi, P.V. (1992) Stretch shortening cycle. In: *Strength and Power in Sport*.

Oxford, UK: Blackwell Scientific, 169–179.

Komi, P.V. (2000) Stretch-shortening cycle: a powerful model to study normal and fatigued muscle. *J Biomech*. 33: 1197–1206.

Morris, C.W. (2015) The Effect of Fluid Periodization on Athletic Performance Outcomes in American Football Players. PhD dissertation, University of Kentucky. Theses and Dissertations – Kinesiology and Health Promotion. 24.

Murtaugh, B. & Ihm, J.M. (2013) Eccentric training for the treatment of tendinopathies. *Curr Sports Med Rep*. 12: 175–182.

Nardone, A., Corra, T. & Schieppati, M. (1990) Different activations of the soleus and gastrocnemii muscles in response to various types of stance perturbation in man. *Exp Brain Res*. 80: 323–332.

Nicol, C. & Komi, P.V. (1998) Significance of passively induced stretch reflexes on Achilles tendon force enhancement. *Muscle Nerve J*. 21: 1546–1548.

Onambélé, G.L., Maganaris, C.N., Mian, O.S., Tam, E., Rejc, E., McEwan, I.M. & Narici, M.V. (2008) Neuromuscular and balance responses to flywheel inertial versus weight training in older persons. *J Biomech*. 41: 3133–3138.

Preuß, P. (2010) Muskuläre Leistung im Krafttraining: Analyse verschiedener Formen der Bewegungsausführung auf die Maximal- und Schnellkraft nach der Methode der submaximalen Kontraktionen bis zur Erschöpfung unter Berücksichtigung akuter hormoneller Auslenkungen. Dissertation. Köln, Germany.

Radcliffe, J.C. & Farentinos, B.C. (1999) *High-Powered Plyometrics*. Champaign, IL: Human Kinetics.

Rassier, D. & Herzog, W. (2005) Force enhancement and relaxation rates after stretch of activated muscle fibres. *Proc Royal Soc B Biol Sci*. 272: 475–480.

Sano, K., Nicol, C., Akiyama, M. et al. (2015) Can measures of muscle–tendon interaction improve our understanding of the superiority of Kenyan endurance runners? *Eur J Applied Physiol*. 115: 849.

Schmidtbleicher, D. & Gollhofer, A. (1985) Einflussgrößen des reaktiven Bewegungsverhaltens und deren Bedeutung für die Trainingspraxis. In: Bührle, M. (Ed.), *Grundlagen des Maximal- und Schnellkrafttrainings*. Schorndorf: Hoffmann, 271–281.

Sialis, J. (2004) Innervationscharakteristik und Trainingsadaptibilitaet im Dehnungs-Verkuerzungs-Zyklus. Stuttgart, Germany: University of Stuttgart.

Spurrs, R.W., Murphy, A.J. & Watsford, M.L. (2003) The effect of plyometric training on distance running performance. *Eur J Appl Physiol*. 89: 1–7.

Tofas, T., Jamurtas, A.Z., Fatouros, I., Nikolaidis, M.G., Koutedakis, Y., Sinouris, E.A., Papageorgakopoulou, N. & Theocharis, D.A. (2008) Plyometric exercise increases serum indices of muscle damage and collagen breakdown. *J Strength Cond Res*. 22: 490–496.

Verkhoshansky, Y. & Siff, M.C. (2009) *Supertraining*. Sixth edition, expanded version. Rome: Verkhoshansky SSTM.

Wathen, D. (1994) Literature review: explosive plyometric exercises. In: National Strength and Conditioning Association (Eds), Position Paper and Literature Review: Explosive Exercises and Training and Explosive Plyometric Exercises, pp.13–16. Colorado Springs: National Strength and Conditioning Association.

Zanon, S. (1989) Plyometrics: past and present. *New Studies in Athletics*. 4: 7–17.

Zatsiorky, V.M. & Kraemer, W.J. (2008) *Krafttraining – Praxis und Wissenschaft*. Third Edition. Aachen: Meyer & Meyer.

Eccentric training: The key for a stronger, more resilient athlete?

Jan Wilke and Håkan Alfredson

In sports and exercise, concentric contraction is often regarded as the superhero of muscle work: basketball and volleyball players are interested in the achieved jump height, sprinters are concerned about their legs' rate of force development, and injured football (soccer) players are cleared for return to play once having restored their pre-injury strength levels, alongside other factors. Despite the unquestionable relevance of these aspects, concentric contraction has a fascinating twin, which rarely enters the spotlight. Eccentric contraction plays a vital role in both injury prevention and sports performance. This chapter provides a comprehensive and practice-oriented review of the basic mechanisms, related training methods and fields of application in sports and exercise.

Basic physiology of eccentric contraction

Eccentric contraction (see Figure 26.1 for an overview of contraction types) is what makes life feel smooth and easy. When descending a flight of stairs or sitting down on a chair, we do not let ourselves fall down passively, which could be painful. Instead, prior to making contact with the ground or an object, we activate our internal "brakes" using this special type of muscle work: in the case of sitting down, the calf, quadriceps and gluteus maximus muscles are stretched while simultaneously developing force in order to decelerate the downward movement. As the

term "decelerate" indicates, it is a hallmark of eccentric muscle work that the amount of force lengthening the muscle exceeds the force output it produces. Using the feedback of the joint proprioceptors (muscle spindle, Golgi tendon-like organ, Ruffini and Pacinian corpuscles), the most crucial task of the central nervous system is to meticulously adapt the required contraction level according to the requirements of each situation in daily life, as well as during exercise. A better understanding of the role of eccentric contraction as a shock-absorbing servo-mechanism is therefore highly beneficial for health professionals and performance coaches.

In the sarcomere, the stretch occurring during eccentric contractions leads to rapid detachments and re-attachments of the cross-bridges between the actin and myosin filaments. On a more macroscopic level, the superordinate functional units (sarcomere, myofibrils, myofibers and the whole muscle) are successively elongated. Experiments in the 1970s revealed an interesting phenomenon: during a contracted stretch, considerable force increases can be registered (Edman et al., 1976). If tissue lengthening ends but muscle activation is maintained (e.g. at the end point of an eccentric movement), one part of this extra force is lost. However, the other part, making the contraction stronger than a normal isometric contraction at the same muscle length, remains until the muscle is relaxed or returned to its resting length. Extensive research has been

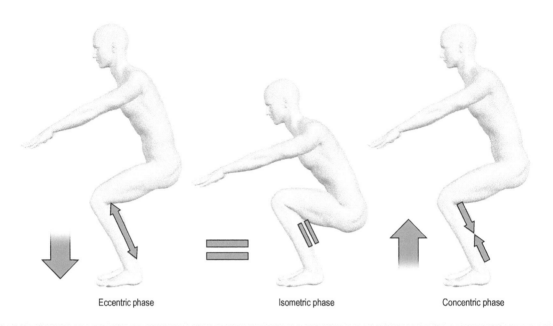

Chapter 26

Eccentric phase Isometric phase Concentric phase

Figure 26.1

Schematic illustration of different contraction types. When eccentrically descending into a deep squat position (left), the gastrocnemius is lengthened. If the deep position is held isometrically for a few seconds (middle), the muscle length remains constant. When returning to the upright position, the gastrocnemius shortens due to the concentric contraction (right).

performed to identify the origin of this effect, which is called residual force enhancement. Although still not understood fully, it is assumed that the elastic properties of the spring-like titin filaments play a key role. Particularly during an active stretch or an eccentric contraction, a specific part of the titin (the PEVK region) is stiffened and stores kinetic energy. The resulting recoil forces pulling the muscle towards its resting length could explain a major part of the increased muscle force (Hessel et al., 2017). Although there is a paucity of research concerning this hypothesis, it can be assumed that the deep fascia also contributes to this rebound effect as it is stretched during the eccentric movement phase. In summary, the observation that eccentric movements allow the handling of

higher weights is attributable to two factors, (1) the nature of this contraction type, which does not aim to accelerate but to decelerate objects, and (2) the residual force enhancement combined with elastic energy storage.

Forms of eccentric training

The most traditional form of eccentric training (ET) is the performance of body weight exercises with a long eccentric contraction phase. Typical examples include lowering the center of mass in squats and push-ups as slowly as possible. For some muscles and joints, and if training progress is made, external weights may be required to achieve sufficient eccentric stimulation. In addition to strength training machines (which are not recommended in most cases because of

293

Eccentric training: The key for a stronger, more resilient athlete?

the limited co-ordination challenge), barbells, dumbbells and kettlebells are well-suited for this purpose. As mentioned above, the maximal training weight is limited by concentric force. Therefore, if weights exceeding the latter are chosen, a training partner can assist during the muscle-shortening phase while not providing assistance in the heavy-loaded eccentric part of the movement. The possibility of imposing higher mechanical stresses to the targeted tissues certainly represents an advantage of this method. However, in real life, eccentric movement is almost always coupled with concentric activity, meaning that exercises with concentric support are less functional. In addition, when seen from a fascial perspective, the effective use of elastic energy stored in the intra- and extra-muscular connective tissue is not trained with this technique. In recent years, specific devices have been designed to optimize muscle loading during ET. Flywheel training is an increasingly popular, instrument-assisted form of isoinertial ET. Connected via a strap, the training individual moves the flywheel with a concentric contraction. In the subsequent eccentric movement phase, resisting the pull of the strap, the rotation of the wheel needs to be decelerated.

Morphological and mechanical adaptations of ET

When performed over a period of several weeks, ET elicits substantial muscle hypertrophy. While it is similarly effective as concentric exercise in this regard, there is an interesting region-specificity: following ET, distal muscle size increases more strongly as opposed to concentric training, where thickness changes predominantly affect the mid-portion of the muscle. Another significant adaptation of ET is a larger increase in type IIx muscle fiber cross-sectional area (Douglas et al., 2017). The fast-type glycolytic fibers are crucial for rapid force development and hence, all athletes who require explosive movement may consider incorporating ET into their exercise routines.

ET can significantly affect the morphological and material properties of the tendon (Chapter 5), inducing increases in the cross-sectional area, stiffness and Young's modulus (Bohm et al., 2015). It further stimulates collagen synthesis, which may explain the observations described above (Kjaer et al., 2009). While all these adaptations are beneficial for athletes and clients, it has to be reiterated that the effect magnitude is not different between ET and concentric training. It is assumed that the training intensity (high loading) is more decisive than the contraction type (Kjaer et al., 2009; Bohm et al., 2015). However, as ET allows the use of higher weights, it may still be the more appropriate choice if sufficient time for progressive load increases is available.

In addition to triggering adaptations in the muscle and the tendon, ET leads to marked changes in the intra- and extra-muscular connective tissue. On days following heavy eccentric exercise until fatigue, a substantial thickening of the deep fascia can be detected using high-resolution ultrasound imaging (Nosaka and Lau, 2018). The results from other studies also suggest a profound mechanical impact on the muscle-associated soft tissue. Raastad et al. (2010) required their participants to perform 300 eccentric contractions of the knee extensors. After the training session, the authors observed increases in tenascin-C and a propeptide of procollagen III. These reflect both high extracellular matrix loading and remodeling. When compared with concentric exercise, ET provides a stronger

Chapter 26

stimulus for the synthesis of intramuscular collagen type I, which may lead to increased connective tissue cross-linking (Heinemeier et al., 2007). While an initial bout of eccentric exercise creates a strong tissue response, repeated training without progressive load increase does not seem to evoke the same adaptations. Mackey et al. (2011) examined the tensascin-C concentration 48 h after both an acute and an identical second electrical eccentric exercise bout (performed 30 days after the first session). In contrast to the initial bout, the repetition did not alter the expression of the protein. Most likely, a protective remodeling process rendered the connective tissue more resilient. This hypothesis is supported by the fact that the thickening response of the deep fascia (as described above), occurring after an unaccustomed bout of eccentric exercise, does not manifest after an identical repeated training session (Nosaka and Lau, 2018).

Effects of ET on performance

Several systematic reviews demonstrate that ET substantially increases absolute strength (Roig et al., 2009). With regard to the different methods, flywheel training represents the most effective type of exercise (Maroto-Izquierdo et al., 2017). A meta-analysis of 15 studies showed similar gains in concentric and eccentric exercise (Roig et al., 2009). However, when exclusively analyzing studies that used higher intensities in the eccentric exercise group than in the concentric exercise group (which is realistic because the former allows the use of higher loads), the increases in total strength were higher for ET. This implies that, as long as developing maximal strength represents the main objective, the highest possible intensity needs to be chosen if ET is used instead of concentric exercise. Not surprisingly,

in addition to maximal concentric strength, ET is more effective in developing maximal eccentric strength. Notwithstanding, this specificity is of utmost importance if an athlete or client needs to be prepared for the mechanical stresses associated with rapid deceleration.

While several studies have examined the effect of ET on maximal strength, there are less data regarding vertical jump height and sprinting speed, which are extremely important in several sports. However, from the evidence available it can be inferred that eccentric exercise, particularly when performed at high movement speeds, seems to improve both parameters more effectively than concentric exercise: in their systematic review, Douglas et al. (2017) reported stronger improvements of stretch-shortening cycle movement following eccentrics compared with traditional concentric exercise. Similar findings were reported by Maroto-Izquierdo et al. (2017), who additionally revealed the superiority of flywheel training over traditional ET with free weights or machines.

Besides improving strength and explosive movement capacities, ET of the lower limb has been demonstrated to enhance flexibility in the ankle, knee and hip joint. The magnitude of this effect is comparable with that of static stretching interventions (Sullivan et al., 2012). Although different factors are discussed, the ROM increases appear to result from the formation of new sarcomeres. Sarcomerogenesis has been confirmed in animal studies and represents an adaptation optimizing the length-tension relationship of the muscle (Sullivan et al., 2012).

ET and musculoskeletal disorders

While ET can increase strength in the long term, a single eccentric contraction does not make you run substantially faster or hit the ball harder.

295

Eccentric training: The key for a stronger, more resilient athlete?

However, its impact in sports cannot be overrated in the short term either. Rapid deceleration, which is based on eccentrics, is key for quick changes of direction and, even more importantly, effective injury prevention. Up to 77% of all non-contact traumas occurring in game sports are due to failed jump landings (Woods et al., 2003). One important strategy to reduce this dramatically high incidence is teaching proper landing techniques based on eccentric contraction (Sinsurin et al., 2016). Imagine the ground contact after a depth jump performed with either extended or flexed knees. With the former, there is no substantial involvement of the leg muscles in the dampening of the impact. By contrast, with dynamic knee flexion, the landing is softened due to the eccentric contraction (from extended to flexed knees) of the glutes and the quadriceps muscle.

Besides improving landing technique (which involves a better acute use of eccentrics within a specific movement), regular eccentric exercise has been shown to be an effective strategy to prevent (myofascial) muscle injuries. Hamstring strains are the most frequent disorder in sports, particularly in football/soccer (Edouard et al., 2015; Ernlund and Vieira, 2017).

ET, when performed regularly, can reduce the injury risk by as much as 65% (Goode et al., 2015). The signature exercise to be used here is Nordic Hamstring Lowering (Figure 26.2).

ET is frequently performed in the rehabilitation of musculoskeletal disorders. Lateral epicondylitis mainly affects tennis players and causes pain that may radiate to the hand and shoulder. A multimodal therapy with ET improves pain, function and grip strength more effectively than interventions without ET (Cullinane et al., 2014). A simple exercise can be performed with small dumbbells (2–5 kg) or a water bottle. Positioning the lower arm on a table, the wrist is extended (with support of the free hand if needed) and then slowly lowered into flexion.

Tendinopathy represents another pathology that is frequently treated by means of ET. An extended description with an exemplary loading protocol for the Achilles tendon is provided at the end of this chapter. One recent meta-analysis concludes that there are still insufficient high-quality data to conclusively judge the effectivity of ET in Achilles tendinopathy compared with other treatments, although it is assumed that ET is more effective than normal physiotherapy (Murphy et al., 2019). In patients

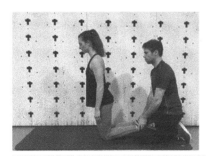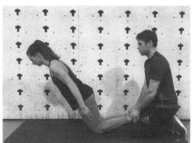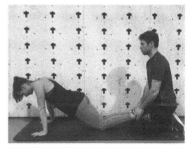

Figure 26.2

The Nordic Hamstring exercise is an excellent method to increase eccentric strength of the dorsal thigh muscles. The movement is initiated in an upright position (left). With the feet fixed (e.g. by a coach) and the hip extended, the body is slowly lowered towards the ground (middle). Only if the movement can no longer be controlled, the arms are used to cushion the fall (right).

Chapter 26

with Patellar tendinopathy, ET performed in conjunction with or without stretching and core stabilization exercises leads to a mean improvement of 61% in subjectively rated symptoms (Everhardt et al., 2017). A suitable exercise to intensify the eccentric loading of the Patellar tendon is the unilateral or bilateral squat using a decline board (Figure 26.3).

ET and the prevention of tendon disorders

In view of the beneficial effects of ET in the therapy of tendinopathy, it seems reasonable to use the method as a prophylactic intervention in asymptomatic individuals. However, available data from prospective studies do not indicate an injury-preventive effect. Based on current evidence, therefore, ET cannot be recommended with regard to primary prevention (Peters et al., 2016).

Important aspects to consider in ET

- ET imposes substantial stresses on the locomotor system. Coaches and therapists should therefore ensure sufficient time for gradual tissue adaptation. When designing training interventions, start with slow concentric and isometric movements and then progress to eccentric movements. Similarly, begin with body weight only, step by step increasing external loads.

- If large strength gains or muscle hypertrophy are desired, controlled single-joint exercises may be an adequate choice. However, from a functional point of view, the additive use of multi-joint movements is essential to transfer and exploit triggered adaptations in the target sport.

- If rapid eccentric movements are intended to be trained, the use of heavy barbells or

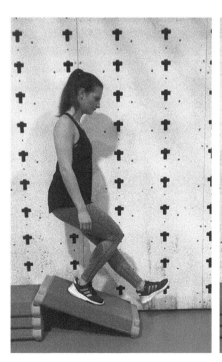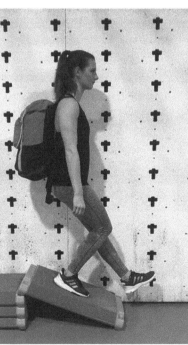

Figure 26.3

A decline board can be used during a conventional squat to increase eccentric loading of the quadriceps femoris muscle. Keeping the body upright, the knee is progressively flexed as far as possible (left). To increase intensity, besides performing the exercise on one leg, a backpack with weights can be worn (right).

297

Eccentric training: The key for a stronger, more resilient athlete?

dumbbells may not be optimal. In this case, elastic bands can provide a workable solution.

- While athletes from multiple sports benefit from lower extremity eccentric exercises (e.g. Nordic Hamstrings, Decline Squats/Lunges), throwers can also effectively develop eccentric strength. For deceleration throws, use small balls of varying weights (start light), instructing the athletes to catch them dynamically, following the direction of the ball. Additionally, traditional exercises (e.g. bench press) can be used to increase eccentric strength.

Conclusion

Performing eccentric exercises is a highly effective method to elicit both functional and structural changes in muscles, tendons and the extramuscular connective tissue. Besides improving performance, it seems to be of value in the prevention and treatment of musculoskeletal disorders and, therefore, the use of ET should always be considered when designing long-term training regimes. If athletes suffer from tendinopathy, ET represents a gold standard method to alleviate the symptoms with minimal use of medication.

Clinical advice from the expert
Håkan Alfredson
Basic rationale for the use of eccentric exercise in tendinopathy

Curwin and Stanish (1986) were the first to raise the theory of eccentric exercises being included in the treatment of painful tendinopathy. They proposed that pain-free eccentric exercises, performed with gradually increased speed, should be used on patients with mid-portion Achilles and patellar tendinopathy. However, no patient material on a specific diagnosis was presented in a scientific study. After trying eccentric exercises on my own chronically painful

Achilles mid-portion, with a modified version including painful heavy eccentric loading and multiple repetitions performed at slow speed, the successful result was the beginning for research projects evaluating large patient cohorts, with the diagnosis of mid-portion Achilles tendinopathy/tendinosis verified by means of ultrasound.

Scientific evaluation of the method

Our treatment was initially tried on patients on our waiting list for, at that time, traditional open tendon surgery (including tenotomy, excision of tendinosis tissue, and a 4-6 months postoperative rehabilitation). In the pilot study, all 15 included patients were satisfied with the treatment, and did not want to have surgery (Alfredson et al., 1998). After 1 year, one patient had regained pain symptoms and this patient was surgically treated. The other 14 patients were still active in Achilles tendon loading activities. Following this pilot study, we performed multiple studies on the effects of ET, including a randomized study and follow-up studies with large sample sizes (Mafi et al., 2001; Fahlström et al., 2003).

An interesting observation is that in successfully treated patients, the tendon thickness is decreased and the structure is sonographically normalized (Öhberg et al., 2004). Consequently, it seems that eccentric calf muscle training has a potential to remodel, and possibly also induce, a regeneration of the previously so-called degenerative tendon.

We have learned that, overall, the results of heavy-load ET are beneficial in about 80% of cases. However, it seems that high-level athletes, especially spike-shoe runners and jumpers, have less positive results with this treatment. Also, it is important that the patients have a correct diagnosis before this treatment is initiated. If eccentric exercises are used on a patient with a partial tendon rupture, there is a high risk of full-thickness rupture, a condition that is very difficult to treat, and may render the patient with permanently reduced calf muscle strength and function.

Chapter 26

Observations during the last 7–8 years have shown that there is a subgroup of patients with mid-portion Achilles tendinopathy that exhibit a plantaris tendon involvement (Alfredson, 2011). The plantaris tendon can be considered as a remnant from earlier human development stages when we were moving on four legs (Spang et al, 2016). This thin tendon, which occasionally develops tendinopathies, thickening and widening at the medial side of the Achilles, has been shown to have multiple different positions in relation to the Achilles tendon. In rare cases it is even invaginated into the medial side of the Achilles. Patients with plantaris involvement frequently have a poor response to ET, and sometimes even a worsening of the pain condition occurs. If plantaris involvement is suspected, coaches and therapists should ask for the exact pain location, as patients typically report complaints at the medial side of the Achilles. The soft tissues in between the plantaris and Achilles tendons have been shown to be richly innervated, alongside the plantaris itself, and, in contrast to the Achilles, have been shown to frequently contain multiple sensory nerves. The plantaris tendon has been shown to mechanically interfere with the medial side of the Achilles tendon, and often requires surgical removal.

Physiology

The mechanisms behind good clinical results in a chronically painful tendon have yet not been fully clarified. There are multiple theories, such as increased type 1 collagen formation, increased calf muscle strength, and altered shearing forces within the tendon. However, patients often experience pain relief within 2–4 weeks from when they begin the exercises, although the time needed for collagen formation and muscle strength increases is much longer. A recent theory suggests that the effects are due to shearing forces between the ventral side of the Achilles tendon and the Kager fat tissue. This shearing mechanism is demonstrated by movement from plantar flexion to dorsiflexion in the tendon, when the ventral fat tissue moves in opposite directions. The theory fits with observations from biopsies, in that the nerves responsible for the pain in this condition are located in the fat tissues close to the ventral side of the Achilles. This has been tested using local anesthetic injections (temporary total pain relief) and surgical scraping procedures (permanent pain relief) outside the ventral side of the tendon.

Eccentric calf muscle training in Achilles tendinopathy

The following tips may be helpful when performing eccentric exercise to alleviate tendon pain:

- Use stable shoes to prevent pain in the plantar fascia, midfoot or toe joints.

- If knee arthrosis or low-back pain is present it may not be possible to do these exercises.

- Start by using the body weight only. If no tendon pain manifests during the exercise, increase the load by using weights in a back pack. Gradually increase the load to reach a new level of "painful eccentric loading".

- The easiest way to perform the exercises is by standing on a staircase, using the bannisters for stability. If high loads are required in the future, a standing weight machine can be used.

- Start from a tip-toe position with all the body weight on the injured side, then slowly lower the heel beneath the step until you reach bottom position (Figure 26.4). Next, support yourself to return to the start position by using the other asymptomatic leg. In bilateral Achilles tendinopathy use both legs.

- Perform 3 x 15 repetitions with straight knees and 3 x 15 repetitions with the knees bent. Carry this out two times each day for a total of 12 weeks.

299

Eccentric training: The key for a stronger, more resilient athlete?

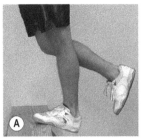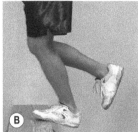

Figure 26.4

Eccentric calf muscle training with (**A**) straight knee and (**B**) bent knee.

References

Alfredson, H., Pietilä, T., Jonsson, P. & Lorentzon, R. (1998) Heavy-loaded eccentric calf-muscle training for the treatment of chronic Achilles tendinosis. *Am J Sports Med*. 26: 360–366.

Alfredson, H. (2011) Midportion Achilles tendinosis and the plantaris tendon. *Br J Sports Med*. 45: 1023–1025.

Bohm, S., Mersmann, F. & Arampatzis, A. (2015) Human tendon adaptation in response to mechanical loading: a systematic review and meta-analysis of exercise intervention studies on healthy adults. *Sports Med Open*. 1: 7.

Cullinane, F.L., Boocock, M.G. & Trevelyan, F.C. (2014) Is eccentric exercise an effective treatment for lateral epicondylitis? A systematic review. *Clin Rehabil*. 28: 3–19.

Douglas, J., Pearson, S., Ross, A. & McGuigan, M. (2017) Chronic adaptations to eccentric training: a systematic review. *Sports Med*. 47: 917–941.

Edman, K.A., Mulieri, L.A. & Scubon-Mulieri, B. (1976) Non-hyperbolic force-velocity relationship in single muscle fibres. *Acta Physiol. Scand*. 98: 143–156.

Edouard, P., Branco, P. & Alonso, J.M. (2016) Muscle injury is the principal injury type and hamstring muscle injury is the first injury diagnosis during top-level international athletics championships between 2007 and 2015. *Br J Sports Med*. 50: 619–630.

Ernlund, L. & Vieira, L.A. (2017) Hamstring injuries: update article. *Rev Bras Ortop*. 52: 373–382.

Everhart, J.A., Cole, D., Sojka, J.H., Higgins, J.D., Magnussen, R.A., Schmitt, L.C. & Flanigan, D.C. (2017) Treatment options for patellar tendinopathy: a systematic review. *Arthroscopy*. 33: 861–872.

Fahlström, M., Jonsson, P., Lorentzon, R. & Alfredson, H. (2003) Chronic Achilles tendon pain treated with eccentric calf-muscle training. *Knee Surg Sports Traumatol Arthrosc*. 11: 327–333.

Goode, A.P., Reiman, M.P., Harris, L., DeLisa, L., Kauffman, A., Beltramo, A., Poole, C., Ledbetter, L. & Taylor, A.B. (2015) Eccentric training for prevention of hamstring injuries may depend on intervention compliance: a systematic review and meta-analysis. *Br J Sports Med*. 49: 349–356.

Heinemeier, K.M., Olesen, J.L., Haddad, F., Langberg, H., Kjaer, M., Baldwin, K.M. & Schjerling, P. (2007) Expression of collagen and related growth factors in rat tendon and skeletal muscle in response to specific contraction types. *J Physiol*. 582: 1303–1316.

Hessel, A.L., Lindsted, S.L. & Nishikawa, K.C. (2017) Physiological mechanisms of eccentric contraction and its applications: a role for the giant titin protein. *Front Physiol*. 8: 70.

Kjaer, M., Langberg, H., Heinemeir, K., Bayer, M.L., Holm, L., Doessing, S., Kongsgaard, M., Krogsgaard, M.R. & Magnusson, S.P. (2009) From mechanical loading to collagen synthesis, structural changes and function in human tendon. *Scand J Med Sci Sports*. 19: 500–510.

Mackey, A.L., Brandstetter, S., Schjerling, P., Bojsen-Moller, J., Qvortrup, K., Pedersen, M.M., Doessing, S., Kjaer, M., Magnussion, P. & Langberg, H. (2011) Sequenced response of extracellular matrix deadhesion and fibrotic regulators after muscle damage is involved in protection against future injury in human skeletal muscle. *FASEB J.*

Mafi, N., Lorentzon, R. & Alfredson, H. (2001) Superior results with eccentric calf-muscle training compared to concentric training in a randomized prospective multi-center study on patients with chronic Achilles tendinosis. *Knee Surg Sports Traumatol Arthrosc.* 9: 42–47.

Maroto-Izquierdo, S., García-Lopez, D., Fernandez-Gonzalo, R., Moreira, O.C., González-Gallego, J. & de Paz, J.A. (2017) Skeletal muscle functional and structural adaptations after eccentric overload flywheel resistance training: a systematic review and meta-analysis. *J Sci Med Sport.* 20: 943–951.

Murphy, M.C., Travers, M.J., Chivers, P., Debenham, J.R., Docking, S.I., Rio, E.K. & Gibson, W. (2019) Efficacy of heavy eccentric calf training for treating mid-portion Achilles tendinopathy: a systematic review and meta-analysis. *Br J Sports Med.* 53(17): 1070–1077.

Nosaka, K. & Lau, W.Y. (2018) Increases in biceps brachii fascia thickness after eccentric exercise of the elbow flexors. *J Bodyw Mov Ther.* 22: 858.

Öhberg, L., Lorentzon, R. & Alfredson, H. (2004) Eccentric training in patients with chronic Achilles tendinosis-normalized tendon structure and decreased thickness at follow-up. *Br J Sports Med.* 38: 8–11.

Öhberg, L. & Alfredson, H. (2004) Effect on neovascularisation behind the good results with eccentric training in chronic mid-portion Achilles tendinosis? *Knee Surg Sports Traumatol Arthrosc.* 12: 465–470.

O'Sullivan, K., McAuliffe, S., DeBurca, N. (2012) The effects of eccentric training on lower limb flexibility: a systematic review. *Br J Sports Med.* 46: 838–845.

Peters, J.A., Zwerver, J., Diercks, R.L., Elferink-Gemser, M.T., van den Akker-Scheek, I. (2016) Preventive interventions for tendinopathy: A systematic review. *J Sci Med Sport.* 19(3): 205–211.

Raastad, T., Owe, S.G., Paulsen, G., Enns, D., Overgaard, K., Crameri, R., Kiil, S., Belcastro, A., Bergersen, L.H. & Hallén, J. (2010) Changes in calpain activity, muscle structure, and function after eccentric exercise. *Med Sci Sports Exerc.* 42: 86–95.

Roig, M., O'Brien, K., Murray, R., McKinnon, P., Shadgan, B. & Reid, W.D. (2009) The effects of eccentric versus concentric resistance training on muscle strength and mass in healthy adults: a systematic review with meta-analysis. *Br J Sports Med.* 43: 556–568.

Sinsurin, K., Vachalathi, R., Jalayondeja, W. & Limroongreungrat, W. (2016) Knee muscular control during jump landing in multidirections. *Asian J Sports Med.* 7: e31248.

Spang, C., Alfredson, H., Docking, S.I., Masci, L. & Andersson, G. (2016) The plantaris tendon. A narrative review focusing on anatomical features and clinical importance. *Bone Joint J.* 98: 1312–1319.

Spang, C., Harandi, V.M., Alfredson, H. & Forsgren, S. (2015) Marked innervation but also signs of nerve degeneration between the Achilles and plantaris tendons and presence of innervation within the plantaris tendon in midportion Achilles tendinopthy. *J Mus Skel Neur Interact.* 15: 197–206.

Woods, C., Hawkins, R., Hulse, M. & Hodson, A. (2003) The Football Association Medical Research Programme: an audit of injuries in professional football: an analysis of ankle sprains. *Br J Sports Med.* 37: 233–238.

Foam rolling and roller massage effects and mechanisms

David G. Behm

Introduction

Massage has been used for millennia as a relaxation technique, to decrease musculoskeletal and myofascial pain, relieve or cure illnesses, increase range of motion (ROM) and enhance performance (Behm, 2018). Historical records of massage originate from China (the Yellow Emperor's *Classic Book of Internal Medicine* was written around 2700 BC), Egypt (Egyptian tomb paintings showing massage as a medical therapy around 2500 BC) and India (records of massage date from 1500–500 BC). The western world adopted these techniques relatively recently, with Per Ling from Sweden incorporating hand stroking into the Swedish Movement System in the early 1800s. Over the last 20 years, foam rollers and roller massagers have become popular as self-massage therapy devices (Figure 27.1) (MacDonald et al., 2013; Sullivan et al., 2013; Halperin et al., 2014; Macdonald et al., 2014; Aboodarda et al., 2015; Bradbury-Squires et al., 2015; Pearcey et al., 2015).

Foam rollers and roller massagers are often branded as "self-myofascial release" devices, reducing or helping to reduce (myo)fascial restrictions. These fascial restrictions are reported to occur in response to injury, disease, inactivity and inflammation (Schleip 2003a,b). It is commonly reported that when fascia becomes inelastic and dehydrated, it binds around the traumatized areas, resulting in fibrous adhesions (Schleip 2003a,b). These myofascial adhesions may generate "hypersensitive tender spots", also known as trigger points. Fibrous adhesions can

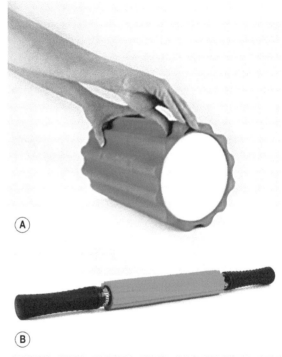

Figure 27.1

Illustrations of **(A)** a foam roller and **(B)** a roller massager, with permission from Performance Health.

be painful, initiate abnormal muscle mechanics (i.e. neuromuscular hypertonicity, decreased strength, endurance and motor coordination) and decrease soft-tissue extensibility, adversely affecting ROM and muscle length (Schleip 2003a,b).

Rolling involves moving over the muscle and fascia with a dense foam roller or roller stick (roller massager), with either small excursions

Chapter 27

or longer movements from the proximal to the distal portion of the muscle or vice versa. Foam rollers now appear in many forms. Some rollers are made from polyvinyl chloride pipe surrounded by neoprene foam while others may be made from closed cell foam. Roller sticks or roller massagers are typically composed of dense foam wrapping around a solid plastic cylinder. There are many types, with some having a ridged design that is supposed to allow for both superficial and deep-tissue massage (Sullivan et al., 2013; Bradbury-Squires et al., 2015). Others have cells (squares or circular shapes) of different sizes and hardness, with recent modifications including vibration.

The few studies examining vibrating rollers have shown some advantages over non-vibrating rollers, such as inducing greater pain tolerance (Cheatham et al., 2017; Han et al., 2017), lower extent of proprioceptive errors (Lee et al., 2018) and some specific improvements in joint ROM (greater hip flexion and internal rotation but similar hip extension and external rotation; Han et al., 2017). Possible mechanisms underlying these effects may be related to vibration-induced increases in tissue temperature, blood flow, or neurogenic potentiation through augmented muscle spindle activity and gamma motoneuron activity. However, more research is needed to investigate this type of hybrid roller.

Rolling-induced pain inhibition

Rolling has been shown to reduce chronic pain such as muscle or myofascial tender spots (Aboodarda et al., 2015; Wilke et al., 2018), relatively short term pain associated with delayed onset muscle soreness (DOMS) (Macdonald et al., 2014; Pearcey et al., 2015) as well as acute pain induced by high frequency, electrical muscle (tetanic) stimulation (Cavanaugh et al., 2017).

DOMS was induced in two similar studies with 10 sets of 10 squat repetitions to failure. Subjects in the first study were examined 24 and 48 h after the exercise-induced muscle damage (Pearcey et al., 2015). In the second study, participants were also measured at 72 h post-squat exercise protocol (MacDonald et al., 2014). In both studies, the experimental group rolled before testing and the controls did not. Rolling decreased pain perception by 18–24% and 16–19% at 24 and 48 h post-exercise, respectively, in both studies. Other performance tests that were impaired by DOMS, such as muscle activation, vertical jump, sprint time and strength endurance, showed less impairment with rolling.

While exercise-induced muscle damage pain may persist for a week in response to muscle damage and inflammatory responses (Behm et al., 2001), muscle tender points may persist for months. Rolling has been demonstrated to also decrease muscle tender point pain. Aboodarda et al. (2015) had a massage therapist find and identify the most sensitive muscle tender point on participants' calf (triceps surae/plantar flexors). The painful calf was then either massaged by the therapist, rolled or not rolled (control). In addition, the contralateral calf was also rolled. Rolling or massaging the affected calf decreased muscle tender point pain sensitivity. Curiously, rolling the contralateral calf also reduced pain sensitivity. Hence, the description of rolling as a self-myofascial release technique cannot possibly explain the full array of mechanisms, if there was no need to even touch the painful calf.

With a similar study, the pain associated with electrically induced (tetanic muscle contractions) high frequency stimulation was also diminished without manipulating the affected limb. Cavanaugh et al. (2017) induced high levels of acute pain by stimulating the tibial nerve (activates plantar flexors) with maximal and sub-maximal (70%) intensity high frequency (50 Hz) electrical stimulation (tetanus). Similar to the previous study, the affected calf was either rolled or not (control), while the contralateral calf was also rolled. Each time muscle stimulation was inflicted, pain sensitivity increased by ~10%. Whether the affected or contralateral limb was rolled, the result was a decrease in pain. It seems evident that a systemic or global neural response contributed to the pain inhibition.

Pain receptors (nociceptors) are widespread in muscle, fascia and skin (Kosek et al., 1995). Even light rolling can increase the sensitivity of superficial nociceptors (Aboodarda et al., 2015). This afferent stimulation, whether applied to the affected limb or a contralateral limb, may be related to the gate control theory of pain (Melzack and Wall, 1965; Moayedi and Davis, 2013), diffuse noxious inhibitory control (Mense, 2000) and parasympathetic nervous system alterations (Weerapong et al., 2005). The gate control theory involves stimulation of lower velocity, myelinated group III and IV afferents nerve fibers (via activation of skin, fascia and muscle mechano-receptors, metaboreceptors and proprioceptors), which transmit the signals from ascending noci-ceptors via small diameter $A\delta$ fibers to the periaqueductal gray nucleus (Moayedi and Davis, 2013). Pain suppression can arise peripherally from the subsequent activation of type I and II (i.e. tactile, pressure, vibration) higher velocity afferents that may impede the transmission of the slower type III and IV afferents (block the gate). Analgesia can also emanate supraspinally by activating opioid receptors, which inhibit pain with serotonergic and noradrenergic neurons (Pud et al., 2009).

A second pain inhibitory pathway could be ascribed to diffuse noxious inhibitory control (DNIC), which can work by counter-irritation activating nociceptive stimuli through mechanical pressure from a non-local tissue. (Your toe hurts, so irritate your hand to decrease pain in the toe). With DNIC, non-local (i.e. if toe hurts activate the hand) receptor activation is transmitted to multi-receptive, wide dynamic range convergent neurons in the cortical subnucleus reticularis dorsalis, where pain transmission is suppressed monoaminergically (i.e. transmitters such as norepinephrine and serotonin). Pain sensitivity is then inhibited, not only with the affected location, but also at distant (non-local) areas (Mense, 2000; Pud et al., 2009).

Parasympathetic activation may also be activated by massage. Pain sensitivity would be modified due to alterations in cortisol, endorphins, serotonin and oxytocin (Weerapong et al., 2005). Suppressed parasympathetic reflexes could minimize the strain on the smooth muscles embedded in the soft tissue, thus inhibiting pain by decreasing myofascial tissue stress. Massage or rolling can lead to acute ischemic compression, which has been shown to result in reduced perceived pain in the upper trapezius muscles (Kostopoulos et al., 2008) and with neck and shoulder muscles (Hanten et al., 2000).

In addition to neural mechanisms, psycho-physiological factors could also contribute to pain inhibition. Magnusson et al. (1996) has proposed that the acute or immediate increase in ROM following stretching is due to an increased stretch or pain tolerance. When an individual feels discomfort or pain for a prolonged period, as with rolling or stretching, persisting with that pain or discomfort results in the individual partially accommodating the painful or uncomfortable sensation. This may be labeled as a psycho-physiological effect, as the mechanisms could be predominately psychological or work in concert with the gate control and DNIC mechanisms.

Chapter 27

Rolling-induced increases in ROM

Rolling can increase ROM (MacDonald et al., 2013; Sullivan et al., 2013; Halperin et al., 2014; Macdonald et al., 2014; Aboodarda et al., 2015; Bradbury-Squires et al., 2015; Markovic, 2015; Pearcey et al., 2015; Skarabot et al., 2015; Vigotsky et al., 2015; Murray et al., 2016) for as long as 20 min (Junker and Stoggl, 2015; Kelly and Beardsley, 2016). Improved joint flexibility has even been demonstrated after 1–2 sets of 5–10 s of rolling (4.3%; Sullivan et al., 2013). Other studies have used an array of rolling durations such as 15, 20, 30, 60, 90 and 120 s. Typically, longer durations show greater increases in ROM than shorter durations. For example, the 10 s of rolling in the Sullivan et al. (2013) study provided a greater sit and reach score than 5 s. Other studies have reported that 60 s of rolling provided greater flexibility results than 20 s (16% vs. 10%, Bradbury-Squires et al., 2015), while 120 s exceeded 60 s with both foam rolling (9.8% vs. 30%) and roller massage (11% vs. 21.9%) (Monteiro et al., 2017a). ROM improvements are quite variable (3–30%) (Grieve et al., 2015; Skarabot et al., 2015). Rolling possesses some of the advantages of static stretching, such as improvements in flexibility, while generally not sharing the disadvantage of impaired performance after prolonged static stretching in isolation (without the inclusion of dynamic activities; Behm and Chaouachi, 2011; Behm et al., 2016). With most rolling studies, there is no adverse effect on subsequent performance such as muscle strength, power and balance (MacDonald et al., 2013; Sullivan et al., 2013; Halperin et al., 2014; Healey et al., 2014; Behara and Jacobson, 2015). An additional positive rolling effect that may or may not contribute to the increased ROM is the report that foam rolling reduces arterial stiffness and improves vascular endothelial function (Okamoto et al., 2014). Hence, there could be other health benefits that

need to be explored further. The effect on performance will be examined in more detail later (Table 27.1).

One of the major factors contributing to rolling-induced increases in ROM are thixotropic effects, which occur when fluids become less viscous or more fluid-like when agitated, sheared or stressed. Rolling adds shearing and compression pressure to the soft tissue and also creates friction. The rolling-induced shear stress and increased friction-related temperature of the soft tissues can decrease the viscosity of intracellular and extracellular fluid, providing less resistance to movement. For example, hyaluronan is a glycosaminoglycan within fascia that provides compression strength, lubrication and hydration, and facilitates fascial movement. It is a highly thixotropic material that, dependent upon its state (either high or low viscosity), can greatly affect fascia's resistance to movement or sliding (Cowman et al., 2015; Fede et al., 2018). An excellent example in daily life is when an individual attempts to pour some ketchup from a container/bottle. Typically, the ketchup will not flow quickly initially. However, if the container is jostled or shaken first, then opened and squeezed, then the ketchup flows smoothly. The stress and shearing action on the ketchup decreases its viscosity making it more fluid-like and thus easier to flow. Similarly, after rolling, the high viscosity fluid-induced resistance to movement is lowered, allowing the myofascia and musculotendinous tissues to elongate or lengthen to a greater degree.

It is also suggested that neural inhibition can contribute to rolling-induced increases in ROM. Myofascia, muscle and skin are densely innervated by sensory neurons (Schleip 2003a,b). Within the various skin layers (i.e. epidermis and dermis), there are a number of mechanoreceptors such as the Merkel receptor, Meissner corpuscle, Ruffini cylinder and Pacinian corpuscles. These mechanoreceptors possess a variety of different-sized receptor fields, adapt slowly or rapidly, and respond to different skin stimulation frequencies. Merkel disks (small receptor field) and Ruffini cylinders (large receptor field) are examples of slowly adapting receptor fields, which respond as long as the stimulus is present, whereas the Meissner (small receptor field) and Pacinian (large receptor field) corpuscles adapt rapidly and respond with a burst of activity at both the beginning and end of stimulation. They respond to a variety of stimulation frequencies ranging from 0.3–3 Hz (Merkel receptor), 3–40 Hz (Meissner corpuscle) and 15–400 Hz (Ruffini cylinder) to 10–500 Hz (pacinian corpuscle). All of these mechanoreceptors respond to slow rolling or massage, with Ruffini cylinders and Pacinian corpuscles also responding to high-frequency vibrations. While the primary responsibilities are proprioception, Ruffini and Pacinian receptors can contribute to sympathetic activity inhibition and thus help to relax the muscles (Wu et al., 1999). Ruffini receptors are more sensitive to tangential forces and lateral stretch, which are common with rolling. Ruffini corpuscle stimulation can decrease sympathetic nervous system activity (Wu et al., 1999). Interstitial type III and IV receptors can also modulate sympathetic and parasympathetic activation (Mitchell and Schmidt, 1977). Interstitial receptors can be thinly myelinated or unmyelinated and originate from free nerve endings with both low and high threshold sensory capabilities. While they can be activated by pain, they can also act as mechanoreceptors responding to tension and pressure. This massage-induced increased relaxation, decrease in heart rate and blood pressure (Ruffini and Pacinian receptors) (Weerapong et al., 2005), in addition to vasodilatory effects (Mitchell and

Schmidt, 1977), contributes to greater flexibility capacity.

Massage (Goldberg et al., 1992; Behm et al., 2013) as well as roller massage (Young et al., 2018) have decreased the Hoffman (H)-reflex to muscle action potential wave (M-wave) ratio, signaling an attenuation of the afferent excitability of the motoneuron. The H-reflex is used as a tool to measure the afferent excitability of the motoneuron. However, this reflex electromyographic (EMG) signal can be influenced by the muscle membrane action potential and thus we cannot be certain whether any changes would be due to changes in the reflex arc (changes in the muscle spindle afferent reflex activity to the motoneuron), or are attributable to changes in the muscle membrane excitability. Thus, by normalizing or comparing the H-reflex to the M-wave, it permits us to evaluate whether the change is peripheral (muscle membrane) or central (afferent reflexes to motoneuron). The suppression of the spinal reflex excitability with the H-reflex when normalized to the M-wave has been attributed to decreased alpha motoneuron excitability and/or increased pre-synaptic inhibition. Massage has suppressed the H-reflex by 40–90% in these studies (Goldberg et al., 1992; Behm et al., 2013, Young et al., 2018).

Golgi tendon organs (GTO) (type Ib afferents) respond to musculotendinous tension and strong stretch, which can result in inhibition. Huang et al. (2010) showed that a single bout of a short-duration (10 or 30 s) massage at the hamstrings' musculotendinous junction improved ROM without an increase in passive muscle tension or EMG activity. Thirty seconds of musculotendinous massage provided greater flexibility than 10 s. It could be assumed that the tension applied to the tendon would activate the inhibitory responses of the GTO, leading to greater muscle relaxation. However, GTO effects persist for only 60 ms after the stressor desists (Trajano et al., 2017). Thus,

Chapter 27

the respective 5.8–11.3% ROM increases found in these studies (Huang et al., 2010, Trajano et al., 2017) immediately after massage could not be due to GTO inhibition.

Further evidence for the neural influence on improved ROM is the crossover or non-local effect of rolling. Similar to the aforementioned contralateral limb pain suppression (Abood-arda et al., 2015; Cavanaugh et al., 2017), ROM improvements after rolling have been reported with non-rolled limbs. Kelly and Beardsley (2016) unilaterally rolled the plantar flexors (3 x 30 s) and found increased dorsiflexion ROM (1.9–5.5%) with the contralateral ankle for up to 10 min post-rolling. Similarly, Killen et al. (2018) had participants perform 10 repetitions of 30 s of unilateral foam rolling of the hamstrings and discovered a small magnitude (effect size = 0.2) improvement in the contralateral hip flexors. In addition, they had a stretching condition, which induced an impairment in the contralateral knee flexion maximal voluntary isometric contraction (MVIC) force, but this was not as apparent following rolling. A recent study by Monteiro et al. (2018) compared 60 and 120 s of foam rolling with proprioceptive neuromuscular facilitation stretching of the quadriceps and hamstrings. The authors found significant shoulder flexion and extension ROM increases from immediate post-intervention to 10 min post-intervention for all protocols (main effect for time) after rolling the lower body. However, not all research consistently demonstrates this effect. Grabow et al. (2017) rolled the plantar surface of the foot but did not find any non-local effects on sit and reach scores or balance. Hence, the bulk of this evidence highlights the possibility of a musculotendinous myofascial rolling-induced global or systemic afferent neural inhibition effect resulting in a lower reflex-induced muscle tonus throughout the body. It could also suggest that the moderate or greater discomfort associated with rolling any part of the body translates into a global pain or stretch tolerance effect permitting the individual to push through a greater ROM independent of the rolled body part.

Thus, ROM improvements with massage and rolling have been attributed to thixotropic factors, neural reflex inhibition, increased parasympathetic relaxation and a greater stretch or pain tolerance. However, the label or term "self-myofascial release technique" used to describe foam rollers and rollers massagers, implying that the major mechanism of foam rolling or roller massage is a physical removal of myofascial restrictions (or trigger points), is contentious. Schleip (2003a,b) proposed that the amount of force needed to remove fascial adhesions could exceed physiological limitations. Hence, the pressure of a body mass on a foam roller or the force applied on a roller massager with the arms would probably not be sufficient to break up these adhesions. More research is needed to investigate this possible mechanism.

Rolling recommendations for ROM

ROM improvements have been demonstrated with as little as 5-10 s of rolling, with 10 s providing significantly greater increases than 5 s (Sullivan et al., 2013). The majority of studies use multiple sets of 30–60 s bouts of rolling and, although the varying durations have not been not directly compared in most studies, 60 s of rolling tends to induce greater ROM improvements (MacDonald et al., 2013; Halperin et al., 2014; Macdonald et al., 2014; Bradbury-Squires et al., 2015; Pearcey et al., 2015). However, Monteiro and Neto (2016) did

Foam rolling and roller massage effects and mechanisms

report greater ROM with 120 s of rolling versus 60 s. The intensity or discomfort of rolling does not have to be high. Grabow et al. (2018) demonstrated that whether rolling was conducted at 5, 7 or 9/10 on a visual analog pain scale, ROM improvements were similar in each case. An earlier study by Curran et al. (2008) showed that a multi-level rigid roller exerted greater pressures on the skin than a biofoam roller, and the authors suggested that the more rigid roller might be more beneficial. However, Grabow et al.'s 2018 study shows that high pressures are unnecessary to achieve greater ROM results. Thus harder, or more unyielding, and possibly more painful, rollers may not provide any greater benefits. In addition, other devices such as balls could also be substituted to provide a stimulus to the tissues (see Figure 27.2 for examples). Furthermore, following a typical warm-up (5 min of aerobic activity, static and dynamic stretching and sport-specific activities), when rolling was performed at 10 min-intervals after the warm-up, the augmented ROM was maintained for 30 min (Hodgson et al., 2017). This result is valuable for athletes who wait on a bench for 10-30 min before entering the game. Continuing to intermittently roll their muscles while sitting on the bench could maintain some of the benefits of the warm-up.

Rolling effects on performance

One of the advantages of rolling compared with prolonged static stretching is the lower incidence of reported subsequent performance impairments. Table 27.1 illustrates that, out of 17 studies, six reported no effect of rolling on subsequent performance (MacDonald et al., 2013; Halperin et al., 2014; Behara and Jacobson, 2015; Jones et al., 2015; Aune et al., 2018; Smith et al., 2018), five examining rolling

demonstrated improved performance (i.e. vertical jump measures, MVIC force, neuromuscular efficiency, shorter electromechanical delay; Macdonald et al., 2014; Peacock et al., 2014; Bradbury-Squires et al., 2015; Monteiro et al., 2017b; MacGregor et al., 2018), and three showed an attenuation of fatigue-induced performance impairments with rolling compared with control (Healey et al., 2014; Fleckenstein et al., 2017; Madoni et al., 2018). Only two studies reported rolling-induced impairments. Monteiro et al. (2017 c) applied 60, 90 and 120 s of rolling between four sets of knee extensions. Whereas 120 s of rolling decreased the number of knee extension repetitions by 14%, the 90 and 60 s of rolling also decreased repetition numbers by 8–9% (Monteiro et al., 2017 c). Cavanaugh et al. (2016) had participants perform three repetitions of 30 s of roller massage on the plantar flexors at 7/10 on a visual analog pain scale, and found that the force produced in the first 200 ms of a knee extension MVIC (F200) decreased by 9.5% and 19.1% post-test and 5 min post-test, respectively.

Summary

Whereas massage has been used for millennia, foam rollers and roller massagers have only recently become popular. Rolling can increase ROM for ~20 min, generally without subsequent performance deficits (with the exception of two studies (Cavanaugh et al., 2016, Fleckenstein et al., 2017)). Mechanisms underlying these ROM improvements may be related to thixotropic effects (decreased visco-elasticity), rolling-induced decreases in sympathetic activity and motoneuron excitability, and increased stretch/pain tolerance. Rolling has also been shown to reduce pain pressure thresholds with

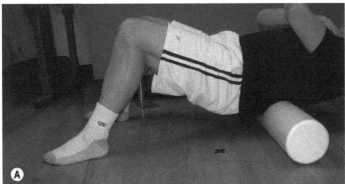

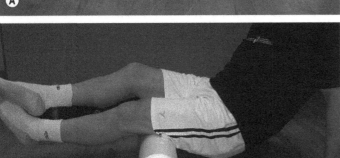

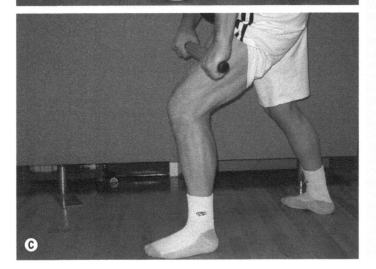

Figure 27.2

Illustrations of sample rolling exercises with foam roller and roller massager: **(A)** lower back, **(B)** hamstrings and **(C)** quadriceps (roller massager).

Table 27.1 Foam rolling (FR) and roller massage (RM) effects on range of motion (ROM) and performance

Reference	Intervention	ROM changes	Performance changes
Aune et al., 2018	FR: 4 weeks of 3 x 60 s on gastrocnemius	↑9% acute ↑7% with training	No change in PF torque or drop jump RSI
Behara and Jacobson, 2015	FR: 1 min each for quadriceps, hamstrings, gluteals and gastrocnemius	↑15.6% hip flexion ROM	No significant change in VJ, KE and KF torque
Bradbury-Squires et al., 2015	RM: 5 x 20 s and 5 x 60 s on quadriceps	5 x 20 s: ↑10% 5 x 60 s: ↑16%	Lunge neuromuscular efficiency ↑3–7%
Cavanaugh et al., 2016	RM: 3 x 30 on PF at 7/10 VAS	Not measured	F200 ↓9.5% and 19.1% post-test and 5 min post-test
Fleckenstein et al., 2017	FR: Before or after fatigue: 30 s on quadriceps, hamstrings, adductors, PF and iliotibial tract	Not measured	↓fatigue-induced losses in KE MVIC. Post-fatigue FR had greater ES than pre-fatigue
Halperin et al., 2014	RM: 3 x 30 s	↑4% ankle	↑8.2% MVIC
Healey et al., 2014	FR: 30 s on quadriceps, hamstrings, latissimus dorsi and rhomboids	Not measured	Fatigue impairments of VJ, MVIC and agility were less after FR vs. planking
Jones et al., 2015	FR: 30 s on quadriceps, hamstrings, gastrocnemius and gluteals	Not measured	No effects on VJ measures
MacDonald et al., 2013	FR: 2 x 60 s on quadriceps	Knee joint ROM 10.3–12.7%↑	No change in voluntary (MVIC) or evoked (twitch and tetanus) muscle properties
MacDonald et al., 2013	FR: 20 min at post-test, post-24 h and post-48 h after EIMD (10 x 10 squats)	↑11–13% quadriceps at post-48 h and 72 h ↑3% hamstrings at post-72 h	↓1–2% EMD at post-24 h and 48 h (beneficial effect) Attenuated VJ impairments ↑1% Impaired evoked contractile properties
MacGregor et al., 2018	FR: 2 min daily for 3 consecutive days	Not measured	↑MVIC force, ↓MVC, EMG and ↑NME with 50% KE MVIC
Madoni et al., 2018	FR: 3 x 30 s on hamstrings	↑2.6% hamstrings	Hamstrings PT ↓3.4–6.1% but decreases less than control
Monteiro et al., 2017 b	FR: 30, 60, 90 and 120 s on lateral thigh	Not measured	90 s of FR↑ overhead deep squat performance vs. 30, 60 or 120 s
Monteiro et al., 2017 c	FR: 60, 90 and 120 s on quadriceps between 4 sets of dynamic KE	Not measured	↓ no. of KE repetitions by 8.6–13.8%
Peacock et al., 2014	Dynamic warm-up vs. dynamic warm-up with FR: 5 strokes x 30 s on back, gluteals, quadriceps, hamstrings, calves and pectorals	No difference between dynamic warm-up and combined	↑performance with combined warm-up for power, agility, strength and speed
Smith et al., 2018	FR: 3 x 30 s on quadriceps, hamstrings and gluteals	FR: ↑9–13.8% Combination of DS/FR: ↑7.2–15.4%	Combination ↑more than FR for VJ No change in VJ with FR
Sullivan et al., 2013	RM: 1–2 sets of 5 + 10 s	↑4.3% sit and reach	No change in MVC force or EMG

Abbreviations: DS, dynamic stretch; EIMD, exercise-induced muscle damage; EMD, electromechanical delay; EMG, electromyography; F200, force produced in the first 200 ms; KE, knee extensors; KF, knee flexors; MVIC, maximal voluntary isometric contraction; NME, neuromuscular efficiency; PF, plantar flexors; RSI, reactive strength index; VAS, visual analog scale for pain; VJ, vertical jump; arrow up, increase; arrow down, decrease.

Chapter 27

acute and longer term discomfort (i.e. myofascial and muscle tender points and delayed onset muscle soreness). It is recommended to perform multiple sets of 30–120 s of rolling, performed below the maximum pain tolerance (50–90%).

Rolling may be combined with static stretching to further enhance ROM as well as applied at 10-min intervals after the warm-up to maintain the increased flexibility achieved with the warm-up (see Figure 27.3 for a summary of rolling effects).

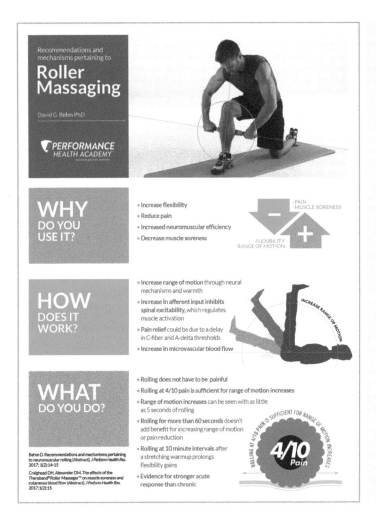

Figure 27.3

Pictograph summary of rolling effects and recommendations.

With permission from Performance Health.

References

Aboodarda, S.J., Spence, A.J. & Button, D.C. (2015) Pain pressure threshold of a muscle tender spot increases following local and non-local rolling massage. *BMC Musculoskelet Disord.* 16: 265.

Aune, A.A.G., Bishop, C., Turner, A.N., Papadopoulos, K., Budd, S., Richardson, M. & Maloney, S.J. (2018) Acute and chronic effects of foam rolling vs eccentric exercise on ROM and force output of the plantar flexors. *J Sports Sci.* 37(2): 138–145.

Behara, B. & Jacobson, B.H. (2017) The acute effects of deep tissue foam rolling and dynamic stretching on muscular strength, power, and flexibility in division I linemen. *J Strength Cond Res.* 31(4): 888–892.

Behm, D.G. (2018) *The Science and Physiology of Flexibility and Stretching: Implications and Applications in Sport Performance and Health.* London, UK: Routledge Publishers.

Behm, D.G., Baker, K.M., Kelland, R. & Lomond, J. (2001) The effect of muscle damage on strength and fatigue deficits. *J Strength Cond Res.* 15: 255–263.

Behm, D.G., Blazevich, A.J., Kay, A.D. & McHugh, M. (2016) Acute effects of muscle stretching on physical performance, range of motion, and injury incidence in healthy active individuals: a systematic review. *Appl Physiol Nutr Metab.* 41: 1–11.

Behm, D.G. & Chaouachi, A. (2011) A review of the acute effects of static and dynamic stretching on performance. *Eur J Appl Physiol.* 111: 2633–2651.

Behm, D.G., Peach, A., Maddigan, M., Aboodarda, S.J., DiSanto, M.C., Button, D.C. & Maffiuletti, N.A. (2013) Massage and stretching reduce spinal reflex excitability without affecting twitch contractile properties. *J Electromyogr Kinesiol.* 23: 1215–1221.

Bradbury-Squires, D.J., Noftall, J.C., Sullivan, K.M., Behm, D.G., Power, K.E. & Button, D.C. (2015) Roller-massager application to the quadriceps and knee-joint range of motion and neuromuscular efficiency during a lunge. *J Athl Train.* 50: 133–140.

Cavanaugh, M.T., Aboodarda, S.J., Hodgson, D. & Behm, D.G. (2016) Foam rolling of quadriceps decreases biceps femoris activation. *J Strength Cond Res.*

Cavanaugh, M.T., Doweling, A., Young, J.D., Quigley, P.J., Hodgson, D.D., Whitten, J.H., Reid, J.C., Aboodarda, S.J. & Behm, D.G. (2017) An acute session of roller massage prolongs voluntary torque development and diminishes evoked pain. *Eur J Appl Physiol.* 31(8): 2238–2245.

Cheatham, S.W., Stull, K.R. & Kolber, M.J. (2018) Comparison of a vibrating foam roller and a non-vibrating foam roller intervention on knee range of motion and pressure pain threshold: a randomized controlled trial. *J Sport Rehabil.* doi: 10.1123/jsr.2017-0164.

Cowman, M.K., Schmidt, T.A., Raghavan, P. & Stecco, A. (2015) Viscoelastic properties of hyaluronan in physiological conditions. *F1000Res.* 4: 622.

Curran, P.F., Fiore, R.D. & Crisco, J.J. (2008) A comparison of the pressure exerted on soft tissue by 2 myofascial rollers. *J Sport Rehabil.* 17: 432–442.

Fede, C., Angelini, A., Stern, R., Macchi, V., Porzionato, A., Ruggieri, P., De Caro, R., & Stecco, C. (2018) Quantification of hyaluronan in human fasciae: variations with function and anatomical site. *J Anat.* 233: 552–556.

Fleckenstein, J., Wilke, J., Vogt, L. & Banzer, W. (2017) Preventive and regenerative foam rolling are equally effective in reducing fatigue-related impairments of muscle function following exercise. *J Sports Sci Med.* 16: 474–479.

Goldberg, J., Sullivan, S.J. & Seaborne, D.E. (1992) The effect of two intensities of massage on H-reflex amplitude. *Phys Ther.* 72: 449–457.

Grabow, L., Young, J.D., Byrne, J.M., Granacher, U. & Behm, D.G. (2017) Unilateral rolling of the foot did not affect non-local range of motion or balance. *J Sports Sci Med.* 16: 209–218.

Grabow, L., Young, J.D., Alcock, L.R., Quigley, P.J., Byrne, J.M., Granacher, U., Skrabot, J. & Behm, D.G. (2018) Higher quadriceps roller massage forces do not amplify range-of-motion increases or impair strength and jump performance. *J Strength Cond Res.* 32(11): 3059–3069.

Grieve, R., Goodwin, F., Alfaki, M., Bourton, A.J., Jeffries, C. & Scott, H. (2015) The immediate effect of bilateral self myofascial release on the plantar surface of the feet on hamstring and lumbar spine flexibility: A pilot randomised controlled trial. *J Bodyw Mov Ther.* 19: 544–552.

Halperin, I., Aboodarda, S.J., Button, D.C., Andersen, L.L. & Behm, D.G.

(2014) Roller massager improves range of motion of plantar flexor muscles without subsequent decreases in force parameters. *Int J Sports Phys Ther.* 9: 92–102.

Han, S.W., Lee, Y.S. & Lee, D.J. (2017) The influence of the vibration form roller exercise on the pains in the muscles around the hip joint and the joint performance. *J Phys Ther Sci.* 29: 1844–1847.

Hanten, W.P., Olson, S.L., Butts, N.L. & Nowicki, A.L. (2000) Effectiveness of a home program of ischemic pressure followed by sustained stretch for treatment of myofascial trigger points. *Phys Ther.* 80: 997–1003.

Healey, K.C., Hatfield, D.L., Blanpied, P., Dorfman, L.R. & Riebe, D. (2014) The effects of myofascial release with foam rolling on performance. *J Strength Cond Res.* 28: 61–68.

Hodgson, D.D., Quigley, P.J., Whitten, J.H.D., Reid, J.C. & Behm, D.G. (2017) Impact of 10-minute interval roller massage on performance and active range of motion. *J Strength Cond Res.* 33(6): 1512–1523.

Huang, S.Y., Di Santo, M., Wadden, K.P., Cappa, D.F., Alkanani, T. & Behm, D.G. (2010) Short-duration massage at the hamstrings musculotendinous junction induces greater range of motion. *J Strength Cond Res.* 24: 1917–1924.

Jones, A., Brown, L.E, Coburn, J.W. & Noffal, G.J. (2015) Effects of foam rolling on vertical jump performance. *Int J Kinesiol Sport Sci.* 3: 38–42.

Junker, D.H. & Stoggl, T.L. (2015) The foam roll as a tool to improve hamstring flexibility. *J Strength Cond Res.* 29: 3480–3485.

Kelly, S. & Beardsley, C. (2016) Specific and cross-over effects of foam rolling on ankle dorsiflexion range of motion. *Int J Sports Phys Ther.* 11: 544–551.

Killen, B.S., Zelizney, K.L. & Ye, X. (2018) Crossover effects of unilateral static stretching and foam rolling on contralateral hamstring flexibility and strength. *J Sport Rehabil.* 28(6): 533–539.

Kosek, E., Ekholm, J. & Hansson, P. (1995) Increased pressure pain sensibility in fibromyalgia patients is located deep to the skin but not restricted to muscle tissue. *Pain.* 63: 335–339.

Kostopoulos, D.N., Arthur, J., Ingber, R.S. & Larkin, R.W. (2008) Reduction of spontaneous electrical activity and pain perception of trigger points in the upper trapezius muscle through trigger point compression and passive stretching. *J Musculoskelet Pain.* 16: 266–278.

Lee, C.L., Chu, I.H., Lyu, B.J., Chang, W.D. & Chang, N.J. (2018) Comparison of vibration rolling, nonvibration rolling, and static stretching as a warm-up exercise on flexibility, joint proprioception, muscle strength, and balance in young adults. *J Sports Sci.* 36: 2575–2582.

Macdonald, G.Z., Button, D.C., Drinkwater, E.J. & Behm, D.G. (2014) Foam rolling as a recovery tool after an intense bout of physical activity. *Med Sci Sports Exerc.* 46: 131–142.

MacDonald, G.Z., Penney, M.D., Mullaley, M.E., Cuconato, A.L., Drake, C.D., Behm, D.G. & Button, D.C. (2013) An acute bout of self-myofascial release increases range of motion without a subsequent decrease in muscle activation or force. *J Strength Cond Res.* 27: 812–821.

MacGregor, L.J., Fairweather, M.M., Bennett, R.M. & Hunter, A.M. (2018) The effect of foam rolling for three consecutive days on muscular efficiency and range of motion. *Sports Med Open.* 4: 26.

Madoni, S.N., Costa, P.B., Coburn, J.W. & Galpin, A.J. (2018) Effects of foam rolling on range of motion, peak torque, muscle activation, and the hamstrings-to-quadriceps strength ratios. *J Strength Cond Res.* 32: 1821–1830.

Magnusson, S.P., Simonsen, E.B., Aagaard, P., Sorensen, H. & Kjaer, M. (1996) A mechanism for altered flexibility in human skeletal muscle. *J Physiol.* 497: 291–298.

Markovic, G. (2015) Acute effects of instrument assisted soft tissue mobilization vs. foam rolling on knee and hip range of motion in soccer players. *J Bodyw Mov Ther.* 19: 690–696.

Melzack, R. & Wall, P.D. (1965) Pain mechanisms: a new theory. *Science.* 150: 971–979.

Mense, S. (2000) Neurobiological concepts of fibromyalgia – the possible role of descending spinal tracts. *Scand J Rheumatol.* 113 (suppl.): 24–29.

Mitchell, J.H. & Schmidt, R.F. (1977) *Cardiovascular reflex control by afferent fibers from skeletal muscle receptors.* Bethesda, MA: American Physiological Society.

Moayedi, M. & Davis, K.D. (2013) Theories of pain: from specificity to gate control. *J Neurophysiol.* 109: 5–12.

Monteiro, E.R., Cavanaugh, M.T., Frost, D.M. & Novaes, J.D. (2017a) Is self-massage an effective joint range-of-motion strategy? A pilot study. *J Bodyw Mov Ther.* 21: 223–226.

Monteiro, E.R. & Neto, V.G. (2016) Effect of different foam rolling volumes on knee extension fatigue. *Int J Sports Phys Ther.* 11: 1076–1081.

Monteiro, E.R., Skarabot, J., Vigotsky, A.D., Brown, A.F., Gomes, T.M. & Novaes, J.D. (2017b) Acute effects of different self-massage volumes on the FMS overhead deep squat performance. *Int J Sports Phys Ther.* 12: 94–104.

Monteiro, E.R., del Melo Fuiza, A.G.F., de Oliviera Muniz Cunha, J.C., da Silva Novaes, G., Vianna, J.M., Behm, D.G. & da Silva Novaes, J. (2018) Quadriceps and hamstrings foam rolling and stretching increases passive shoulder range-of-motion. *J Perform Health Res.* 2: 14.

Monteiro, E.R.V.A., Skarabot, J., Brown, A.F., del Melo Fiuza, A.G.F., Gomes, T.M., Halperin, I., da Silva Novaes, J. 2017c Acute effects of different foam rolling volumes in the interset rest period on maximum repetition performance. *Hong Kong Physiother J.* 36: 57–62.

Murray, A.M., Jones, T.W., Horobeanu, C., Turner, A.P. & Sproule, J. (2016) Sixty seconds of foam rolling does not affect functional flexibility or change muscle temperature in adolescent athletes. *Int J Sports Phys Ther.* 11: 765–776.

Okamoto, T., Masuhara, M. & Ikuta. K. (2014) Acute effects of self-myofascial release using a foam roller on arterial function. *J Strength Cond Res.* 28: 69–73.

Peacock, C.A., Krein, D.D., Silver, T.A., Sanders, G.J. & Carlowitz, KA. (2014) An acute bout of self-myofascial release in the form of foam rolling improves performance testing. *Int J Exerc Sci.* 7: 202–211.

Pearcey, G.E., Bradbury-Squires, D.J., Kawamoto, J.E., Drinkwater, E.J., Behm, D.G. & Button, D.C. (2015) Foam rolling for delayed-onset muscle soreness and recovery of dynamic performance measures. *J Athl Train.* 50: 5–13.

Pud, D., Granovsky, Y. & Yarnitsky, D. (2009) The methodology of experimentally induced diffuse noxious inhibitory control (DNIC)-like effect in humans. *Pain.* 144: 16–19.

Schleip, R. (2003a) Fascial plasticity - a new neurobiological explanation: Part 2. *J Bodyw Mov Ther.* 7: 104–116.

Schleip, R. (2003b) Fascial plasticity - a new neurobiological explanation: Part I. *J Bodyw Mov Ther.* 7: 11–19.

Skarabot, J., Beardsley, C. & Stirn, I. (2015) Comparing the effects of self-myofascial release with static stretching on ankle range-of-motion in adolescent athletes. *Int J Sports Phys Ther.* 10: 203–212.

Smith, J.C., Pridgeon, B. & Hall, M.C. (2018) Acute effect of foam rolling and dynamic stretching on flexibility and jump height. *J Strength Cond Res.* 32: 2209–2215.

Sullivan, K.M., Silvey, D.B., Button, D.C. & Behm, D.G. (2013) Roller-massager application to the hamstrings increases sit-and-reach range of motion within five to ten seconds without performance impairments. *Int J Sports Phys Ther.* 8: 228–236.

Trajano, G.S., Nosaka, K. & Blazevich, A.J. (2017) Neurophysiological mechanisms underpinning stretch-induced force loss. *Sports Med.* 47(8): 1531–1541.

Vigotsky, A.D., Lehman, G.J., Contreras, B., Beardsley, C., Chung, B. & Feser, E.H. (2015) Acute effects of anterior thigh foam rolling on hip angle, knee angle, and rectus femoris length in the modified Thomas test. *Peer J.* 3: e1281.

Wilke, J., Vogt, L. & Banzer W. (2018) Immediate effects of self-myofascial release on latent trigger point sensitivity: a randomized, placebo-controlled trial. *Biol Sport.* 35: 349–354.

Weerapong, P., Hume, P.A. & Kolt, G.S. (2005) The mechanisms of massage and effects on performance, muscle recovery and injury prevention. *Sports Med.* 35: 235–256.

Wu, G., Ekedahl, R., Stark, B., Carlstedt, T., Nilsson, B. & Hallin, R.G. (1999) Clustering of Pacinian corpuscle afferent fibres in the human median nerve. *Exp Brain Res.* 126: 399–409.

Young, J.D., Spence, A.J. & Behm, D.G. (2018) Roller massage decreases spinal excitability to the soleus. *J Appl Physiol.* 124: 950–959.

Fascial stretching

Ann Frederick, Frieder Krause and Chris Frederick

Introduction

Stretching is but one of multiple activities that athletes, fitness enthusiasts and movers of all persuasions may engage in before, during and after training or event participation. It may be performed by a person alone, with partners, with a team, or performed in an assisted fashion with a trainer or a therapist. There are several concepts and methods of stretching, from passive, static stretching of isolated muscles to dynamic or ballistic stretching during multi-joint movements to name just a few. Research in the last 2 decades has shown that most stretching methods are able to improve flexibility and joint ROM (Harvey et al., 2002; Decoster et al., 2005; Thomas et al., 2018). However, static stretching of longer durations seems to hamper neuromuscular performance, while dynamic and active stretching methods improve performance (Behm and Chaouachi, 2011; Kay and Blazevich, 2012; Opplert and Babault, 2018).

In this chapter, a specific and comprehensive approach called fascial stretching is introduced and described. When integrated into a complex training regimen, such a method may assist in improving movement ability and athleticism while potentially speeding up recovery and reducing risks of injury (Schleip and Müller, 2013). Applied together with manual and movement therapy for rehabilitation after injury or surgery, we believe that fascial stretching can be used for relief from common subjective complaints of pain, soreness, stiffness and tightness.

Stretching and the fascial system

Flexibility has long been seen as a matter of muscle extensibility only. However, our modern understanding of flexibility now also includes neurophysiological factors (Weppler and Magnusson, 2010), as well as other non-muscular components such as peripheral nerves and the fascial system (Wilke et al., 2016; Nordez et al., 2017). A fascial approach to stretching uses the same principles and philosophy that all types of fascia-oriented training are based on. It is well-established that functional outcomes in movement, sport and fitness are greatly improved when incorporating whole body participation, in contrast to an isolated focus on single muscles and body parts.

Fascial stretching has been described as one of the four essential elements necessary to help build, repair and maintain connective tissue health and fitness for optimal movement (Schleip and Müller, 2013). Stretching can provide the necessary stimulus to affect tissue remodeling in the connective tissue (Benhardt and Cosgriff-Hernandez, 2009), entailing improved mechanical properties of fascia. This includes helping muscles to efficiently contract, lengthen and expand. Dynamic forms of stretching can both mentally prepare and physically "warm-up" the

Chapter 28

entire neuromyofascial system for imminent activity. Traditionally, static stretching has been used to aid cool down, repair stress, strain and injury from activity and restore normal function, although many of its claimed effects remain under question (Herbert and Gabriel, 2002; McHugh and Cosgrave, 2010; Herbert et al., 2011).

Stretching based on function

As pointed out, more research on applied stretching is needed to showcase the broad and deep spectrum of possibilities in prescribing personalized parameters for individual athletes and patients. This challenge is multiplied when considering how to apply stretching parameters to the broad spectrum of flexibility variations commonly found among groups or teams.

Therefore, function-based stretching depending solely on task participation lacks an important component unless a person's mobility type is also considered. In addition to several other factors like anthropometrics or genetic muscle fiber composition, the degree of mobility also often determines what sport or fitness activity an athlete engages in. For example, we will see lean people participate in rock climbing and solid people engage in power lifting.

If we use the extreme ends of the "flexibility in humans" spectrum as examples of how to apply stretching to improve connective tissue fitness and health, we come up with what have been described as the Viking and the Dancer types (Schleip and Bayer, 2017). Briefly, the Viking can be described as the least mobile but strongest type of person. These large, wide people are built more for stability than mobility and participate in sports and activities where their size and strength are an asset (e.g. weightlifting and athletic field sports such as the shot put and hammer).

The other extreme is the Dancer, who is extremely flexible and supremely mobile. Naturally, the approach which either one of these extreme types takes when stretching must be different, based on whether they (1) tend to be less or more mobile and (2) on their function. Other important considerations are that the Viking must not have increased flexibility at the expense of their functional stability otherwise they may lose power and strength. Likewise, the Dancer must not gain joint stiffness or myofascial tightness that decreases their functional flexibility to perform aerial splits.

While both extremes of the flexibility spectrum—the Viking and the Dancer—are commonly seen, there are many more people who fall somewhere in between these two extremes. Some people may be half Viking and half Dancer, with some individuals being one or the other in the top half as opposed to the bottom half of the same body!

The stretch spectrum

The variety of the different methods, techniques, parameters and applications of stretching is vast. For the limits of this chapter we will discuss active stretching, used for warm-up before activity and for post-activity recovery.

Activity preparation (warm-up)

Depending on the individual needs and the desired sport, it is generally advised that a warm-up consists of a period of aerobic exercise, followed by dynamic stretching, and ending with a period of movement similar to the upcoming activity (McGowan et al., 2015).

The National Strength and Conditioning Association describes two basic phases of the warm-up (Sands et al., 2012). The first is a gen-

Fascial stretching

eral warm-up period. In sport this may consist of five minutes of slow aerobic activity such as jogging, skipping, or cycling. The second phase, activating and mobilizing, is analogous to the stretching component of a typical warm-up. The focus on mobility, or actively moving through a range of motion, requires a combination of motor control, stability, and flexibility and more closely relates to the movement requirements an athlete will face. Typically, this phase lasts between ten and twenty minutes, with the shorter time periods being more common (Sands et al., 2012).

Activity recovery

The goal of post-activity recovery is to return the athlete back to a pre-activity level of optimal performance. A plethora of strategies are used in everyday practice, including sleep and nutritional strategies as well as active recovery such as light aerobic movement or stretching (Nédélec et al., 2013; Calleja-González et al., 2016). Although scientific data suggests that there is no effect for stretching to reduce muscle soreness (Herbert et al., 2011), it is still widely used as a recovery tool after exercise.

The Great 8 Stretch to Win® program

The Great 8 stretches (Figure 28.1) are one example of a global core mobility program of fascial stretches that integrate well with core dynamic stability programs commonly performed by athletes and fitness enthusiasts before activity participation.

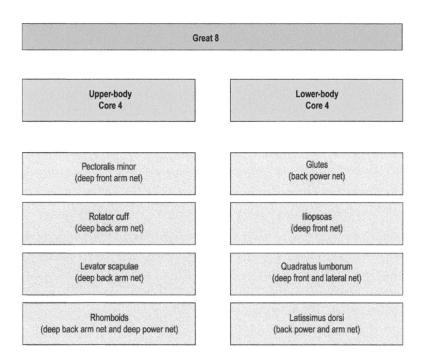

Figure 28.1

Structure and components of the Great 8

Chapter 28

We believe that achieving balanced mobility in the core regions of the body before training for stability will provide results that are more effective. This is because the program also serves as a self-assessment for the athlete. It empowers them to self-correct any imbalances that are discovered, which hopefully results in a decreased risk of micro-trauma, such as localized strain or stress accumulation.

The program is divided into the Core 4 of the lower body and the Core 4 of the upper body and target tissues lying within and around long chains or nets of fascia (see Figure 28.1). In contrast to other established approaches of myofascial chains we chose to use the term "fascial nets" (Frederick and Frederick, 2017).

For instance, the back power net (posterior diagonal line) includes the connection between the gluteal muscles and the contralateral lats.

While each stretch has the intent to mobilize and stretch a specific fascial net, it is also associated with a key local myofascial unit that (in our experience with athletes) is most directly responsible to improve functional movement.

Our focus for this chapter is on the Core 4 lower body part of the Great 8, because many sports and fitness activities engage these fascial nets to generate the power required for optimal performance.

What we call the Core 4 of the lower body anatomically includes the lumbar-pelvic-hip area. In terms of muscles, this would be all the core muscles and fasciae in the region of the lumbodorsal or thoracolumbar fascia, transversus abdominis, obliques, deep and superficial back extensors, iliopsoas, glutes and deep hip rotators. Our focus is on four key myofascial regions, which aim to improve mobility in professional athletes:

- Iliopsoas in the deep front net
- Glutes in the back power net
- Quadratus lumborum (QL) in the deep front, lateral and spiral net
- Latissimus dorsi in the back power net.

Lateral and back power nets: glute complex (Figure 28.2)

1. Sit on the floor and bend both knees, placing one leg in front and one behind.
2. Bring the front foot inward until the foot touches the back knee if possible.
3. Position your weight so you are sitting more on the glute of the front leg. Make any adjustments for comfort.
4. Place your hands in front of you in a push-up position with the arms straight to begin.
5. Lengthen your whole spine out from the top of your head as you inhale. Exhale moving down and forward over the knee into the stretch, keeping your spine long.
6. Flex, rolling up through spine to the upright start position. Repeat, taking the torso

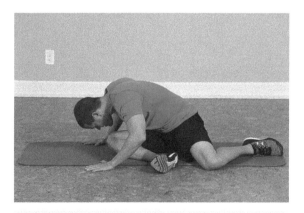

Figure 28.2
Glute complex within back power net.

Fascial stretching

forward to the left and right of knee at different angles targeting the different glute fibers.

7. Tip: Breathe, moving in and out of the stretch until you feel your tissues release. Drop your body down closer to the floor and move from side to side.

Spiral and lateral net: QL (Figure 28.3)

1. From the glute stretch, start walking your hands back until you feel a slight stretch in your back, hips or legs.

2. Keeping your hands still, lean to the front hand and inhale.

3. Exhale as you lean into the back hand, slightly bending the elbow.

4. Tip: Walk your hands slightly further away with each repetition to progress the stretch.

Deep front net: hip flexors (Figure 28.4)

1. From your last position, place your forearm back on the ground and find a stable position to balance, so there is full weight on that arm.

2. Slide your forearm to the rear as your back starts to arch and stop when a mild stretch is felt.

3. Slightly leaning forward on both hands (not shown), inhale.

4. Exhale while arching back, looking up to ceiling. Repeat.

5. Tip: Lean further back to progress the stretch. Turn your chest towards the floor then to ceiling to stretch different angles. Find the stretch by arching your back, not by twisting.

Back power net: Latissimus dorsi (Figure 28.5)

1. Moving from the last position, inhale and then reach your arm up overhead.

2. Extend the arm out from the hip as you reach up and overhead, as though you are swimming in the air.

3. Exhale as you rotate your chest towards the floor, reaching your arm out.

4. Circle your arm down and back up overhead to repeat.

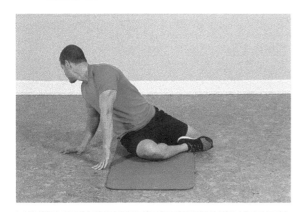

Figure 28.3
Quadratus lumborum within spiral and lateral nets.

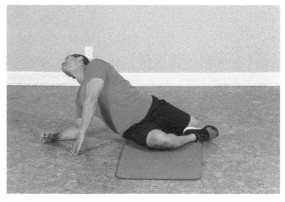

Figure 28.4
Hip flexors within the deep front net.

Chapter 28

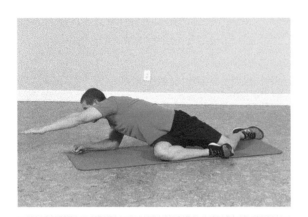

Figure 28.5
Latissimus dorsi within back power net.

5. Tip: Keep reaching your arm throughout the stretch for maximal effect. Try to get your chest increasingly parallel to floor with each rep.

Fascial stretch technique

The difference in technique between traditional and isolated muscle stretching and that of fascial stretching can be summed up in a term we named The Stretch Wave™, which incorporates the following principles:

- Initiate and terminate body movement with eye movement
- Exhale on the stretch, inhale on the recoil
- Lead the stretch by breath volume and duration, not counting
- Perform tempo of stretch movement that matches the phase of training
- Undulate through the fascial net
- Oscillate across adjacent fascial nets
- Train elastic recoil by extending the fascial net movement intent.

Initiating and terminating body movement with eye movement may encourage full neuromyofascial engagement from the mechanoreceptors in the skeletal eye muscles. They are connected to the deep neck muscles via the galea capitis and the superficial fascia of the neck (Stecco and Hammer, 2014). Potentially, this fascial connection can mediate an effect of eye movement on the neck and shoulder muscles, and encourages incorporating them into a holistic stretching and training program.

Exhale on the stretch, inhale on the recoil coordinates proper breathing with movement versus movement preparation.

Lead stretch by breath volume and duration, not counting encourages the athlete to experience a deeper, more interoceptive sense of timing. It uses the breath with the movement rather than just counting seconds. So, when the athlete performs slower breathing to match slower stretch movements, it may help shift the nervous system to the parasympathetic for better recovery. By contrast, faster, more dynamic movements accompanied by faster breathing better prepares the athlete sympathetically for imminent activity.

Perform tempo of stretch movement that matches phase of training parallels the description above in Lead stretch by breath volume and duration, not counting. In mimicking the movement velocity and amplitude according to the desired movement, the stretch serves as an optimal warm-up to enhance performance.

Undulate through the fascial net ensures full fascial engagement along the part of the net that is moving as well as being transmitted beyond.

Oscillate across adjacent fascial nets ensures that adjacent nets along septa and other connections between myofasciae are included for a full fascial net experience.

Fascial stretching

Train elastic recoil by extending the fascial net movement intent encourages the athlete to maximize the extent of the specific movement to help train fascia's efficiency at storing potential energy and releasing kinetic energy in movement. This is carried out within the parameters specific to the activity so that any unnecessary stretching or overstretching is avoided. It also incorporates all of the previous techniques.

Below follows an example of how you would use the principles of fascial stretching described above. It is particularly effective at improving or maintaining maximum functional flexibility potential. Focus moving one key myofascial region at one attachment, release it then focus on moving the other attachment. Finish by combining both attachments for a full fascial net stretch, until there is no more gain in range of motion for that movement. Then move on to adjacent nets as indicated by your coach or practitioner, or based on your own self-assessment.

See the photographs and instructions below for an example of fascial stretching for the back net of the leg, targeting key muscles, hamstrings and gastrocnemius:

Proximal net focus (Figure 28.6)

- Use a bench, table or the floor, which facilitates a body position without tension or stretch in the target tissues. The foot is fixed on the chosen surface and the ankle is in a neutral position to start.
- Inhale to prepare then exhale as you perform a gentle anterior pelvic tilt until a mild stretch is felt at a proximal attachment

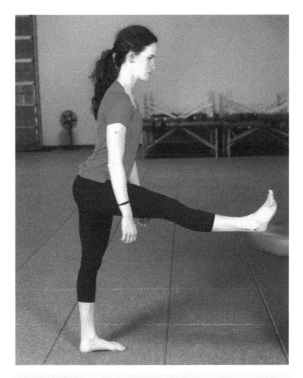

Figure 28.6
Proximal net stretch focus.

region. Avoid any other movement through the hip or spine. Inhale as you come out of the stretch then exhale as you repeat, until no further gain in movement is possible.

Distal net focus (Figure 28.7)

- Inhale to prepare then exhale and allow your pelvis to relax passively into a posterior pelvic tilt as you lean forward, flexing your spine and hip and lowering your head toward your knee until a mild stretch is felt. Inhale as you come out of the stretch then exhale as you repeat, until no further gain in movement is possible.

Chapter 28

Full net focus (Figure 28.8)

- Gently combine and simultaneously perform the previous proximal and distal stretches together. Inhale to come out of the stretch then exhale as you repeat, until no further gain in movement is possible.

Spread the stretch and add adjacent nets.

- Spread the stretch to access more of the target tissue: add options to include adjacent septa of connecting myofascial regions, by including gentle and small triplanar movements with circular undulations and/or oscillations.

- Add foot-ankle dorsiflexion and/or head-neck flexion one at a time or in combination for an even more comprehensive fascial stretch. (Note: that while this more extreme stretch may be appropriate and indicated with athletes like gymnasts, it will be contraindicated or unnecessary for most athletes because it is not part of their functional movement patterns. One example of a contraindication, among many, is a diagnosis of sciatica or any spinal disc lesion).

Repeat for all key muscle nets in the Core 4 or Great 8 program as needed or indicated.

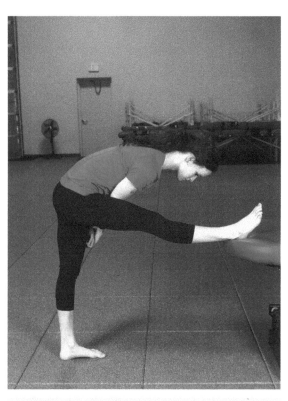

Figure 28.7
Distal net stretch focus.

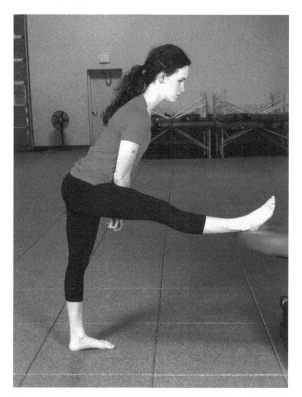

Figure 28.8
Full net stretch.

Fascial stretching

Other important principles and concepts

- Experience a slow awareness of stretch without ever feeling pain. This will be more pronounced or apparent during slow tempo recovery phase stretching than pre-activity dynamic stretching.

- Creating a little extra space by tractioning your joints during recovery-phase stretching will increase the effectiveness and prolong the benefits of the stretch. Do this by gently lifting, reaching and/or expanding out before moving directly into a stretch.

- Do as many repetitions of a stretch as it takes before you no longer realize a gain in pre-activity or functional movement. Otherwise, try 3–6 progressive repetitions of each position. This can vary from side to side and from stretch to stretch.

- If there is any imbalance experienced like one-sided (unilateral) restriction to mobility, then it is advised that you correct it with more repetitions and/or duration of stretch movement until your reassessment shows the imbalance is resolved (see more details below).

How to correct functional imbalances in your fascial net

Stretching does not permanently alter muscle or connective tissue length. However, as chronic stretching leads to increased stretch tolerance, functional flexibility asymmetries can be resolved. Often, you can easily and quickly correct imbalances discovered when you mobilize or stretch yourself. We have found that one of the easiest and quickest ways is to first test the stretch on each side to determine if one side is less mobile. Then start and end with the less mobile side, so that you get a 2-to-1 ratio. In other words, the tighter side gets a double dose. Over time, when you assess that both sides have the same mobility, you can go back to stretching at a 1-to-1 ratio for maintenance.

If the imbalance persists, increase the duration of the stretch. For instance, if you were using a slow stretch wave tempo then switch to a very slow stretch wave tempo so you spend more time releasing restrictions while you move through the stretch.

Also, keep in mind that with fascial stretching, sometimes the source of the problem is not locally, where you may feel pain or restriction, but is likely more distal or on the contralateral side.

A persistent imbalance also suggests that you add self-myofascial release like foam rolling, after you assess where you need to focus. This is described in more detail in Chapter 27. Table 28.1 lists self-stretch program parameters to help you design and integrate what you need for any phase of movement activity.

Table 28.1 Self-stretch program parameters

Stretch program	Technique	Tempo	Intensity	Duration	Reps	Sets	Frequency	Notes
Preparation	Stretch Wave fast	Moderately fast	Light to moderate	Short exhale (1-2 counts)	3	1	Pre-training	• Adjust any parameter as needeed. • Reps and sets are per side or for the whole body. • Adjust the program to what the body needs that day. • See Chapter 7 for self-programs and Chapter 8 for assisted programs.
Recovery and maintenance	Stretch Wave slow	Moderately slow	Moderate	Long exhale (3 counts)	3 or until there are no futher gains in mobility	1	Pre-training	• Adjust any parameter as needeed. • Reps and sets are per side or for the whole body. • Adjust the program to what the body needs that day. • See Chapter 6 for self-programs and Chapter 8 for assisted programs.
Restoration and correction	Stretch Wave very slow	Very slow	Moderate	Long exhale (3 counts)	3 or until there are no futher gains in mobility	1	Every day until functional mobility goals are met	• Reps and sets are per body region. • Adjust the program to what the body needs that day. • If stretching increases pain, try stretching other regions of the same or nearby fascial nets, and then reassess. • If stretching increases tenderness, decrease all parameters and move more gently, and then reassess.

Reprinted by permission from A. Frederick and C. Frederick, *Stretch to Win*, 2nd ed. Champaign, IL: Human Kinetics, 2017, 91.

References

Behm, D.G. & Chaouachi, A. (2011) A review of the acute effects of static and dynamic stretching on performance. *Eur J Appl Physiol.* 111: 2633–2651.

Benhardt, H.A. & Cosgriff-Hernandez, E.M. (2009) The role of mechanical loading in ligament tissue engineering. *Tissue Eng Part B Rev.* 15: 467–475.

Calleja-González, J., Terrados, N., Mielgo-Ayuso, J., Delextrat, A., Jukic, I., Vaquera, A., et al. (2016) Evidence-based post-exercise recovery strategies in basketball. *Phys Sportsmed.* 44: 74–78.

Decoster, L.C., Cleland, J., Altieri, C. & Russell, P. (2005) The effects of hamstring stretching on range of motion: a systematic literature review. *J Orthop Sports Phys Ther.* 35: 377–387.

Frederick, A. & Frederick, C. (2017) *Stretch to Win*, 2nd edition. Champaign, IL: Human Kinetics.

Harvey, L., Herbert, R. & Crosbie, J. (2002) Does stretching induce lasting increases in joint ROM? A systematic review. *Physiother Res Int.* 7: 1–13.

Herbert, R.D. & Gabriel, M. (2002) Effects of stretching before and after exercising on muscle soreness and risk of injury: systematic review. *BMJ.* 325(7362): 468.

Herbert, R.D., de Noronha, M. & Kamper, S.J. (2011) Stretching to prevent or reduce muscle soreness after exercise. *Cochrane Database Syst Rev.* 7: CD004577.

Kay, A.D. & Blazevich, A.J. (2012) Effect of acute static stretch on maximal muscle performance: a systematic review. *Med Sci Sports Exer.* 44: 154–164.

McGowan, C.J., Pyne, D.B., Thompson, K.G. & Rattray, B. (2015) Warm-up strategies for sport and exercise: mechanisms and applications. *Sports Med.* 45: 1523–1546.

McHugh, M.P. & Cosgrave, C.H. (2010) To stretch or not to stretch: the role of stretching in injury prevention and performance. *Scand J Med Sci Sports.* 20: 169–181.

Nédélec, M., McCall, A., Carling, C., Legall, F., Berthoin, S. & Dupont, G. (2013) Recovery in soccer. *Sports Med.* 43: 9–22.

Nordez, A., Gross, R., Andrade, R., Le Sant, G., Freitas, S., Ellis, R., et al. (2017) Non-muscular structures can limit the maximal joint range of motion during stretching. *Sports Med.* 47: 1925–1929.

Opplert, J. & Babault, N. (2018) Acute effects of dynamic stretching on muscle flexibility and performance: an analysis of the current literature. *Sports Med.* 48: 299–325.

Sands, W., Wurth, J. & Hewit, J. (2012) The National Strength and Conditioning Association's (NSCA) Basics of Strength and Conditioning Manual. NCSA. https://www.nsca.com/contentassets/116c55d64e1343d2b264e05aaf158a91/basics_of_strength_and_conditioning_manual.pdf.

Schleip, R. & Bayer, J. (2017) *Fascial fitness. How to be resilient, elegant and dynamic in everyday life and sport.* Chichester, UK: Lotus Publishing.

Schleip, R. & Müller, D.G. (2013) Training principles for fascial connective tissues: scientific foundation and suggested practical applications. *J Bodyw Mov Ther.* 17: 103–115.

Stecco, C. & Hammer, W.I. (2014) *Functional Atlas of the Human Fascial System.* E-Book: Elsevier Health Sciences. https://books.google.de/books?id=8eDTBQAAQBAJ.

Thomas, E., Bianco, A., Paoli, A. & Palma, A. (2018) The relation between stretching typology and stretching duration: the effects on range of motion. *Int J Sports Med.* 39: 243–254.

Weppler, C.H. & Magnusson, S.P. (2010) Increasing muscle extensibility: a matter of increasing length or modifying sensation? *Phys Ther.* 90: 438–449.

Wilke, J., Niederer, D., Vogt, L. & Banzer, W. (2016) Remote effects of lower limb stretching: preliminary evidence for myofascial connectivity? *J Sports Sci.* 34: 2145–2148.

Food for the fascia: Molecular and biochemical processes

Kurt Mosetter

How to puzzle a fascia

Within the living myofascial system, some pieces are always degraded and some others are newly built all the time. Beside the inherent genetic and structural pattern, environmental conditions can have a huge influence. Factors such as food and nutrition, shear forces and mechanical overload have strong effects on quality and fine tuning of tissue puzzling.

The characteristics of the soft tissue are regulated according to the individual requirements. External stimuli help to create the structural details of the required synthesis with tailor-made adjustments. There are a number of further checkpoints, including the availability of all essential building materials, sufficient energy for the work of synthesis, turnover from restructuring and breakdown, as well as the activities of the stress axis with signal effects on post-translational epigenetic fine tuning.

The tissue's capacity for regulation, elasticity, stress and shear-force tolerance, deformation capacity, resilience, inflammatory status, homeostasis, dynamic reciprocity, capacity for recycling and new synthesis, are all critical parameters for human health. They are also major criteria for the strategy and success of each therapist, doctor, trainer, bodyworker and dancer working in this dynamic puzzle, and therefore concern areas of pain, the locomotor system, regeneration and the immune response.

The detailed biochemistry of our internal architecture offers far-reaching insight into a deeper understanding of the function, quality and dysregulation of fascia. This backdrop also points the way towards developing differentiated concepts for the rational and physiological nourishment of connective tissue structures.

The essential ingredients for high-performing fascia can be readily understood based on the principles of anatomy and biochemistry. Basically, any tissue in the body consists of two main components: cells and the extracellular matrix (ECM). While the cells are responsible for the synthesis of the ECM, the latter itself consists of fibers (providing tensile strength), water and ground substance. Primarily, ground substance is built up of water, galactose, mannose, glucosamine, omega-3 and amino acids.

There are several specific amino acids that are required for the synthesis of the large protein family of collagens. Additional requirements include vitamins B, C and D, plus minerals such as magnesium, calcium, manganese, zinc, selenium, copper, sulfur, silicon and phosphorus, as well as secondary plant substances.

The ground substance

The ground substance and its milieu are existential requirements for life with respect to nutrition, control, signaling activity, and the basic nature of cellular processes, both physiological

Chapter 29

and pathological. Thus, extracellular processes affect and control the cells themselves through contact with the cell surface, ligands and biochemical pacemaker processes. The intercellular substance is a critical element for understanding bacterial and viral infections, the pathways of carcinogenesis and metastasis, inflammatory processes, and neurodegenerative changes. Beginning from the earliest developmental stages of the central nervous system, structures of the extracellular matrix are essential for maturation, growth, migration and cell control, differentiation of neurons and glial cells, and organization of the connective tissues and fasciae.

In addition, the activity and complex regulatory functions of nerve cell growth factors, target-region dependent growth factors, and growth factors for collagen would not be possible without the fundamental functions of the substances located in the extracellular matrix.

Special features of the extracellular space

The ground substance is made up of a jelly-like substance that holds cells together and provides pathways for the diffusion and transport of nutrients, signal carriers, oxygen and messenger substances. It consists of an interwoven network of proteins and monosaccharides, which are called proteoglycans and glycosaminoglycans (Lindahl et al., 2017).

Looking at their architecture and microstructure, these components are sponge-like, consisting of many branches, looking like fern or fir branches. They are imbued of water, hydrogen bonds and minerals. They provide resistance against different types of compression, shear forces, shock absorbance, elasticity, as well as tear strength. These qualities

are guaranteed by special networks, in which monosaccharides and proteins are connected and interwoven. Typical examples include proteins such as collagen, elastin, fibronectin, syndecans and the glycocalyx. The glycocalyx is the frosted-like surface of all cells.

All of the synthetic pathways for these sugar-amino-sugar molecules (glycosaminoglycans and proteoglycans) depend upon galactose (Lehninger et al., 2005). As a monosaccharide, galactose is the key substance, the building block, the dynamic adhesive and the key puzzler inside the surface antenna of all compounds within the ground substance, providing the signaling properties at the surface of all cells (see Figure 29.1). The surface of the cell can be seen as an interface and field of micro-antennas that are essential for all processes of cell to cell communication (Bibb and Nestler, 2006).

The process of how monosaccharides are combined to each other is akin to putting the pieces of a puzzle together, and is called glycosylation. The synthetic pathway also represents a critical biochemical genetic regulatory mechanism. This process involves large numbers of essential substrates, hormones, enzymes, messenger substances, receptors and life-sustaining components of the intra- and extra-cellular space. In conjunction with signal communication and cell recognition, monosaccharides like galactose play a vital role in cell adhesion, cell signal cascades, immune regulation, neuroregeneration and neurobiochemical processes.

Beside galactose, sulfate groups and sulfur-containing amino acids such as cysteine and methionine are essential key factors.

The three-dimensional (3D) network in soft tissue is designed to regulate metabolic acidosis and buffer pH levels.

Food for the fascia: Molecular and biochemical processes

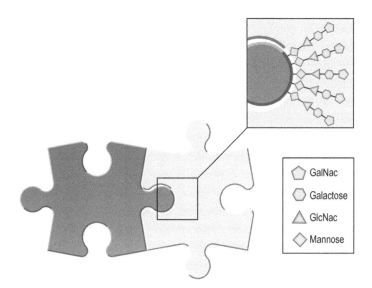

Figure 29.1

In the picture of the puzzle we talk about the arms and hands of the puzzle pieces. The biochemical metabolic pathways for galactose and mannose show how these terminal components of all heteroglycans or puzzle pieces represent the substrate for cellular biosynthesis. They act as metabolic and functional cell-to-cell anchors and communicators in the intercellular space of the ground substance.

GalNac

Galactose

GlcNac

Mannose

Typical examples of glycosaminoglycans include hyaluronan, which serves as a lubricant in joint synovial fluid. In addition, their interactions with the extracellular matrix assure tensile strength and elasticity in cartilage, tendons and connective tissue.

Chondroitin sulfate is responsible for the tensile strength of cartilage, tendons and connective tissue. Dermatan sulfate assures the suppleness of skin, vessels and heart valves. Keratin sulfate is found in cartilage and bone as well as in the cornea and the nails. In the extracellular matrix, the network of proteoglycans and glycosaminoglycans mature to become a functional series of small molecular cytokines, growth factors and chemokines. They reside in the extracellular matrix and contribute to its spatial 3D structure while also serving as a standby reservoir in the proteoglycan receptors of syndecans. These components are highly dynamic, depend on the rule of offer and demand, and can be regulated by functional changes and requests. Therapists in the fields of osteopathy, yoga and myoreflex therapy, as well as teachers of Pilates,

Thai Chi and Qi Gong, claim to observe changes in these fields by activating processes of regulation within the ground substance.

These structures assure super-fast information processing along with fine regulation of the ground substance and endocrine control of cell response.

Glycosylation helps to determine almost all of the fine structures and functions of living tissues. Glycosylated proteins and lipids are essential structural components of cell membranes and help to shape cell interactions. Thus, glycosylation presents enormous biological storage capacity, greatly exceeding that of classical information carriers such as nucleic acids and proteins.

Non-disrupted biological glycosylation ensures physiological folding, functional protein conformation, seamless intracellular transport (protein targeting) and exocytosis, the stability of lipids and proteins, affinity for binding partners (such as the insulin receptor), and protects from proteolytic breakdown.

Chapter 29

"Together, the extracellular matrix and cells form a viscoelastic system, which maintains a self-stabilizing structure when impacted by external forces ('tensegrity'). Therefore, the extracellular matrix represents an attractor for all external and internally acting forces similar to a coupled spring, whereby small causes can have very large effects." (Heine, 2005)

Inside the puzzle of sugar-amino-sugar molecules building the ground substance, the family of fibroblast growth factors (FGF) are the clue in between the pieces of the puzzle (Landreth, 2006). To understand the activity of fibroblasts and to balance their physiological activity, nutritional factors and exercise are key factors.

The ground substance is also populated by cytokine families. "Sleeping" within this ground substance are myoblasts, fibroblasts, glial cells, chondroblasts, osteoblasts and mast cells, all of which are activated, transported and regulated according to need in building a fitting picture. There is a complex balance between situationally directed tissue restructuring, on one side by potent inflammatory substances, and on the other side by growth factors, including transforming growth factor beta (TGF-ß) and nerve growth factor.

The large group of TGF-ß growth factors regulates the synthesis of ground substance proteins, stimulating the breakdown of bone, connective tissue, muscle and the skin. They are essential for the stability of the bone matrix as well as for wound healing.

Immobilization and inflammation caused by junk food may result in impaired growth, bone growth disorders, chronic inflammation and infections, and can even cause the malignant transformation of cells.

In this setting, pro-inflammatory messenger substances such as prostaglandins, histamine, proteases and leukotrienes are key factors for understanding a wide range of disease states. These processes can be balanced by training and exercise.

The ground substance and signal control

Integrins function as multidirectional nodal points and modify their docking behavior inside the soft tissue. Indeed, they look like the telescopes of a submarine. They communicate actively in all directions: similar to a mobile phone, they are able are receive, send and modulate messages, and can be online in the body network all the time.

The interaction of cells and their surface structures with components of the extracellular space has a profound impact on the development and behavior of individual cells.

Signals related to mechanical stress and associated burdens from the outside shape the living world of this ground substance. Depending on the nature of the signals, very different forms and types of connective tissue can be synthesized. Depending on use and activation, these signals will induce production of collagen and elastin or the synthesis of myofibroblasts. Even those structures that appear more solid and self-contained, such as bones and joints, are thus highly dependent upon function at the cellular level. And even in the context of severe developmental restrictions and dysplasia, they remain shapeable and modifiable well into advanced age. Many years of therapeutic experience and clinical progress show that myofascial back pain is often related to changes like edema, swollen and thickened areas, and inflammation in the thoracolumbar fascia. Different functional demands caused by active resistance stretch training (Mosetter and Mosetter, 2016; Mosetter 2017, 2018) induces different signals through transduction of a wide

Food for the fascia: Molecular and biochemical processes

spectrum of glycoproteins. These are able to regulate the synthesis of the type of collagen. Inflammatory parameters decrease and elasticity is regained. In systemic sklerosis, sklerodermia and lupus, stretching leads to anti-inflammatory activities, changing the composition of soft tissue (Berrueta et al., 2016; Xiong et al., 2017). In osteogenesis imperfecta, an active stretch with KiD and intense training on a vibrating platform (Galileo) are translated through glycoprotein signals in soft tissue and bone remodeling. Even the inner structure of the bones is changed in 3D architecture (Sa-Caputo et al., 2017). Density in corticalis is reduced to almost normal conditions and inner stability in inner architecture is switched on. Skin and soft tissue remodeling and recovery are also translated by these cross-talks.

The form, development, growth, polarization, movement and, at times, the nature of individual cells and their functions typically reflect corresponding shifts in the cellular environment.

Interactions and water binding between glycosaminoglycans and proteoglycans also generate fluctuations in charge and electrical and chemical gradients, which open information bridges and transport pathways. This mobility of the ground substance helps to maintain the proper organization of connective tissues, fasciae, the cytoskeleton, and biochemical communication cascades.

The synthesis of connective tissue

Collagen is synthesized in a series of multiple intracellular and extracellular steps (Figure 29.2).

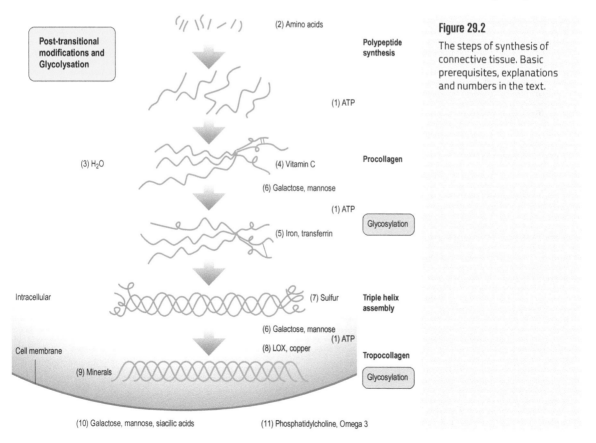

Figure 29.2

The steps of synthesis of connective tissue. Basic prerequisites, explanations and numbers in the text.

Chapter 29

Basic prerequisites

1: ATP

In each step of synthesis, turnover and repair of collagens are dependent on energy in the form of ATP, which is produced in the mitochondria. The more economical the function of mitochondria is, the more ATP is available, and then less metabolic acidosis, oxidative stress and inflammatory signals disturb the process of repair and regeneration.

2: Amino acids and proteins

Amino acids are essential block substances for all collagens and proteoglycans. In particular, lysine, proline, hydroxyproline, glycine, glutamine, GABA, ß-leucine and arginine are very important. Deficiencies in the supply of amino acids impair physiological synthesis.

The individual amino acids are configured like pearls into a chain. Folding, which consumes ATP, results in the formation of 3D figures, spirals and custom-configured complex, helix-shaped structures. Through specific charging of the amino acid bonds and crosslinked attractive and repulsive forces, these pro-collagens are hardened, gaining tensile strength to become stabilized into stiff or elastic fibers.

3: Water and hydrogen bonds

Water molecules are an important component of this network system, with their specific lattice structures, their interconnections through hydrogen bonds, and their bridge formations with ions and minerals. The best nutritional source is still water (CO_2 in the water may disturb the processes because organic acids enforce metabolic acidosis).

4: Vitamin C

To create fibrillar collagen 1, which is responsible for the strength of bones, cartilage, tendons, ligaments, fascia, the dermis, sclerae, cornea and dentine, proline and lysine are hydroxylated with the assistance of vitamin C to hydroxyproline and hydroxylysine. Good sources are fruits low in glucose and fructose and high in fibers, such as berries, lemons, apricots, the old sort of apples, and papaya.

5: Iron and transferrin

Iron ensures the hydroxylation of proline, which is essential for stabilization of the tropocollagen spirals and triple helices. High concentrations of iron are found in organic, unprocessed red meat, fish, wholegrain products, cacao, nuts, almonds, sesame and poppy seeds.

6: Galactose and mannose

The hydroxylation of lysine is a precondition for the important steps that follow: through the adherence of monosaccharides, signal antennae are configured for task specificity, lifespan, contact behavior and 3D structure, etc. This critical process is known as glycosylation. Fine tuning takes place by means of building, dismantling and reconfiguring these small components by means of glycosyl transferases.

In the steps for fine adjustment of collagen to the milieu conditions of the microenvironment, the collage is tuned by the amino acids asparagine, serine, lysine and threonine with monosaccharides such as mannose and galactose.

Through the aggregation of several spirals, in the final intracellular step, complex triple-helix shapes are built with disulfide bridges.

High amounts of galactose and mannose are found in lentils, blackberries and vegetables.

7: Sulfur-containing amino acids

For the next step in the synthesis, through the appendage of sulfur (sulfating), secretion into the extracellular space is initiated. After secretion, the propeptides are split off by small shears (peptidases). In this way, water-insoluble tropocollagens are created. The stringing together of different tropocollagen units ensures the formation of microfibrils, which ultimately are built up into fibrils by way of fibrillar collagen (Lindahl et al., 2017).

Eggs, fish, red organic meat, cashew, almonds, beans, chickpeas, lentils, pecorino and millet are all good sources.

8: Copper

Lysyl oxidase (LOX) is a copper-dependent enzyme that initiates wiring and crosslinking of elastin, fibronectin and collagen in the ground substance. LOX activity can be regulated by secondary plant substance, green tea, vitamin D, beta-carotene, vitamin B6 and *Calendula officinalis* (Kothapalli and Ramamurthi, 2009).

Good sources include artichokes, sprouts, cacao, cashew, lentils, beans and chickpeas.

9: Minerals

Minerals such as magnesium, manganese, copper, iron and zinc always act in their ionic-colloidal form within the gel-like network of charges; in fact, this is generally the only form in which they can be utilized by the body.

Calcium and magnesium are particularly important for bone formation, but phosphate, arsenate, vanadate and silicate are also built into the corresponding collagen structures.

Salads, herbs, celery, vegetables, red and black rice, nuts, peas, lentils, oatmeal, sesame and wholegrains are all good sources.

10: Sulfur, galactose, mannose, charging the GAG

Extracellular proteins typically occur in glycosylated form. Glycans, typically hydrophilic and acidic from the negatively charged sialic acids, contribute substantially to the water solubility of proteins.

Eggs, fish and organic red meat contain sulfur. Still water as well as cranberry, goji berries and lentils support these processes.

11: Omega-3 fatty acids and phosphatidylcholine

Intracellular transport pathways across the dynamic border-layers of the cell membrane (via diffusion, active transport, vesicles, tubules and rafts) and normal contact behavior (adhesion, deformability) to the cytoskeleton require several additional substances, primarily omega-3 fatty acids, vitamin D and phosphatidylcholine/serine.

Good sources are wild deepwater fishes, seaweed, chia seeds, hemp oil, linseed oil and cod liver oil.

The enemies of ground substance

Mechanical overload and pain

Asymmetrical muscular-biomechanical leverage effects in fascia lead to corresponding chronic overloads. Along with the non-physiological forces, this causes metabolic, mechanical and molecular restructuring of the connective tissue with loss of function, resulting in pain (Eekhoff et al., 2018).

The ground substance of the fascia, with its glycosaminoglycans, is filled with free nerve endings, and has specific pain receptors for substance P and, in addition, is extensively innervated by branch connections from the sympathetic nervous system.

The ensuing problems include myofascial trigger points, hardened muscles and increased density of the fascial structures with a loss of elasticity. Fibroblasts, an especially agile cell type, respond to mechanical, molecular and metabolic stress with edema, synthesize smaller amounts of elastic collagen 1 and larger amounts of dysfunctional collagen 3, as well as a series of inflammatory mediators, including TGF-ß 1, IL-1 ß, IL-6 and TNF-α, thereby charting the course to fibrosis. Small blood vessels and nerve plexuses arise within the points of intersection in the fascia under shear stress. Vasoconstriction, ischemia, activation of pain messenger substances, and over-reactivity of the sympathetic system with neural pain sensitization, aggravate the crisis. Conditions of insulin resistance, metabolic acidosis, and low levels of coenzyme Q10, NADH, vitamin B3 and ATP, may all impair the rate of synthesis and the ultimate quality of collagen connective tissue and GAGs.

The flexibility from dynamic tensegrity, with its equilibrated tension-band system, becomes progressively impaired. Inflammation, excessive acidity, loss of water, slagging (reaction remains with deposit of waste, inflamed proteins which destroy the sponge of ECM), mineral and amino acid deficiencies, over time lead to coarse inflammatory thickening of the tissues, and fibrosis,

the deposition of advanced glycation end products (AGE) with pathological saccharification, oxidative stress and pain-generating excesses of ammonia, spread out through the connective tissue matrix.

The overconsumption of sugar

It is now generally agreed that the most destructive enemies of connective tissue are sugar, short-chain carbohydrates and trans fats (DiMauro and De Vino, 2006). Unphysiological excesses of sugar lead to sugar being burned with proteins in the process known as the Maillard reaction, and to increased production of AGE along with free radicals, which cancel out protein synthesis. The levels of glycine, proline, lysine, glutamine, GABA and acetylcholine fall.

As the causative agent for bad "aging" and diseases of civilization, one significant mechanism is a biochemical reaction which was already understood in 1912. When sugar reacts with proteins, so-called "glycation" products are produced. The biochemist Louis Maillard described the precise process by which sugar and milk proteins caramelize and burn in the cooking pot. Too much sugar in the blood sticks together and caramelizes not only hemoglobin in the red blood cells, but also nerves, blood vessels, essential fats, messenger substances, signal proteins, and hormones as well as their docking sites, nucleic acids, the extracellular matrix, and the connective tissues.

The larger the quantity of caramelized glycation products that are produced, the more widespread are advanced, complex burnt AGE. This preventable escalating metabolic process represents a catastrophe for the entire body and all of its cells (Ott et al., 2014).

The damage runs even deeper. The increased AGE lead to a rise in the corresponding binding

Food for the fascia: Molecular and biochemical processes

sites and receptors for AGE, known as RAGE. Through these receptors, sabotage signal cascades are initiated in the interior of cells, including abnormal cell nuclear activation. Oxidative stress, mitochondrial dysfunction, disorders of the autophagosomes and degenerative processes are the biological consequences (Chen et al., 2017; Peng et al., 2018).

AGE significantly induce macrophages to express IL-6 and TNF-α. M1 macrophage markers such as iNOS and surface markers are significantly upregulated (while M2 macrophage markers such as Arg1 and CD206 remain unchanged after AGE stimulation.) AGE significantly increase RAGE expression in macrophages and activate NF-κB pathway. Together with m-Tor signaling, the cytokines TGF-1 ß, IL-1 ß, IL-6 and TNF-α are all chronically upregulated (Derk et al., 2018). Post-translational modification and glycosylation are severely undermined by AGE!

The overconsumption of short-chain carbohydrates and sugar, with associated hyperglycemic states with AGE, insulin resistance conditions with oxidative stress, ATP deficiency, shortage of energy, metabolic acidosis, toxic breakdown products, excessive ammonia, chronic inflammatory changes, as well as crisis-dependent insulin and AGE/RAGE signal cascades, all lead to degeneration of connective tissue along with the related cell groups (Bierhaus, 2004; Chang et al., 2014; Serban et al., 2015)

At the same time, disruptions of energy metabolism, stress metabolism and states of emergency lead to the interruption of all regenerative metabolic pathways. The pathways for repair and synthesis of fascia, connective tissue, skin and neuronal repair are all inhibited. The consequences are injuries to the fascia, ligaments, muscle and joints. Painful muscles, fascia, and joints, inflammatory swelling of the connective

tissue, fibrotic degeneration, striae, stress fractures, rheumatic conditions, osteoporosis, and periosteal pain may all be sequelae of malnutrition and a deficient diet. Chronic activation of the sympathetic nervous system in the terminal portion of the extracellular matrix and the myofascial connective tissues intensify the spiral of pain and inflammation. Increasing levels of TNF-α, TGF-1 ß, IL-1 ß and IL-6 all culminate in degenerative changes.

Insulin resistance and hyperglycemia also inhibit physiological glycosylation, and, additionally, expose the soft tissues to stress-associated modifications (O-glycosidic acetylation, O-GlcNac). These processes set the stage for degeneration and block natural autophagosomes (Zhu et al., 2018).

What to do? An overview

The elimination of toxic overloads and nutritional medical care by means of natural eating, in particular, a glycoplan (Mosetter, 2018) and ketogenic diet (Wilson et al., 2017), can set in motion turning points for regeneration. Enhancing energy metabolism, especially in those hubs of ATP metabolism, the mitochondria, boosts the processes of collagen synthesis, rapidly synchronized protein folding, functional diversity, and—of critical importance in this context—their regular breakdown, economical digestion and tailor-made recycling.

Helpful essential replacement therapy with NADH, coenzyme Q10, ribose and creatine prepare the organism for a new start. They promote elimination and digestion of waste, while at the same time they can also facilitate the start of reparative processes and new synthesis. Glucosamine and galactose are first aid instruments in the repair toolkit and provide critical assistance.

Chapter 29

Endogenous detoxification

Irreversible ammonia production that occurs in stress metabolism, and causes damage to ion channels, receptors and nerve cells, can be redirected along an alternative metabolic pathway (Butterworth, 2006).

Amino acids are formed with galactose from toxic metabolites and ammonia as well as ammonia equivalents. In this process, detoxification takes place in the form of endogenous detoxification with a recycling feature. Moreover, mediators that are required for normal brain function can be synthesized from the amino acids (Mosetter, 2018). The body's endogenous detoxification steps can benefit from the broad activities of galactose through so-called pump glycoproteins with respect to structure, recognition and ATP-dependent performance.

Anabolic metabolism

The situation of catabolic degradative metabolism of protein with amino acid loss can be categorically diverted into constructive anabolic pathways.

In the metabolism of ammonia and ammonia equivalents, amino acids are produced from a portion of the galactose. This process takes up toxic ammonia produced by the stressed organism (in stress metabolism). Thus, detoxification is achieved in this simple protective pathway. The amino acids formed in this way can serve in the formation of valuable proteins. By metabolizing ammonia, galactose ensures the synthesis of alpha-ketoglutarate, glutamic acids, glutamate and aspartate (Yudkoff, 2006). In situations of insulin resistance, galactose can induce the activity of osteoblasts.

Supplementing the anti-oxidative protection program with zinc, selenium, magnesium, alpha

lipoic acid, ribose and glutathione further aids these measures.

Phosphatidylcholine and omega-3 fatty acids are utilized in the regenerative processes in the cell membrane.

The individualized rebalancing of deficient amino acid levels using a broad spectrum of essential amino acids (glycine, proline, leucine, lysine, glutamine, GABA) provides the raw materials for potential new synthesis.

The sulfur-containing amino acids methionine and cysteine have anti-oxidative properties while the sulfate groups are also co-factors in collagen synthesis.

Vitamin C, vitamin D, basic minerals, and metals, particularly iron, copper, zinc, magnesium and selenium, manganese, calcium, silicon and phosphorus, ensure good nutrition and energy supply of the fascia and also ensure that they do not become matted.

Provision of the monosaccharides, galactose, mannose and sialic acid, along with glucosamine, facilitates essential metabolic pathways of glycosylation (see above).

Omega-3 fatty acids and the spectrum of omega-3 fatty acids also bring into play so-called "resolving factors" (Zhang et al., 2017).

The 2016 Nobel Prize in Medicine has underscored the essential role of the mitochondria for successful autophagy, and proves that the activation of mitochondria, intermittent fasting, ketogenic diet, natural eating with the glycoplan and moderate training can fundamentally promote these processes.

The large family of myokines is capable of regulating fibroblasts as well as the structure of connective tissue. Stroma, cartilage and bone metabolism may thereby be reset towards a reparative function. Fibroblast growth factor-21 (FGF-21), BDNF, IL-15, IL-6 and IL-1β are associated with increased soft tissue repair (Kaji, 2018; Guo et al., 2017).

Important actuators of successful repair are activated through the bowel and the microbiome.

Using prebiotics and probiotics, through the successful metabolism of dietary fiber and superfoods, well-synchronized gut bacteria can synthesize short chain fatty acids, which are key substances for intestinal health, the immune system, and also for the metabolism of the fascia. In particular, the healthy bacteria Faecalbacterium prausnitzii and Akkermansia muciniphila support all manner of tissue repair, especially in the ECM. These factors include butyrate, folic acid, biotin, vitamin B3, propionate and acetate.

The 2016, 2017 and 2018 Nobel Prizes for Medicine highlight the potential for self-healing powers through intrinsic bodily repair mechanisms, that is, the essential role of the mitochondria for successful autophagy, the activation of internal rhythmicity (mindfulness), as well as the reparative capacities of immune and regeneration metabolism. Intermittent fasting, a ketogenic diet, natural eating with the glycoplan, supplementation, KiD (strength through stretch training) and moderate training can fundamentally promote all reparative processes.

Major protective anti-inflammatory factors can also be activated through resistance and muscle-fascia length training (Bouffard et al., 2008; Berrueta et al., 2018; Guzzoni et al., 2018) and active resistance stretch training (Mosetter and Mosetter, 2016; Mosetter 2017, 2018).

The most recent insights of pioneers in the field of fascia research help to confirm experience, concepts and hypotheses regarding Yoga, Tai Chi, Qi Gong, Pilates and active resistance stretch training. Form follows function. The better you move, the less you will suffer from inflammation.

References

Berrueta, L., Bergholz, J., Munoz, D., Muskaj, I., Badger, G.J., Shukla, A., Kim, H.J., Zhao, J.J. & Langevin, H.M. (2018) Stretching reduces tumor growth in a mouse breast cancer model. *Sci Rep.* 8: 7864.

Berrueta, L., Muskaj, I., Olenich, S., Butler, T., Badger, G.J., Colas, R.A., Spite, M., Serhan, C.N. & Langevin, H.M. (2016) Stretching impacts inflammation resolution in connective tissue. *J Cell Physiol.* 231: 1621–1627.

Bibb, J.A. & Nestler, E.J. (2006) Serine and Threonine Phosphorylation/Intercellular signalling. In: Siegel, U.A. (Hrsg.), *Basic Neurochemistry*. Amsterdam, the Netherlands: Elsevier, 391–413.

Bierhaus, A. (2014) RAGE - Das Geheimnis des Alterns. UGB-Forum 6/04, 296–299.

Bouffard, N.A., Cutroneo, K.R., Badger, G.J., White, S.L., Buttolph, T.R., Ehrlich, H.P., Stevens-Tuttle, D. & Langevin, H.M. (2008) Tissue stretch decreases soluble TGF-beta1 and type-1 procollagen in mouse subcutaneous connective tissue: evidence from ex vivo and in vivo models. *J Cell Physiol.* 214: 389–395.

Butterworth, R.F. (2006) Metabolic Encephalopathies. In: Siegel, G.J., Albers, R.W., Scott, T.B. & Price, D.L. (Eds), *Basic Neurochemistry. Molecular, cellular and medical aspects* (seventh edition). Amsterdam, the Netherlands: Elsevier, 593–602.

Chang, P.C., Tsai, S.C., Jheng, Y.H., Lin, Y.F. & Chen, C.C. (2014) Soft-tissue wound healing by anti-advanced glycation end-products agents. *J Dent Res.* 93: 388–393.

Chen, Y.S., Wang, X.J., Feng, W. & Hua, K.Q. (2017) Advanced glycation end products decrease collagen I levels in fibroblasts from the vaginal wall of patients with POP via the RAGE, MAPK and NF-kappaB pathways. *Int J Mol Med.* 40: 987–998.

Cretoiu, D., Xu, J., Xiao, J. & Cretoiu, S.M. (2016) Telocytes and their extracellular vesicles - evidence and hypotheses. *Int J Mol Sci.* 17: 8.

Derk, J., et al. (2018) The receptor for advanced glycation endproducts

(RAGE) and mediation of inflammatory neurodegeneration. *J Alzheimers Dis Parkinsonism.* 8(1): 421.

DiMauro, S. & De Vino, D.C. (2006) Diseases of Carbohydrate, Fatty Acid and Mitochondrial Metabolism. In: Siegel, U.A. (Ed.), *Basic Neurochemistry.* Amsterdam, the Netherlands: Elsevier, 695–712.

Eekhoff, J.D., Fang, F. & Lake, S.P. (2018) Multiscale mechanical effects of native collagen cross-linking in tendon. *Connect Tissue Res.* 59: 410–422.

Guo, B., Zhang, Z.K., Liang, C., Li, J., Liu, J., Lu, A., Zhang, B.T. & Zhang, G. (2017) Molecular communication from skeletal muscle to bone: a review for muscle-derived myokines regulating bone metabolism. *Calcif Tissue Int.* 100: 184–192.

Guzzoni, V., Ribeiro, M.B.T., Lopes, G.N., de Cassia Marqueti, R., de Andrade, R.V., Selistre-de-Araujo, H.S. & Durigan, J.L.Q. (2018) Effect of resistance training on extracellular matrix adaptations in skeletal muscle of older rats. *Front Physiol.* 9: 374.

Heine, H. (2005) Die extrazelluläre Matrix als Attraktor für Verschlackungsphänomene. [The extracellular matrix as an attractor for slagging phenomena.] *Ärztezeitschrift für Naturheilverfahren.* 46: 236–266.

Ibba-Manneschi, L, Rosa, I. & Manetti, M. (2016) Telocytes in chronic inflammatory and fibrotic diseases. *Adv Exp Med Biol.* 913: 51–76.

Kaji, H. (2018) Body weight and bone/calcium metabolism. Muscle, myokines and bone/calcium metabolism. *Clin Calcium.* 28: 919–926.

Kothapalli, C.R. & Ramamurthi, A. (2009) Lysyl oxidase enhances elastin synthesis and matrix formation by vascular smooth muscle cells. *J Tissue Eng Regen Med.* 3: 655–661.

Landreth, G.E. (2006) Growth Factors. In: Siegel, U.A. (Ed.), *Basic Neurochemistry.* Amsterdam, the Netherlands: Elsevier, 471–484.

Lehninger, A.L., Nelson, D.L. & Cox, M. (2005) *Biochemie.* (3. Auflage). Berlin, Heidelberg, New York: Springer.

Lindahl, U., et al. (2017) *Proteoglycans and Sulfated Glycosaminoglycans.* https://www.ncbi.nlm.nih.gov/books/NBK453033/.

Mosetter, K. (2017) Fascias are creating a furore. *Sport Medicine* newspaper, 8–9.

Mosetter, K. (2018) *Myoreflex Therapy – experienced biography.* Konstanz: Vesalius.

Mosetter, K. & Mosetter, R. (2016) Schneller schmerzfrei mit der KiD-Methode. Beweglich in Muskeln und Faszien. [2008, überarbeitete Neuausgabe.] Ostfildern: Patmos.

Ott, C., et al. (2014) Role of advanced glycation end products in cellular signaling. *Redox Biol.* 2: 411–429.

Peng, Y., Kim, J.M., Park, H.S., Yang, A., Islam, C., Lakatta, E.G. & Lin, L. (2016) AGE-RAGE signal generates a specific NF-kappaB RelA "barcode" that directs collagen I expression. *Sci Rep.* 6: 18822.

Sa-Caputo, D.C., Dionello, C.D.F., Frederico, E., Paineiras-Domingos, L.L., Sousa-Goncalves, C.R., Morel, D.S., Moreira-Marconi, E., Unger, M. & Bernardo-Filho, M. (2017) Whole-body vibration exercise improves functional parameters in patients with osteogenesis imperfecta: a systematic review with a suitable approach. *Afr J Tradit Complement Altern Med.* 14: 199–208.

Serban, A.I., Stanca, L., Geicu, O.I., Munteanu, M.C., Costache, M. & Dinischiotu, A. (2015) Extracellular matrix is modulated in advanced glycation end products milieu via a RAGE receptor dependent pathway boosted by transforming growth factor-beta1 RAGE. *J Diabetes.* 7: 114–124.

Wilson, J.M., Lowery, R.P., Roberts, M.D., Sharp, M.H., Joy, J.M., Shields, K.A., Partl, J., Volek, J.S. & D'Agostino, D. (2017) The effects of ketogenic dieting on body composition, strength, power, and hormonal profiles in resistance training males. *J Strength Cond Res.*

Xiong, Y., Berrueta, L., Urso, K., Olenich, S., Muskaj, I., Badger, G.J., Aliprantis, A., Lafyatis, R. & Langevin, H.M. (2017) Stretching reduces skin thickness and improves subcutaneous tissue mobility in a murine model of systemic sclerosis. *Front Immunol.* 8: 124.

Yudkoff, M. (2006) Disorders of Amino Acid Metabolism. In: Siegel, G.J., Albers, R.W., Scott, T.B. & Price, D.L. (Eds), *Basic Neurochemistry. Molecular, cellular and medical aspects* (seventh edition). Amsterdam, the Netherlands: Elsevier, 667–683.

Zhang, Q., Zhu, B. & Li, Y. (2017) Resolution of cancer-promoting inflammation: a new approach for anticancer therapy. *Front Immunol.* 8: 71.

Zhu, Y., Shan, X., Safarpour, F., Erro Go, N., Li, N., Shan, A., Huang, M.C., Deen, M., Holicek, V., Ashmus, R., Madden, Z., Gorski, S., Silverman, M.A. & Vocadlo, D.J. (2018) Pharmacological inhibition of O-GlcNAcase enhances autophagy in brain through an mTOR-independent pathway. *ACS Chem Neurosci.* 9: 1366–1379.

Walking: The benefit of being on two legs

James Earls

Introduction

Many palaeontologists have a rare point of agreement on the importance of upright gait as a major, if not the main, impetus for evolution of the *Homo sapiens* lineage (Lieberman, 2012). Obligate bipedalism was one of the most significant evolutionary developments as locomotor economy allowed the diversion of metabolic resources to "expensive tissues", such as the brain. However, despite new fossil finds, increasing clarity of comparative anatomy and better research all round, the origins of bipedalism are still not yet fully understood (Osborn, 1928; Lieberman, 2012; Pontzer, 2017). The fossil record indicates bipedal adaptations probably began 6–7 million years ago (MYA), but it was not until around 2 MYA that locomotor efficiency was fully developed through a suite of anatomical refinements (Pontzer, 2017).

This chapter will blend comparative and functional anatomy with paleontological research to provide a unifying understanding of why and how our ancestors made the change from some form of quadrupedalism to our unique upright bipedal locomotion. Such an approach should provide a better appreciation of whole-body mechanics and the intricate interaction between form and function for various tissue types. Finally, it aims to illustrate some new ideas on clinical reasoning for movement dysfunctions and various pathologies.

Efficiency

There is general consensus that upright walking is metabolically cheaper than staying down on all four limbs (Figure 30.1). In a world were calories were the only currency, being able to move between food sources, shelter, mating potentials and safety with as little metabolic cost as possible confers significant evolutionary advantage. Sockol et al. (2007) (Figure 30.1) compared the cost of locomotion of a number of individual chimps and humans. In each case, the humans were significantly more efficient in their gait regardless of whether the chimps walk on two or four limbs. Human bipedalism was found to be up to 75% less costly in comparison.

While human fascial tissues are undoubtedly involved and part of the reason for economical propulsion, we must first explore some of the other contributing factors that facilitate their exploitation.

Skeletal changes

Aligning the center of gravity directly above our feet is not as simple as just standing up. Our vertical stability is facilitated by the lumbar lordosis and posteriorly extended ischial tuberosities that provide leverage for the hamstrings even when the hip is extended. As seen in Figure 30.1, chimps do not fully straighten their lower limbs when adopting a bipedal posture and have to

Chapter 30

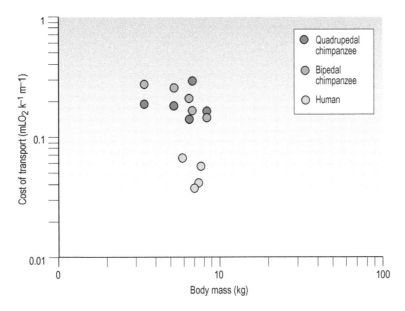

Figure 30.1

Net cost of transport (ml of O$_2$ kg^{-1} m^{-1}) for chimpanzee quadrupedal walking (purple), chimpanzee bipedal walking (orange) and human walking (yellow).

Adapted from Sockol et al. (2007).

maintain bent knees and hips. The chimps' lower limb flexions are not due to limited range in their hips or knees, they are necessary because of limited lumbar extension and reduced support from the hamstrings when upright due to an inferiorly extended ischial tuberosity.

Limited space prevents a fuller exploration of each plane and nuance of gait but we should at least acknowledge the abductors' contribution to frontal plane stability. In contrast to our primate cousins, our ilia face laterally allowing the gluteals to provide frontal plane stability during single leg support. Being able to support our center of mass during single-leg stance without pitching our trunk from side-to-side allows us to move forward more smoothly. Frontal plane support provided by the gluteals resulted from the most notable shape change in the pelvis as it evolved to turn the gluteals from backward-facing extensors to lateral stabilizers by changing the orientation of the iliac blades.

Lateral stability and our upright stance facilitate a longer stride but only when coupled with

parasagittal range from the ankle and toes. Taking fewer strides to cover a distance is beneficial and many adaptations occurred in the foot. The foot morphed from a climbing tool and became an adaptable rigid lever to aid efficient walking. To assist a long stride the great toe changed from its adducted grasping position and toe extension increased at each metatarsal phalangeal joint (MTP). Both modifications, alignment of the hallux and increased MTP extension, were coupled with the development of an arched foot. The intricate multi-joint arrangement of the foot created a locomotor base that can be stable at heel-strike, unlock and adapt to the surface while absorbing ground reaction forces during stance phase.

During the gait cycle, the human foot experiences two peaks of ground reaction forces, one following heel-strike and the other towards toe-off. It appears advantageous to have a skeletally stable foot at these points and a mobile foot in between which allows some force to be absorbed by the plantar tissues and facilitates the foot's adaptation to the substrate. The half-domed arch of the human foot allows the foot to alter its state from being more stable (supinated) to relatively mobile (pronated) and return to a stable, supinated condition in readiness for the release of energy toward toe-off (McKeon et al., 2014) (Figure 30.2A).

Re-supination of the foot prior to toe-off is enhanced by MTP extension (Fernández et al., 2018). As the toes extend, the plantar tissues (plantar fascia, long and short toe flexors) are tensioned to draw the foot's many bones together. Tensioning of the plantar tissues forms part of the "windlass mechanism" that stiffens the foot in preparation for propulsion at toe-off (Holowka and Lieberman, 2018). The supinated foot provides the stable platform for the release of energy and has formed as a result of the parasagittal progression over the foot; deviating to either side will negatively affect supination.

Parasagittal movement over the foot is facilitated by the adducted great toe and toe extension changes discussed above. We fail to see these two peaks of reaction forces in the gait pattern of other primates (Figure 30.3). Our ape cousins lack the functional combination of an adaptable rigid lever, adducted great toe and enhanced toe extension lack and hence detour into other planes during stance phase.

The net result of the skeletal changes was that *Homo* could expend less energy working against gravity and, as we explore below, could capture and recycle kinetic energy from momentum. Coupled hip and low back extension and an adaptable foot allowed the development of a longer, straight-legged stride. Using four rockers with the foot and ankle complex—heel, ankle, forefoot and toe—allows a straight-leg heel-strike and for the trunk to then vault over a dynamically reactive foot. The new skeletal alignment and joint ranges reduced the need for muscle work to

resist gravity and deal with impact forces but also brought new possibilities in how humans (*Homo sapiens*) could use their soft tissues.

Soft tissue mechanics

The locomotor system incorporates elastic soft tissue elements that exchange energy within the environment. Recruitment of elastic elements provides an efficiency which is enhanced by the increased joint ranges outlined above. The greater joint range allows more strain of the elastic tissues, which again profits locomotor efficiency through a number of mechanisms outlined below.

Muscle and the deep fascia that holds it in place form a symbiotic relationship that can optimize efficiency during movement. Various researchers have shown the interplay between in-series and in-parallel collagenous tissues and the contractile tissues when experiencing repeated rhythmical movement and how the system optimizes to reduce eccentric and concentric and concentric muscle contractions (Fukunaga et al., 2002; Sawicki et al., 2009). For example, the in-series tendons of the plantar flexor group uses the body's momentum as it "vaults" over the foot to correct and bring the foot out of pronation (the windlass effect) while the tendons simultaneously lengthen and the muscles isometrically contract. While it is necessary to understand the properties and resultant interactions between tissues of varying stiffness (Fukunaga et al., 2002), doing so is extremely difficult because of the problems in separating the energy contribution of one from the other (Roberts, 2016).

As seen above, toe extension facilitates the windlass mechanism of the foot by tensioning of the plantar tissues and toe flexors. The plantar flexors and toe flexors are tensioned neurologically and by stretch during the latter moments

Chapter 30

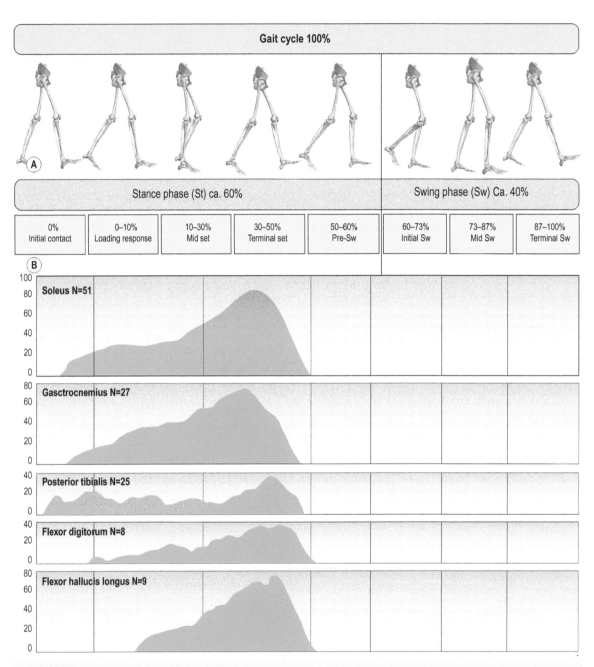

Figure 30.2

(A) Gait cycle phases and percentage portion of each. Heel strike is represented as "initial contact" and occurs at 0% and 100%, toe-off occurs at 60%. **(B)** Quantified electromyography readings are shown as a percentage of maximum manual muscle test value (dark shading) and are aligned to the relevant phase of gait.

of stance phase as the ankle dorsiflexes and the toes extend (see Figures 30.2A and B, mid- to late-stance). The body's forward momentum has to be decelerated by the plantar soft tissues, which tend to be pennate muscles. By arranging shorter muscles fibers at angles, pennated (feathered) muscle architecture provides maximum force production for the least amount of volume.

Pennation is an important feature of distal limbs muscles as it reduces their volume without sacrificing potential force output. Feet and legs move furthest during locomotion and reducing inertia pennation provides another energy-saving design (McNeill Alexander, 2002; Biewener, 2016; Roberts, 2016). Interestingly, pennation may have been selected for in our ancestry purely as a weight-saving device (Biewener, 2016), but other primates do not appear to have unlocked the full elastic potential of this arrangement.

Utilization of elastic energy benefits from a number of anatomical features and is enhanced by the correct myofascial architecture: pennated muscles with long in-series tendons. There must also be enough momentum involved to strain the tendons an appropriate degree, but not so much momentum that the muscles cannot control it. Achieving tendon stretch also requires associated joints to have a range of movement that allows lengthening of the tissues, hence why the development of a long stride and its associated joint extensions are so important.

Muscles act eccentrically to control movement, commonly in the opposite direction of their listed "actions". We saw this above as part of the windlass mechanism: the plantar and toe flexors are tensioned by dorsiflexion and toe extension. This apparent reversal of function can initially make EMG readings confusing but in Figures 30.2A and B we can see that the plantar

flexors are stimulated to control the lower leg as it progresses over the foot into dorsiflexion from mid- to late stance prior to toe-off.

Muscle force combined with momentum will lengthen, or strain, tendons, and it is the strain that provides the mechanism to capture, store and then release kinetic energy. Tendons can strain to 5%; failure is said to occur at 7–12% of strain (although it often experiences more), and it can recover 97% of the energy used to stretch it (McNeill Alexander, 2002). One can sometimes experience this build-up of energy when it is inadvertently released walking over a patch of ice or sand on a pavement. Loss of friction for the foot as it extends gives a premature release of captured energy and the foot flicks rapidly backwards before reaching full toe-off position.

It is this author's belief that captured energy is held within the system during gait because of friction between foot and ground, and as the body progresses over the foot into the series of extensions a catapult-like mechanism is created. Catapult and trigger mechanisms are well-known within the animal kingdom, especially for ballistic feeders and high jumpers like the flea, but each of these usually have an obvious locking mechanism that allows the build-up of muscle tension to lengthen the elastic springs (Vogel and and DeFerrari, 2013). Ballistic feeders and athletic jumpers of the animal kingdom release the locks to unleash the energy and, I believe, we roll over our toes to achieve the same end.

As the collagenous elastic tissues capture energy the muscles associated with any tendon can be contracting eccentrically, concentrically or isometrically, depending on the associated forces and the stiffness inherent within the tendon. For example, if the tendon is more compliant and momentum is high the muscle may

Chapter 30

need to shorten to control the movement and, conversely, if the tendon is stiff the muscle will need to lengthen to allow an appropriate range of movement to occur. Efficient loading of calf musculature requires enough range of the ankle and toe joints but being able to take a long enough stride to facilitate the stretch also recruits the ranges of the same-side knee, hip and lumbar spine (Whittington et al., 2008).

Loss of extension in any one of these joints (toes, ankle, knee, hip or lumbar spine) will influence the extension and/or the alignment of the others. A simple experiment of walking with a restriction in one of them will reaffirm the important interrelationships through the body: we must be able to couple each of those joint extensions simultaneously to maximize the efficiencies within the myofascial system. In performing the experiment one often feels the extra workload placed on the musculature around the hip and low back. The loss of range into extension creates a need for more active concentric positive work.

The hip flexors tension during hip extension as the limb progresses into late stance toward toe-off, thereby providing deceleration and control of the movement while also loading elastic strain into the anterior hip region (Figure 30.3). Although the hip does not have the same collection of long tendons available to the foot and ankle, it has been calculated that up to 40% of the net negative work during extension is performed by passive elastic tissues (single and two-joint

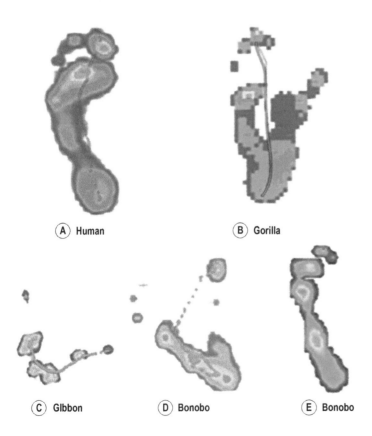

(A) Human   (B) Gorilla

(C) Gibbon   (D) Bonobo   (E) Bonobo

Figure 30.3 Pressure pad readings from a number of primate species.

(A) Human shows a heel strike followed by lateral to medial translation of body weight with an overall parasagittal progression. Two peaks of pressure are seen, one at heel strike and another at toe-off.
(B) Gorilla pressure readings show a wide distribution with only small peaks in the mid/fore-foot region.
(C) The gibbon shows a change of almost 90 degrees during weight transfer.
(D & E) The bonobo demonstrates two general strategies, one with a strong lateral to medial transfer, and the other **(E)** a roll over the lateral aspect of the foot. Peak pressures are seen through the mid-foot in both cases.

Adapted from Crompton, Vereecke and Thorpe, 2008

muscles, joint capsule, ligament and skin; Silder et al., 2007), and that they provide ~50% of the net positive work during the hip flexor power burst during toe-off (Whittington et al., 2008).

Achieving the idealized toe-off position (seen at 60% of gait cycle in Figure 30.3) requires the interplay between a number of joint ranges and tissue tensioning. Immediately prior to toe-off, the toes, knee, hip and lumbar spine are all extended. The increased range at each joint has loaded an amount of energy into the fascial tissues and they are all ready to release that load at toe-off. The amount of passive energy being produced is difficult to calculate and figures vary within the literature. There are many estimates for the contribution of the Achilles tendon, but individual contribution is almost meaningless in a system of this complexity as many fascial tissues contribute to efficiency of human gait.

Muscle force and timing

Just as joint ranges are interdependent during gait, so too is the interaction between muscle and fascial tissue length. Muscle-tendon mechanics were investigated by Rubenson et al. (2012) and fascicle length was found to be optimized for force production during walking and running to within a narrow range on the ascending limb of its force-length curve. Rubenson et al. concluded that the regulation of muscle strain is probably regulated by tendon stretch.

Similar conclusions are drawn from the work of Sawicki et al. (2009), who showed that elastic tissue strain appears attuned to fascicle length in a complex system that optimizes force production. This relationship is significant because force output is reduced when muscle fibers contract from shortened and lengthened positions, and there is a mid-range in which myosin and actin fibrils are optimally aligned to produce force. Maintaining the Goldilocks length of both

elastic and contractile tissues will minimize metabolic cost while optimizing force output.

Muscle force output is also affected by speed of contraction with slower speeds generally producing higher forces. It is known that elastic loading allows a slower contraction of the muscle when the load is released (Vogel, 2013). The initial momentum of the movement is produced by elastic energy released from the fascial tissues and the muscle can then contract at a speed which maximizes its force-velocity relationship, that is, a muscle contracting at speed is less able to produce force for the movement. Elastic recoil not only contributes directly to movement but also increases the efficiency within the associated muscles.

The long stride of *Homo sapiens* therefore further adds another two muscle dynamics: force-length and force-velocity ratios are both enhanced by elastic tissue stretch. If we now contrast the long stride to our primate cousins' bent knee and bent hip gait patterns, the gulf in metabolic costs of locomotion becomes clearer. Our efficiency results from a mosaic of factors that include better alignment with gravity and a long stride, an adaptable foot that allows heel-strike and toe-off, hips and lumbar spines that facilitate extension; and each range of motion assists the simultaneous loading and release of kinetic energy in a range of elastic tissues which, in turn, also optimizes muscle force output.

Cyclical movement, such as walking, provides the human movement system with a range of energy efficiencies. Many muscles, especially those which are pennated, benefit from a stretch-shorten contraction cycle (Biewener, 2016). The lengthening of the tissue activates the muscle tendon unit, which increases force development and provides for elastic capture and storage to increase the potential for work output with reduced metabolic energy consumption.

Chapter 30

Therefore, we have to assume that removing the stretch-shortening cycle reduces those benefits and their loss must be compensated for through concentric muscle work. Future research may give further insight to myofascial pain and dysfunction generated through compensatory overuse.

Efficiency versus endurance

Due to the attention given to long-distance running in recent years, it is worth noting the difference between efficiency and endurance and their role in gait. In terms of a locomotor strategy, walking is more efficient for moving our mass over long distances and incurs a much lower metabolic cost than running. Endurance running is metabolically costly but may have been beneficial in creating new, more successful hunting strategies, which helped create calorie surplus.

The ability to endurance run, while unmistakeably instilling an evolutionary advantage, required physiological changes such as hair loss and sweating for heat management. Although endurance running may use a number of energy-efficient mechanisms, human running, by weight comparison, is actually less efficient than for other species.

Much of the extra cost associated with running compared with walking is due to the bent knee and hip necessary to reduce shock load. Ground impact with joint flexion reduces the mechanical advantage at these joints and increases muscle load. While elastic efficiencies can still be achieved with the correct running mechanics and tempo, the change from the elastically assisted straight leg vault of walking to elastically assisted flexed hip and knee running is a leap in metabolic cost.

The inefficiency of running does not undermine any of the endurance running claims but emphasizes the need to understand the intricate interplay between joint and ground reaction force alignment in context with momentum and tissue dynamics. The important evolutionary element is that the net increase in calorie supply created by endurance running allowed the expensive brain tissue to develop. Importantly, we see many anatomical changes that enhance locomotor efficiency and endurance around 2 MYA, coinciding with expansion of cranial capacity and the transition to a more modern human body plan (Pontzer, 2017).

Elastic walking – a user's guide

The late Leon Chaitow summarized the causes of soft tissue dysfunction as being due to "overuse, misuse, disuse and abuse" (Chaitow and DeLany, 2008), and it is this author's belief that we have created numerous effective modalities for the assessment and treatment of the dysfunctions but we have yet to fully understand the complexities involved in the correct use of soft tissues. For example, as alluded to above, we need to explore the implications of restricted or deviated toe extension on hip flexors and many other similar interdependent relationships that play out in the moving body, whereby the loss of one range affects the potential efficiency of another area. In the first edition of this text, Adjo Zorn outlined his thoughts on the benefits of "elastic walking". By following some of that advice, it is hoped we can find the correct use of our soft tissues to minimize the chances of "overuse, misuse, disuse or abuse".

Through a series of tips, Zorn outlined several ways in which we can help maximize elastic contribution to gait; some of these follow below:

1. Walk with straight legs: heel-striking with a straight leg is our natural strategy but requires the ability to heel-strike on the

Walking: The benefit of being on two legs

forward leg and extend through the posterior limb. Our calcanei have adapted to absorb the shock at impact with an appropriate arrangement of the trabeculi and the natural curve of the heel facilitates the forward roll to enhance forward momentum. We then vault over the other rockers of the foot using a combination of elastic and muscle force.

2. Take long steps: the ability to heel-strike on a straight leg allows long steps, and long steps are required to transfer kinetic energy into the elastic tissues. The stretch tensions the tendon and assists the force output of the muscles. However, there are many factors that could shorten the stride. If one cannot heel-strike on the forward leg, ankle dorsiflex or extend the toes, knee, hip or lumbars on the side of the trailing limb, the stride will shorten and lose some stretch-shorten cycle benefits. Further, if we lose parasagittal range, we may compensate by using another less ideal movement strategy. This often recruits and exaggerates movement in another plane, which may influence the vector of stretch into the anterior hip, pelvis and lumbars.

However, stride length must be matched with the extension abilities of each joint. Simply striding out as far as one can will likely lead to compensations. For example, lack of toe extension prevents loading of the front of the hip but if one tries to overstride, the foot is likely to rotate and the effect will be to take the momentum to the inside of the hip rather than the front. In this case, if toe extension is irretrievable, some form of assisted toe rocker might be prescribed, either in the form of enhanced toe spring or custom orthoses, and these will allow load of the hip flexors.

I will fall short of biomechanical determinism in stating the potential for pain and dysfunction if stride length is challenged, however, clinically, it may be useful to consider the functional range throughout both limbs when confronted with seemingly localized issues. It is more scientifically defendable to predict that tissue efficiency will be reduced. The degree to which efficiency is affected is probably variable and may correlate to age, tissue health, and degree or style of movement compensation.

3. Pressure with the ball of the foot: Adjo Zorn and I differ in this advice. Zorn recommends pushing into the ground in preparation for toe-off. I totally agree if you need to speed up or walk uphill.

I have deliberately referred to toe-off in this chapter in preference to the more common "push-off". As outlined above, should we get the mechanics correct during a normal-paced flat walk, we can swing our legs from a predominately elastic strategy. The active cue to push will incur metabolic cost through the concentric contraction it creates and, I believe, is a misunderstanding caused by the pressure readings, as seen in Figure 30.3. The increased pressure reading under the ball of the foot is naturally interpreted as part of push-off but it can also be the natural result of plantar flexor tensioning as the foot and ankle complex extends.

To get a sense of this, try putting the palm of both hands together in front of your trunk as if praying. Now, bring one elbow higher to create wrist extension on that side and feel the response on the opposing fingers. The simple act of lengthening the wrist and finger flexors created a flexion force on the side of the rising elbow. If your passive hand represents the ground and the extending wrist your foot, I hope you get a sense of the push that is created by the plantar flexor tendons around the pulley of the talus.

The cue to actively push could be a useful intervention for those with hypermobile first rays or lacking in supination, but could also interfere with the timing of the anterior hip. An active push-off could inhibit full extension of the metatarsophalangeal joint and thereby prevent full hip extension. The active push-off may therefore undermine but compensate for the lack of loading of the anterior hip.

4. Carry your pelvis: Zorn advocates the support of the pelvis from above using the tensioning of the abdominal tissues. It is an unfortunate side effect of anatomy that we have to speak of individual joints and tissues and rarely talk of overall, complete body patterns. Above, I have mentioned the coupling of hip and lumbar extension, and these will coincide with an overall anterior tilting of the pelvis. Multi-joint reaction is all one normal response through a continuous and necessarily reciprocal system. Our tissues are aligned to control movement and we need enough to facilitate the efficiency mechanisms mentioned above but not so much movement that it creates impingements elsewhere due to tissue weakness and lack of control. Functional movement is the balance between enough and not too much range. There are two dynamics at play—the need for the pelvis to tilt enough to stimulate the rectus abdominis (RA) and the ability of the RA to respond—in the ongoing dance between mobility and stability, and the need for enough and not too much of either.

As we progress through mid-stance (see Figure 30.2A), the hip begins to extend, the pelvis is drawn into an anterior tilt and the RA will tension. RA and many hip flexors are often considered antagonists in their control of the pelvis: RA will posteriorly tilt it and the flexors will anteriorly tilt it. But, I believe, in gait they should be considered synergists, as they all control the overall extension through the body to create an elastic line along the front of the body.

A balance must be struck between the mobility of the ankle, the front of the hip and lumbar spine and the strength of each associated tissue needed to control those events. Ideally, they should be in harmony with one another, and it requires full clinical investigation to reveal, for example, if an overly lordotic spine is due to weak abdominals or restricted hip extension. As Zorn recalls, "true strength is not hardening; it is resilience, adaptability, stability. It is characterised by elasticity" (Rolf, 1989).

There are many such functional couplings, triplings and more through the body and it is my hope that true functional anatomy will filter further into clinical literature to enhance assessment and reasoning skills.

5. A sideline: elastic breathing: Zorn suggests uses a diaphragmatic breath and not letting the abdomen protrude forward. I can concur and encourage thinking of the whole system as one tensioning unit; if we lose tone and tension in one area it will influence elasticity in another. Full, normal breaths allow the thorax to support itself and, in turn, support the resiliency of other structures around it.

6. Move your upper body: there is considerable debate over the contribution of arm swing during gait. Perry and Burnfield (2010) describes the trunk as a "passenger"

responsible only for its own postural integrity. While that integrity will assist the elasticity of the lower body, it does not assist with the image and, I hope, reality of the contribution to gait from the trunk. Trunk rotation, side flexion and extension will all contribute elasticity, it is a natural feature by which lengthening of the soft tissue can add efficiency into the system. If we lock that movement down, we have to find other sources to recoup lost potential energy.

Along with the tensioning (but not the prevention of movement) of the thorax through the breath, the side flexion, extension and rotations that travel up through the trunk from the pelvis during gait will tension the intercostals, abdominals and spinal tissues. Each joint movement and separation of bones created by the body's natural response to the forces traveling through it has the potential, not to create more work for the body but, judged on the work focused on lower limb tissues, should actually increase efficiency of the moving body when it is considered as a whole and not separated into units, as suggested by Perry and Burnfield.

7. The arms are important, too. Contralateral arm swing is part of the natural reaction during gait and, by creating a counterbalancing rotation, helps create tension through the system. The counter-swing of the shoulder complex seems to contain the rotations from the pelvis to cause a wringing effect that appears oriented to the oblique tissues of the abdominals and intercostals.

Of particular interest to Zorn is the more superficial relationship from one latissimus dorsi through the thoracolumbar fascia to the opposite gluteus maximus. By tensioning this oblique line he suggests we create a sling to capture energy across the back of the trunk and pelvis and help propel it forward. This "posterior oblique sling" described by Vleeming et al. (2012) is one of many long chains of tissues that may be tensioned during and thereby assist with gait.

If we take a moment to analyze the woman in Figure 30.4 (Zorn, 2015), we could spend considerable time mapping out lines of tension and stretch that have been created by the extensions on one side and the flexion on the other. This woman is making the best of her "resonant elastic system" (Snyder and Foley, 2011 in Roberts, 2016) as she progresses forward.

Summary

The full body tensioning we see, has been allowed by the anatomical changes made over time, which have allowed movement at one joint to couple into another. The long strides with straight legs are the outcome of a number of skeletal changes in some form of primate ~7 MYA. Alterations of joint angles allowed numerous joints to be simultaneously extended to stretch the tissues crossing each of them prior to toe-off, whereby they contribute to the forward swing of the leg. The changes in joint orientation and range have led to the evolution of a metabolically efficient biped. *Homo sapiens'* optimization of fascial tissues to capture kinetic energy diverted calorie usage from locomotion to feed a larger brain.

We have focused on the back leg as it prepares for toe-off but similar, less well researched dynamics will be at work for the forward leg as it swings through to heel-strike. The lively propulsion captured in Figure 30.4 results from joints ranges developed through our hominin lineage, and those interrelated ranges grant us an ability

Chapter 30

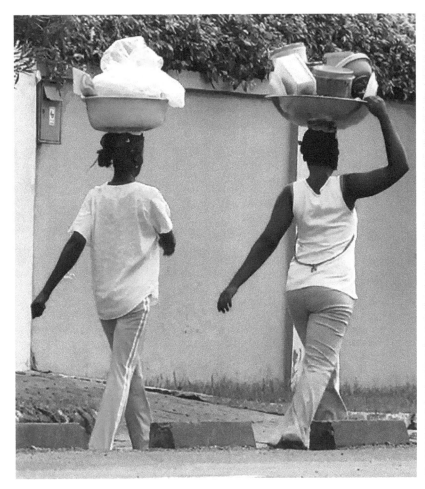

Figure 30.4

The long stride and contralateral arm swing helps tension the whole body in angles appropriate for dealing with forces following heel-strike (front limb, note the forward swing of the opposite arm to help tension the posterior oblique sling), and for the preparation for toe-off on the posterior lower limb.

to tension elastic and contractile tissues optimally on the front and back legs during gait to minimize muscle work and its resultant metabolic cost. If overuse is a cause of soft tissue dysfunction, understanding how it should be optimally loaded is essential knowledge for any therapist as they strive to understand the complexities of the presenting client.

Developing a wider view of tissue and joint interactions is essential when considering soft tissue dysfunctions; as described above, the foot, hip and spine are all interdependent for their appropriate loading. Joint interrelationships are particularly important during the retraining of healthy movement patterns, especially when using any forms of environmental intervention such as orthoses or changes in footwear, in which cases the therapist must consider the knock-on effects further along the chain.

References

Biewener, A. (2016) Locomotion as an emergent property of muscle contractile dynamics. *J Exp Biol.* 219: 285–294.

Chaitow, L. & DeLany, J., 2008 *Clinical Application Of Neuromuscular Techniques*. Edinburgh: Churchill Livingstone Elsevier.

Crompton, R., Vereecke, E. & Thorpe, S. (2008) Locomotion and posture from the common hominoid ancestor to fully modern hominins, with special reference to the last common panin/hominin ancestor. *Journal of Anatomy.* 212(4): 501–543.

Fernández, P., Mongle, C., Leakey, L., Proctor, D., Orr, C., Patel, B., Almécija, S., Tocheri, M. and Jungers, W. (2018) Evolution and function of the hominin forefoot. *Proceedings of the National Academy of Sciences.* 115(35): 8746–8751.

Fukunaga, T., Kawakami, Y., Kubo, K. & Kanehisa, H. (2002) Muscle and tendon interaction during human movements. *Exerc Sport Sci Rev.* 30: 106–110.

Holowka, N. & Lieberman, D. (2018) Rethinking the evolution of the human foot: insights from experimental research. *J Exp Biol.* 221: 1–10

Lieberman, D. (2012) Those feet in ancient times. *Nature.* 483: 550–551.

McKeon, P., Hertel, J., Bramble, D. & Davis, I. (2014) The foot core system: a new paradigm for understanding intrinsic foot muscle function. *Br J Sports Med.* 49: 290.

McNeill Alexander, R. (2002) Tendon elasticity and muscle function. *Comparative Biochemistry and Physiology Part A: Molecular & Integrative Physiology.* 133: 1001–1011.

Osborn, H. (1928) The influence of bodily locomotion in separating man from the monkeys and apes. *Scientific Monthly*, 385–399.

Perry, J. & Burnfield, J. (2010) *Gait Analysis.* Thorofare, NJ: SLACK.

Pontzer, H. (2017) Economy and endurance in human evolution. *Curr Biol.* 27: R613–R621.

Roberts, T. (2016) Contribution of elastic tissues to the mechanics and energetics of muscle function during movement. *J Exp Biol.* 219: 266–275.

Rolf, I.P. (1989) *Rolfing: Reestablishing the natural alignment and structural integration of the human body for vitality and well-being.* Rochester, VT: Healing Arts Press.

Rubenson, J., Pires, N., Loi, H., Pinniger, G. & Shannon, D. (2012) On the ascent: the soleus operating length is conserved to the ascending limb of the force-length curve across gait mechanics in humans. *J Exp Biol.* 215: 3539–3551.

Sawicki, G., Lewis, C. & Ferris, D. (2009) It pays to have a spring in your step. *Exerc Sport Sci Rev.* 37: 130–138.

Silder, A., Whittington, B., Heiderscheit, B. & Thelen, D. (2007) Identification of passive elastic joint moment–angle relationships in the lower extremity. *J Biomech.* 40: 2628–2635.

Vleeming, A., Schuenke, M., Masi, A., Carreiro, J., Danneels, L. & Willard, F. (2012) The sacroiliac joint: an overview of its anatomy, function and potential clinical implications. *Journal of Anatomy.* 221(6): 537–567.

Vogel, S. & DeFerrari, A. (2013) *Comparative biomechanics*. Princeton, NJ: Princeton University Press.

Whittington, B., Silder, A., Heiderscheit, B. & Thelen, D. (2008) The contribution of passive-elastic mechanisms to lower extremity joint kinetics during human walking. *Gait Posture.* 27: 628–634.

Zorn, A. (2015) Elastic Walking. In: Schleip, R. & Baker, A. (eds), *Fascia in Sport and Movement*. Edinburgh, UK: Handspring.

Functional training methods for the runner's myofascial systems

Wilbour Kelsick

Introduction

Running is big business and preparation is paramount to success in the sport. Participation has increased exponentially in the last 3 decades at both the amateur and the professional level. On average, runners cover ~110–130 km a week but, at times, can be thwarted by a variety of injuries. First, it should be mentioned that running is a complex elastic/spring-like movement involving the whole body's gait mechanism. An improved efficiency or energy-saving motion can be achieved when close to ideal elastic bounce in the running or walking gait is attained (Chapter 8). The beauty of functional myofascial training is that it can not only prevent injuries but can also increase running efficiency and myofascial tissue fatigue resistance.

This chapter focuses on how functional myofascial training can address the elastic strength and coordination components of the running and walking mechanism (Chapter 30). Reference will also be made to the principles of biotensegrity (Chapters 11 and 36) as a means of explaining the mechanism of running and the behavior of the body tissues, which allow it to happen. Briefly, biotensegrity explains how the principles of tensegrity (Chapter 11) manifest in biological systems: from viruses to cells and tissues of living systems (i.e. plants and animals). Biotensegrity integrates complex anatomy and biomechanics to make sense of living systems as a functional unit. From a biotensegrity perspective, any body movement (including walking, running and sprinting) is a continuous balancing dance of tension and compression forces within the body systems (Levin, 2002; Scarr, 2014).

Running injuries are related to poor running technique and coordination, minimal or poor elastic bounce, muscle (myofascial complexes) weakness (e.g. hip abductors, quadricep/knee mechanism), myofascial complexes imbalances in running structure (e.g. pelvic trunk myofascial complexes), biomechanical faults (over-pronation of feet, valgus of the knee), micro-trauma from overuse, an inadequately trained elastic myofascial net, low resistance to tissue fatigue and overall diminished body global strength relative to impact cyclic loading. All of the above can influence each other, creating a collage of epidemiological causes for running injuries. Studies show that the majority of running injuries can be summed up as micro-trauma to collagenous tissues (Stanish, 1984; Elliott, 1990).

It has been well documented that over 70% of recreational runners will sustain an injury during a 1-year period (Caspersen et al., 1984; Rochcongar et al., 1995; Ferber et al., 2009). For instance, more than eight out of 10 running injuries are below the knee, suggesting some common mechanism might be the culprit (Ferber et al., 2009). Based on the biotensegrity model, evidence does not support any one segmental region but more a global involvement of myofascial-skeletal running structures. Excessive pronation as a causative factor in overuse injuries is well documented (Clarke et al., 1983; Messier et al., 1991; Ferber et al., 2010.). Also, hip and pelvic complex mecha-

Chapter 31

nism weakness and imbalance, or poor stabilization, are now believed to be one of the major links to lower body running injuries: for example, iliotibial band compression syndrome and patella femoral syndrome (Horton and Hall, 1989; Livingston, 1998; Fredericson et al., 2000; Mizuno et al., 2001; Witvrouw et al., 2000). The aforementioned studies indicate that the causes of the majority of running injuries are related, or have some link to, inefficiency in the structural integrity of the running mechanism (the myofascialskeletal system). It is, therefore, clear that the prevention, pre-habilitation and rehabilitation of such injuries must address these causes in a practical manner. This leads to the proposed functional approach to train the runner's fascia from a global prospective.

However, at this point, the following questions must be addressed:

- What are the principles of running and how do they relate to global functional training?
- What do we mean by functional training?
- What is the purpose of strength training for runners?
- What do we mean by myofascial training?
- What functional myofascial training is specific to runners?

What are the principles of running and how do they relate to global functional training?

Walking, running and sprinting are complex elastic movements involving the entire body. They involve a cyclic exchange between potential and kinetic energy (a storage and release mechanism). The bones, tendons and ligaments are some of the stiffest springs in the body. The movement in such activities is not incremental or segmental but involves the entire body in simultaneous global action. Hence, training runners and sprinters cannot merely include exercises, which target segmental body parts (e.g. muscle groups- hamstrings, calves or core-meaning abdominal muscle strength; i.e. six-pack look). Evidence has shown that such exercises do not target the true bio-movements of running and sprinting in an effective and functional manner. In fact, this type of segmental training creates more myofacial and biotensegral imbalances setting up a platform/environment in the body's structure/architecture making it more prone to injury and substandard performance (Huijing et al., 2007; Stecco et al., 2013; Myers ,2009; Ferber et al., 2009). The concept of global functional training (GFT) is geared to address biotensegrity in the body's myofascia architecture. Since the myofascial net infiltrates the entire body, and its elastic and sensorimotor properties are crucial to running, it makes sense that the GTF method of training is an effective and efficient approach (Kram and Dawson, 1998; Kubo et al., 2003; Schleip, 2003; Kjaer et al., 2009).

What do we mean by functional training?

Functional training is exercise that is specific to the body movement you are attempting to execute.

In more detail, functional training describes the concept of using multi-joint exercise (i.e. sports-specific exercises) which more closely reproduces the movement pattern of a sport (in our case running) and can be modulated to improve the sum of parts, all of the biomechanical movement pattern or physiological profile of the sport. For example, in running, the biomechanical pattern would be stride distance or frequency and the physiological profile would be aerobic power for a distance runner. In functional training, exercise must be global (i.e. using

Functional training methods for the runner's myofascial systems

the whole body as much as possible) and not addressing isolated body regions.

In summary, functional training could be any sport-specific activity that moves an injured, deconditioned athlete or physically dysfunctioning individual towards safe return to sport or activities as soon as feasible.

What is the purpose of strength training for runners?

Running performance is dependent not only on a combination of aerobic and anaerobic capabilities, which vary based on the distance of the event, but also on other factors related to lower and upper body power and strength (Hudgens et al., 1987), speed and coordination.

It has been documented that force and power are strongly correlated with running performance for short distances (i.e. sprints, hurdles) (Meylan and Malatesta, 2008; Kale et al., 2009; Mikkola et al., 2011). For example, plyometric (Meylan and Malatesta, 2008) resistance (Mikkola et al., 2011) and explosive strength training (Spurrs et al., 2003; Buchheit et al., 2010) have shown significant improvements in sprint training performance (sprinting is not just about speed but strength, endurance, balance, etc.).

From observation, I firmly believe that strength training can help improve trunk pelvic complex, hip and lower extremity strength both concentrically and eccentrically, enhancing the structural integrity of the body's biotensegral architecture, thus improving running efficiency and performance.

The mechanism for this improved performance in distance runners is thought to be related to improved muscle (Dumke et al., 2010; Fletcher et al., 2010) and tendon stiffness (Dumke et al., 2010) and the elastic properties of the fascial net (Schleip, 2003; Huijing and Langevin,

2009; Tapale et al., 2010; Chapter 7). Therefore, the evidence for adapting exercises that train the fascial tissue net, as well as muscles and tendons, is paramount in decreasing and preventing running injuries and improving running economy. It should be noted that speed of running is a function of strength and coordination.

Sport-specific strength training for running must take into consideration sensorimotor factor and movement pattern behaviors (i.e. using global approach to exercise design) to guarantee the most transferrable effect of the training (Franklin and Wolpert, 2011; Smirniotou et al., 2008).

By contrast, middle and long distance running have received (have undergone or conducted) few studies that suggest force and power improve performance. However, a few well-designed studies have recently revealed that explosive strength training can improve the running economy of middle and long distance runners to a significant degree (Mikkola et al., 2007; Kelly et al., 2009; Ferraut et al., 2010) and also strengthen elastic elements like fascia, tendons and ligaments thus making more robust to withstand repetitive loading and injury (Arampatazis et al., 2007; Arampatazis et al., 2010; Hrysomallis, 2012; Kubo K et al., 2007).

What do we mean by myofascial training?

In the past, training for athletes focused mainly on conventional cardiovascular fitness, muscular strength, power and neuromuscular coordination. The classical biomechanical tradition of considering the body as functioning in separate segments, with attached levers, and concepts of linear mechanics is no longer feasible in the light of new research on myofascial function in the whole body (Schleip, 2003; Desmouliere et al., 2005; Huijing, 2007; Kubo et al., 2006). Humans

Chapter 31

like other species are complex biological and biotensegral systems (Levin, 2002). You cannot train body parts in isolation and expect to have efficient global functioning.

Running, in its true form, is mostly an elastic event (Bosch and Klomp, 2001; Legramandi et al., 2013). The mechanism of running involves the storing of energy during the deceleration or breaking phase (during foot ground contact) and instantaneous releasing energy during the lift-off phase initiated by ground reaction force (GRF) (Figure 31.1) (Legramandi et al., 2013). Using an elastic recoil technique (Chapter 7) will allow the runner to be more efficient, placing less stress on the musculoskeletal system and eventually decreasing injury risk. Training for runners must be elastically functional and global in its approach, inclusive of the entire body, and not just the lower extremities or individual muscle groups. It should be considered as complex training targeting neural adaptation, coordination, strength and proprioception modes.

There is evidence to support that different myofascial elements are affected by different loading styles and that fascia has an important role in maintaining muscle function (Steven et al., 1981; Ingber, 2008). Typical weight training loads the muscle in its normal range of motion, therefore strengthening fascial tissues arranged in series with active muscle fibers (Mackey et al., 2008; McBride et al., 2009). This type of loading has minimal effect on the intramuscular fibers that are arranged in parallel to active muscle fibers and also extra-muscular fascia (Huijing, 1999; Latrides et al., 2003; Fukashiro et al., 2006). This evidence reinforces that, during functional training of the runner's fascial net, exercises must have a dynamic varied loading pattern with rhythm to have an effect on the elastic components and resilience of the body's myofascial net.

The concepts of global functional training for the runner arise from these insights. The global functional training program, designed in this context, will address the running mechanism from a global perspective with exercises geared to train the runner's elastic myofascial component as well as the muscle, ligaments, bone and tendons. The functional myofascial exercise protocol for the runner is carried out with a certain amount of rhythm and an explosive component. Special attention is paid to the sport-specific movement pattern for running.

In maintaining form, or activated structural integrity, the body is able to set up its own internal and external anchor to create the dynamic stability needed as one segment generates power and the other stabilizes (Ingber, 2008; Kelsick 2006). This creates the alternate movement pattern biology designed for running. This patterning is classified as the concentric/eccentric; dynamic structural stability power/generating switching mechanism (between concentric and eccentric myofascial contraction) required for alternate body segmental movement in walking and running (Chapter 30). As previously described, running and walking are a simultaneous balancing dance between tension and compression in harmony with concentric and eccentric movement patterns of the entire body myofascial net and other supporting tissues. This tension and compression mechanism is always engaged during static or dynamic activity based on the principles of biotensegrity (Figure 31.1). In addition the body's tissues (which are soft matter) exhibit auxetic properties (i.e. they expand when tensioned (stretched) as opposed to shrinking-narrowing).

What global functional fascia training is specific to runners?

It has been documented that the manner, slow or fast, in which connective tissue is loaded

Functional training methods for the runner's myofascial systems

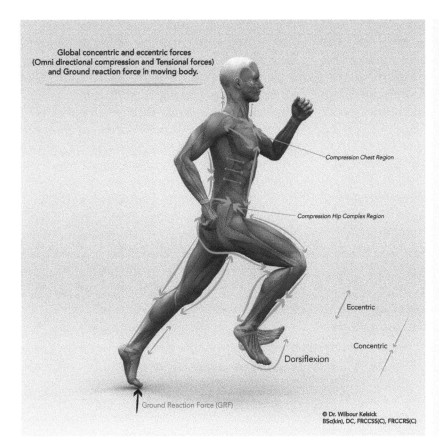

Global concentric and eccentric forces
(Omni directional compression and Tensional forces)
and Ground reaction force in moving body.

Compression Chest Region

Compression Hip Complex Region

Eccentric

Concentric

Dorsiflexion

Ground Reaction Force (GRF)

© Dr. Wilbour Kelsick
BSc(kin), DC, FRCCSS(C), FRCCRS(C)

Figure 31.1 Some key global and compression omini directional external forces in a moving body

In terms of biotensegrity, a body in motion (walking, running, climbing, swimming, etc.) is a continuous well balanced harmonic dance between tension and compression of its global myofascial net and other supporting tissues.

will determine whether the tissue will become more elastic or react with hypertrophy (i.e. volume) (Kubo et al., 2003; Kjaer et al., 2009; Chapter 14).

In nature, kangaroos and gazelles are excellent examples of elastic storage and the release of energy during their movement patterns (Kram and Dawson, 1998; Chapter 8). The human myofascial net seems to have similar elastic behavior (i.e. kinetic energy storage and release) in our daily activities of walking, running or jumping (Chino et al., 2008; Sawicki et al., 2009). This justifies the approach of global functional training for the runner's myofascial net using explosive, rhythmic type exercise movement patterns (Fukunaga et al., 2002; Kawakami et al., 2002).

The functional fascia training concept

The elastic behavior of human fascia is now documented (Kubo et al., 2006; Chino et al., 2008). It stores energy and returns it quickly, as seen in cyclic movements like walking and running (Chapter 29; Kubo et al., 2006; Chino et al., 2008; Legramandi et al., 2013).

Running elastically uses less muscle power, that is, less metabolic energy (glucose) and more of the elastic fascia feature of the tissue, thus storing and returning energy back during propulsion. Global functional training for runners' fascia is designed to train the elastic myofascia net of the entire body (i.e. muscle, tendons, ligaments, bones). The modes of exercise include bouncing or plyometric movements, preparatory

Chapter 31

countermovement, unilateral movement patterns, coordination drills, and other exercises which mimic the mechanism of running (e.g. single leg hops, single leg squats, etc.). The exercise protocol avoids slow, jerky-type movement patterns, repetitive constant-angled movements, movement with mono tempo/rhythm, muscular dominant movement, segmental isolation-type movement pattern and minimizes constant loading thus encouraging variable loading of the runner's body. This is in line with research suggesting that the fascial system is better trained by use of a variety of vectors/angles, loads and rhythm (Huijing, 2007; Chapter 24).

We cannot delve into this topic without mentioning the importance that running, coordination posture and technique play in enhancing running efficiency and performance. In a correct sprinter's posture, for example, the athlete is at a considerable height off the ground in the flight phase, with a well-positioned body preparing for the landing phase (a very important body position to maximize horizontal distance travel through the air). Although it is not possible to discuss the concept of running technique in this context in this chapter, it should be noted that it is a crucial piece of the puzzle in preventing running injuries and improving performance.

Exercise protocol for training the runner's myofascia net

Sports conditioning programs need to be optimally individualized and specific because the limits of peak performance are highly variable even within the same discipline of sport. As described above, the purpose of appropriate exercises is geared to enhance sensorimotor coordination and to strengthen the elastic components of the runner's myofascial net. Energy is stored in the eccentric phase of motion and immediately released on the concentric phase.

The exercises are preceded by an eccentric pre-stretch (counter movement) (Chapter 24) that loads the muscle, tendon and fascia, preparing it for the ensuing concentric contraction. This coupling of the eccentric concentric muscle contraction is known as the stretch-shortening cycle, which physiologically involves the elastic properties of the connective tissues (fascia, tendon) and proprioceptive reflexes (Radcliffe and Farentinos, 1985; Tippett and Voight, 1995). The fact that connective tissue has a high capacity of adaptability and resilience makes it ideal for this type of training where loading forces, shearing and strain are highly variable. Connective tissue has the ability to continuously remodel its fibrous network when specific functional strain or load is applied to it (Chen et al., 1997; Langevin et al., 2010; Chapter 4).

In designing any exercise strengthening program, there are some basic exercise prescription guidelines which must be taken into consideration and a few important questions that need to be asked: Why are you doing the activity? What is the goal of the activity? Is it for fitness maintenance or for competition? Note that the basic principles of training will also apply here (i.e. principles of adaptation [acute and chronic], specificity, overload, and progressive overload, stress-rest, contraction, control, coordination, ceiling, maintenance, symmetry and overtraining) (Kraemer, 1994; Fleck and Kraemer, 1997). In this context we cannot address all these principles but they are found in detail in physiological texts on training (Fleck and Kraemer, 1997).

First, exercise prescription must consider the total demands of the program and ensure that the volume of exercise is not excessive, which can negatively interfere with the optimal physiological adaptation and performance. It should also consider the activity movement pattern, since complex systems like our bodies do not move in a linear manner or pattern.

Functional training methods for the runner's myofascial systems

To ensure an effective prescription (Kraemer and Koziris, 1992; Tippet and Voight, 1995; Fleck and Kraemer, 1997), the following should be taken into consideration:

- the concept of periodization of the training program and goals of training
- developing a well-planned exercise recovery and rest protocol by using the principles of periodization
- understanding the balance between strength/power (intensity), coordination and aerobic and anaerobic (volume) training.

In addition, the key resistance training program components should be considered when designing functional fascia-type exercises (Kraemer, 1994; Fleck and Kraemer, 1997). These components are:

1. **Needs analysis**: this addresses questions about the myofascial net, whole-body segments to be trained, the energy/metabolic systems involved (aerobic, anaerobic), the type of muscle action (eccentric or isometric). Also the principle that the body is a complex biological system and is non–linear.

2. **Acute program variables**: this deals with choice, order, number of sets, rest period between sets and amount of load (intensity).

3. **Chronic program manipulation**: this addresses the principles of periodization as a means of designing long-term programs.

4. **Administrative concerns**: this deals with equipment needs in the gym (free weights, machine-assisted resistance isokinetics, jump platforms, etc.).

Exercise posture

These exercises are geared more towards middle distance and recreational runners, taking into consideration the concepts of transfer training and exercise specificity. The concept of practicing one movement pattern to improve the efficiency of another movement pattern is known as "transfer of training". For example, a runner will get little benefit from doing high-intensity seated rowing. Split squats or walking lunges, which are more similar to the movement pattern of running, would be more beneficial. When exercise movement patterns are similar, this principle is known as "exercise specificity". Specificity in athletic or any type of training is paramount and a main guarantee that one can achieve transfer of training. (Franklin and Wolpert, 2011). Due to space constrains in this chapter, only eight exercises have been documented.

All exercises are performed in a "closed kinetic chain" posture to increase joint compressive forces, improve joint congruency and myofascial co-contraction/activation, which will overall enhance the dynamic stability of the body segments targeted (modified from Lefever, 2011) although the entire body is involved (the global approach). The concept of transfer of training and exercise specificity is taken into consideration. Proper foot placement is paramount. The ankle should be in a "locked" position attained by dorsi-flexion. This allows a stiff but dorsiflexed forefoot to contact the ground, instantaneously transmitting the GRF up the kinetic chain. This well-timed, coordinated action of the foot creates the stiffness in the lower extremity chain required to create reactive strength to receive the GRF (Winkler, unpublished data). Such action ensures a pre-stretch and engages the elastic components of calf. Engagement/activation of the neuromuscular components of the trunk, pelvis, pelvic floor and lower extremities is also necessary. The exercises are not segmental but address the entire body running movement pattern.

Exercise mode

All exercises are performed explosively with quick repeated rhythm/tempo to enhance the elastic effect on the muscular and fascial tissues.

Chapter 31

Pre-exercise preparation

This preparation should be about 15 min and consists of the following to enhance general body mobility, ankle and foot ground reactiveness:

- 3–5 min jogging
- Upper body alternating arm action (simulating arms during running) with rhythmic breathing
- Low amplitude ankle/foot bouncing with initial active dorsiflexion and plantar flexion when landing on ground
- Standing lower extremity swings from hips
- Walking lunges with quick tempo
- Sideway scissors runs – lower extremity crossovers
- Double and single ankle hops with dorsiflexion of foot landing on balls of the feet
- Hip mobility drills – flexion and extension hip swings.

Functional training exercises

Some of these exercises were developed in collaboration with the coach, Gary Winckler. These exercises are designed to target and exploit the elastic components in the fascia net, muscle and tendon tissues. Execution must be explosive, rhythmic and reactive. Attention to global body posture and technique execution is crucial to achieve the full benefits.

1. Extended arm overhead with resistance: rectus abdominis and anterior compartment eccentric strengthening (Figure 31.2)

Purpose

To build anterior trunk anchoring eccentric strength for abdominal and lateral wall muscles (transversus, internal and external obliques), which transmit forces from the back structures

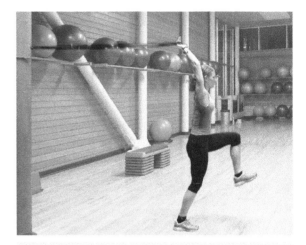

Figure 31.2
Over-head pull: eccentric resistance for anterior abdominals/trunk.

(mainly the thoraco-lumbar fascia). The rectus abdominis, pelvis and hip complex all work eccentrically to improve balance, coordination and force transmission during the single leg stance in the walking movement of this exercise.

Position/posture

Stand upright, engage trunk anterior and posterior musculature, pelvic floor and hip structures. Hands are overhead with extended elbows.

Start position

Stand facing away from anchor of elastic tubing or pulley weight cables, which is anchored at the height of extended forearm overhead. Alternatively, you can use an individual assistant (as an anchor) to hold the tubing.

Movement technique

- Flex one hip with flexed knees (e.g. like running stance) with your thigh in midline and your pelvis level.
- Check your alignment then begin to march or walk against the overhead resistance.

- Lift the chest and chin up and look slightly upward so you feel the tension in the anterior abdominal wall complex.
- Increase pace from a walk to a slow jog maintaining tension on the elastic strap at all times.

The key is to be as upright as possible and to try not and over-extend the spine/trunk but maintain good tension of the elastic strap as you move forward. You can also use cable pulley weights for this exercise.

Dosage

Set: 3–6

Reps: 10–20 steps

Rest: 1–2 min

2. Quick step-ups

Purpose

This is a close kinetic-chain movement to strengthen trunk, pelvis, hip, knee, ankle and foot, and to improve coordination and balance in single leg stance.

Position/posture

Stand upright and engage anterior and posterior trunk musculature, pelvic floor, hip structures.

Start position

Stand facing a step or box.

Movement technique

- Your front leg on the step/box (12–14") with your thigh in midline and your pelvis level back leg on ground.
- Check your alignment then quickly push with the back leg, lifting it off the ground and pushing your body straight upward.
- Step off with the leg, which was first on the box.
- Repeat alternating your legs.
- The key is to push off with the back leg/leg on the ground and not the front leg/leg on the box.

Dosage

Set: 3–6

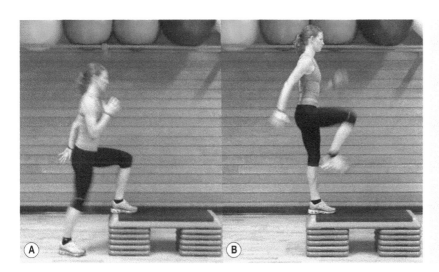

Figure 31.3

(A) Quick step-ups and **(B)** walking step-ups.

Chapter 31

Reps: 10–20

Rest: 1–2 min.

3. Low amplitude double leg hop over mini-hurdles

Purpose

A plyometric drill, which initiates the stretch-shortening cycle of the lower extremity complex. This drill assists in developing elastic strength, speed and explosive power of the lower leg and the pelvis, especially the gluteals, hamstrings, quadriceps and gastrocnemius-ankle complex. Enhances the elastic fascial components in the trunk, pelvis, hip, knee, ankle and foot.

Position/posture

Stand upright and engage the trunk's anterior and posterior musculature, pelvic floor, hip structures. Step up two mini-hurdles 6–12 inches high about one stride length apart.

Start position

Stand upright about half a stride length in front of the hurdles with shoulders slightly forward, head up. Elbows should be at 90° and hands at your sides with thumbs up.

Movement technique

- Begin by performing a counter-movement downward and jump as high as possible, flexing legs so the feet arrive under the buttocks. Bring the knees up medium high and forward for each jump to ensure maximum lift.

- To land, ensure the ankle is dorsiflexed. Jump forward again with the same cycle of leg and foot pattern.

- Execute as rapidly as possible, always moving forward.

- The key is to gain moderate height and maximum distance without affecting repetition rate.

Dosage

Set: 3–6

Reps: 10–20

Rest: 1–2 min.

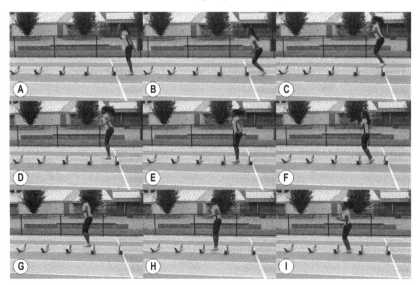

Figure 31.4
(A–I) Double leg hops over mini-hurdles.

4. Double leg ankle hops (Figure 31.5)

Purpose

A plyometric drill, which initiates the stretch-shortening cycle of the lower extremity complex. It helps develop elastic strength, speed and explosive power of the lower leg and gastrocnemius-ankle complex. It enhances the elastic myofascial components of the lower knee, ankle and foot.

Position/posture

Stand upright and engage trunk anterior and posterior musculature, pelvic floor, hip structures.

Start position

Stand upright with both feet on the ground and hands by your side.

Movement technique

Push off the ground and immediately dorsiflex the ankle joint. The knee should be in extension. On landing, ensure your foot is dorsiflexed and land on the balls of your feet. Repeat the sequence rapidly, maintaining an extended knee. Remain basically in the same spot.

Dosage

Sets: 4

Reps: 15–30

Rest: 2 min.

5. Single leg ankle hops (Figure 31.6)

Purpose

A plyometric drill, which initiates the stretch-shortening cycle of the lower extremity

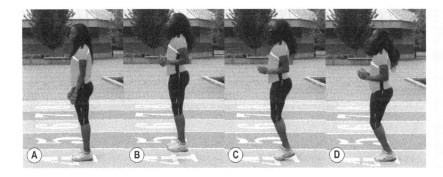

Figure 31.5
(A–D) Double leg ankle hops.

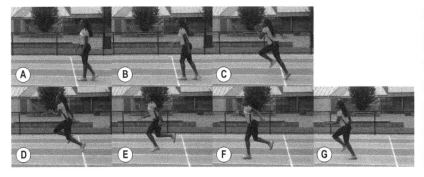

Figure 31.6
(A–G) Single leg ankle hops.

Chapter 31

complex. It helps develop elastic strength, speed and power of the lower leg and gastrocnemius-ankle complex. It enhances the elastic fascial components of the lower knee, ankle and foot.

Position/posture

Stand upright and engage the trunk's anterior and posterior musculature, pelvic floor, hip structures.

Start position

Stand upright with both feet on the ground and hands by your side.

Movement technique

Push off the ground on one leg, only leaping forward and immediately dorsiflexing the ankle joint. Try to land one stride length ahead on the ball of your foot. The knee should be in extension. On landing, ensure your foot is dorsiflexed and land on the push-off leg on the ball of your feet. Repeat the sequence rapidly, maintaining an extended knee and alternating legs.

Dosage

Sets: 4

  Reps: 15–30

  Rest: 2 min.

6. Double leg jumping split lunges on the spot (Figure 31.7)

Purpose

A plyometric drill, which initiates the stretch-shortening cycle of the hip and lower extremity complexes. This drill helps to develop elastic strength, speed and power of the lower leg and pelvis, especially the hip flexors, gluteals, hamstrings, quadriceps and gastrocnemius-ankle complex. It enhances the elastic strength of fascial components in trunk, pelvis, hip, knee, ankle and foot complexes. The goal is to attain maximum height.

Position/posture

Stand upright and engage trunk anterior and posterior musculature, pelvic floor, hip structures, as in the previous exercises.

Start position

From a standing parallel foot position and shoulder width apart get into lunge posture. Step forward with say the **right** leg knee at 45–90° at the hip and 45–90° and hip flex about the same degree and your **left** back hip is now extended (to a comfortable near maximum range of motion) and knee of back **left** leg also flex at 45–90°. In this position you are maintaining an upright/ erect and engaged trunk and pelvis. Your arm positioning is important. The arm (left) on the opposite side of the leg that's in the back (extended hip) should be flexed 90° at shoulder and elbow. The arm (right) on the same side of the leg that's in front (flexed hip) should be extended about 50–60° and 90 degrees flexion of the elbow (basically your posture should be the running stance).

Movement technique

The goal is to jump into the next lunge position landing on the same area/spot by pushing off the back leg explosively lifting your body into the air and again landing in a lunge position. Using counter-movement technique, drop down into a lunge position and stop that movement subsequently exploding upward as far as you can with a scissor-like motion. Note while in the air you need to execute a scissor action. Quickly bring the **right** hip which was in flexion in extension

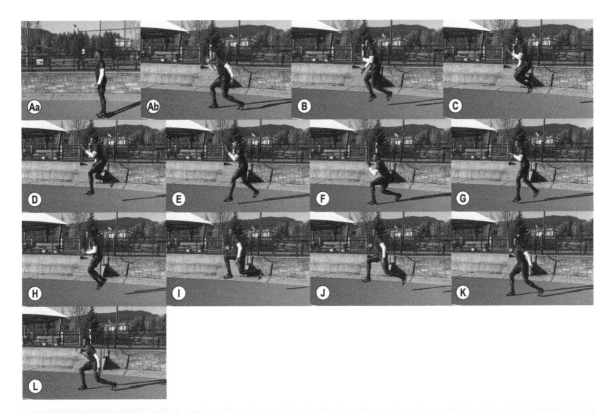

Figure 31.7

(A–L) Double leg jumping split lunges on the spot

and the extended **left** hip into flexion before landing again in a lunge posture but this time your **left** hip and leg is now in front (flexed **left** hip) and your **right** hip and leg are now in the back (extended **right** hip). This scissors movement (alternating leg position front and back) is repeated continuously for desired number of reps. It is important during landing (should be on ball of feet) and pushing off that the ankle complex is held in dorsiflexion posture as much as possible. This exercise can be performed by moving the forward covering distance but is much more demanding (as for quick walking lunge) for desired number of repetitions.

Dosage

Sets: 4

Reps: 5–1

Rest: 2 min.

7. Quick walking lunge (Figure 31.8)

Purpose

This is a close kinetic-chain movement in lower extremity complex. It helps to develop the elastic strength, speed and power of the lower leg and pelvis, especially the hip flexors, gluteals,

Chapter 31

hamstrings, quadriceps and gastrocnemius-ankle complex. It enhances the elastic strength of myofascial components in trunk, pelvis, hip, knee, ankle and foot. The goal is to attain a good rhythm.

Position/posture

Stand upright and engage the trunk's anterior and posterior musculature, pelvic floor, hip structures as in the previous exercises.

Start position

Place feet shoulder width apart, bend one leg to 90° at the hip and 90° at the knee, attaining more or less a running stance.

Movement technique

Lunge forward quickly with the unsupported leg. As soon as contact is made with the ground, recover the hind leg and use it to repeat the lunge.

Land with feet/ankle in dorsiflexion so you land on the balls of the feet in a split lunge position and immediately repeat the sequence, initiating the pushing phase on the front leg to propel the body forward. Cover about 30–40 m.

Dosage

Sets: 4

Reps: 15–30 (30–40m)

Rest: 2 min.

8. Alternate leg box jumps (Figure 31.9)

Purpose

A plyometric drill, which initiates the stretch-shortening cycle of the lower extremity complex. This drill helps to develop the elastic strength, speed and explosive power of the lower leg and

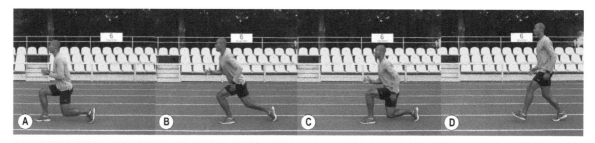

Figure 31.8

(A–D) Quick walking lunge.

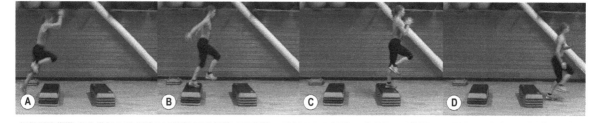

Figure 31.9

(A–D) Alternate leg box jumps.

pelvis, especially the hip flexors, gluteals, hamstrings, quadriceps and gastrocnemius-ankle complex. It enhances the elastic fascial components in the trunk, pelvis, hip, knee, ankle and foot.

Position/posture

Stand upright and engage trunk anterior and posture musculature, pelvic floor and hip structures.

Start position

Stand upright on one leg, with one leg in front of the other, as if taking a step. Shoulders are oriented slightly forward and head faces upwards. Arms are at the sides.

Movement technique

Begin the exercise by pushing off with the back leg. Drive the knee up to the chest to achieve maximum height and distance before landing. Quickly extend the driving foot outward. Cycle the arms in contra-lateral motion in the air for balance. Repeat the sequence using alternate legs on landing.

Dosage

Sets: 2–4

Reps: 8–12 (40 m)

Rest: 2 min.

Summary

Speed is a composite of strength and coordination. Walking, running and sprinting are movements in complex biological systems where the principles of biotensegrity (internal omni-directional forces, tension and continuous compression) function in a harmonic dance of balance, to maintain the integrity of the body's architectural systems during motion. In addition these internal forces prepare the body's closed kinetic chain system to absorb, transmit and create movement from the external GRF. Effective training for runners must address complex global movement pattern similar to running and not individual muscle groups. Training the myofascia net re-enforces strength and enhances elasticity of the biotensegral architecture of the running body systems. This, in turn, results in improved running economy and efficiency and decreases running injuries.

References

Arampatziz, A., Karamanidis, K., Albracht, K. (2007) Adaptational responses of the human achilles tendon by modulation of the applied cyclic strain magnitude. *J Exp Biol.* 210: 2743–2753.

Arampatzis, A., Peper, A., Bierbaum, S., Albracht K. (2010) Plasticicty of human Achilles tendon mechanical and morphological properties in response to cyclic strain. *J Biomech.* 43(16): 3073–3079

Bosch, F. & Klomp, R. (2001) *Running-Biomechanics and exercise physiology in practice.* Churchill Livingstone.

Buchheit, M., Mendez-Villanueva, A., Delhomel, G., Brughelli, M. & Ahmaidi, S. (2010) Improving repeated sprint ability in young elite soccer players: Repeated shuttle sprints vs. explosive strength training. *J Strength Cond Res.* 24: 266–271.

Caspersen, C.J., Powell, K.F., Koplan, J.P., Shirley, R.W., Cambell, C.C. & Sikes, R.K. (1984) The incidence of injuries and hazards in recreational and fitness runners. *Med Sci Sports Exerc.* 16: 113–114.

Chen, C.S., Mrksich, M., Huang, S., Whitesides, G., Ingber, D. (1997) Geometric control of cell life and death. *Science.* 276: 1425–1428.

Chino, K. Oda, T., Kurihara, T., Nagayoshi, T. (2008) In vivo fascicle behaviour of synergistic muscles on concentric and eccentric plantar flexion in humans. *J Electromy Kines.* 18: 79–88.

Clarke, T.E., Frederick, E.C. & Hamill, C.L. (1983) The effects of shoe design parameters on rearfoot control in running. *Med Sci Sports Exerc.* 15: 376–381.

Desmouliere, A., Chapponier, C. & Gabbiani, G. (2005) Tissue repair, contraction, and the myofibroblast. *Wound Repair Regen.* 13: 7–12.

Dumke, C.l., Pfaffenroth, C.M., McBride, J.M. & McCauley, G.O. (2010) Relationship between muscle strength, power and stiffness and running economy in trained male runners. *Int J Sports Physiol Perform.* 5: 249–261.

Elliott, B.C. (1990) Adolescent overuse sporting injuries: a biomechanical review. *Aust Sports Commission Program.* 23: 1–9.

Ferber, R., Davis, I.S., Noehren, B. & Hamill. J. (2010) Competitive female runners with a history of iliotibial band syndrome demonstrate atypical hip and knee kinematics. *Journal of Orthopaedic & Sports Physical Therapy.* 40 (2): 52–58.

Ferber, R., Hreljac, A. & Kendall, K. (2009) Suspected mechanisms in the cause of overuse running injuries: a clinical review. *Sports Health.* 3: 242–246.

Ferrauti, A., Bergerman, M. & Fernandez-Fernandez, J. (2010) Effects of a concurrent strength and endurance training on running performance and running economy in recreational marathon runners. *J Strength Cond Res.* 24: 2770–2778.

Fleck, J., & Kraemer, W.J. (1997) Designing resistance training programs. *Library of Congress Cataloging-in-Publication Data.* 4: 88–106.

Fletcher, J.R., Esau, S.P. & Macintosh, B.R. (2010) Changes in tendon stiffness and running economy in highly trained distance runners. *Eur J Appl Physiol.* 110: 1037–1046.

Franklin, D.W. & Wolpert, D.M. (2011) Computational mechanism of sensorimotor control. Review Article. *Nueron.* 72: 425–442.

Fredericson, M., Cookingham, C.L., Chaudhari, A.M., Dowdell, B.C.,

Oestreicher, N. & Sahrmann, S.A. (2000) Hip abductor weakness in distance runners with iliotibial band syndrome. *Clin J Sport Med.* 10: 169–175.

Fukashiro, S., Hay, D.C. & Nagano, A. (2006) Biomechanical behavior of muscle-tendon complex during dynamic human movements. *J Appl Biomech.* 22: 131–147.

Fukunaga, T., Kawakami, Y., Kubo, K. & Kanehisa, H. (2002) Muscle and tendon interaction during human movements. *Exerc Sport Sci Rev.* 30: 106–110.

Horton, M.G. & Hall, T.L. (1989) Quadriceps femoris muscle angle: normal values and relationships with gender and selected skeletal measures. *Phys Ther.* 69: 897–901.

Hudgens, B., Scharafenberg, J., Travis Triplett, N., & McBride, J.M. (1987) Relationship between jumping ability and running performance in events of varying distance. *J Strength Cond Res.* 27: 563–567.

Huijing, P.A. (1999) Muscle as a collagen fiber reinforced composite: a review of force transmission in muscle and whole limb. *J Biomech.* 32: 329–345.

Huijing, P. (2007) Epimuscular myofascial force transmission between antagonistic and synergistic muscles can explain movement limitation in spastic paresis. *J Biomech.* 17: 708–724.

Huijing, P.A., & Langevin, H. (2009) Communicating about fascia: history, pitfalls and recommendations. In: P.A. Huijing, Hollander, P., Findley, T. (Eds) *Fascia Research II: Basic Science and Implications for Conventional and Complementary Health Care.* Munich, Germany: Elsevier GmbH.

Ingber, D. (2008) Tensegrity and mechanotransduction. *J Bodyw Mov Ther.* 12: 198–200.

Hrysomallis, C. (2012) The effectiveness of resisted movement training on sprinting and jumping performance. *J Strength Cond Res.* 26: 299–306.

Kale, M., Alper, A., Co‚skun, B. & Caner, A. (2009) Relationship among jumping performance and sprint parameters during maximum speed phase in sprinters. *J Strength Con Res.* 23: 2272–2279.

Kawakami, Y., Muraoka, T., Ito, S., Kanehisa, H. & Fukunaga, T. (2002) In vivo muscle fibre behaviour during countermovement exercise in humans reveals a significant role for tendon elasticity. *J Physiol.* 540: 635–646.

Kelly, C.M., Burnett, A.F. & Newton, M.J. (2010) The effects of strength training on three-kilometer performance in recreational women endurance runners. *J Strength Cond Res.* 23: 1633–1636.

Kjaer, M., Langberg, H., Heinemeier, K., Bayer, M.L., Hansen, M., Holm, L., Doessing, S., Konsgaard, M., Krogsgaard, M.R. & Magnusson, S.P. (2009) From mechanical loading to collagen synthesis, structural changes and function in human tendon. *Scand J Med Sci Sports.* 19: 500–510.

Kraemer, W.J. (1994) *The physiological basis for strength training in mid-life. In sports and exercise in midlife.* In S.L. Gordon (Ed), 413–433. Park Ridge, IL: American Academy of Orthopaedic Surgeons.

Kraemer, W.J. & Koziris, L.P. (1992) Muscle strength training. Techniques and considerations. *Phys Ther Pract.* 2: 54–68.

Kram, R. & Dawson, T.J. (1998) Energetics and biomechanics of locomotion by red kangaroos *(Macropus rufus). Comp Biochem Physiol B.* 120: 41–49.

Kubo, K., Kanehisa, H., Miyatani, M., Tachi, M. & Fukunaga, T. (2003) Effect of low-load resistance training on the tendon properties in middle-aged and elderly women. *Acta Physiol Scand.* 178: 25–32.

Kubo, K., Ohgo, K., Takeishi, R., Yoshinaga, K., Tsunoda, N., Kanehisa, H., Fukunaga, T. (2006) Effects of series elasticity on the human knee extension torque-angle relationship in vivo. *Res Q Exercise Sport.* 77(4): 408–416.

Kubo, K., Marimoto, M., Komuro T., (2007) Effects of plyometric and weight training on muscle-tendon complex and jump performance. *Med Sci Sports Exerc.* 39: 1801–1810

Langevin, H. et al. (2010) Fibroblast cytoskeletal remodeling contributes to connective tissue tension. *J Cell Physiol. E-pub ahead of publication.* Oct. 13, 2010.

Latrides, J. et al. (2003) Subcutaneous tissue mechanical behavior is linear and viscoelastic under uniaxial tension. *Connect Tissue Res.* 44: 208–217.

Hall, C. (1999) *Therapeutic Exercise – Moving Toward Function.* Lippincott William & Wilkins. 18: 313–317.

Legramandi, M.A., Schepens, B. & Cavagna, G.A. (2013) Running humans attain optimal elastic bounce in their teens. *Sci. Rep.* 3: 1310.

Levin, S.M. (2002) The tensegrity-truss as a model for spine mechanics: biotensegrity. *J Mech Med Biol.* 2: 375–388.

Livingston, L.A. (1998) The quadriceps angle: a review of literature. *J Orthop Sports Phys Ther.* 28: 105–109.

Mackey, A.L., Heinmeier, K.M., Koskinen, S.O. & Kjaer, M. (2008) Dynamic adaptation of tendon and muscle connective tissue to mechanical loading. *Connect Tissue Res.* 49: 165–168.

McBride, J.M., Blow, D., Kirby, T.J., Haines, T.L., Dayne, A.M. & Triplett, N.T. (2009) Relationship between maximal squats strength and five, ten and forty yard sprint time. *J Strength Cond Res.* 23: 1633–1636.

Messier, S.P, Davis, S.E. & Curl, W.W. (1991) Etiologic factors associated with patellofemoral pain in runners. *Med Sci Sports Exerc.* 23: 1008–1015.

Meylan, C. & Malatesta, D. (2008) Effects of in-season plyometric training within soccer practice on explosive actions in young players. *J Strength Cond Res.* 23: 369–403.

Mikkola, J., Rusko, H., Nummela, A., Pollari, T. & Hakkinen, K. (2007) Concurrent endurance and explosive type strength training improves neuromuscular and anaerobic characteristics in young distance runners. *Int J Sports Med.* 28: 602–611.

Mikkola, J., Vesterinen, V., Taipale, R., Capostango, B., Hakkinen, K. & Nummela, A. (2011) Effect of resistance training regimens on treadmill running and neuromuscular performance in recreational endurance runners. *J Sports Sci.* 29: 359–1371.

Mizuno, Y., Kumagai, M. & Mattessich, S.M. (2001) Q-angle influences tibiofemoral and patellofemoral kinematics. *J Orthop Res.* 19: 834–840.

Myers, T. (2009) *Anatomy Trains: Myofascial Meridians for manual and movement Therapists.* New York: Churchill-Livingston.

Radcliffe, J. & Farentinos, R. (1985) Plyometrics: Explosive power training. *Library of Congress Cataloguing-inPublication Data.* 5: 30–72.

Rochcongar, P., Pernes, J. & Carre, F. (1995) Occurrence of running injuries: a survey among 1153 runners. *Sci Sports.* 10: 15–19.

Sawicki, G.S., Lewis, C.L. & Ferris, D.P. (2009) It pays to have a spring in your step. *Exerc Sport Sci Rev.* 37: 130–138.

Scarr, G. (2014) *Biotensegrity: The Structural Basis of Life.* Pencaitland, UK: Handspring Publishing.

Schleip, R. (2003) Fascial plasticity – a new neurobiological explanation. *J Bodyw Mov Ther.* 7(1): 11–19, 7(2): 104–116.

Schleip, R. & Klingler, W. (2007) Fascial strain hardening correlates with matrix hydration changes. In: Findley, T.W. & Schleip, R. (Eds), *Fascia Research – Basic science and implications to conventional and complementary health care.* Munich: Elsevier GmbH. 51.

Smirniotou, A., Katsikas, C., Paradisis, G., Argeitaki, P., Zacharogiannis, E. & Tziortzis, S. (2008) Strength-power parameters as predictors of sprinting performance. *J Sports Me Phys Fitness.* 48: 447–454.

Spurrs, R.W., Murphy, A.J. & Watsford, M.L. (2003) The effect of plyometric training on distance running performance. *Eur J Appl Physiol.* 89: 1–7.

Stanish, W.D. (1984) Overuse injuries in athletes: a prospective. *Med Sci. Sports Exerc.* 16: 1–7.

Stecco, A., Gilliar, W., Hill, R., Fullerton, B. & Stecco, C. (2013) The anatomical and functional relation between gluteus maximus and fascia lata. *J Bodyw Mov Ther.* 17(4): 512–517.

Steven, R. et al. (1981) Role of fascia in maintaining muscle tension and pressure. *Appl Physiol: Respirat Environ Exercise Physiol.* 51: 317–320.

Tapale, R.S., Mikkola, J., Nummela, A., Vesterinen, V., Capostango, B., Walker, S., Gitonga, D., Kraemer, W.J. & Hakkinen, K. (2010) Strength training in endurance runners. *Int J Sports Med.* 3: 468–476.

Tippett, S. & Voight, M.L. (1995) Functional progressions for sports rehabilitation. *Library of Congress Cataloging inPublication Data.* 6: 74–75.

Witvrouw, E., Lysens, R., Bellemans, J., Peers, K. & Vanderstraeten, G. (2000) Open versus closed kinetic chain exercises for patellofemoral pain: a prospective, randomized study. *Am J Sports Med.* 28: 687–694.

Further reading

Bissas, A. & Havenetidis, K. (2008) The use of various strength-power tests as predictors of sprint running performance. *J Sports Med Phys Fitness.* 48: 49–54.

Chaudhry, H., Schleip, R., Ji, Z., Bukiet, B., Maney, M. & Findley, T. (2008) Three-dimensional mathematical model for deformation of human fasciae in manual therapy. *J Am Osteopath Assoc.* 108: 379–390.

Cichanowski, H.R., Schmitt, J.S., Johnson, R.J & Niemuth, P.E. (2007) Hip strength in collegiate female athletes with patellofemoral pain. *Med Sci Sports Exerc.* 39: 1227–1232.

Duffey, M.J., Martin, D.F., Cannon, D.W., Craven, T. & Messier, S.P. (2000) Etiologic factors associated with anterior knee pain in distance runners. *Med Sci Sports Exerc.* 11: 1825–1832.

Fagan, V. & Delahunt, E. (2009) Patellofemoral pain syndrome: a review on the associated neuromuscular deficits and current treatment options. *Br J Sports Med.* 43(4): 310–311.

Ferber, R. & Kendall, K.D. (2007) Biomechanical approach to rehabilitation of lower extremity musculoskeletal injuries in runners. *J Athl Train.* 42: S114.

Hennessy, L. & Kilty, J. (2001) Relationship of the stretch shortening cycle to sprint performance in trained female athlete. *J Strength Cond Res.* 15: 326–331.

Hunter, J.P., Marshall, R.N. & McNair, P.J. (2005) Relationship between ground reaction force impulse and kinematics of sprint-running acceleration. *J Appl Biomech.* 21: 31–43.

Grinnell, F. (2008) Fibroblast mechanics in three dimensional collagen matrices. *J Bodyw Mov Ther.* 12: 191–193.

Grinnell, F. & Petroll, W. (2010) Cell motility and mechanics in three-dimensional collagen matrices. *Ann Rev Cell Dev Biol.* 26: 335–361.

Hrysomallis, C. (2012) The effectiveness of resisted movement training on sprinting and jumping performance. *J Strength Cond Res.* 26: 299–306.

Hudgens, B., Scharafenberg. J., Travis Triplett, N. & McBride, J.M. (2013) Relationship between jumping ability and running performance in events of varying distance. *J Strength Cond Res.* 27: 563–567.

Kraemer, W.J. (1982) Weight training: what you don't know will hurt you. *Wyoming Journal of Health, Physical Education, Recreation and Dance.* 5: 8–11.

Langevin, H. (2006) Connective tissue: A body-wide signaling network? *Med Hypo.* 66: 1074–1077.

Myers, T.W. (1997) The Anatomy Trains. *J Bodyw Mov Ther.* 1: 91–101.

Shoes or no shoes during locomotion and exercise: Training potential for fascial structures of the lower extremity

Thorsten Sterzing and Torsten Brauner

Introduction

It is one of the most controversial and vivid discussions in the world of sport and exercise: Should I wear "regular" sports shoes, shoes with added material components, shoes with reduced material components, or no shoes at all during locomotion? While wearing shoes is generally considered to add a certain functionality, it may also prevent the foot from unfolding its full natural potential based on its sophisticated anatomy. Furthermore, wearing shoes may even prevent the foot from receiving beneficial training stimuli suited to enhance its functional capability. This chapter focuses on the effect of wearing shoes, or not, during locomotion and exercise. Until now, these considerations have been widely linked to movement kinetics and kinematics, as well as aspects of muscle activity. However, they have not been linked to the structural disposition or the functional performance of the fascial network or the individual fasciae of the lower extremity. As the role of fascia for human performance and well-being draws increasing attention, it is beneficial to understand how the fascial tissue of the lower extremity is affected by different types of shoes (or not) during activities of daily life, athletic training or physical therapy. Recommendations follow how to implement specific stimulation of fascial tissue of the lower extremity during locomotion and exercise training regimens of individuals, athletes and patients. These should aid interested individuals, as well as coaches and therapists, in considering another worthwhile component for their training or rehabilitation regimens.

Why athletic shoes are worn

Shoes form an artificial interface between the foot and the ground. Thereby, they influence the way people walk, run, or execute other types of locomotion and exercise. Importantly, not only the shoe, but also the ground can be varied during locomotion and exercise by using different surfaces present in natural environments, or by arranging different surface conditions in specific athletic conditioning or therapeutic environments. The whole body, but in particular the foot and the lower extremity, is affected by the combination of shoe and surface, which determine the functional circumstances individuals, athletes and patients cope with when contacting the ground during locomotion and exercise. While shoes and surfaces may be easily changed, the foot and the lower extremity with their formed anatomical structures and functional characteristics need to be trained over a longer period of time. Bio-positive stimulation eventually leads to a higher structural and functional level, while bio-negative stimulation, due to acute or accumulated overloading, eventually leads to trauma or overuse injuries.

For a number of sports or disciplines, shoes are an inherent necessity or provide an obvious advantage for their execution and related performance. Examples include ice hockey, soccer, or track and field sprinting. In activities where shoes are not a necessity, however, what are the reasons an artificial shoe interface is preferred over the more direct foot-to-ground contact experienced being barefoot?

The four core functional aspects, comfort, performance, injury prevention and training, sum up the main reasons for wearing athletic shoes during locomotion and exercise (Figure 32.1). Whereas comfort and performance provide instantaneous benefits to the individual, injury prevention has an acute component, when supporting the avoidance of traumatic injuries, and a remote component, when supporting the avoidance of overuse injuries. Additionally, certain shoes are regarded as specific training devices, when designed to provide enhanced stimuli for a bio-positive development of the musculoskeletal system of the wearer, which is not provided by regular athletic shoes. In this sense, barefoot, as the no-shoe condition, may be regarded as a training option, too.

When referring to athletic shoes as training devices, two well researched and also extensively marketed concepts are footwear minimization (Sinclair, 2014) and footwear instability (Apps et al., 2017) (Figures 32.2 and 32.3). Footwear instability concepts commonly feature additions to or variation of the shoe midsole and outsole construction, or reshaping of

midsole and outsole geometry, to create functional instability during the stance phase of locomotion and exercise. Thereby, it is intuitive that actual performance when wearing less stable shoes is decreased as a trade-off in creating increased training stimuli compared with regular athletic shoes. Footwear minimization concepts commonly feature a reduction of shoe material, involving components of the shoe upper and the shoe sole. This results in lower shoe weight but also in reduced comfort, mainly due to decreased cushioning, while on the other hand it induces more lateral stability, by bringing the foot closer to the ground, thereby reducing the lateral lever arm. Furthermore, footwear minimization concepts free the foot to a certain degree, allowing the numerous foot segments to act more individually, fostering pronounced

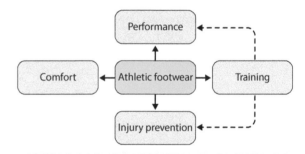

Figure 32.1

Core functions of athletic footwear, enhanced from Sterzing (2015), emphasizing the influence of the training function on functions of performance and injury prevention.

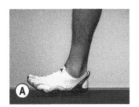 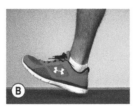 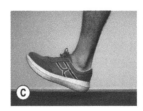

Figure 32.2

Examples of differing shoe concepts from various brands during running, ~20–30 ms before ground contact: **(A)** minimalistic footwear, **(B)** regular running footwear and **(C)** elastic instability footwear.

Shoes or no shoes during locomotion and exercise: Training potential for fascial structures of the lower extremity

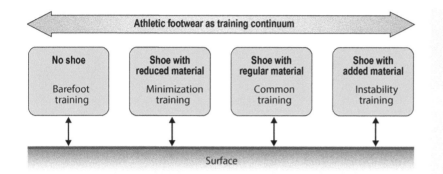

Figure 32.3
Material aspect of athletic shoes from a training shoe continuum perspective.

gripping of the ground. In this sense it is argued that the more "minimal" our footwear, the more we expose the foot to its sophisticated natural potential and therefore improve its functionality.

The current debate about the benefits of wearing athletic shoes, or not, covers direct biomechanical effects during locomotion and exercise. It also addresses if and how such biomechanical adaptations affect anatomical and physiological structures of the foot and the lower extremity in the mid and long term, in the sense of functional training. With regard to training effects due to the wearing of shoes, to date the structural and functional characteristics of fascia tissue have been ignored.

Biomechanical effects of barefoot, minimization and instability movement

In order to delve into the potential consequences of biomechanical adaptations to the shoe and surface type on fascial tissue of the lower extremity, we need to illustrate the main biomechanical alterations from barefoot, minimization, and instability locomotion and exercise. The effects are explained in comparison to locomotion and exercise using regular athletic shoes, as they resemble the "habitual" standard. While most of the available insights are related to analyses of walking and running, gym class or

dance movements should also be considered, as they often include variations of walking and running, like lunges, or steps and jumps in various directions.

Barefoot and minimization locomotion and exercise

During shod walking and shod endurance running, the rear-foot strike is the overwhelmingly applied foot-strike pattern. In walking, the rear-foot strike is widely maintained irrespective of shoe or surface type, as forces and regional pressures are comparatively low, and thus discomfort and pain levels are bearable in most scenarios (Fong Yan et al., 2013), even though they are reported to be close to the individuals' pain thresholds (Wearing et al., 2014). In running, the rear-foot strike is often changed to a more moderate rear-foot strike and, quite frequently, even to a mid-foot or fore-foot strike when running barefoot or wearing minimization shoes, as forces and regional pressures are twice as high in heel striking than in fore-foot striking (Shih et al., 2013). Adopting a mid-foot or fore-foot strike pattern during barefoot or minimization running is considered a balance between avoiding high pressure under the heel and bearing higher energetic expenditure. Consequently, a consistent application of fore-foot strike during barefoot or minimization running is rarely

Chapter 32

seen among general individuals. Differences in ground pressures for running with and without shoes are displayed, allowing visualization of the altered ground contact development between running barefoot and in regular shoes at moderate speed (Figure 32.4).

To avoid increased discomfort and pain during barefoot or minimization running, runners adapt their foot-strike patterns in an individual manner. Some apply a more moderate rear-foot strike, some use a mid-foot strike, while some exhibit a fore-foot strike. While these terms seem discrete in nature, we need to be aware that within the range of a pronounced rear-foot strike and a pronounced fore-foot strike, numerous variations of strike-type execution may take place, depending on the runner. Interestingly, changes in foot-strike behavior can also be executed purely voluntarily for the purpose of variation of training regimens, which becomes important when aiming to induce certain training stimuli for the fascial network of the lower extremity. Due to the strike type applied, the force transmission from the ground to the foot, and on to the lower extremity, changes its nature influencing respective effects on the muscular-skeletal system, as well as on the fascia network of the lower extremity. Whenever impacts are created by ground contacts, or propulsion forces need to be transmitted through the foot, these principles may be applied as they result in similar consequences for the tissues of the leg, and therefore on the fascia network (Figure 32.5). Being aware of these principles allows strike-type variation to be systematically implemented into training regimens by the individual, the coach, and the therapist.

Instability locomotion and exercise

Instability locomotion and exercise can be executed by wearing instability shoes during both everyday and athletic training movements, or by just executing such movements on unstable surfaces. Therefore, the instability induced can

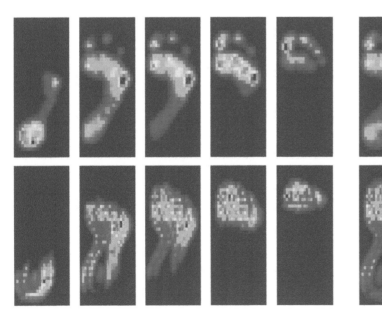

Figure 32.4

Ground pressures during barefoot (top) and shod (bottom) endurance running at moderate speed on a hard surface at 10%, 30%, 50%, 70% and 90% of stance (left), and peak pressures across stance (right). Barefoot running shows a less pronounced rather moderate rear-foot strike and an earlier foot flat during stance, while exhibiting high localized peak pressures across the foot sole, due to the anatomical foot structure not being shielded by the shoe. Shod running ground pressures are smoothened due to being distributed across the whole shoe sole.

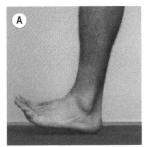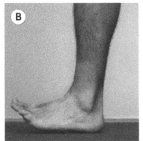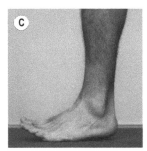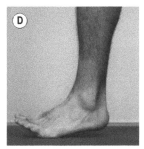

Figure 32.5
Initial ground contact during barefoot running with differing foot-strike patterns to illustrate the dominant ground reaction force attack location during **(A)** pronounced rear-foot strike, **(B)** moderate rear-foot strike, **(C)** mid-foot strike and **(D)** fore-foot strike.

have different forms. The basic form is referred to as constant instability. This is induced by shoes that do not change their instability properties, such as those featuring an outsole rocker or a soft outsole padding, and on surfaces that have consistent properties, like soft mats or sand. The advanced form can be referred to as varied or random instability. This may also be induced by shoes, artificial treadmill surfaces or natural surfaces, like trails. A commonly accepted effect of instability shoes is an enhanced activation of the small muscles surrounding the ankle, in response to ankle instability induced during exercise (Landry et al., 2010). Frequent use of instability shoes has also indicated an increased amount of movement variability: a factor considered beneficial, as it requires the wearer to negotiate different types of movement execution. However, it has also been shown that such movement variability decreases as wearers become increasingly familiarized with this constant instability stimulus (Stöggl et al., 2010). As a result, varied instability movements are endorsed, by proposing random instability footwear, or by movement execution on artificial or natural instability surfaces, for example, specifically adapted treadmills or trails. This means the individual does not become familiar with the instability stimuli induced (Apps et al., 2017).

Mechanisms of fascia stimulation and fascia response

Probable underlying mechanisms to be considered when addressing the effect of barefoot locomotion and exercise (as well as wearing minimization or instability shoes during locomotion and exercise, and when executing locomotion and exercise on instability surfaces) might be:

- Distal shift of plantar force during foot strike, causing increased fascia stimulation
- Increased foot segment activity, causing increased muscle, tendon, and fascia stimulation
- Increased ankle instability, causing increased muscle, tendon, and fascia stimulation.

Distal shift of plantar force

As illustrated in Figure 32.5, the plantar force attack location during pronounced rear-foot strikes and during moderate rear-foot strikes is beneath the heel. This results in predominantly bony force transmission, primarily originating at

Chapter 32

the calcaneus, leaving the fascial network of the lower extremity to some extent at rest. This scenario is changed when the plantar force vector attack location shifts distally, under the mid-foot during mid-foot strikes, or under the balls of the feet during fore-foot strikes. In these cases, which can be fostered by barefoot locomotion or minimization shoe running, increased loading and tensile stretch of muscles, tendons and fasciae on the plantar side of the foot occurs, as well as of the posterior side of the shank and of the knee extensors. In these areas, the higher stress during foot strike needs to be absorbed by the muscles, tendons and fascia, and can therefore be considered as an eccentric training of these structures. Under such circumstances, the myofascial structures lengthen during eccentric muscle contraction due to high external loads. By contrast, shod running predominantly fosters rear-foot or moderate rear-foot striking and, thus, the loading is primarily transferred through bones and absorbed by cartilage within the ankle and the knee joint. It is concluded that foot-strike alteration modifies the stimulation of the fascial network when the plantar force vector attack location is shifted from the rear-foot to the mid-foot or onto the fore-foot. Such a shift can be expected to occur more often when reducing shoe material or during barefoot locomotion and exercise.

Increased foot segment activity

Barefoot and minimization footwear locomotion increases the mobility of individual foot segments which, in turn, increases the activity of intersegmental muscles and connective tissues of the foot. While this intersegmental mobility causes extra activity of these structures during the complete stance phase, it is of specific importance during terminal stance until push-off. During this phase, forward and upward propulsion is generated. To transfer this force, which is generated at the ankle joint and transmitted towards the fore-foot region, the foot needs to stiffen. During barefoot locomotion, this stiffness is mainly produced by the intrinsic foot muscles and the plantar fascia, whereas during shod locomotion the stiffness of the foot/shoe unit is partially provided by the shoe. It is assumed that the stiffer the shoe construction the less stiffness needs to be generated by the foot structures, thus reducing the physiological incentive for the muscle and fascia tissue to be heavily involved. Consequently, it is concluded that long-term shod walking and shod running does not train intrinsic foot muscles and connective tissues as much as barefoot locomotion does, thus also having less beneficial effects on the functional structure of the foot arch (Hollander et al., 2017)

Increased ankle instability

Changes in ankle stability and related muscle, tendon, and fascia stimulation are well investigated for the muscle tendon complex during standing, walking and running (Apps et al., 2017). It is concluded that a decrease of ankle stability induced by wearing instability footwear benefits the stimulation of the fascial network around the ankle joint and the shank, alongside the previously mentioned stimulation of the small muscles of the lower extremity around the ankle joint.

Footwear training effects on the general fascial network and specific fasciae

As with all training, structural and functional adaptations of the bony and the musculoskeletal system, due to locomotion and exercise, need time to develop, as will potential structural and functional fascial adaptations. General effects on the fascia network are described below, followed by effects on specific fascial structures. At this point, such adaptations are only considered

Shoes or no shoes during locomotion and exercise: Training potential for fascial structures of the lower extremity

potentially, as sound scientific evidence of the proposed adaptations is not available yet.

Footwear effects on the general fascia network

In the following, wearing of shoes or being barefoot is analyzed for the effects of fascial structure and function. Biomechanical adaptations in response to differing loading scenarios show some already well-investigated effects on bones, ligaments, muscles and tendons. Two comprehensive reviews (Guadalupe-Grau et al., 2009; Karlsson et al., 2008) demonstrate that high-impact physical activities have higher osteogenic (bone-building) effects than low-impact physical activities, such as swimming. While less investigated, it seems reasonable that fascial tissue is also affected by these adaptations as the above-mentioned structures are permeated by the fascial network: the number of collagen fibers in fasciae, and also their orientation, is highly adaptable and reacts directly to applied loads. Consequently, in fasciae that are regularly exposed to increased loading, the number of collagen fibers along the load axis is increased and their orientation is in better alignment with the predominantly applied force vectors, whereas fibers of less mobilized fasciae show a markedly irregular orientation with respect to the predicted most important force vectors in locomotion (Stecco, 2015). Despite these insights into fascial structure and functionality, the complexity of the fascial network and the wide variation of fascial tissue have impeded sound scientific evidence regarding the relationship of physiological fascial structure in response to the loads applied.

Footwear effects on specific fasciae

Alongside the effects on the general fascia network, focusing on specific fascial structures allows further potential effects to be proposed.

In particular, specific fascial impairments are addressed as locomotion and exercise form a substantial part of prevention and rehabilitation regimens. While such regimens routinely consider the individual circumstances of a patient, reflected in the therapeutic motor tasks and their doses, little attention is awarded to the aspect of the shoe type worn during the execution of such prevention and rehabilitation sessions.

Plantar fascia

Two different fascia types, superficial and deep, are referred to. The network of the deep fasciae of the foot and shank are of particular importance functionally. The plantar fascia (aponeurosis plantaris) resembles a fusion of superficial and deep fascial layers. The combination of these two layers results in a fascial structure exhibiting high stiffness, due to the functional alignment of the deep-layer fibers in longitudinal foot direction, alongside high proprioceptive capacity, due to its connection to the skin of its superficial layer fibers. The plantar fascia is a key structure as it spans over the foot's whole plantar side, connecting the tuberosity of the heel bone (calcaneus) and the heads of the metatarsal bones, the balls of the foot. In this sense, the plantar fascia is strongly exposed to the ground reaction forces experienced during foot strike and push-off.

Several functions are attributed to the plantar fascia. Its main function is the stabilization of the longitudinal foot arch by absorbing and distributing loads along the longitudinal axis of the foot. Hicks (1954) has described it as beam and truss, as it is subject to bending during propulsion while absorbing energy during landing and over general stance (Benjamin, 2009). The forefoot strike pattern uses this load absorption and propulsion mechanism of the plantar fascia for transferring loads through the longitudinal axis of the foot. Several investigations link exposure of the plantar fascia to high loading with an

Chapter 32

increase of its stiffness, thus strengthening the longitudinal arch of the foot. It therefore is assumed that by fostering mid- or fore-foot strike patterns, running barefoot or with minimization footwear stiffens the plantar fascia, and consequently has stabilizing effects of the longitudinal arch of the foot. A study comparing the foot arch of 425 habitually shod children with 385 habitually barefoot children supports this assumption by observing higher foot arches in habitually barefoot children (Hollander et al., 2017).

High loading and lengthening stimuli of the plantar fascia are reported to have bio-positive effects in the treatment of plantar fasciitis, a common inflammatory pathology among athletes, usually experienced at the transition area of the plantar fascia and the calcaneus. This is interesting in the context of barefoot versus shod running, as the fore-foot strike pattern induced by running barefoot, or applied voluntarily during shod running, corresponds to eccentric training of the intrinsic foot muscles and the plantar fascia. Whether barefoot running should be applied as a therapy in people suffering from plantar fasciitis is, however, controversially discussed and extreme views on both side of the spectrum are put forward. Traditionally, people suffering from plantar fasciitis are told to avoid walking and running barefoot on hard surfaces as the high loads might increase the inflammatory response, whereas barefoot promoters assume that arch strengthening will eventually reduce stress on the plantar fascia and cite anecdotal evidence of reduced injuries in barefoot runners (Lieberman et al., 2010). Thus, further prospective investigations are needed to provide solid recommendations in this regard.

Achilles tendon

A further aspect of the plantar fascia needs to be mentioned in the context of potential footwear influence. There is compelling evidence that the plantar fascia is continuous with the Achilles tendon and, thus, not only transfers stress and loading between hind and fore-foot, but is also involved in the movements within the ankle joint (Stecco, 2015). This is meaningful because it has been shown that pathologies of the Achilles tendon should not be seen in isolation but in context with the disposition of the plantar fascia. Therefore, the tightness of the plantar fascia has to be evaluated and, where necessary, treated in patients suffering from tendinopathies of the Achilles tendon (Chapter 14). High eccentric loading is considered the gold standard for treating pathologies of the Achilles tendon and, as pointed out previously, is a direct effect of forefoot striking, which is promoted by barefoot running. Thus, biomechanical adaptations induced by barefoot locomotion are assumed to contribute positively to the treatment of tendinopathies of the Achilles tendon.

Patella tendon

The knee joint is another area of high axial loading, especially the Patella tendon, as the structure bearing the high loads generated by the quadriceps femoris plays a vital role in force distribution during locomotion. Interestingly, the Patella tendon is surrounded by a complex network of fascial tissue. In animal cadaver studies, it was shown that 15–20% of the longitudinal force at the knee joint is not transferred through the Patella tendon but through the surrounding fascial network (Yousefi et al., 2013). This finding draws attention within the context of footwear as footwear changes movement patterns not only at the ankle but also at the knee region, and thus intensely affects the fascial network surrounding the knee. In his study of the biomechanical effects of barefoot running on the knee joint, Sinclair (2014) concludes that the change in loading response might attenuate the risk of running-related knee injuries.

Epimysial fascia

Besides these distinct local fascial structures being affected, effects on the whole and complex fascial network, especially epimysial fascia, can be expected. Epimysial fascia surrounds and permeates muscles and is considered to contribute majorly to load transfer within and between muscles (Zügel et al., 2018). Similar to the function of the plantar fascia, epimysial fascia distributes and transfers load longitudinally. This aspect is of high importance in the foot, shank and thigh, as during locomotion high loads are transferred along the long axis of the leg. As illustrated previously, the fore-foot strike pattern causes high eccentric loads that have to be absorbed by the muscles of the foot and shank and, consequently, by the epimysial fascia, too. Recent findings suggest that micro-tearing of epimysial fascia and the presence of free nerve endings may contribute to the phenomenon of delayed onset of muscle soreness, often following the application of eccentric training stimuli (Chapter 16). Research of these mechanisms, however, are at an early stage and further progress should be expected in the near future.

Muscle septa

In addition to the aforementioned fasciae that contribute to the longitudinal load distribution, there is also stiff aponeurotic fascia tissue (septa), whose main function is the separation, connection and shaping of muscles and muscle groups from each other (Figure 32.6). Especially at the shank, these compartments need to be included in training considerations, as changes in locomotion are known to affect them. Namely, the interosseous membrane of the leg, the anterior intermuscular septum, the transverse

intermuscular septum and the posterior intermuscular septum, which divide the muscles of the shank into the anterior, lateral, deep posterior and superficial posterior compartments.

While these septa may not, or may only very slightly, be affected by the footwear type worn, they play a vital role, as sudden changes in footwear can result in painful consequences. The high eccentric loading of the shank muscles caused by fore-foot striking creates an effective training stimulus resulting in muscle hypertrophy, an increase in muscle thickness. Muscle hypertrophy is a mechanism happening at a fast rate, exceeding the rate the fascial tissue of the septa can adjust. Thus, the growing muscle within the septa induces compression forces that affect blood vessels and nerves traveling within the septa. This phenomenon is referred

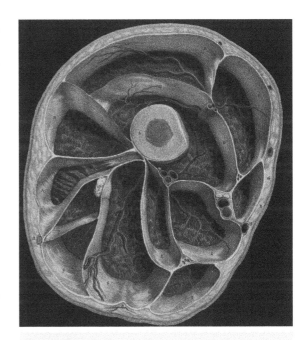

Figure 32.6

Muscle septa of the thigh shape the muscle compartments (Bourgery, 1832).

Chapter 32

to as chronic compartment syndrome and creates painful sensations due to nerve irritations and oxygen undersupply of the muscle tissue. To avoid the onset of a chronic compartment syndrome as a consequence of sudden changes towards barefoot or minimization footwear, a slow transition from regular footwear towards barefoot or minimization footwear is advised. Such a slow transition will allow the fascial tissue of the septa sufficient time to adjust to the growing muscle volume.

Movement coordination

Alongside the biomechanical aspects referred to, and linked to force absorption and force transfer, physiological sensation and subjective perception are worthwhile aspects to examine. There is a lack of studies specifically addressing the effects of footwear and their influence on physiological sensation and subjective perception within fascial tissue. There are, however, possible scenarios where footwear, or the absence of footwear, might alter subjective perception. In general, fascial tissue is highly innervated as various types of free and encapsulated nerve endings, including Ruffini and Pacinian corpuscles, are found inside. In particular, the epimysial fascia and the fascial network surrounding the Achilles and Patella tendons may contribute to the subjective perception of body posture and movement coordination. Running barefoot or in minimization footwear shifts the load absorption during foot strike from bony tissue towards the fascial tissue, as well as tendons and muscles of the foot and shank. Consequently, force absorption is directly connected to the tension of these tissues, while higher impact forces lead to higher tension. The highly innervated fascia network may therefore contribute to an increased awareness of changes in loading circumstances and joint angle position and can support movement

coordination control (Altman and Davis, 2012). Anecdotal reports of increased body feeling and control when running barefoot underpin the proposed effect.

Recommendations for individuals, coaches and therapists

While beneficial training effects on the fascia network and single fasciae have been illustrated, we need to be aware that no training magically changes body composition from weak to strong or from painful to pain-free. This also applies to the stimulation induced on the fascial network or single fasciae. Furthermore, while individuals, athletes and patients often have profound sensation of the disposition of bones, ligaments, muscles and tendons, less is known regarding their sensory awareness of their fascial network. While they clearly perceive better muscular strength relating it to the core contractile element of the muscle, this is different with regard to the tensile fascia components during muscular activity. Therefore, the success or failure of fascial training in healthy individuals and athletes is difficult to estimate due to inconclusive subjective perception and the lack of practical objective measures for respective validation. This differs when referring to patient groups, who are treated when subjectively experiencing inflammation and/or stiffening of the fascial network or single fasciae, frequently accompanied by perceivable discomfort or pain. The vanishing of such discomfort or pain then marks therapeutic success, also leading to an objectively measurable more efficient locomotion, alongside the regained practical ability to participate in standard physical exercise regimens.

Regarding training effectiveness, the dose of the stimuli applied to individuals, athletes and patients needs to be considered. While doses

Shoes or no shoes during locomotion and exercise: Training potential for fascial structures of the lower extremity

below a certain threshold will not result in bio-positive fascial tissue adaptation, applying doses above a certain threshold may result in an overload to the fascial tissue, which, similar to the more prominent passive (bones, cartilage and ligaments) and active (muscles and tendons) human skeletal structures, may be damaged as well. In this respect, the general training advice to increase training stimuli slowly and in response to the adapted tissue should prevail. When meeting these general recommendations, the likelihood to acquire a new and persisting injury are relatively small (below 3%) according to a study on 509 runners (Hryvniak et al., 2014). Furthermore, when teasing out further beneficial effects, 69% of the runners of that same study reported that their previous injuries vanished after switching to barefoot running. Research is also necessary to examine to what extent the fascial network adapts to the above training mechanisms, and to get an idea of threshold levels separating bio-positive from bio-negative fascia tissue adaptation.

Ultimately, it is not as simple as whether wearing shoes (or not) triggers beneficial structural and functional effects on the fascial network. It rather needs to be considered which type of shoe has which kind of effect. Based on the training or therapy objectives of individuals, athletes or patients, respective treatments should be executed, and certain shoes should be worn or taken off. In practical terms the use of instability footwear is recommended to stimulate the fascia network of the lower limb, especially the fascial network surrounding, crossing or inserting at the ankle region. By contrast, instability footwear, which sometimes appears bulky due to added material to the midsole and outsole, does not overly stimulate the intrinsic fascia tissue of the foot. Thus, for the latter, minimization footwear usage or barefoot locomotion is

recommended, which can be complimented by exercising on soft surfaces.

Finally, while it is easy to observe what type of shoe is worn or which type of surface locomotion and exercise are carried out on, this does not allow us to judge whether the physical activity executed is adding structural or functional stimulation to the fascial network. Such assessment needs to be based on the actual execution of walking, running or other training exercises. Using minimization shoes or moving barefoot will only additionally stimulate the fascial network when the foot-strike behavior is considerably changed and mid-foot or fore-foot strikes are applied, as otherwise the force attack location remains at the bony calcaneal region. In this sense, minimization footwear and barefoot locomotion can act as a trigger to execute strike types beneficial for facial tissue; however, these are not the purpose and effect by themselves. It has been shown that when barefoot, people often still apply rear-foot strikes, just in a rather moderate style (Sterzing et al., 2010).

Conclusion and perspective

This chapter has introduced three mechanisms of locomotion and exercise adaptation assumed to be beneficial for bio-positive stimulation of the fascial network and single fasciae of the lower extremity. These mechanisms are fostered by wearing different types of shoes or by not wearing shoes at all. Namely, they are (1) a distal shift of foot-strike location during walking and running triggered by minimization footwear or barefoot activities, (2) an increase in intrinsic muscular and fascial tissue activity present during barefoot locomotion, (3) an increase in ankle joint movement triggered by instability footwear. The topic of training stimulation of the fascial network by footwear is innovative,

Chapter 32

therefore this chapter has a derivative nature. The combination of future practical experience and scientific research is needed to verify the proposed mechanisms and, furthermore, to subjectively and objectively quantify respective structural and functional effects on the fascial network and single fasciae when incorporated in training regimens. For evidence-based guidance of individuals, athletes and patients, as well as of their respective coaches and therapists, to induce positive footwear-related effects on fascial tissue, the following information is needed: type of footwear, type of movement, time period of stimulation, and also certain characteristics of the individual. To date, sound scientific evidence is lacking to provide most of this information.

The effects of barefoot running, and especially the effects of mid- and fore-foot running patterns, on muscles and tendons, are already known (Altman and Davis, 2012). These effects will likely be transferable to the fascial network surrounding these structures. Thus, the eccentric training stimulus created by mid- to fore-foot strike patterns that are usually induced by barefoot locomotion exposes the fascia tissues of the leg, especially the foot and posterior shank, to high loading stress. This seems to provide the necessary stimulus for the fascial tissue to increase the number of collagen fibers and to adjust their alignment towards the applied force vector. Both adaptations increase the stiffness of the fascial structures and may contribute to foot arch stabilization and treatment of various pathologies of the plantar fascia, Achilles tendinopathy, and anterior knee pain. While we see these potential positive effects promoting at least a sporadic, if not general, inclusion of barefoot or minimization footwear locomotion into the training regime of athletes and physically active people, it has to be pointed out that research in this area is in its infancy and that future research is mandatory to provide therapists and coaches with the necessary information for standardized applications.

References

Altman, A. & Davis, I. (2012) Barefoot running: biomechanics and implications for running injuries. *Curr Sports Med Rep.* 11: 244–250.

Apps, C., Sterzing, T., O'Brien, T., Ding, R. & Lake, M. (2017) Biomechanical locomotion adaptations on uneven surfaces can be simulated with a randomly deforming shoe midsole. *Footwear Sci.* 9: 65–77.

Benjamin, M. (2009) The fascia of the limbs and back-a review. *J Anat.* 214: 1–18.

Bourgery, J.M (1832) Anatomie Descriptive Ou Physiologique -Traite Complet de L Anatomie de L Homme. In C.

Delaunay (Ed.), Tome 1-2: *Anatomie Descriptive Et Physiologique.*

Fong Yan, A., Sinclair, P.J., Hiller, C., Wegener, C. & Smith, R.M. (2013) Impact attenuation during weight bearing activities in barefoot vs. shod conditions: a systematic review. *Gait Posture.* 38: 175–186.

Guadalupe-Grau, A., Fuentes, T., Guerra, B. & Calbet, A.L. (2009) Exercise and bone mass in adults. *Sports Med.* 39: 439–468.

Hicks, J.H. (1954) The mechanics of the foot: II. The plantar aponeurosis and the arch. *J Anat.* 88: 25–30.

Hollander, K., Villiers, J. E. de, Sehner, S., Wegscheider, K., Braumann, K.-M.,

Venter, R. & Zech, A. (2017) Growing-up (habitually) barefoot influences the development of foot and arch morphology in children and adolescents. *Sci Rep.* 7: 8079.

Hryvniak, D., Dicharry, J. & Wilder, R. (2014) Barefoot running survey: evidence from the field. *J Sport Health Sci.* 3: 131–136.

Karlsson, M.K., Nordqvist, A. & Karlsson, C. (2008) Physical activity increases bone mass during growth. *Food Nutr Res.* 52.

Landry, S.C., Nigg, B.M. & Tecante, K.E. (2010) Standing in an unstable shoe increases postural sway and muscle activity of selected smaller extrinsic foot muscles. *Gait Posture.* 32: 215–219.

Lieberman, D.E., Venkadesan, M., Werbel, W.A., Daoud, A. I., D'Andrea, S., Davis, I.S., Mang'Eni, R. O. & Pitsiladis, Y. (2010) Foot strike patterns and collision forces in habitually barefoot versus shod runners. *Nature*. 463: 531–535.

Shih, Y., Lin, K.-L. & Shiang, T.-Y. (2013) Is the foot striking pattern more important than barefoot or shod conditions in running? *Gait Posture*. 38: 490–494.

Sinclair, J. (2014) Effects of barefoot and barefoot inspired footwear on knee and ankle loading during running. *Clin Biomech*. 29: 395–399.

Stecco, C. (2015) *Functional atlas of the human fascial system*. Edinburgh, UK: Churchill Livingstone.

Sterzing, T., Brauner, T. & Milani, T.L. (2010) Laufen: Barfuß vs. Schuh – Kinetische und kinematische Adaptationen der unteren Extremität, Biomechanik – Grundlagenforschung und Anwendung, dvs Schriften der Deutschen Vereinigung für Sportwissenschaft, Edition Czwalina. Hamburg, Germany: Feldhaus Verlag, 26–32.

Sterzing, T. (2015) Athletic footwear research: Effects of shoe construction and relationships of evaluation parameters. Habilitation Thesis, Faculty of Educational Sciences, University of Duisburg-Essen, Essen, Germany.

Stöggl, T., Haudum, A., Birklbauer, J., Murrer, M. & Mueller, E. (2010) Short and long term adaptation of variability during walking using unstable (Mbt) shoes. *Clin Biomech*. 25: 816–822.

Wearing, S.C., Hooper, S.L., Dubois, P., Smeathers, J.E. & Dietze, A. (2014) Force–deformation properties of the human heel pad during barefoot walking. *Med Sci Sports Exer*. 46: 1588–1594.

Yousefi, H., Baniasadi, M. & Rostami, M. (2013) The role of fascia around the patellar tendon in force transmission: an experimental study on sheep stifle joint. *Biomed Eng Res*. 71–78.

Zügel, M., Maganaris, C.N., Wilke, J., Jurkat-Rott, K., Klingler, W., Wearing, S. C., Findley, T., Barbe, M.F., Steinacker, J.M., Vleeming, A., Bloch, W., Schleip, R. & Hodges, P.W. (2018) Fascial tissue research in sports medicine: from molecules to tissue adaptation, injury and diagnostics: consensus statement. *Brit J Sports Med*. 52: 1497.

Further reading

Bramble, D.M. & Lieberman, D.E. (2004) Endurance running and the evolution of Homo. *Nature*. 432: 345–352.

Nigg, B.M. (2010) *Biomechanics of sport shoes*. Calgary, Alta: University of Calgary.

Overarm throwing in humans

Christian Puta, Thomas Steidten and Martin S. Fischer

Evolutionary aspects

Overarm throwing is a concert of single motions of almost all the muscles and fascia from the tip of the hallux to the tip of the index. Throwing conforms to an individual program: no two people throw in exactly the same way. It is a matter of talent, and even top athlete throwers can enhance their performance by just 10% (Thomas Röhler, personal communication). Throwing also shows the highest gender difference in a motion performance.

Overarm throwing has always been an effective long range weapon to keep predators at distance or injure possible prey. The oldest known javelins are only ~400 000 years old (Thieme, 1997). The so-called Schöninger examples were about 2.20 m long, 3–5 cm in diameter and extremely pointed. They weighed 600–800 g. Experienced javelin throwers can reach distances of up to 100 m with replicas of these oldest known javelins (Milks et al., 2019). Depth of penetration is similar to modern javelins with a spearhead and best when thrown at a distance of 15–25 m. Why do these evolutionary aspects matter? They give us an idea of the relatively short time of change, in evolutionary terms, which occurred to reshape the human body allowing the new action of overarm throwing.

Gender differences in throwing

As overarm throwing has been the basis of hunting in humans and, therefore, was essential for survival, it is interesting to learn about possible gender differences in this motion. Gender differences in bipedal locomotion (sprinting, marathon running and walking) are non-existent in prepubescent humans and times differ between only 6–10% after puberty (Bhambani and Singh, 1985). By contrast, the differences in overarm throwing are already significant in boys and girls and increase to 30% in post-pubescent men and women (Young, 2009). Four-year-old boys accelerate a tennis ball up to 42 km/h while girls achieve 20 km/h (-30%). Thirteen-year-old boys show a mean acceleration of 85 km/h while girls of the same age achieve 61 km/h (-30%), with the exception of Aborigine girls (-22%) (Thomas et al., 2010). No other action shows a greater gender difference than overarm throwing.

Biomechanics of overarm throwing

In experienced javelin throwers, it takes around 150 ms from the moment of the contralateral foot touching down before the javelin leaves the fingertips (Valeala, 2012). The javelin is accelerated to more than 100 km/h. The internal rotation of the arm generating the largest impulse lasts only a few milliseconds and is the fastest known action of the human body. The timing for a target-oriented throw is around 3 ms in experienced throwers and 10 ms in those who are less experienced. We distinguish three phases for the throwing action of non-athletes. First, the contralateral foot touches down. During arm-cocking the hip starts rotating, followed by the

Chapter 33

rotation of the shoulder. The arm finally acts like a whip and delivers the object (at the end of the acceleration phase). Figure 33.1A outlines the arm-cocking phase and the acceleration phase of the overhand throw during javelin. Figure 33.1B depicts a series of photographs showing the arm-cocking phase and the acceleration phase from a nearly perfect javelin throw.

Female throwers often start with the ipsilateral foot, which prevents body rotations, and the action mainly comes only from the arm.

In addition to the torso rotation in the waist, anatomical pre-requesites for a successful overarm throw are a close to double shoulder (biglenoidal width) than pelvic width (biacetabular width), and a reorientation of the shoulder glenoid that points to the side (greater abduction is possible), and which is no longer cranial as in apes. Finally, the humerus has 10–20° lower torsions than in apes. Together, all three components enable greater range and momentum.

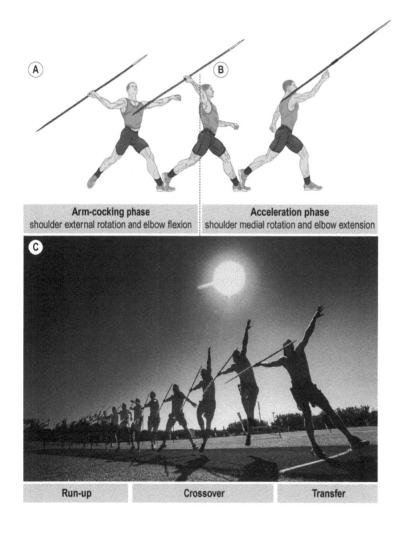

| Arm-cocking phase
shoulder external rotation and elbow flexion | Acceleration phase
shoulder medial rotation and elbow extension |

| Run-up | Crossover | Transfer |

Figure 33.1

(A, B) Arm-cocking and acceleration phases of the overhand throw, the relative timing of the cocking motions **(A)**, and the relative occurrence of the opposing acceleration motions **(B)**, adapted from Roach et al. (2013). **(C)** After run-up, crossover and transfer **(C)**, arm-cocking phase **(A)** and acceleration phases **(B)** follow. The nearly perfect throwing of Thomas Röhler, Olympic champion, 2016.

Torques are generated at each joint from the hallux to the fingertip, accelerating segment masses and creating angular movements. Internal (medial) rotation around the long axis of the humerus makes the greatest contribution to projectile velocity and is the fastest known motion in humans (Hirashima et al., 2007) shoulder internal rotation, elbow extension, and wrist flexion in all speed conditions. The study participants adjusted the angular velocities of these four motions to throw the balls at three different speeds. We also analyzed the dynamics of the 3D multijoint movements using a recently developed method called \"nonorthogonal torque decomposition\" that can clarify how angular acceleration about a joint coordinate axis (e.g., shoulder internal rotation. However, it is not the result of immediate muscular action, but rather of power amplification due to elastic energy recoil (Roach et al., 2013). According to the authors, the energy storage occurs during the arm-cocking phase, starting with the pre-delivery stride: "The positioning of the shoulder and elbow at this time increases the mass moment of inertia around the long axis of the humerus, causing the forearm and hand to lag behind the accelerating torso. Furthermore, a flexed elbow during the cocking phase enables passive inertial forces to externally counter rotate the arm, stretching the short, parallel tendons, ligaments and elastic components of muscles that cross the shoulder, potentially storing elastic energy in the large aggregate cross-sectional area of these structures. When the biceps deactivate and elbow extension begins, the arm's moment of inertia is reduced, allowing these stretched elements to recoil, releasing energy and helping to power the extremely rapid internal rotation of the Humerus." (Roach et al., 2013). Storage of elastic energy is a matter of connective tissue and, in the form of a dense meshwork, fascia in particular.

Soft tissue aspects of throwing

The role of fascial soft tissue in sports performance is underestimated. It is not only a passive tissue with the ability to store elastic energy. Containing contractile cells, free nerve endings and mechanoreceptors, it has an active role in proprioception and mechanics (Wilke et al., 2016).

As mentioned previously, overarm throwing involves torque generation throughout the whole body. Thereby, energy is stored using the stiffness of fascial tissue. Although it appears that fascial tissue should be very stiff, too much stiffness inhibits joint mobility, leading to impairment in the arm-cocking and acceleration phase, resulting in decreased acceleration distance and throwing performance. The torque generation does not happen in every muscle or muscle-soft-tissue complex separately. It is generated and transmitted through myofascial chains (see Chapter 13), involving muscles and soft tissue throughout the whole body (Wilke et al., 2016). Eleven myofascial chains have been described by Myers (2014), based on the principle of continuity of direct linear connection between two muscles. A recent review (Wilke et al., 2016), which addressed evidence-based findings about myofascial chains, showed that not all myofascial chains could be "approved". Analyzing findings for six myofascial meridians (i.e. superficial backline, superficial frontline, back functional line, front functional line, spiral line and lateral line), only the superficial back line, back functional line and front functional line showed strong evidence. In addition, moderate evidence was found for the spiral line and lateral line. This reveals that fascia and muscles are arranged in a body-wide network with the capability to transmit pain perception, stiffness regulation and torque transmission. With regards to overarm throwing, the functional frontline (M. (musulus) adductor

Chapter 33

longus, M. rectus abdominis, M. pectoralis major) is of special interest (Tittel, 2012). Each transition in the functional frontline (M. adductor longus–M. rectus abdominis and M. rectus abdominis–M. pectoralis major), could be approved by two studies with high consistency (Wilke et al., 2016; 2019). In addition to the functional frontline, the spiral line is also important for overarm throwing. Evidence could only be found for the cranial transitions above the iliac crest (M. obliquus internus abdominis, M. obliquus externus abdominis, M. serratus anterior, Mm. rhomboideus major et minor, M. splenius capitis), but not for the caudal transitions (Wilke et al., 2016). For high performance in overarm throwing, the ability to contract and stretch is very important in those functional systems. Disorders in these myofascial networks can cause functional impairments such as thoracic outlet syndrome, which is a common issue in "throwing athletes".

Thoracic outlet syndrome in overarm throwing

The thoracic outlet is anatomically defined as the area through which the neural and vascular structures pass from the neck to the armpit. It was first described by Adson and Coffey (1927) as scalenus anticus syndrome. As a kind of entrapment syndrome, thoracic outlet syndrome (TOS) is characterized by a nerve, venous or arterial compression (Archie and Rigberg, 2017). The neurogenic TOS (nTOS) is the most common diagnosis, accounting for 95% of all TOS incidences (Weaver and Lum, 2017). The compression of the brachial plexus can occur in two key sections, the areas above (sca lenus aperture) and (more rarely) under the clavicle involving M. pectoralis minor (Sanders and Annest, 2017). The diagnostic for nTOS is subjective in nature, creating controversy about its validity (Weaver and Lum, 2017). The preliminary diagnosis criteria for nTOS

are presence for a minimum of 12 weeks without being satisfactorily explained by other incidences, the symptoms being different to the distribution of a single cervical nerve root or peripheral nerve, and meeting at least one symptom in four out of five categories (Table 33.1).

Further assistive techniques for diagnostics are computed tomography and magnetic resonance imaging to identify bony or fibromuscular abnormalities, which may predispose one to nTOS. Another technique to assess surgical outcomes is scalene injection as a predictive tool. However, it is not clear if there is genetic predisposition to nTOS (Weaver and Lum, 2017). Other forms of TOS, such as venous TOS and aterial TOS entrapments, may be additionally present in patients with nTOS, affecting the arms when in abducted positions (Orlando et al., 2016). In overarm throwing in particular, this is a crucial aspect of diagnostics and has to be examined alongside the symptoms for nTOS.

Therapeutic range from surgical management to medical management

Although medical management has a high success rate with minimal complications, medical management is effective in about 70% of nTOS patients (Weaver and Lum, 2017). As well as for diagnostic purposes, anterior scalene injection is also used as treatment for nTOS, with a better response over a shorter symptom duration (Lee et al., 2011). With regard to athletes with nTOS, full function can be restored in one third by the use of physiotherapy only (Chandra et al., 2014).

Functional therapeutic aspects: scapula alata

In general, being upright against gravity within the first year after birth is related to the release of the upper extremities from the postural support

Table 33.1 Symptoms of neurogenic thoracic outlet syndrome (nTOS) according to Weaver and Lum (2017)

Categories	Symptoms
Principal symptoms	(1A) Pain in the neck, upper back, shoulder, arm and/or hand (1B) Numbness, paresthesias and/or weakness in the arm, hand or digit
Symptom characteristics	(2A) Pain/paresthesias/weakness exacerbated with elevated arm positions (2B) Pain/paresthesias/weakness exacerbated with prolonged or repetitive arm/hand use or by prolonged work on a keyboard or other repetitive strain (2C) Pain/paresthesias radiates down the arm from the supraclavicular or infraclavicular space
Clinical history	(3A) Symptoms began after occupational, recreational or accidental injury of the head, neck or upper extremity, including repetitive upper extremity strain or overuse activity (3B) Previous clavicle or first rib fracture or known cervical rib(s) (3C) Previous cervical spine or peripheral nerve surgery without sustained improvement (3D) Previous conservative or surgical treatment for TOS
Physical examination	(4A) Local tenderness on palpation over scalene triangle or subcoracoid space (4B) Arm/hand/digit paresthesias on palpation over scalene triangle or subcoracoid space (4C) Weak handgrip, intrinsic muscles, or digit 5, or thenar/hypothenar atrophy
Provocative maneuvers	(5A) Positive upper limb tension test (5B) Positive 1- or 3-min elevated arm stress test

function used in crawling. This functional process supports the gripping function of the hand and increased upper limb mobility for manipulation. The transition from multiple contact points (e.g. crawling) to two major contact points (bipeds) leads to a reversal of the punctum fixum and the punctum mobile concerning hand and shoulder girdle. For example, in crawling or climbing, punctum fixum is the hand (e.g. touching the ground or the fixation of a grip in climbing) and the shoulder girdle is the punctum mobile (e.g. moving the thoracic region forward). Conversely, with the hand upright for manipulation (e.g. grasping), the shoulder girdle works as punctum fixum to secure the manipulative function of the hand (punctum mobile). The gripping function of the hand must be postural when secured in the shoulder girdle. The shoulder girdle works as punctum fixum. The important basis for this free functioning of the hand is related to the myofascial control of the scapula position.

What does this mean for overarm throwing in humans? For example, as depicted in Figure 33.1, javelin throwing needs efficient torque production "from proximal to distal" (acceleration of the upper extremities while the lower extremities and the trunk are stable) for optimal performance and injury prevention (von Laßberg and Rapp, 2015). This concept was introduced as the "punctum fixum–punctum mobile model": the "punctum fixum" is defined as the part of the body that is fixed at the rotational axis, and the "punctum mobile" is defined as the free part of the body located most distant from the rotational axis. From a clinical point of view, inadequate myofascial control of the body part that is fixed at the rotational axis (e.g. shoulder girdle and scapula during javelin) is often associated with signs of neurogenic thoracic outlet syndrome. One other clinical sign of inadequate postural security of the scapula is the so-called "scapula alata" (Figure 33.2). The following functional changes are often related to the scapula alata:

Chapter 33

protraction of the shoulder, painful tension of the m. pectoralis major and m. pectoralis minor and the neck muscles, and an anteversion of the head. This malfunctional adaptation is often related to sternosymphysal syndrome (Brügger, 1986). Overarm throwing in humans needs the best possible myofascial functional positioning of the scapula as a pre-requisite for acceleration in overarm throwing.

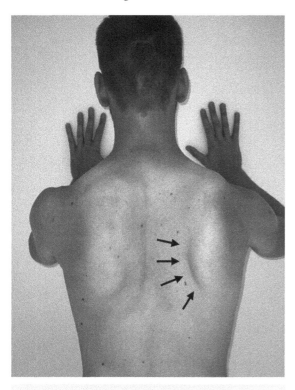

Figure 33.2 Clinical picture of impingement syndrome of the right shoulder. Note: Arrows mark the insufficient scapular fixation on the right side (scapula alata)

Credit: Christian Puta.

Overarm throwing is characterized by strong one-sided flexors, adductors and interior rotator activity in the acceleration phase, leading to hypertension, for example in the M. pectoralis minor and major. By contrast, extensors, abductors and exterior rotators are functionally inhibited. Figure 33.3 outlines four relevant myofascial and muscular connections (Benninghoff, 2008): (1) craniocaudal connection (M. trapezius pars ascendens–M. levator scapulae); (2) transversal connection (M. serratus anterior pars divergens and superior–M. trapezius pars transversa); (3) upper diagonal connections (M. trapezius pars descendens–M. pectoralis minor); and (4) lower diagonal connection (M. serratus anterior pars convergens–Mm. rhomboidei). As shown in Figure 33.3, hypertension of the M. pectoralis minor causes shoulder depression and reflective tension in the M. trapezius pars descendens. Consequently, the cervical spine is forced into lateral flexion and rotation inhibiting its stabilizing muscles (Mm. scaleni and M. splenius capitis). Because of fast shoulder protraction, high acceleration force in the cervical spine and the associated demand for shoulder and spine stability, muscles like the M. pectoralis minor, M. serratus anterior and Mm. scaleni are key, and are predominantly involved in functional impairments in overarm-throwing athletes (Figure 33.3).

In addition, shoulder stability is affected by M. serratus anterior inhibition. Therefore, it is recommended to implement extensors, abductors and external rotators exercises with a ratio of 2:1 towards their antagonists to prevent functional disorders in the context of overarm throwing in

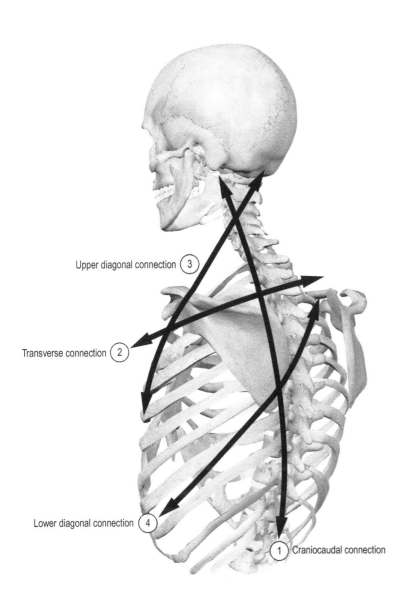

Upper diagonal connection (3)

Transverse connection (2)

Lower diagonal connection (4)

(1) Craniocaudal connection

Figure 33.3 Functional muscular connection of the shoulder girdle (Adapted from Benninghoff, 2008)

(1) Craniocaudal connection (M. trapezius pars ascendens–M. levator scapulae); (2) Transversal connection (M. serratus anterior pars divergens and superior–M. trapezius pars transversa); (3) Upper diagonal connections (M. trapezius pars descendens–M. pectoralis minor); (4) Lower diagonal connection (M. serratus anterior pars convergens–Mm. rhomboidei).

humans. Because of its importance to shoulder stability, special attention should be paid to neuromuscular training involving the M. serratus anterior as one functional main "positioner" of the scapula. As mentioned earlier, the functional front line and the spiral line are involved in overarm throwing by stretching and contraction. To restore myofascial function and prevent or treat TOS, myofascial release techniques are recommended to decrease disorders in those myofascial chains.

Chapter 33

References

Adson, A.W. & Coffey, J.R. (1927) Cervical rib: a method of anterior approach for relief of symptoms by division of the scalenus anticus. *Ann Surg*. 85: 839–857.

Archie, M. & Rigberg, D. (2017) Vascular TOS—creating a protocol and sticking to it. *Diagnostics*. 7(2): 34.

Benninghoff, Drenckhahn, Anatomie (2008) Makroskopische Anatomie, Histologie, Embryologie, Zellbiologie. Band 1: Zelle, Gewebe, Entwicklung, Skelett- und Muskelsystem, Atemsystem, Verdauungssystem, Harn- und Genitalsystem. Drenckhahn, Detlev (Herausgeber). 17. Auflage. Urban & Fischer Verlag/Elsevier GmbH.

Bhambhani, Y. & Singh, M. (1985) Metabolic and cinematographic analysis of walking and running in men and women. *Med Sci Sports Exerc*. 17: 131–137.

Brügger, A. (1986) *Die Erkrankungen des Bewegungsapparates und seines Nervensystems*. Urban & Fischer Verlag.

Chandra, V., Little, C. & Lee, J.T. (2014) Thoracic outlet syndrome in high-performance athletes. *J Vasc Surg*. 60(4): 1012–1017.

Hirashima, M., Kudo, K., Watarai, K. & Ohtsuki, T. (2007) Control of 3D limb dynamics in unconstrained overarm throws of different speeds performed by skilled baseball players. *J Neurophysiol*. 97(1): 680–691.

Lee, G.W., Kwon, Y.H., Jeong, J.H. & Kim, J.W. (2011). The efficacy of scalene injection in thoracic outlet syndrome. *J Korean Neurosurg Soc*. 50(1): 36–39.

Milks, A., Parker, D. & Pope, M. (2019) External ballistics of Pleistocene hand-thrown spears: experimental performance data and implic ations for human evolution. *Sci Rep*. 9.

Myers, T.W. (2014). *Myofascial Meridians for Manual and Movement Therapists*. 3rd ed. New York: Churchill Livingstone.

Orlando, M.S., Likes, K.C., Mirza, S., Cao, Y., Cohen, A., Lum, Y.W., et al. (2016) Preoperative duplex scanning is a helpful diagnostic tool in neurogenic thoracic outlet syndrome. *Vasc Endovascular Surg*. 50(1): 29–32.

Roach, N.T., Venkadesan, M., Rainbow, M.J. & Lieberman, D.E. (2013) Elastic energy storage in the shoulder and the evolution of high-speed throwing in Homo. *Nature*. 498: 483–486.

Sanders, R.J. & Annest, S.J. (2017) Pectoralis minor syndrome: subclavicular brachial plexus compression. *Diagnostics*. 7(3): 46.

Thieme, H. (1997) Lower Palaeolithic hunting spears from Germany. *Nature*. 385: 807–810.

Thomas, J.R., Alderson, J.A., Thomas, K.T., Campbell, A.C. & Elliott, B.C. (2010) Developmental gender differences for overhand throwing in Aboriginal Australian children. *Res Q Exercise Sport*. 81: 432–441.

Tittel, K. (2012) Das Ganzheitssystem in der körperlichen Bewegung. *Beschreibende und funktionelle Anatomie*. Munich, Germany: Kiener, 245–279.

Valleala, R. (2012) Biomechanics in Javelin Throwing. KIHU Research Institute for Olympic Sports Jyvaskyla, 2nd World Javelin Conference, Kuortane, Finland, 7-9 November, 2012. www.kihu.fi/tuotostiedostot/julkinen/2012_val_biomechani_sel72_42228.pdf.

von Laßberg, C., Beykirch, K.A., Mohler, B.J. & Bülthoff, H.H. (2014) Intersegmental eye-head-body interactions during complex whole body movements. *Plos One*. 9: e95450.

von Laßberg, C. & Rapp, W. (2015) The punctum fixum-punctum mobile model: a neuromuscular principle for efficient movement generation? *Plos One*. 10: e0120193.

Benninghoff, Drenckhahn, Anatomie (2008) Makroskopische Anatomie, Histologie, Embryologie, Zellbiologie. Band 1: Zelle, Gewebe, Entwicklung, Skelett- und Muskelsystem, Atemsystem, Verdauungssystem, Harn- und Genitalsystem. Drenckhahn, Detlev (Herausgeber). 17. Auflage. Urban & Fischer Verlag/Elsevier GmbH.

von Laßberg, C., Rapp, W. & Krug, J. (2014) Patterns of anterior and posterior muscle chain interactions during high performance long-hang elements in gymnastics. *J Electromyogr Kines*. 24: 359–366.

Weaver, M. & Lum, Y. (2017) New diagnostic and treatment modalities for neurogenic thoracic outlet syndrome. *Diagnostics*. 7(2): 28.

Wilke, J., Krause, F., Vogt, L. & Banzer, W. (2016) What is evidence-based about myofascial chains: a systematic review. *Arch Phys Med Rehabil*. 97: 454–461.

Wilke, J., Krause, F. (2019) Myofascial chains of the upper limb: a systematic review of anatomical studies. *Clinical Anatomy*. 32: 934–940.

Young, R.W. (2009) The ontogeny of throwing and striking. *Hum Ontogenet*. 3: 19–31.

The secret role of fascia in the martial arts

Sol Petersen

Introduction

We live in two worlds, one on either side of our skin. The very survival of the Ninja or the hunting wild cat is dependent on their alertness and presence in both worlds. Body-Mindfulness is the term I use to refer to this embodied awareness and aliveness. It is both a state and a skill to be developed. Awareness of the body is the ground floor, the entry portal to mastery of the martial arts. Body-Mindfulness is a calm, yet alert, open state of present-time awareness of inner and outer body experiences, including sensory stimulations such as pressure, touch, stretch, temperature, pain, tingling, physical movement and position in space, visual, auditory, taste and olfactory impressions and even our inner organ and gut feelings. The care and curiosity required to refine this skill naturally develops a deeper mindfulness of the mind and heart, with all its inherent complexities.

The quest for ultimate power and awareness in martial arts is ancient. Two thousand years ago, Shaolin and Tai Ji masters training tendon power knew something intuitively that science has only recently validated. The masters recognized the vital importance of the appropriate conditioning and strengthening of the fascia and connective tissues to build and protect the body's Qi (life force). They operated from the assumption that the Qi of the universe and the Qi of the individual are one and that we can recharge our Qi directly from the universal source. They cultivated the power of the physical body but also trained to circulate the Qi as light in the three Dan Tiens, the head, heart and gut centers. They studied to support the body's own healing wisdom with touch transmission, herbal concoctions and acupuncture. Science now recognizes these centers as our three brains.

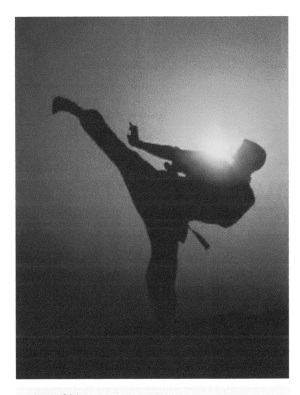

Figure 34.1

Shaolin Kung Fu training develops fascial strength.

SiFu Pierre Yves Roqueferre.

Chapter 34

What has not been appreciated about fascia until recently is how much we have to learn about its contractile properties, its elastic potential, and its important role as a global connector as well as a sensory awareness tissue. Research has confirmed that the body's extensive network of appropriately tensioned fascial sheets, tubes, membranes, wrappings, and fine and powerful cords, is not only the main connector for the functional fraemwork but the fascia is "how" our body holds its form, senses, and achieves its function in stillness and in movement. It is the architectural tissue of the body and, in many ways, the home of our innerness, our self-sensing.

As most musculo-skeletal injuries involve inappropriate loading of the fascia and connective tissues, rather than the muscles, the fascia must be considered an important factor in training, peak performance and rehabilitation.

The new fascia researchers define fascia more broadly than traditionally. They recognize fascia as permeating the entire human body as one interconnected tensional network, including tendons, ligaments, joint and organ capsules, membranes, dense sheets and softer collagenous layers (Chapter 1). In the new fascia training there is an emphasis on developing elasticity, of acknowledging the stress-responsive nature and tensional integrity of fascial tissue, of conditioning and hydrating the fascia for appropriate stress-loading, as well as appreciating its proprioceptive and interoceptive qualities (Chapter 15).

This chapter explores current insights into the role of fascia in martial art training. Fascia's new sensory attributes elevates this previously unappreciated tissue to a much more significant role in our body-wide awareness and explains why fascial awareness is one of the secrets for success in martial arts mastery and for a successful human life.

The mindful heart and the right technology

The Qi generated and expressed in martial arts practice follows the deepest intention of our hearts and minds, and, according to Chia, our fascial planes. "The fasciae are extremely important in Iron Shirt Chi Kung; as the most pervasive tissue they are believed to be the means whereby Qi is distributed along acupuncture meridians" (Chia, 1988).

How do we explain an event where a light-framed woman somehow lifts a car to save her child? Her shock and desperate belief enabled

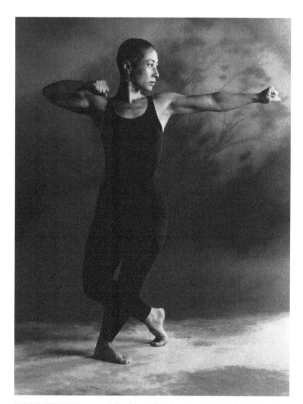

Figure 34.2

The Qi follows the intention of the heart and mind.

Harumi Tribble, dancer and choreographer.

her to transcend her usual capacity. Her muscles were not strong enough to lift the car. How did she do it? Perhaps, like a kangaroo, which does not have enough muscle strength to jump very far but can spring great distances with tendon and fascia power (Chapter 8), her focused mind, coupled with tendon power, took her beyond what we would consider possible.

Lee Parore, former trainer for world heavyweight boxer, David Tua, sees awareness as primary: "Technology is the key to high performance but we are often looking at the wrong technology. The key isn't machine training or muscle bulk. It is awareness and then self-awareness. It is a fire inside us that awakens the power in the Lower Dan Tien Energy Centre, below the navel. The lower abdominal musculature is double-layered because it's the main switch box for absolute Qi power. This life force floods all the conductive fascial channels in the entire body for vitality and regeneration" (Parore, 2013).

Fascial awareness – Is our fascia feeling our muscles?

Schleip considers the connective tissues as the global connecting network, a listening system for the whole body: "Science now recognizes this richly innervated body-wide fascial web as the seat of our interoception, exteroception, kinesthesia and proprioception, and hence the sensory base for our experience of embodiment" (Schleip, 2013). In fact, the fascia is six times more richly innervated than our muscles. So, when we say that our muscles are sore, it may be that we are feeling our fascia or that our fascia is feeling our muscles (Chapter 15).

Cirque du Soleil acrobat, Marie Laure, related that her refined body awareness was even more important than her core strength and endurance,

in her performances with her partner. One might assume that her impressive muscular power would translate into rigidity in her fascial and muscle tissue. On the contrary, as a therapist, I experienced her myofascial tissue to be surprisingly supple and her physique hardly bulked. McGill says, "The hallmark of a great athlete is the ability to contract and relax a muscle quickly and to train the rate of relaxation" (McGill, 2004).

"Measuring top mixed martial arts competitors, the ones who hit the hardest were not the ones with the biggest muscles. When a muscle contracts it creates force and stiffness- stiffness slows motion and velocity. The most powerful athletes use skilled strategic muscle pulses to create the highest speed and most effective force. These pulses are potentiated with strategic storage and recovery of elastic forces into the fascial system. A tuned fascial system is essential for high performance. The fighters with big muscles 'pushed' their punches and had less impact" (McGill, 2018).

Fascial awareness enables the martial artist to self-tune the muscles and fascia and maintain high alertness in their internal and external worlds. This is a practice of feeling with the whole body, sensing nuances in the balance of the other's body and then manipulating or deflecting the other's expressed energy to their own advantage.

Huang Sheng Shyan was famous for his powerful issuing of the Tai Ji-Jin elastic force. His training method involves precise attention to the internal changes of muscles, tendons and fascia. Patrick Kelly, Tai Ji teacher and author, speaks about this awareness, where internal relaxation means every muscle in the body elongates and actively stretches under the pressure, rather than contracts and shortens (or holds unchanged) in

Chapter 34

a tense resistance. "We can say that the basis of the secret is: Tai Ji-Jin is motivated by the Yi (mind intention) energised by the Qi, issued from the root and transmitted through the body in a wave of stretching muscles" (Kelly, 2007). Intense physical training, without self-awareness, will not produce the best results. There are many stories of masters stopping an opponent with their mind intention alone. This is the inner art. If we do not develop our inner and outer sensing, we will not achieve awareness of the space around us, of our opponent, or of the sword we hold. Quite simply, our fascia is a vital sensory organ in movement and martial training.

Building fascial resilience and fascial armoring

Iron Shirt is an ancient Kung Fu method that profoundly takes advantage of the stress-responsive nature of the bones and fascia. Wolff's law states that bone, in a healthy person or animal, will adapt to the loads under which it is placed. If loading increases, the bone remodels itself over time to become stronger. Iron Shirt strengthens muscles, tendons, fascial sheaths and bones, by subjecting them directly and gradually to increasing stress. The important detail here is "gradually". Internal energy visualization, combined with breath and body conditioning, are used to cultivate the Qi. "The Qi that is generated is then stored in the fascial layers where it works like a cushion to protect the organs" (Chia, 1988).

This concept of Qi between tissue layers helps to explain an experience I had with a Singaporean Tai Ji master in 1981. I was waiting at a table to ask if I could study with him. He walked out, smiled, reached across, pinching the skin of my forearm between his thumb and forefinger, rolling it back and forth in different places for about 10 seconds. "Yes," he said, "I can see you have

been practicing Tai Ji for a while. Good practice creates elasticity between the tissue layers."Lau Chin-Wah was a senior student of Master Huang. I studied with him in Kuching, Malaysia. Our practice centered on refining the form, Pushing Hands and White Crane Quick Fist. Sometimes Chin-Wah would throw his arm, as if it was an enormous wet rag or rope, against a stone wall, apparently not hurting himself at all. He said the secret was to totally relax the muscles and fascia of the arm and to condition and harden the bones to become like steel, by training with a partner, hitting bony forearms and shins against each other. This is extremely painful initially but becomes easier and may transform even the marrow and substance of the bones and soft tissues (Chia, 1988). Chin-Wah spoke of the cultivated Qi inside him, gathering, without his will, to meet the force of an attack. He said that when he was centered in his structure, his body and energy field, his fascia, bones and soft tissues became like impenetrable armor, enabling him to have a heavy roof tile broken over his head as if it were nothing. Our fascial system is capable of great adaptation to precise and progressive loading.

Fascia power training keys

Training for speed depends on our capacity to relax

In boxing drills, fighters need to become experts at letting go of all muscle tension. A system that is genuinely relaxed does not need to overcome tension to ignite itself for immediate response. "You don't want muscle bulk for true speed and strength in boxing but resilient fascia like Spiderman" (Parore, 2013). In Tai Ji Pushing Hands, the players must be willing to be pushed over and invest in loss, to learn to use elastic fascia force instead of relying on muscular

The secret role of fascia in the martial arts

strength to combat force. Master Huang was simultaneously totally relaxed yet totally stable. To push him was to feel drawn into empty space and then be sent flying.

Bruce Lee, the famous Kung Fu master, was not a big man. At only 1.7 m and 68 kg, he often defeated opponents who were both larger and much heavier. One day, he demonstrated his one-inch punch to a skeptical, burly man, who was astonished as he flew back 5 m into the swimming pool. McGill's perspective on this was that Bruce Lee did not hit with only the mass of his fist, but rather that his entire body hardened into an effective mass, so the fascia allowed him to hit his opponent with 68 kg (McGill, 2018).

When Lee himself was asked how he had done it, he said, "To generate great power you must first totally relax and gather your strength, and then concentrate your mind and all your strength on hitting your target" (Hyams, 1982).

The body's mind modifies your peripersonal space

Neuroscientists call the space around the body peripersonal space (Rizzolatti et al., 1997). Recently, brain mapping techniques have confirmed what my first Tai Ji Master said to me: "You must extend your feeling sense out around your body. When you move the sword through space, feel the length of it and the tip, as if it was part of your body" (Mak Ying Po, 1976). Similarly, in *The Body Has a Mind of Its Own* the Blakeslees, say, "Your self does not end where your flesh ends, but suffuses and blends with the world, including other beings. Thus when you ride a horse with confidence and skill, your body maps and the horse's body maps are blended in shared space" (Blakeslee and Blakeslee, 2007). The kick-boxer and the Kung Fu master both rely on the sensing mechanism of their body-wide fascial network to feel both their own self and the other. This enables them to respond without hesitation to the slightest change in their peripersonal space. As Master Huang said, "If you are thinking, it's too late" (Huang Sheng Shyan, 1980). The most profound training takes us beyond thinking to a new automatic responsiveness.

Tensegrity strength: stabilizing the myofascial framework

Those studying the fascial matrix have compared the body to a bio-tensegrity structure, a living structure of tensional integrity. Unlike a pile of bricks, our bones do not touch each other but are spaced by cartilage or soft tissues and the skeletal relationships are maintained by the tension and span of the global architecture of the myofascial system, in some ways like a tent. The concept of spreading the stress and tension throughout the whole body may shed light on how barefoot runners may endure less shin splints than runners in protective shoes (Warburton, 2001). Barefoot runners strike the ground more gently with more forefoot than runners in conventional shoes. This reduces the stress transmitted to the shinbones and joints and spreads it throughout the entire fascial and skeletal framework, where it is stored as elastic energy (Chapter 32). Balance exercises, such as slack line, wobble board, Swiss ball, and rock climbing, challenge and train our fascia and internal strength to develop spontaneous tensegral adaptability.

I observed Cirque du Soleil acrobats maintaining their core stabilization through "animal-like" stretches and play, consistent practice of their art, and specific exercises to strengthen the flexors, extensors, lateral torso and hip muscles for balance of myofascial tone in all three functional planes. They rarely seemed to train with machines. This core stabilization and core

Chapter 34

stiffening is essential for hyper-mobile acrobats to avoid injury. The capacity for a resilient yet mobile whole body stabilization is paramount for martial artists.

The no inch punch: preparatory counter movement at its most subtle

In boxing and Wing Chun punching training, much like the golf swing, we see the value in spring-loading and pre-tensioning to unleash the explosive punch. In fighting, it is vital that our intention is not telegraphed to our opponent. Perhaps the alert poise of the kick-boxer could be seen as a sustained pre-stretching of the fascial network, where the muscles prevent the release of recoil-power until the precise moment for the perfect delivery (Chapter 8).

Alan Roberts, Aikido teacher said, "In Aikido, Cheng Hsin and Jiu Jitsu, much of the purpose of the internal training is to develop the ability to strike with immediacy and power. This is even more of a concern in the sword arts, where efficiency, speed, accuracy and the unexpected are highly prized" (Roberts, 2013).

Huang was known throughout the Chinese martial arts world for his capacity to effortlessly throw opponents many meters. Not only was he not extending his hands and arms to do so, but, paradoxically, his hands almost appeared to be withdrawing as the person flew back, as if from an electric shock. In Tai Ji, the deep stance, focused breath and cultivation of Qi in the lower Dan Tien, as the weight is shifted, is a systematic spring-loading, ready to explode the issuing force.

Peter Ralston, author of *Cheng Hsin: The Principles of Effortless Power* (1989), when asked about Bruce Lee's one-inch punch, placed his hand on the questioner's chest and said, "You don't need an inch," then knocked him 6 m across the room, with little visible movement.

Actively stretching the fascia

Stretching is often seen as an important part of training. Yet how shall we best stretch? The classic holding of long passive stretches is not something we observe much in powerful primates or other animals. Naturally and spontaneously, animals roll, actively stretch against, scratch, push and rub their soft tissues and joints against the ground or trees, to neutralize built-up stress, and possibly to nourish and rehydrate their myofascial systems (Bertolucci, 2011). Interestingly, no other large primates in the wild appear to suffer as much from osteoarthritis or rheumatoid arthritis as much as modern-day humans do.

Our body is designed for active loading, walking, running, carrying, digging, climbing, etc. "We are hard-wired to move, for survival, pleasure, creative self-expression and optimal function. The body has an inherent vocabulary of movement patterns that develop naturally and concurrently with brain development and practiced coordinated movements. I refer to these as primary movements and postures. In cultures where people squat, sit cross-legged on the floor as a matter of course and walk barefoot at least sometimes, they cultivate their internal strength and fascial flexibility, which lasts into old age. On the other hand, many Westerners, even in their teens and certainly as they get older, struggle to squat flat-footed and sit upright on the floor. This loss of primary postures, movements and healthy fascial functioning is more and more evident in our chair-based society" (Petersen, 2009).

Our movement repertoire is locked into the myofascial mechanisms of our breathing patterns. Each breath is a physical and energetic impulse into the entire fascial network (Chapter 8). In martial arts, abdominal, reverse abdominal and conscious breathing is an integral part of a practice. The master realizes we are "breathed"

The secret role of fascia in the martial arts

by the universe and entering the universe of the breath is a prominent path within all meditation methods. Training of a powerful range of motion of the arm, spinal and leg myofascial chains in kicks, punches, blocks and evasive movements, amplifies the fascial elasticity and tone in both the core, the powerhouse of our internal strength, the extension of the three chains, and in the engine of our entire breathing mechanism.

Many trainers suggest not stretching immediately before demanding exercise but to warm up and mobilize the joints and tissues instead. Experience suggests that fast, dynamic stretching, which occurs in many kicks and punches, is beneficial for the fascia when performed correctly: soft tissues should be warm and abrupt movements avoided. Rhythmic controlled bouncing at the end range may also be effective, but for the elastic recoil, not the muscles (Chapter 8).

"Fascia research highlights the fusion of passive and active tissue. Tuning the interaction of these tissues is a higher concept than simply stretching. This enables optimal strength, speed, and power while reducing injurious stress concentrations. For example, when jumping: if the hamstrings are overstretched, only the active component of the muscle can create force. But great jumpers often have tighter hamstrings where they can time the muscle recoil with the elastic recoil of fascia and connective tissue, creating a higher resultant force. Thus more stretching is not the answer. Enough mobility is needed for the task but no more. The muscle creates force and so does tuned fascia. Consequently we have a better result" (McGill, 2013).

Train the fascia through Kata or Forms for total warrior fighting strength

"To prepare for mixed martial arts or real fight situations, it is important to realize, that functional strength can only be developed through exercises that not only work major muscle groups but also improve the condition and flexibility of the fascial planes," says 8th degree black belt Grand Master, Lance Strong. "Kata or Forms training has a huge effect on developing fascial strength and your ability to apply that strength in many different directions, while still maintaining your body's center and balance. Virtually no form of exercise, other than kata, tai ji or yoga, and some cross-training exercises, develops this ability" (Strong, 2013).

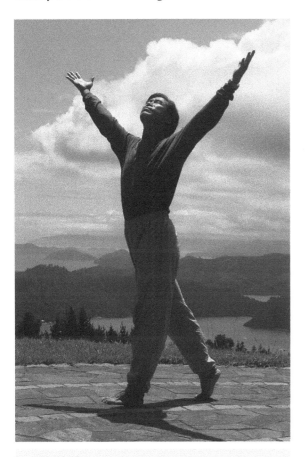

Figure 34.3

Demonstrates energizing the Qi in long anterior myofascial chains

Master Li Jun Feng.

Chapter 34

Conditioning the fascial body

It takes time to build fascial resilience: "It takes two to three years to build an aikido body that is elastic and strong enough for the training practice. Most injuries occur in the tendons and ligaments and are caused by over-training too early or trying to practice techniques more roughly than is appropriate" (Roberts, 2013).

The Shaolin monks knew that, for positive results and to avoid injury, they could only do the intense bone conditioning every second or third day. We now know that collagen has a slow renewal cycle with a half-life of approximately 1 year. Fascial tissues, particularly tendons, have a very slow renewal cycle. We may have little to show initially but then more after 6 to 12 months (Chapter 1). In fascia training, appropriate loading, and in particular eccentric loading, may be more important than repetition. With free weights or kettle bells (Chapter 22), medium weights are used to train the fascia, and heavier weights are used for the muscles.

To achieve the best results, fascia training is limited to two or three times per week. On the other hand, daily exercise has great value for our brains, muscles and cardiovascular systems. So we need to be careful with short intense boot camp trainings, as this often propagates compartment syndromes and fascial inflammation. We evolved to be physically active endurance athletes. So our new recognition of the potential of the fascia in movement and exercise should not distract us from appreciating the importance and absolute necessity of training our muscles. The fascia and the muscles are married, totally connected. To embody our physical potential, we must train throughout our life the whole myofascial network and nurture the whole body-being.

"If tolerated by the joints, training should include a component that demands 100% neural drive to the muscles. This is usually accomplished by training at speed. The actual static load need not be that great. Good form in all exercise promotes sparing of the joints but ensures optimal tensioning all along the musculoskeletal linkage" (McGill, 2013). McGill gives the example of a slow grinding bench press versus standing and falling into a push-up position, where the hands are on a low box, then immediately exploding back up to the standing position. The box height is adjusted so that this is barely possible. The neural drive is exceptional, as is the tuning of the fascia, passive tissue and active muscle tissue.

Finding the gift in an injury

In *Gift of Injury*, McGill documents a champion power-lifter, brought to his deepest despair with a damaged spine and sacrum, who applied the principles of rebuilding and repairing his skeletal and myofacial system to regain world-class performance. Many recognize the importance of assessment to guide appropriate training. When the system is weakened through illness or injury, a new motivation and a new training regime is required.

Finding the optimal dose of stimulation and stress (magnitude, duration, repetition and rest) is critical. Too little stimulation creates no effect and too much stimulation causes stress that damages cells. "Great clinicians hone the art of training to create the best adaptation for athletes at all levels" (McGill, 2018). "Mindfulness practice has a strong correlation with pain reduction making it an important skill in rehabilitation and trauma recovery" (Schleip, 2018).

Healthy fascia for a healthy body

The fascial web, rather than the muscles alone, provides a framework for storage and release of kinetic energy (Chapter 10). It governs the spring-loaded joint mechanisms for the leg, arm, spinal chains, the internal organs and the entire system. Without good nutrition and hydration, the fascia will let you down.

"The foundation for top performance has to be health. So before serious training with an athlete, I test the liver, heart, blood, and immune response and get the nutrition right so the Qi can move through the body. The fascia is a piezo-electric conductive collagen network, that when coupled with water, is the body's battery for energy. The highest concentration of mitochondrial DNA is housed in the brain, the heart, and the immune system within our gut – the three classic Dan Tien energy centres. The mitochondrial DNA are the power plants of our cells with the nuclear DNA being the structural blueprint" (Parore, 2013).

The body's acid/alkaline balance, hormonal influences, lymph and blood flow all have a strong effect on the fascia and this affects our fitness. We rehydrate fascia with an inclusion of appropriate resting times for tissue and viscoelastic recovery. Vitamin C is important in collagen formation. Scurvy, a connective tissue disease, occurs when there is a deficiency. An active life and light nutrition support the fascia and muscles better than a sedentary lifestyle. On a heavy red meat diet with saturated fats and refined sugar products, we may cultivate stress hormones and chronic inflammation.

Fascial restrictions and scarring can affect and inhibit a martial arts practice (Chapter 2). For self-care maintenance and injury healing, foam rollers, massage balls and self-massage can be helpful to release restrictions that can compromise our function. Some therapists use stone massage tools or powerful herbal liniments to reduce fascial scarring. New interventions such as injecting medical ozone, vitamin cocktails and prolotherapy assist in fascial strengthening

and recovery. Adhesions can also be released with integrative myofascial approaches such as osteopathy, acupuncture, integral aquatic therapy and structural integration.

Body-Mindfulness – training for the art of life

The path of the ultimate warrior is a path of awareness, service, love and protection for our community. It demands one to access the deepest qualities of the warrior: focus, energy, perseverance and dedication to a cause bigger than oneself. This heart, this spirit, is the essence of the internal power of the martial arts. It is essential for reaching peak performance, recovering from an injury, or building resilience to deal with the inherent challenges of life. The Buddha said, "Mindfulness is the sole path to freedom" (Goldstein, 1976). He outlined four pillars for the practice of mindfulness. The first two focus on mindfulness of the body, with the fascia now highlighted as the means of our proprioception, kinesthesia, exteroception and interoception. The second two pillars are mindfulness of the mind: the functioning mind we identify as the "me" and mindfulness of the path beyond "me" to the true Tai Ji – unity consciousness.

Contemporary Western culture and the media tend to draw us away from deeper body awareness. A committed martial arts practice is a daily returning to our self. True masters are rare beings who have achieved the ultimate physical expression and the deepest Body-Mindfulness, with the consequent fascial awareness and peace of mind. This is built step-by-step during a lifetime of training as they integrate their art into every dimension of their life and well-being. As Master Huang said, "Eat, sleep and practice Tai Ji" (Huang Sheng Shyan, 1980).

Chapter 34

Be assured, Body-Mindfulness need not be a serious task. To expand your myofascial repertoire is to become elastically playful. It involves bringing a new creative attitude, not only to your martial arts practice but also to simple everyday activities like standing on one leg to brush your teeth, getting comfortable with sitting on the floor, studying stretching with a local cat, and regular practice of the flat-footed squat. It is never too late to begin training. My student Stella started Tai Ji aged 85. She struggled to climb the stairs to the practice room and to accomplish basic movements. At 88, her practice had lightness and flow, and her balance had improved impressively. By 93 she carried her success in every step, reminding us of the adaptability of the neuro-myofascial body, even in old age.

In conclusion, to bring awareness to our fascia is to become more present and more Body-Mindful. This foundation of attention naturally leads us to more consciousness of our mental, emotional and spiritual selves. Cultivating Body-Mindfulness in a martial arts practice brings a fresh aliveness, an enthusiastic resilient energy, and a generous self-care attitude: tools we all need for a long and healthy life.

References

Bertolucci, L. (2011) Pandiculation: nature's way of maintaining the functional integrity of the myofascial system? *J Bodyw Mov Ther.* 15(3): 268–280.

Blakeslee, S. & Blakeslee, M. (2007) *The Body Has a Mind of its Own.* New York: Random House.

Chia, M. (1988) Bone Marrow *Nei Kung.* Thailand: Universal Tao Publications, 32.

Goldstein, J. (1976) *The Experience of Insight.* Boulder, CO: Shambala Press.

Huang Sheng Shyan (1980) Personal interview.

Hyams, J. (1982) *Zen in the Martial Arts.* New York: Bantam.

Kelly, P. (2005) *Spiritual Reality.* New Zealand: Taiji Books.

Kelly, P. (2007) *Infinite Dao.* New Zealand: Taiji Books.

Mak Ying Po (1976) Personal interview.

McGill, S. (2004) *Ultimate Back Fitness and Performance.* Waterloo, Canada: Wabuno.

McGill, S. (2013) Personal interview.

McGill, S. (2018) Personal interview.

Parore, L. (2013) Personal interview.

Petersen, S. (2006) *How Do I Listen?* Missoula, Montana: The Yearbook of IASI.

Petersen, S. (2009) *Cultivating Body-Mindfulness.* Missoula, MT: The IASI.

Ralston, P. (1989) *Cheng Hsin: The Principles of Effortless Power.* Berkeley, CA: North Atlantic Books.

Roberts, A. (2013) Personal interview.

Schleip, R, (2013) Personal interview.

Strong, L. (2013) Personal interview.

The world as a playground: Ninja and parkour training

Robert Heiduk

Introduction

A welcome side effect of the increased interest in targeting the connective tissue by means of physical activity is the comeback of traditional exercises with swinging and bouncing movements seen in German gymnastics in the 19th century. Reviewing historical documents, the reappearance of different exercise modes uncovers that only the sociocultural frame has changed: the new is only the reinvention of the forgotten. In order to understand a big picture we have to revisit the term "sport" as a complex sociocultural construct (Heinemann, 2007).

Over the decades and centuries, there have been substantial changes in social interaction of our bodies that are strongly embedded into the sociocultural background of the society. Many movement cultures have their roots in the preparation of warriors and religious rituals. The development and differentiation of modern sports in the 19th century replaced the ancient movement cultures with new intentions, like health promotion, alongside social, political and economic functions (Scheid and Prohl, 2012).

For example, the theme of the ninja warrior currently is used in an international sports entertainment television show, in which 100 competitors attempt to complete a four-stage obstacle course. The ninja warrior appearance in TV sports entertainment would fit into the part of the economic and entertainment orientation

of our society. Another rediscovery of the ninja warrior theme can be identified in the parkour movement culture. This urban subculture is characterized by the goal of getting from point A to B in the most efficient and straightforward way by using only the body's skills. In this context, overcoming any obstacle is a main characteristic of parkour, which shares common ground with the characteristic of the ninja warrior theme. Both movement cultures have in common that the connective tissue is used and trained to maximize movement efficiency.

In contrast to the economic orientation of the sports entertainment television show and other obstacle race mass events, parkour serves as a non-commercial countermovement to our profit-oriented highly technical society, one leading us to bodily dissociation and disembodiment, independent of physical abilities. It is also worth mentioning that other modern movement cultures (e.g. hardcore bodybuilding) serve to replace absent physical labor (Klaeber, 2014). The perspective of historical sport science shows that ninja training overlaps with sports such as climbing, and street-based subcultures like calisthenics, with their classical branch of gymnastics, alongside Georges Hébert's Méthode Naturelle.

The aim of this chapter is to use a bottom up approach to identify fascia friendly movement patterns in ninja style training and to illustrate how the involvement of connective tissues supports movement efficiency.

Chapter 35

Basic considerations

Ninja style training or parkour lead to a reinterpretation of our environment. A gym is not necessary, you simply use what the environment provides. In contrast to standardized movements, such as those found in gymnastics, yoga, and pilates, ninja-style movements must adapt to the changing environment. Depending on the dimensions, surface and shape of obstacles, single movement phases are extremely variable. Thus, an exact standardization is not possible and there is never just one and only way of overcoming an obstacle. Creativity plays a vital role, but the scope for creativity is strongly dependent on individual skill, strength, body awareness, perception of the environment, willingness to reflect on one's own actions, and an adequate estimation of one's own abilities. The fascination of effortlessness in overcoming obstacles is the result of deliberate practice. Besides prolonged mental and strength training, the internalization of movements plays an essential role to make movements unconsciously available in different situations. From a perspective of motor learning, the internalization of a movement aligns with using less strength, increased efficiency, fluidity and control, because of better coordinated motor programs (Hirtz et al., 2003). From a biomechanical point of view, if less force is used then more elastic energy storage must be used, as seen in Kenyan endurance runners (Sano et al., 2015) or good animal movers like kangaroos, which use their tendons to save energy and require less muscle work.

The following sections provide some basic cues on what you have to focus upon to become an efficient mover using the properties of fascia connective tissues. Before we start with practical analysis of some movement patterns, some general guidelines are important:

- **Safety**: Ninja training is not kamikaze training. Movement control is paramount. Never go beyond your abilities.
- **Sustainability**: Injury and long-term overload for joints and myofascial tissues should be avoided by using the approach of small steps. Sometimes a step back is a step forward. A movement accomplished once does not denote mastery. Practice movements on both sides to prevent imbalances. It pays off to train your weak or unnatural side to challenge your tensegral network and motor control in a new way.
- **No competition**: Our society and many sports educate us to become competitive at an early age. This ignores the individual foundations, learning and adaptation curves of each individual. The rejection of the competitive idea serves to prevent destructive behavior.
- **Efficiency**: The goal is to lower the investment of your resources to accomplish a movement task. Efficiency stands in contrast to effectiveness, where you invest all available resources to reach a goal.
- **Control**: Movement control is strongly related to safety. A controlled movement is fluid, smooth and silent.

Ninja movement patterns

Ninja movements can be classified as jumping, landing, falling, hanging, supporting, pulling up, rolling on the ground, swinging, turning, balancing, moving hand over hand, sliding, and quadrupedal movements. Together, these movements cover all possible human locomotion and, in ninja training, they are used on a regular basis. The following examples represent a small excerpt of the comprehensive movement

The world as a playground: Ninja and parkour training

repertoire in ninja parkour training. The selection focuses on light to medium skills that, to a certain extent, can be incorporated into a regular fascial fitness program.

Balancing

A pre-requisite for all ninja skills is balance. This is the foundation that permeates the whole spectrum of ninja movements. Different situations require very specific balance skills: to improve your balancing skill, many structures and techniques are beneficial. There are, however, differences compared with classical balancing skills, like those seen in rope artists in the circus. These artists usually turn their heels inwards. If you are balancing on rails or similar structures then this is not recommended because subsequent movements are restricted in the ankle joints. An increase in balancing speed can lead to increased balance in the short term but at the expense of control.

The physiology of balancing is based on the integration of inputs from the visual, vestibular and proprioceptive system. Looking at different people and their balancing strategies, it can be concluded that the relative contribution of these systems seems very individual. If someone has poor vision, it can be compensated to a certain degree by relying more on using proprioception. If we keep in mind that fascia is one of our most important organs for proprioception (Findley and Schleip, 2007), then working on your balancing skills can be considered as working on fascia as a sensory organ (see Figure 35.1).

Jumping off

To overcome obstacles, a parkour ninja must be able to jump off and achieve a large jumping distance. In this case very basic biomechanics come into play. Jumping distance can be significantly increased by utilizing a countermovement. The assumed physiological mechanisms behind the performance enhancement using a countermovement are described in more detail in Chapter 25.

Warm up for an experiment, then do three jump-offs from a standing position. In the first attempt bend your knees only a little (Figure 35.2A), in the second attempt jump from a deep squat (Figure 35.2C), and in the third attempt from a half squat position (Figure 35.2B). You will notice that the medium position (Figure 35.2B) shows the best result in jumping distance. In practice you have to find your optimal interaction of acceleration path and joint angles. When it feels good, then it is right. This is also

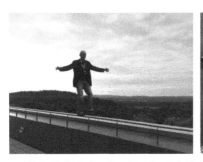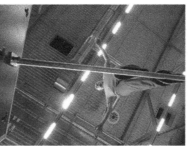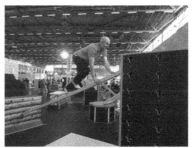

Figure 35.1
Balancing on a handrail in bipedal or quadrupedal mode is a valuable exercise to develop proprioceptive perception.

Chapter 35

dependent on your individual anthropometrics of the lower limbs and muscle fiber composition. A fluid coordination of single movement phases and body parts leads to another increase in jumping distance, like a perfectly integrated arm swing. If the timing of the double arm swing is inappropriate, then you do not achieve an increase in jumping distance compared to a jump off without using a double arm swing.

Landing and falling

Falling means that the body is in a downward motion that ends with an impact. Do not jump before you have learned how to land. Depending on the task, a parkour ninja must be able to land silently in precisely any position they want. This is of great importance in the precision jump, where a very small landing surface must be hit as accurately as possible without losing balance. The mechanical stress on the body for untrained individuals is very high in the precision jump (see Figure 35.3) because the landing is finished in a deep squat position on the balls of the feet. The sound intensity of the landing gives you a precise feedback of the landing quality.

A derivation for the purpose of fascial health is to perform barefoot precision jumps for short distances on different surfaces. Besides the mechanical properties, this form of exercise promotes proprioceptive feedback and a differentiated interaction with your body.

In order to prevent harm, the aim of controlled falling (e.g. after a depth jump) is the amortization of the energy of the accelerated body. Landing technique is of great importance for

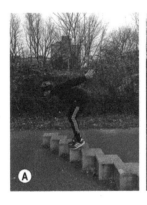
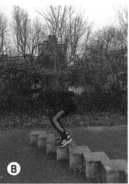
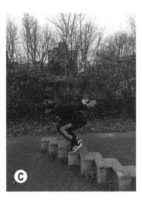

Figure 35.2

Jumping with different countermovement lengths. For each individual there is an optimal angle that leads to the best jumping performance.

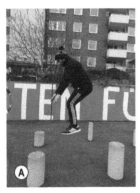
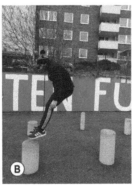
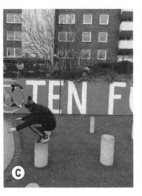

Figure 35.3

Precision jump on small landing surface with landing on the balls of foot.

amortization of the downward motion into a forward motion. There are different unrolling and bounced landing techniques to master this movement task. For example, the impact of a bounced landing (see Figure 35.4) is cushioned by a shift of the body's center of gravity and distribution of the amortization on arms and legs. By using the reactive force (Chapter 25), the vertical energy can be transferred into a locomotion movement. Note that when using the elastic properties of connective tissues, the ground contact time has to be very short, so that you avoid contact with your heels. A long "sit down" position would prevent force distribution and lead to high peak forces in the joints due to unfavorable joint angles (Luksch, 2009).

Hanging

All hanging movements can be considered as fascia-friendly exercises, because gravity provides a strong stretch stimulus on the whole body in every hanging position. They also represent very basic movement patterns that serve as a foundation for a number of skills. These additional skills promote complex flexibility and the movement skill of a ninja. There is no correct way of hanging when we focus on health aspects of fascia. The infinite degrees of freedom are the basic principle here. Thus, you can repeatedly change body

angles to target the desired fascial tissue areas. For example, take a deep squat position and hang up on a balustrade (see Figure 35.5). While you keep tension in the upper body, you begin to bounce in this position. In a ninja parkour progression this is the introduction to the cat leap or arm jump, in which the ninja jumps from the run-up onto the wall.

Monkey bars

When swinging from bar to bar like a monkey, grip strength is the limiting factor to mastering this skill. There is a ninja secret that uses the principle of an inverted pendulum in deviation movements: if you bend your upper arms, you are cutting off body-wide force transmission, using unnecessary upper arm muscles, so you are wasting strength. Bar to bar movements you should consider as a one-handed swing instead. Watch a gibbon's elegant swinging from branch to branch; they hardly bend their elbows in horizontal deviation movements. The same is true for children in the playground. They are able to catch bar to bar, but as a result of their lack of upper arm strength, they are unable to bend their elbows. Nevertheless, in order to train fascia you definitely need strong muscles. This gives us a hint for the importance of muscular strength training as a pre-requisite in order to exercise fascia connective

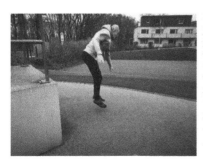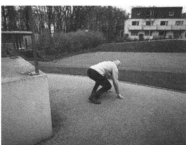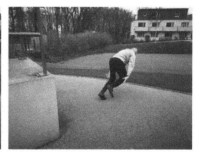

Figure 35.4
Example of a bounced landing technique with amortization into a forward locomotion.

Chapter 35

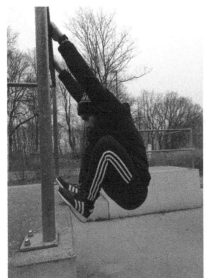
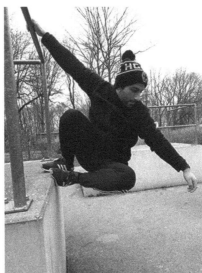

Figure 35.5
Examples of hanging exercises.

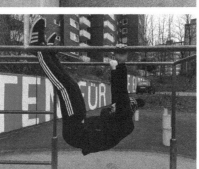

tissues properly. The muscles involved work in a quasi-isometric contraction mode while using the ape-style swing from bar to bar. Interestingly, the muscle's isometric contraction mode can also be observed in other movement patterns, where the elastic properties of fascia predominantly come into play (Chapter 25).

Bar swing, release and catch

In the bar swing, a classical movement from gymnastics, the momentum provides an additional mechanical stimulus for the connective tissues. For the ninja, it is the basic stage before progression to other bar exercises. From the swing it is possible to release the bar and to catch another object (see Figure 35.6). This technique takes time to learn, not only to find optimal timing, moreover to prepare the upper extremities for the high eccentric load and deceleration skill that puts tremendous load on the tissues. It is advisable that training volume and frequency are chosen carefully to ensure sufficient recovery for

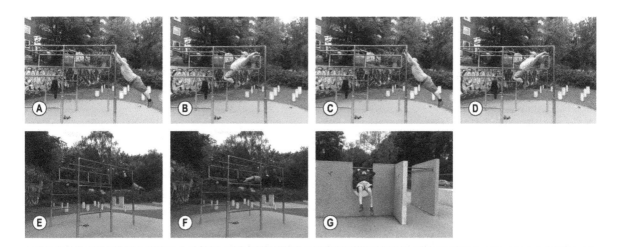

Figure 35.6

(A, B) Flying from bar to bar is a skill that even overweight people can master. (C, D) The difference to more advanced individuals is movement dynamics and the range of movement due to a superior strength-bodyweight ratio. (E, F) Using an underwing can be used in a breakthrough situation (G).

injury prevention. In the beginning you should focus on learning to control the deceleration in the eccentric phase. This can be achieved by eccentric exercises like lowering the body from the bar. Start with small jump distances of 10 to 20 cm, then gradually increase the distance. Mastering this skill requires lots of grip and shoulder strength, a clear example that you need strong muscles first to exercise fascia connective tissues effectively.

Supporting movements

In order to overcome obstacles supporting movements are fundamental and they are extremely rich in variations. Figure 35.7 illustrates a creative variant of the monkey or kong vault. We can observe three supporting contacts on the table that lead to a 180 degree turn of the body and a backwards landing. After the jump off the supporting contacts start in the first third of the table leading to short walking-style hand movements.

Summary

The inductive approach in this chapter demonstrates that exercise and the fitness of fascia can take many forms. Although there are no scientific studies elucidating its effectivity in this regard, ninja style or parkour training contains many components that may be able to trigger significant adaptations in the fascial connective tissue. In this sense, the high scalability and variability could make parkour movements a true fascial fitness exercise mode. Even although these urban subcultures seem to appeal more to teenagers to date, they could be a useful endeavor for adults wanting to break out of their usual movement patterns and habits.

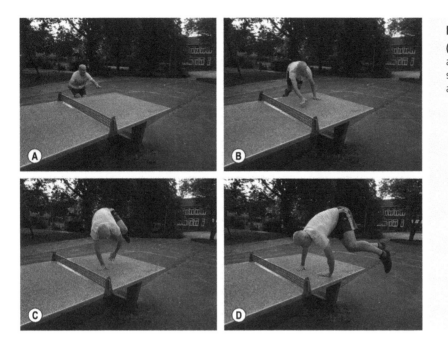

Figure 35.7

(A–D) Creative variation of an obstacle jump with three supporting hand contacts on a ping-pong table.

References

Findley T.W, Schleip R. (eds) (2007) *Fascia Research: Basic Science and Implications for Conventional and Complementary Health Care*. Munich, Germany: Elsevier Urban & Fischer.

Heinemann, K. (2007) *Introduction to the Sociology of Sport: Basics for Studies, Training and Work*. Schorndorf, Germany: Hofmann-Verlag GmbH & Co.

Hirtz, P. (2003) Koordinationstraining. In: Schnabel G., Harre, D., Krug, J., *Trainingswissenschaft: Leistung – Training – Wettkampf*. Germany: Meyer + Meyer Fachverlag.

Kläber, M. (2014) *Modern Muscle Cult: On the Social History of Bodybuilding*. Bielefeld, Germany: transcript Verlag.

Luksch, M. (2009) *Tracers Blackbook: Techniken im Parkour Training*. Germany: ParkourONE.

Sano, K., Kunimasa, Y., Oda, T., Nicol, C., Komi, P.V., Locatelli, E., Ito, A., Ishikawa, M. (2014) Achilles tendon moment arm for Kenyan runners. *Scand J Med Sci Sports*. 24: e269–e274.

Scheid, V., Prohl, R. (2012) *Sport and Society*. 7. Wiebelsheim, Germany: korrigierte Auflage.

Anatomy Trains in motion

Thomas Myers

Introduction

Given the new understanding of what Schleip has termed the "neuro-myo-fascial web" (Schleip, 2003) (Chapter 1), let us now turn our attention to functional chains of myofascia, known as "myofascial meridians" or the Anatomy Trains, to explore some implications of this point of view for movement training (Myers 2001, 2009, 2013, 2020).

Muscle limitations

For the last 400 years, our guiding light in understanding movement has been the concept of "a muscle" (Vesalius, 1548). Movement has been understood to be an interplay between the forces in the surrounding universe—gravity, inertia, friction, momentum—and the force generated by the ~600 named muscles working in concentric, eccentric or static contraction across joints limited by bone shape and ligamentous restriction (Hamilton et al., 2011). Muscle actions have been principally defined in terms of their origin to insertion on bony attachments (Muscolino, 2002).

Thinking more systemically, in the light of recent research (Barker et al., 2004; Vleeming and Stoeckart, 2007), the concept of a muscle working only to draw together its ends appears to be a limited metaphor: useful for getting here but now so outdated that it requires several caveats. For example, it is now clear that muscles also attach to other muscles along their sides

(Huijing, 2007). The far-reaching implications to force transmission and muscle mechanics are just being explored (Maas, 2009). The elasticity of large connective structures, such as tendons, changes our thinking about force transmission and efficient movement (Kawakami et al., 2002). Muscles also attach to and affect nearby ligaments (Van der Wal, 2009). The epimysium also attaches to nerves and neurovascular bundles which serve that muscular tissue (Shacklock, 2005).

Thus, the origin-to-insertion standard theory of muscle action misses out on (at least) the following four aspects, which we now know need active consideration:

1. Force transmission via intermuscular fascia to nearby muscles.
2. The ability of muscle tension to reinforce nearby ligaments.
3. The pull on nearby neurovascular bundles.
4. Force transmission from segment to segment via fascial continuities spanning the joints (Tietze, 1921; Franklyn-Miller et al., 2009).

Fascial neurology

On the neurological side, the nervous system appears to be about six times more sensorially interested in what goes on in the fascial matrix than it does in detecting changes in the muscle itself (Van der Wal, 2009; Grunwald, 2017).

Chapter 36

In other words for each muscle spindle detecting length changes, there is an order of magnitude more stretch receptors in the fascia that, depending on their arrangement, can detect load, stretch, vibration, pressure, shear, or convey pain.

Furthermore, no representation of individual muscles has been found within the sensory or motor cortex of the brain. The nervous system works in terms of a cybernetic, or self-regulating system, managing individual neuro-motor units governing in the order of 10–100 muscle cells within a muscle (Williams, 1995). The brain organizes movement in terms of coordinating these individual units, but not as our anatomy books do, in terms of individually named muscles. This means that the topology of contraction and fascial plane movement within muscles (perimysium) and between them (intermuscular septa) during any motion are far more complex than we have previously assumed (Fukunaga et al., 2010).

Biotensegrity

Another limitation to our current thinking is indicated by the "biotensegrity" model, which has been applied to the whole body (Fuller, 1975; Levin, 2003; Myers, 2009; Scarr, 2008), and to cellular structure and peri-cellular mechanotransduction (Ingber, 1998; Horowitz, 1999). This engineering model allows us to go beyond the usual Newtonian thinking in terms of the forces and vectors of muscles on joints, and enables us to see how our 70 trillion cells hang together in one organism as an "adhesome" (Zaidel-Bar et al., 2007; Zamir and Geiger, 2001), and how the "neuromyofascial web" accommodates movement as a self-adjusting whole. The Anatomy Trains maps out

a set of connected tissues in the parietal myofascia that essentially form the outer tensional network, which pulls in on the skeleton to help keep it erect and in the proper relationship (or not, in dysfunction).

> In summary, from either a fascial, neurological or biomechanical point of view, the ubiquitous concept of "a distinct muscle" turns out to be an artifact of our common dissection method, and is neither a biomechanical nor a neurological reality. This idea has yet to penetrate the professional populace working with the public in either rehabilitative or training terms.

Once we reject the old idea, the significance of all these new findings taken together can be summed up in one word: resilience. All the factors named above contribute to the resilience of human tissue and to rapid global and local distribution of strain and differentiated response of the organism as a whole. The "isolated muscle theory" that has predominated our thinking has limited our perception of this body-wide "give" that is essential to resilience.

Anatomy Trains

The Anatomy Trains myofascial meridians map is one small aspect of this larger vision, and concerns consistent longitudinal connections within the singular fascial webbing. It posits myofascial force transmission, at the very least in the stabilizing of movement and in postural compensation, from one myofascial unit to another along these lines. To construct the Anatomy Trains map, we look for consistent fiber direction and fascial plane level. In this light, 12 myofascial meridians, each of at least three muscles, have been described.

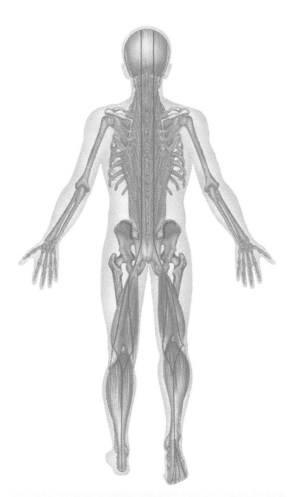

Figure 36.1 Superficial back line

The superficial back line, which traverses the posterior aspect of the body from toes to nose, operates functionally to bring our eyes up to positions that satisfy our curiosity, and lifts our body upright and keeps it posturally stable.

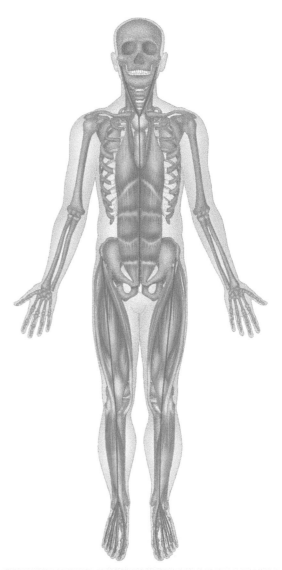

Figure 36.2 Superficial front line

The superficial front line, which traverses the anterior surface of the body, protects the ventral cavity and is thus associated with the startle response, and creates trunk flexion with leg extension.

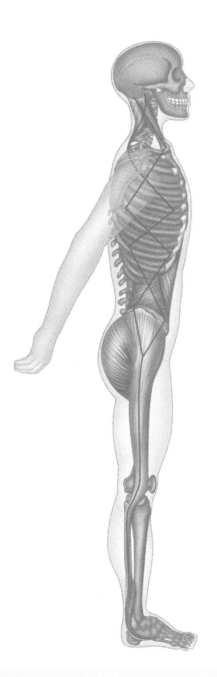

Figure 36.3 Lateral line

The lateral line, which runs from outer arch to ear, operates to create lateral bends or to prevent lateral bends to the opposite side. Thus, the lateral line operates to maintain stability during locomotion.

Trikonasana

Although difficult on the printed page, let us put the anatomy trains map into motion, by looking at a common but complex yoga pose, Trikonasana (or triangle pose), in terms of the Anatomy Trains lines (see Figure 36.8). A good analysis would require seeing the pose executed to both right and left, to see the differences from right to left. Based on this one photograph, we can see good form in the legs, with the lateral line on the left side being evenly elongated from the outer ankle to the hip, and the deep front line up the inside back of the right leg up to the pelvic floor on that side.

In the upper body, we see more compensation, not in the upper lateral line, but in the upper spiral line. From her right anterior superior iliac spine (ASIS), the internal and contralateral external oblique and the serratus anterior on the left ribcage is sufficiently short to pull the left ribcage forward so that the breastbone faces down towards the ground. The extra twist is required as compensation in the neck and in resisting the left shoulder coming forward.

Conversely, the left spiral line, from the left ASIS passing down and under her right ribcage to the right scapula and on to the left side of the head, could be considered to be too weak and in need of some strengthening to bring the right ribs further forward and allow the twist in the torso to straighten. We can wager that, if it is an imbalance in the spiral line, the pose would look significantly different on the other side.

Perhaps our premise is wrong and the inability to rotate the torso is not due to an imbalance in the spiral line but is in the rotational muscles closer to the spine, perhaps the psoas complex in the front or the multifidus complex in the back. We would test this with palpatory or movement assessments to isolate whether the restriction was in either the neuro-motor patterning or the fascia connected to the spiral line, superficial back line, or the deep front line. Any or all of these together could be the cause of this appar ent limitation in movement. Of course, it is possible

(Continued)

that the compensation is due to a structural anomaly within the spine, which we could detect by "end-feel" in the movement assessment.

The author makes no claim as to the exclusive nature of the Anatomy Trains. Firstly, those with significant deviance from the usual structure, as in a significant scoliosis or alteration from trauma, may create their own fascial "lines of transmission". Secondly, the actuality of force transmission along the myofascial meridians is strongly suggested by some literature (Vleeming and Stoeckart, 2007; Franklin-Miller et al., 2009) but has yet to be proven by scientific research. The author is confident that something of this nature will prove to be the case, but meantime *caveat lector* (reader beware).

Proportional movement

In the stability/mobility (stiffness/control) modeling of human movement, the anatomy trains contribute to both. The key to the difference can be summed up as "proportional movement".

All biological structures are granted a bit of "give". Even living bone demonstrates resilience, although it reduces as the body grows older. Every softer tissue, from cartilage to ligament to tendon to fascia to nerve to every other named tissue, will bend or stretch or deform either a little or a lot before it tears or breaks.

In movement, tissues are commonly taken beyond their resting length into a process of stretch. The stretch is translated into both the cells, of all tissues along the line, as well as the

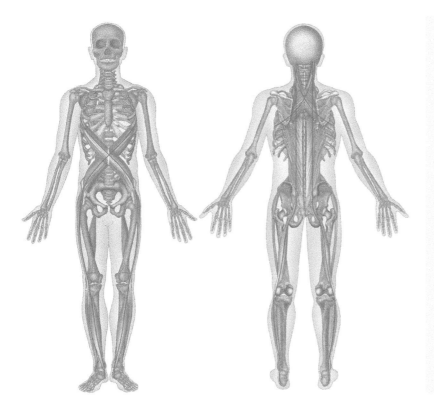

Figure 36.4 Spiral line (front and back view)

The spiral line winds around the body through the previous three cardinal lines, creating and modulating rotational and oblique movements in gait and sport.

Chapter 36

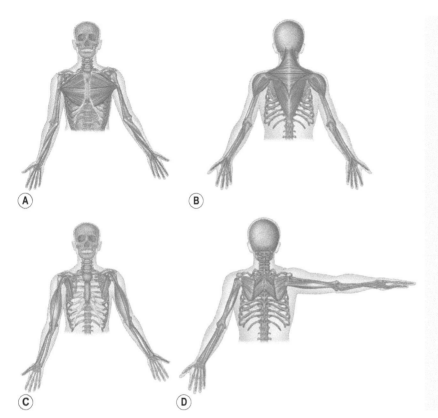

(A)

(B)

(C)

(D)

Figure 36.5 Arm lines
The four arm lines stabilize and move the arms and shoulders through their wide range of motion.

fibers and gels of the interstitia (Ingber, 2006; Langevin et al., 2006).

Given that the bearing point between the bones, at any given moment, constitutes the fulcrum for such tissue stretch, and given that the exogenous forces bearing on the tissues are within that tissue's ability to stay intact, then we can logically conclude that the largest movement will be near the skin, farthest away from that axial point. The rim of the wheel moves more than the hub. Therefore, the sensory endings in the skin will be most sensitive to initiated movement.

Also, if we accept the notion that the body will distribute such strain both laterally and longitudinally, then there must be a slight "give" or resilience in the tissues around the joints.

These tissues are called "muscle attachments" in classical theory, or more generally "peri-articular tissues". In the Anatomy Trains metaphor we call them "stations" to indicate that, even although the connective tissues in those areas are stuck down to the underlying joint capsule or periostea, there is a fundamental continuity of the connective tissue fibers in both direction and plane into the next segment and often onto a different muscle.

Anatomy Trains in motion

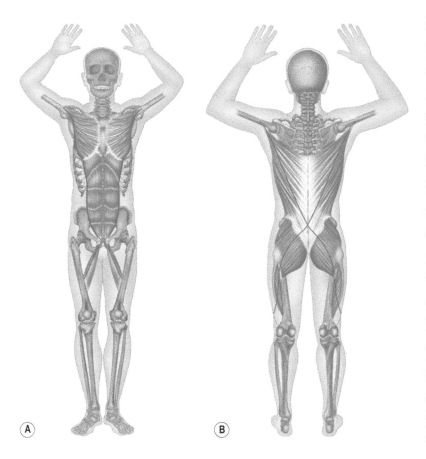

(A)　　(B)

Figure 36.6 Functional lines
The three functional lines stabilize the shoulders to the contralateral and ipsilateral legs, extending the lever arms of the limbs through the trunk.

Resilience

As an example of resilience, the spiral line posits a continuity from the tibialis anterior of the anterior crural compartment with the anterior portion of the iliotibial tract, which in turn connects to the tensor fasciae latae and thus to the anterior superior iliac spine.

The lateral line suggests a connection from the long fibularis muscle (peroneus longus) across the fibular head at the superior end of the lateral compartment onto the central part of the iliotibial tract and up via the aponeurosis of gluteus medius to a wide attachment on the iliac crest. Deep to this line would be the lateral collateral ligament (LCL), connecting the fibular head to the lateral condyle of the femur just above the joint capsule. Deep to the LCL would be the joint capsule itself, which includes the cruciate ligaments.

Although these fascial structures are identified separately, the outside of the knee is a fascial continuity from skin to bone, so all of these structures are connected. There is no discontinuity in

Chapter 36

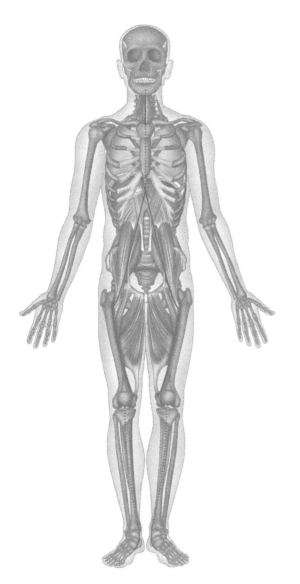

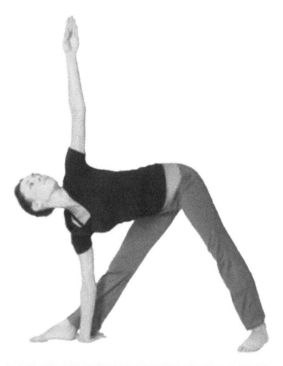

Figure 36.8 Analysis of a yoga pose

Putting our hands just below the bra line on either side and encouraging the ribcage toward a left rotation will reveal which tissues are restraining the motion, so that specific and appropriate movement cues or manual therapy may be applied to create even tone along the line.

Figure 36.7 Deep front line

The deep front line, which runs from the inner arch to the underside of the skull and includes all of what could be termed the body's core, supports the stability and axial-appendicular extension in all our movements.

the tissue (Guimberteau, 2004). So the following question arises: In day-to-day functional movement, or in more strenuous high-performance movement occasioned by sport, dance, or an impending injury, can the tissue "give" enough to allow the force to be distributed more widely or will all the force be focused on a particular structure, which is then more likely to fail?

Obviously, too much "give" in these structures would contribute to joint instability and

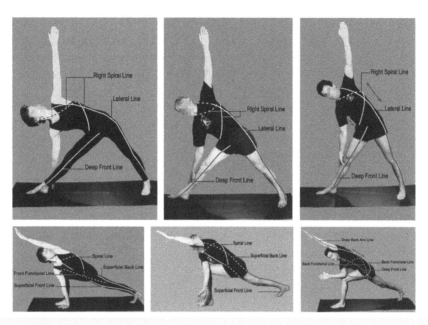

Figure 36.9 Yoga photographs from anatomy trains

Reproduced with kind permission from Thomas Myers.

In the pictures, we can see a teacher, an experienced student, and a neophyte, all performing the same poses. We can readily see how the lines become straighter and more even in tone with developing practice. This palintonicity is a hallmark of elongated and balanced posture, stabilized functional movement, and provides the greatest access to resilience along and deep to the lines.

those with "ligamentous laxity" can experience joint subluxation or malalignment fairly easily (Milhorat et al., 2007). Less obviously, too much stiffness means more strain localization, which can contribute to local structures, the LCL, medial collateral ligament or anterior cruciate ligament, for instance, being strained to the point of tearing.

The ideal lies somewhere in the middle: enough give to allow for strain distribution but not enough to allow for too much joint play. The factors involved in the ideal set point depend on the genetic predisposition to fascial build-up within the individual, as well as their training and performance demands.

If we could magically observe, in a healthy living body, a cross-layer slice from the skin down to the outside of the knee capsule during a long lateral reach, like the top of a tennis serve, we would see each successive layer moving on the one below from the surface down to the nearly immoveable bone-to-bone layer. This resilience, or lack thereof, can be felt when placing the hands inside and outside a knee when such a movement is performed. By doing this, with a number of different subjects, it is easy to tell where the resilience is too tough, so non-compliant as to lead to a tearing injury in some nearby weaker tissue, or too tender and overly compliant, thus likely to lead to joint displacement.

Chapter 36

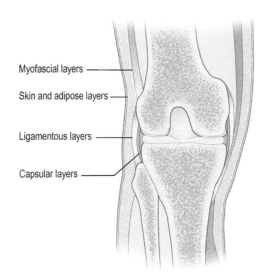

Myofascial layers

Skin and adipose layers

Ligamentous layers

Capsular layers

Figure 36.10
Tissue resilience.

In the case of too tough, specified sustained precise stretching or manual work is called for to increase the resilience across these anatomy trains stations that link the muscles across the joints. Cases that show too compliant tissues would require increased muscle tone in the myofascial tracks that support the stations, in this case the extensions of the abductors and the fibular muscles. This serves simply as an example of a process going on throughout the body. We could imagine a vertical view from the gluteus maximus to the deepest part of the sacrotuberous ligament in a forward bend or the ubiquitous yoga asana, Downward Dog. We would expect:

- the gluteus to give way easily into an elastic stretch
- the superficial part of the sacrotuberous ligament to link and distribute strain from the hamstrings up to the 'myofascialature' of the thoracolumbar area

- the deep portion to maintain the necessary relationship between the sacrum and ischium, allowing only a little give in the sacroiliac joint for the couple of degrees of movement required.

Excess chronic muscle tension or fascial adhesion anywhere in this linked chain could skew the distribution of these forces, creating the conditions for injury, postural compensation, known to trainers as "bad form", or chronic overuse of tissues, leading to inflammation and pain.

As another example: in a side bend, can you see or palpate the progressive movement from the lateral abdominal obliques through the lateral edge of the iliocostalis lumborum, and the lateral raphé of the abdominals through the quadratus lumborum to the intertransversarii, to the intertransverse ligaments near the spine? Lack of resilience in any of these structures will create functional aberrations. The skilled practitioner will apply manual or movement therapy to the precise structures needing either more resilience or more tone.

Give a little

Small movements in the profound tissues allow the big movements closer to the surface. The movement of the dural membranes commonly palpated in cranial osteopathy (Sutherland, 1990) or the mobility of the organs assessed in visceral manipulation (Barrall and Mercier, 1988) are other common examples of small inner movements that have a significant effect on the large outer movements if they are missing or aberrated.

In the parietal myofascia, which is the domain of the Anatomy Trains, most trainers, physiotherapists, and manual therapists observe this effect in the tiny adjustments in the sacroiliac joints, which have a wider impact on the larger movement of the body as a whole. With too little sacroiliac movement, there is a large compensatory pattern in the gait and thus a tendency to "export" the problems to the lumbar spine. With laxity and too much sacroiliac movement, the outer body strives to compensate for too much inner movement by using the outer myofascialature as straps.

Across the entire body, from the spine to the limbs and across all the anatomy trains lines, we are looking for that "Goldilocks" feeling of being "just right". This varies between subjects depending on natural fascial tone. It requires on-the-job training in accurate palpation of the anatomy trains stations in the relative movement of inner structures to set the stage for the proper movement of the outer structures.

Returning to our knee example, soccer players require stability generation on the inside and outside of the postural leg when planting it in preparation for kicking a football with the opposite foot. As that foot lands, and the player seeks stability, differences in the turf or the player's angle require near instantaneous adjustability in the foot, ankle, knee and hip.

As a test for this adjustability and resilience through the knee, have the player stand in front of you as you kneel and cup your hands around the inside and outside of the knee, covering the lateral line tissues on the outside, and the deep front line tissues (from the pes anserinus down to the medial collateral ligament) on the inside. Have your client, while using the other foot or a handhold for balance and keeping the planted foot on the ground, slowly translate their pelvis laterally from left to right. This will naturally create abduction and adduction at the hip, and inversion and eversion at the subtalar joint at the ankle.

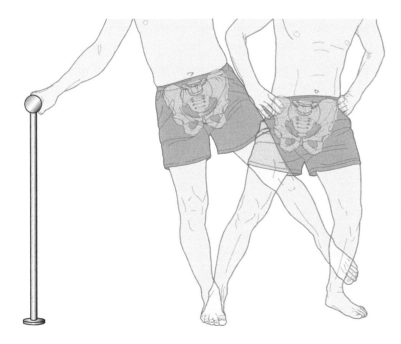

Figure 36.11 Hands on knee

To test myofascial resilience, put your hands on the medial and lateral side of an athlete's knee (in this case, his right) to feel the "give" in the layers between your hands and the middle of the joint as he or she moves from side to side while maintaining the foot on the floor.

Perform this test on a dozen to a hundred people to clearly detect which tissues are deficient in either a resistant or lax condition.

Chapter 36

The knee is supposedly simply maintaining its extension between these two lateral movements at the joints above and below. But what do you feel inside and outside the knee in between as they carry out this movement? In a resilient body, you will feel a slight give in the tissues under your hand. In a healthy body, the skin will move the most, the underlying tissues of the anatomy trains (parietal myofasciae) will manifest some give, and, at the ligamentous level, a very slight give can be felt. With a little practice, you will be able to tell at which level there is too much give in the tissues or too little. With a little more practice you will be able to identify which layer within the leg is not coordinating with the rest, and apply to those tissues whatever treatment form is at your command.

Clinical summary

The new research on the properties of fascial tissues, the cybernetic nature of neural plasticity and the biotensegrity model of the actual engineering relationship between the soft and bony tissues, all suggest that holistic modeling of training results is required to supplement the individual structure model used for the last few centuries. The Anatomy Trains myofascial meridians map provides a model for measuring resilience and total body participation in movement that leads to long-term health. Learning to measure resilience and to recognize where tissue "give" is not occurring will allow the trainer to make adjustments, often at some distance from the site of stress or pain, which will promote maximum performance with minimum injury.

References

Barker, P.J., Briggs, C.A. & Bogeski, G. (2004) Tensile transmission across the lumbar fascia in unembalmed cadavers: effects of tension to various muscular attachments. *Spine*. 29: 129–138.

Barrall, J.P. & Mercier, P. (1988) *Visceral Manipulation*. Seattle, WA: Eastland Press.

Earls, J. & Myers, T. (2010) *Fascial Release for Structural Balance*. Chichester, UK: Lotus Publishing.

Franklyn-Miller, A., et al. (2009) The Strain Patterns of the Deep fascia of the Lower Limb. In: Schleip, R., Huijing, P.A., Hollander, P. & Findley, T.W. (Eds), *Fascial Research II: Basic Science and Implications for Conventional and Complementary Health Care*. Munich, Germany: Elsevier.

Fukunaga, T., Kawakami, Y., Kubo, K. & Kanehisa, H. (2002) Muscle and tendon interaction during human movements. *Exerc Sport Sci Rev*. 30: 106–110.

Fuller, B. (1975) *Synergetics*. New York, NY: Macmillian, Chapter 7.

Grunwald M. (2017) *Homo hapticus: Why we cannot live without a sense of touch*. Munich: Droemer.

Guimberteau, J.C. (2004) *Strolling under the skin*. Paris, France: Elsevier.

Hamilton, N., Weimar, W. & Luttgens, K. (2011) *Kine-siology: Scientific Basis of Human Motion*, 12th ed. NY: McGraw-Hill.

Horwitz, A. (1997) Integrins and health. *Scientific American*. May: 68–75.

Huijing, P. (2007) Epimuscular myofascial force transmission between antagonistic and synergistic muscles can explain movement limitation in spastic paresis. *J Biomech*. 17: 708–724.

Ingber, D. (1998) The architecture of life. *Scientific American*. January: 48–57.

Ingber, D. (2006) Mechanical control of tissue morphogenesis during embryological development. *Int J Dev Biol*. 50: 255–266.

Kawakami, Y., Muraoka, T., Ito, S., Kanehisa, H. & Fukunaga, T. (2002) In vivo muscle fibre behaviour during countermovement exercise in humans reveals a significant role for tendon elasticity. *J Physiol*. 540: 635–646.

Langevin, H.M., Bouffard, N.A. & Badger, G.J. (2006) Subcutaneous tissue fibroblast cytoskeletal remodeling induced by acupuncture: evidence for a mechanotransduction-based mechanism. *J Cell Biol*. 207: 767–744.

Levin, S. (2003) The tensegrity-truss as a model for spine mechanics. *J Mech Med Biol.* 2: 374–388.

Maas, H. & Huijing, P. (2009) Synergistic and antagonistic interaction in the rat forelimb: acute after-effects of coactivation. *J Appl Physiol.* 107: 1453–1462.

Milhorat, T.H., Bolognese, P.A., Nishikawa, M., McDonnell, N.B. & Francomano, C.A. (2007) Syndrome of occipitoatlantoaxial hypermobility, cranial settling, and chiari malformation type I in patients with hereditary disorders of connective tissue. *J Neurosurg Spine.* 7: 601–609.

Muscolino, J. (2002) *The muscular system manual.* Redding, CT: JEM.

Myers, T. (2001, 2009, 2013) *Anatomy Trains.* Edinburgh, UK: Churchill Livingstone.

Scarr, G. (2008) A model of the cranial vault as a tensegrity structure, and its significance to normal and abnormal cranial development. *Int J Osteopath Med.* 11: 80–89.

Schleip, R. (2003) Fascial plasticity: a new neurobiological explanation. *J Bodyw Mov Ther.* 7(1): 11–19; 7(2): 104–116.

Shacklock, M. (2005) *Clinical Neurodynamics.* Burlington, MA: Butterworth-Heinemann.

Sutherland, W.G. (1990) *Teachings in the Science of Osteopathy.* Portland, OR: Rudra Press.

Tietze, A. (1921) Concerning the architectural structure of the connective tissues of the human sole. *Bruns' Beitrage zur Klinischen Chirurgie.* 123: 493–506.

Van der Wal, J. (2009) The architecture of connective tissue in the musculoskeletal system. In Schleip, R., Huijing, P.A., Hollander, P. & Findley, T.W. (Eds), *Fascia Research II, Basic Science and Implications for Conventional and Complementary Health Care.* Munich, Germany: Elsevier.

Vesalius, A. (1548) De fabrici corporis humani pub in 1973. NY: Dover Publications.

Vleeming, A. & Stoeckart, R. (2007) The role of the pelvic girdle in coupling the spine and the legs: a clinical-anatomical perspective on pelvic anatomy. In Vleeming, A., Mooney, V. & Stoeckart, R. (Eds), Chapter 8, *Movement, stability and lumbo-pelvic pain.* Edinburgh, UK: Elsevier.

Williams, P. (Ed.) (1995) The Anatomical Basis of Medicine and Surgery. In *Gray's Anatomy*, 38th ed. Edinburgh, UK: Churchill Livingstone, 753.

Zaidel-Bar, R., Itzkovitz, S., Ma'ayan, A., Iyengar, R. & Geiger, B. (2007) Functional atlas of the integrin adhesome. *Nat Cell Biol.* 9: 858–867.

Zamir, E. & Geiger, B. (2001) Molecular complexity and dynamics of cell-matrix adhesions. *J Cell Sci.* 114: 3583–3590.

Fascial form in yoga

Joanne Avison

Introduction

Yoga is not about stretching (Chapter 9). Yoga is about fostering balance in the length and tension relationships in the body. This approach preserves one of the most valuable features of the fascial matrix: its elasticity. Stretching is but one aspect of promoting elasticity. We are, essentially, designed for storing the potential energy of recoil (Chapter 7). In practice, stretching is not always the way to do that.

Certain body types, or body histories, can mean that stretching for length is the last thing some people need. The kind of stretching that simply pulls on the tissues (Richards, 2012) can be potentially harmful to the integrity of the whole. Yoga and fascia are both beautifully designed to honor everyone's ability to manage movement forces, as distinct from forced movements.

True elasticity is one of several fundamental principles of the fascial matrix profoundly enhanced by the appropriate practice of yoga. It incorporates a reciprocal relationship, such as the balance of tension and compression offers (Chapter 11). The growing understanding of the fascial tensional network makes sense of yoga, in all its potential for health and vitality. The optimization of tensional integrity of the tissues including the whole body, soft-tissue architecture can be depleted by efforts that over-stretch,

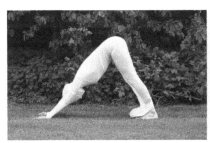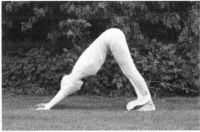

Figure 37.1 Tensional integrity or biotensegrity, is expressed as a whole, in the round

Forcing one part beyond its elastic limits (i.e. by stretching beyond "biotensegral range") can compromise another part. Whatever the pose, the fascial forms that we are made of animate (or are animated by) the whole body in the round. Thus, we take a global approach to overall integrity to enhance elastic recoil potential in individual ways for each individual – whatever the posture. The difference between these two images is that on the left Helen is inhaling, while on the right she is exhaling. There is a subtle, global effect. The tube is used as a metaphor, to imply global change without forcing stretch, facilitating an intimate balance through the relationship between breath and form.

Reproduced with kind permission from: model, Helen Eadie; photographer, Amy Very; tube design/styling, Joanne Avison.

Chapter 37

just as appropriate types of stretching can invigorate and strengthen it (see page 430).

The unifying experience

Yoga did not develop under the classical laws of Cartesian reductionist theory that have dominated Western anatomy, physiology, biomechanics and psychology for centuries. As an art and science, it was only ever based on the unifying experience of mind, body and being. Its ancient wisdom had no history of treating these aspects of "humans being" and "humans doing" separately.

Reducing "humans doing" (be it yoga or any movement modality) to functions and actions of muscles, bones, nerves and linear theories of biomechanical levers sits awkwardly with our fully animated and instinctive experience on the yoga mat. The properties of the fascia, as a ubiquitous sensory tensional network of tissues, throughout the rounded wholeness of our entire form, make perfect sense of it. In many ways it could be considered to perfectly express the biotensegrity principles of tension and compression (Chapter 11) united as volume; to incorporate the wholeness we express, whatever we are doing.

The yoga postures (asanas) in all their rich variety of shape and position, range and dynamics, are a means to explore balance and restore energy to those tissues, if we remain awake to their tensional integrity. Therein lies the containment of energy, the natural elasticity of compliance and our vitality. Even in Corpse Pose (*Shivasana*), the body rests as a pre-tensioned architecture (Van der Wal, 2009). We do not turn into an amoebic puddle on the mat when we are not moving, nor do we take the shape of the postures.

"A recognised characteristic of connective tissue is its impressive adaptability. When regularly put under increasing physiological strain, it changes its architectural properties to meet the increasing demand."

Schleip (2011).

We have considerable power over the nature of the demand we put on the tissues. If we place no strain on them at all, it is the demand for inertia that effectively causes its own "lack of" strain patterns. This can lead to a requirement to tension the tensional network rather than stretch a relatively untensioned one. That is not to say that certain types of stretching are not valuable to all bodies. Consider instinctive stretching or pandiculation (Bertolucci, 2011). This can wake up sedentary tissues and relieve tight ones. However, it is distinct from the kind of stretching for which yoga sometimes has a reputation, one in which reaching for maximum length for its own sake can be considered a worthy goal to "achieve" a posture.

Some yoga practices are dedicated to long sequences, which also suit the development of elastic momentum. However, there is a caveat under the fascialogical theme of tensional integrity (Chapter 11). If a dynamic series is repeated at very regular and frequent intervals all in one direction of strain, for example, flexion biased, it is likely to have a cumulative effect that can potentially encourage a particular strain pattern, which can cost elasticity in the longer term. However, if it is regularly counterbalanced with a series that is, for example, extension biased, then this pattern can be balanced and be more beneficial to the whole. The fascial matrix is a refined force transmission system

(Langevin, 2006) and will respond according to the forces put through it (Schleip, 2011, see the above quotation).

It is possible to ensure an equally refined balance of forces to optimize the elastic capacity and recoil facility of the body (Chapter 11) without overstraining it in one particular direction. Once we understand the polarities involved and the definition of elasticity, we can accumulate the benefits of increased resilience, compliance and spring loading throughout our systems. It gives us moment-to-moment and movement-to-movement balance at naturally instinctive speed, appropriate to the individual and tissue type (Avison, 2015).

Three key points

There are three key points that contribute to understanding elasticity and stretching of the fascial form in yoga practice:

1. **Terminology**: What exactly is elasticity?
2. **Tensional integrity**: How does this work in the whole body?
3. **Energy storage capacity**: How is it optimized in practice?

Once these points are clarified, we can begin to see the foundation of **elasticity** as a valuable attribute of the whole tissue matrix. Then the advantages can be suitably derived from all variations of Hatha yoga styles (Ashtanga, Restorative, Vinyasa Flow, Kria, Iyengar, etc.).

Terminology

Elasticity is the capacity of a material to change shape (deform) under external force and resist internally, thereby returning to previous form (reform). This is measured as the difference between the stiffness (resistance to deformation) and the elastic return (reformation).

A common misunderstanding in the classroom seems to be that (a) something has to be made of elastic to display elasticity and (b) when we let go of an elastic band or elasticated fabric, as it lies at rest, we are modeling our body at rest. Both of these ideas are inaccurate.

Stiffness is the resistance to deformation, but stiff springs (think of car parts) can have more elasticity than weaker springs (think of a slinky toy) because they store more energy and rebound more efficiently. Hard steel ball bearings bounce better than rubber balls (Levin, 2013). A material does not have to be made of elastic to demonstrate elasticity or have the capacity to store elastic energy.

We rest pre-tensioned, or pre-stiffened, by the architectural design of our bones and soft tissues, that is as a volume in space. Our elasticity does not just refer to the amount we can stretch. It refers to the ability or capacity to restore a change in shape. That is a suitable balance between stiffness (i.e. resistance to deformation) and elasticity (i.e. the ability to reform or restore the original shape). We are poised between the extremes of either state when we are relaxed. When we take up a yoga pose, to the extent that we can form the shape of the pose (deformation), it is counterbalanced by our ability to release it without imposition. If we force a stretch, then the ability of the tissues to restore (reformation) might be compromised.

The question is of a balance between these two states, rather than a focus on maximum flexibility for its own sake (Chapter 19). Appropriate counter poses, and respect for the elastic limit, invite an overall balance to the whole practice.

Chapter 37

When you pull on an elastic band or fabric you are measuring its stiffness (deformation capacity). When you release the band, the extent to which it immediately restores its original shape, is a measure of its elasticity (reformation ability). In fact our tissues rest pre-stiffened or pre-tensioned, poised for movement. If we go beyond the elastic limit, it is a different state: that of plasticity (Avison, 2015).

Plasticity: Beyond elasticity is a point where reformation is no longer possible. The so-called stretch is irreversible. The material does not spring back when you let it go and it retains the shape of the deformation. Between that point, the elastic limit, and the breaking or tearing point, is termed "plasticity": when the new shape stays there. The subsequent changes are distinguished in terms of malleability and ductility or brittleness. All of these are properties of different types of materials.

Viscoelasticity is a characteristic of the living body: a solid-and-fluid medium.

"Viscoelasticity is a property of all tensegrity structures. It is a non-linear time dependent deformation. It is called 'viscoelastic' because when stressed it first behaves as if it were a liquid, then behaves as an elastic solid, not because it is made up from those two states. When stress is removed, it does it backwards and there is a splashdown (soft landing)."

Levin (2013).

These different qualities of stiffness to softness are different values or properties that, in combination within the tissues, make for a variety of tensional possibilities throughout the entire fascial forms in the overall architecture, whatever

the yoga position. Car springs have "dampers" on them to slow down the rate of elastic return (or reformation, see above). The fluids in our tissues act somewhat like dampers and give them so-called "viscoelastic properties", which regulate the rate of resistance and reformation (Richards, 2012).

At every level of detail there is a balance of stiffness and elasticity in response to how we load or use them and how intelligently we accumulate useful adaptations, over those which may be less than optimal (such as forcing a stretch, for example, when the body is neither ready, nor able to counter it). Altogether, this exquisitely detailed matrix forms and develops the collagen matrix according to loading and the timing/frequency of that accumulated movement history. Habitual or deliberate strain patterns profoundly affect tissue morphology and mobility. Forced stretching can compromise the tissues' innate ability to spring back if it isn't counterbalanced, or sufficiently stiffened to optimize elasticity. This ability is expressed on the mat as a balance between appropriate stiffness, length and flexibility or compliance, for the individual.

Tensional integrity

One of the main features of our structural balance in motion is based upon the architectural principles of biotensegrity (Levin, 2012). This is the basis of our architecture. Unlike the elastic band resting on the table (untensioned), we remain tensioned all the time, to enclose and occupy space. By the basic laws of biotensegrity, every movement affects the whole and is transmitted through it.

Fascial form in yoga

"Tensegrity structures are omni-directional, independent of gravity, load distributing and energy efficient, hierarchical and self-generating. They are also ubiquitous in nature, once you know what to look for."

Levin (2009).

As biotensegrity (living tensegrity-based) structures, we have the ability to squeeze and draw in our structure and tissues as a whole, besides being able to stretch and fill or expand them, omni-directionally, for example, as in the filling and emptying of our bladders or lungs. The fascial fabric, bones, myofascia, organs, joints, vessels and cavities of our architecture are, paradoxically, held together and apart simultaneously, as volumes. They are globally contained through the tension/compression principles of biotensegrity architecture (Levin, 1990; Ingber, 1998; Flemons, 2006; Martin and Levin, 2012).

This is the basis of "primordial biologic structure" (Levin, 1990). Such a design is organized for stored energy capacity through the balance of stiffness to elasticity in the entire architecture on every scale. It is a foundational principle of human, indeed living, form, and one that we naturally explore in every yoga pose (asana) at the macrocosmic level of our whole form. Essentially, we seek to preserve and promote elastic integrity throughout the body.

Energy storage capacity

We constantly work under three phases of elastic range, not one. We can stretch and release, we can squeeze and release, and we can rest in a pre-tensioned state (neither squeezing nor releasing). The breath is the first place to recognize this law in motion. We breathe in and breathe out in the inhale/exhale rhythm. However, we can then exhale more to empty or squeeze and release by inhaling. It is a three-phase process, with a pausing place in between, and one intent of yoga is to maintain this at a suitable balance. Dynamic sequences, slower restorative practice and the stillness of meditation are designed to explore this range and accumulate a resource of actively contained energy storage capacity throughout the body. This is enhanced by many of the yogic breathing practices of *pranayama*.

For the whole body, an overemphasis on softening, stiffening or stretching will not necessarily result in optimum elasticity in movement, whatever the activity (Chapter 8). The focus in yoga is on the refined transition and continuity along the spectrum either side of resting tension, to restore the phases of length-tension balance to the whole (see Figure 37 .5).

While this may seem like an obvious statement shown in diagrammatic form, it is not always understood when applied practically. Even in yoga classes, breathing exercises are often performed without the distinctions of their value in preserving and promoting compliance and energy storage ability in the tissues. They have global implications of accumulating and fine-tuning elasticity throughout the fascial forms, in all aspects of the yoga practices, especially if the full range of the "breath mobius" is encouraged (Avison, 2015).

If we train the body in any one aspect, i.e. just squeezing (stiffening), just stretching or just softening (releasing), or in one direction or plane (i.e. just flexion), we can compromise overall elastic integrity. If we counter-pose and counteract to maintain that tensional balance, we frequently

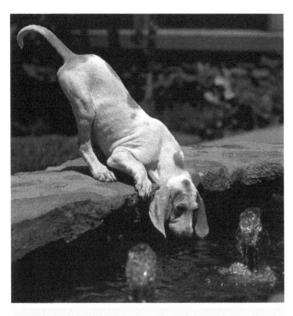

Figure 37.2

The tensional integrity of the whole body can be seen being used for balance. From nose tip to tail tip, this puppy reached out as part of a whole body-balancing act to drink from the pool, extending the tensional integrity to the tip of its tongue.

Reproduced with kind permission from Shane McDermott (www.wildearthilluminations.com).

load the tissues for optimum tensional integrity and range in all degrees of potential. Stretching becomes a feature of balance and suitable control, rather than a purpose for its own sake.

Instinctive stretching

This is a way of stretching that does not seem to compromise the tissues and which naturally regulates the dangers of overstretching globally. Animals can provide us with some clues.

Consider the cheetah, for example. Wild and domestic cats can rest and relax, stretch at a suitable time, move at great speed and pounce on prey. At rest, they become languid and serene. When they have rested, they frequently yawn-stretch their whole body to wake up their tissues after releasing them for a period of time. This particular type of stretching is called pandiculation (Bertolucci, 2011). It is what we call a "lengthening contraction" in yoga. It is a feature of movement with a purpose in nature, to reactivate the tissues after resting them and reorganize, or prime, the internal bonds and fluids ready for mobility (Chapter 9).

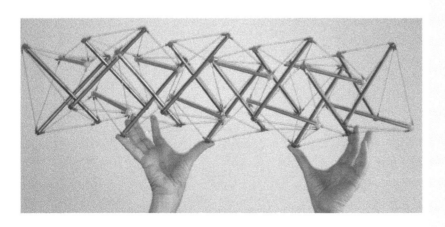

Figure 37.3

A tensegrity mast; originally presented by Kenneth Snelson as a system called "floating compression", the term "tensegrity" was coined by Buckminster Fuller as "tensional integrity" and developed since by Dr Stephen Levin into biotensegrity (see Further information). It is an elastic architecture, balanced between stiffness and elasticity. It bounces and resists deformation, retaining its three-dimensional form.

Model by Bruce Hamilton (see Further information).

Fascial form in yoga

When a cheetah anticipates prey (peak performance), the last thing they do is stretch. They prime their tissues by "squeezing" or stiffening them:

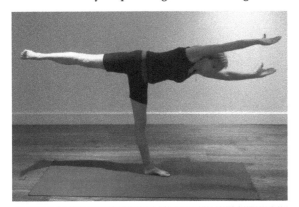

Figure 37.4

A classical model of the spine might suggest that it is a stacked column. This posture would not be possible if that were the case. Nor is it the muscular strength of Katie's standing foot that is holding her up. Her ability to hold and modify this pose is based upon the tensional integrity of her balance as a whole; or the "energy storage capacity", which is the elasticity, perfectly poised in mutual tension/compression balance.

Reproduced with kind permission from Katie Courts (www.yoga-nutco.uk).

they stalk. They are ready to deploy the potential to pounce or sprint as required, maximizing their catapult capacity by tightening the global tissue matrix. Even their fur stands on end, perhaps for super-sensitivity to the task. Cheetahs, like many other mammals, focus and draw their tissues in to make them fit for purpose, globally. There is a time and a place, a dose and a degree, for stretching.

Research in British Columbia (see Further information) regarding how hibernating bears survive a winter of sleep without osteoporosis or degenerative conditions affecting their muscles after months of inertia, revealed an interesting instinctive habit. The bears get up around midday every day and perform 20–40 min of natural movement. They do gentle yoga-type movements, yawning-stretches in all directions, yawning and wriggling and pacing around, reanimating the tissues, before they settle back and sleep and hibernate for the next 24 h.

"Stretching is part of our nature, particularly when accompanied by yawning. This wholeheartedly reflects the 'felt' sense of tension and compression,

Figure 37.5

Resting tension is the middle phase, between the breaths. Inhalation is the stretch to expand and exhale restores resting tension. The "exhale plus" is the ability to squeeze and contain the breath, which restores resting tension by inhaling (Avison, 2014).

Reproduced with kind permission from Art of Contemporary Yoga Ltd.

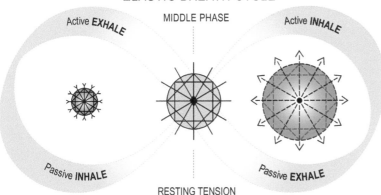

ELASTIC BREATH CYCLE

Active **EXHALE**

MIDDLE PHASE

Active **INHALE**

Passive **INHALE**

RESTING TENSION

Passive **EXHALE**

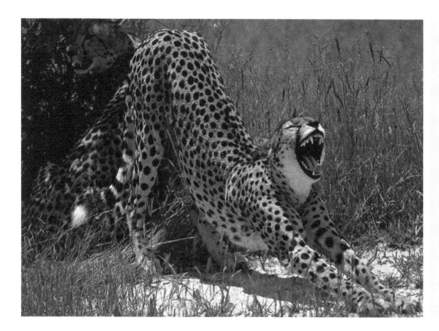

Figure 37.6 Yawning stretch or pandiculation

A wild cheetah in up-down dog pose, its own version of Adho-Urdhva Muhka Svanasana. Notice the beautiful side bend of the cheetah in the background.

Reproduced with kind permission from Shane McDermott (www. wildearthilluminations.com).

or biotensegrity, in the system. It facilitates stretch-and-squeeze simultaneously and naturally self-regulates the tissues."

Bertolucci (2011).

How often do we remember to yawn-and-stretch after rest considering the time we spend in planes, trains and automobiles, not to mention sitting at our desks. Do we counterbalance them with yawning stretches? No cat, dog or bear would forget to do this after a period of inertia. It is instinctive to many animals. We, on the other hand, will force-stretch to reach the most extraordinary shapes as if that is the purpose of yoga.

Building a repertoire in the body of cumulative "enquiries" and "balances" is a clear advantage in improving vitality and may have distinct therapeutic value (Broad, 2012). It also speaks to issues of inertia that research shows to play a key role in many degenerative diseases (Henson et al., 2013). However, it is optimally used in a very

instinctive way, in order to explore those shapes for a given individual and maintain their value in enhancing true elasticity (recoil capacity). If someone is super-bendy or super-soft then they might find improved elasticity in tensioning, or stiffening, their network, rather than typically stretching it.

An example in practice: dog pose

Rather than forcing the stretch, time is taken to compress (stiffen) the body first, contain and gather it in (i.e. squeeze) to find the ground or base of support. This allows the heels, in the given example of Dog Pose (*Urdhva Muhka Svanasana*; Figure 37.7) to explore their tensional relationship throughout the back of the body, and invites the movement towards the ground, rather than forcing or reaching towards it, as if "stretching" is the goal. This, in turn, facilitates the knee to be opened naturally, without pushing it back or hyperextending the joint (Figure 37 .7).

Fascial form in yoga

This "listening approach" ensures that the fold at the hip does not pull the pelvis into a posterior tilt, which would, in turn, compromise the lumbar spine (lordosis), thus pulling on the shoulders or neck, and leaving Alexander straining to stretch to "achieve" the pose (Figure 37.8).

Balancing the tensional components includes the whole body at all its folding potentials (joints),

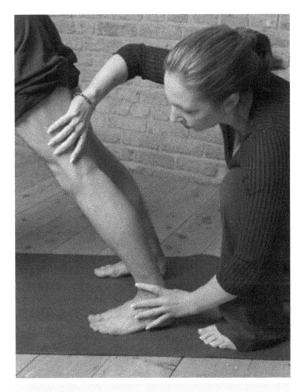

Figure 37.7

Once a principle ballet dancer, Alexander is more than capable of "stretching" his body in Dog Pose, heels to the ground. However, to optimize elasticity, every joint is seen for its role in the tensional balance of the whole. This includes the relationship of the back to the front and the continuity throughout their longitudinal organization, from fingertips to feet and coccyx to crown.

Model: Alexander Filmer-Lorch. Reproduced with kind permission from Charlie Carter Photography.

gathering in the continuous integrity of the tensional matrix. It naturally facilitates Alexander's ability to squeeze/contain throughout the architecture and then "fill" the pose in 360 degrees, through an actively loaded stretch (Chapter 33) (or lengthening contraction), rather than strain for it through pulling on any particular aspect of the posterior tissues (Myers, 2009) (Chapter 35). Then he can explore the posture intelligently to his own elastic (or biotensegral) limit (Chapter 10) as a global gesture or expression to maintain a body-wide "biomotional integrity" (Avison, 2015). This is quite distinct from forcing the heel down or pushing the knee joint to "stretch into the pose" in a fight for length at all costs, which may be implied by stretching. This can cost natural elasticity (see earlier).

The key clue to this, or any other posture, is in the ease and flow of the breath and the subtle

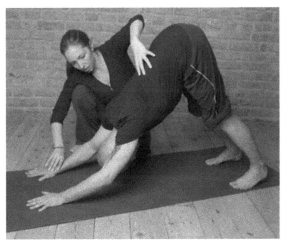

Figure 37.8

Subtle adjustment gives feedback to tension the pose in suitable balance at each of the joints, breathing in to the potential length as it unfolds, without forcing stretch. Model: Alexander Filmer-Lorch.

Reproduced with kind permission from Charlie Carter Photography.

Chapter 37

ability to transmit the breathing motion through the whole pose and body, rhythmically. That is through the expansion, release, squeeze, release cycle mentioned earlier, innate to a biotensegrity architecture (Chapter 11). When this is not compromised there is no need for extraneous, unnecessary tightness, floppiness or strain, only a suitable containment of the whole, to move or hold a pose, any yoga posture.

For the more dynamic practice, it encourages containment and thereby fostering spring-loaded tension or potential: the stored energy capacity for the next posture in a flowing sequence (Chapter 10). Thus it primes the tissues for effortless and contained transition between asanas at the variable speeds. We can, by fostering elasticity over stretching, nourish our loading history, through this conscious process of expansion and impansion of the global fascial matrix, whatever yoga forms we are seeking to morph into and practice. In any yogasana, we can adapt to the speed and transitions of differing styles. This invites us towards the yogic philosophy behind seeking "*sthiram* and *sukham*", the balance between the steady and the sweet if we invite the balance between tension and compression, in multidirectional (or omni-directional) wholeness. We accumulate balance in the elastic recoil potential and invite *sthiram/sukham* to the pose, as well as to the overall practice. We begin by accumulating balance, poise and adaptability, from speed to stillness and beyond.

Summary

Yoga practice is an exploration of balance and integration on many levels. Our fascial form rests in the neutral potential that we call "relaxed", although the fascial tissues are biotensegrally orchestrated and always poised in tensional integrity for potential movement. As a force transmission system with innate elastic properties, dependent upon how we use the body and respect this unifying feature, the fascial matrix (and the forces it transmits) and yoga express and enhance each other in all their variety and possibility.

References

Avison, J. (2015) *YOGA: Fascia, Form & Functional Movement.* Edinburgh, UK: Handspring.

Bertolucci, L.F. (2011) Pandiculation: nature's way of maintaining the functional integrity of the myofascial system? *J Bodyw Mov Ther.* 15: 268–280.

Broad, W.J. (2012) *The Science of Yoga.* New York, NY: Simon & Schuster.

Flemons, T. (2006) *The Geometry of Anatomy.* www.intensiondesigns.com.

Henson, J.J., Yates, T., Biddle, S.J.H., Edwardson, C.L., Khunti, K., Wilmot, E.G., Gray, L.J., Gorely, T., Nimmo, M.A. & Davies, M.J. (2013) Associations of objectively measured sedentary behaviour and physical activity with markers of cardiometabolic health. *Diabetolgia.* 56: 1012–1020.

Ingber, D.E. (2006) The Architecture of Life. *Scientific American*, January 1998. http://time.arts.ucla.edu/Talks/ Barcelona/Arch_Life.htm.

Langevin, H.M. (2006) Connective tissue: a body-wide signaling network? *Med Hypotheses* 66: 1074–1077.

Levin, S. M. (1990) The primordial structure. In: Banathy, B.H. & Banathy, B.B. (Eds), *Proceedings of The 34th Annual Meeting of The International Society for the Systems Sciences.* Portland, vol. II, 716–720. [This article explores the icosahedron as the primordial biologic structure, from viruses to vertebrates, including their systems and sub-systems; www.biotensegrity.com.]

Levin, S.M. (1995) The importance of soft tissues for structural support of the body. *Spine.* 9: 357–363.

Levin, S. (2006) Tensegrity, the New Biomechanics. In: Hutson, M. & Ellis, R. (Eds), *Textbook of Musculoskeletal Medicine.* Oxford, UK: Oxford University Press. Updated http://www.biotensegrity.com/tensegrity_new_biome-chanics.php.

Levin, S.M. (2012) Comments on Fascia Talkshow, Episode 7, Biotensegrity

(Avison) www.bodyworkcpd.co.uk (19.09.12 webinar). [See Further information below.]

Levin, S. (2013) Comments on biotensegrity and elasticity. Personal correspondence. [See Further Information below.]

Martin, D.C. & Levin, S.M. (2012) Biotensegrity: the mechanics of fascia. Chapter 3.5. In: Schleip, R., Findlay, T.W., Chaitow, L. & Huijing, P.A. (Eds). *Fascia: The Tensional Network of the Human Body.* Edinburgh, UK: Elsevier. [See Further information below.]

Myers, T.W. (2009) The Superficial Back Line. *Anatomy Trains.* Chapter 3. Edinburgh, UK: Elsevier.

Richards, D. (2012) University of Toronto, Assistant Professor Medical Director, David L. MacIntosh Sport Medicine Clinic: Doug Richards on Stretching: *The Truth.*

Schleip, R. (2003) Fascial plasticity – a new neuro-biological explanation; Part 1. *J Bodyw Mov Ther.* 7: 11–19.

Schleip, R. (2011) Principles of Fascia Fitness. Issue 7. www.terra-rosa.com.au.

van der Wal, J. (2009) The architecture of the connective tissue in the musculoskeletal system-an often overlooked functional parameter as to proprioception in the locomotor apparatus. *Int J Ther Massage Bodywork.* 2: 9–23.

Further information
Bears at Grouse Mountain

At Grouse Mountain in Vancouver (http://www. grousemountain.com/wildlife-refuge) there is a BearCam facility and it is possible to watch Coola and Grinder in hibernation. Researchers and rangers in the park run a blog and films about the bears (and other wildlife at the reserve) and their hibernating habits.

Carter, C., photography.

Further reading

Courts, K. see www.yoga-nut.co.uk.

Eadie, H. see www.heleneadieyoga.com.

Filmer-Lorch, A. (2012) *Inside Meditation.* Leicester, UK: Troubador Publishing.

Guimberteau, J. see handspringpublishing.com and http://www.guimberteau-jc-md.com/en/.

Hamilton, B. see www.tensegrity.com for tensegrity models.

Ingber, D.E. (1993) Cellular tensegrity; defining new rules of biological design that govern the cytoskeleton. *J Cell Sci.* 104: 613–627.

Jager, H. & Klinger, W. (2012) Fascia is alive. In: Schleip, R., Findlay, T.W., Chaitow, L. & Huijing, P.A. (Eds), *Fascia: The Tensional Network of the Human Body.* Chapter 4.2. Edinburgh, UK: Elsevier.

Levin, S. see www.biotensegrity.com for a variety of articles and papers and instructional video material.

McDermott, S. see *Wildlife Conservation Photography* at www.shanemcdermottphotography.com for images of animal behavior and movement in their natural habitat.

Schmidli, S. see www.samirayoga.co.uk

Snelson, K. see http://kennethsnelson.net/articles/. TheArtOfTensegrityArticle.pdf.

Very, A. see http://amyvery.com for photography.

Yin yoga as a fascia-oriented practice

Paul Grilley

Introduction

In the modern era, authors use "bullet points" to highlight the logical structure of their writings. The bullet points of ancient India were terse statements that were easy to memorize. Each statement was called a "sutra". In this chapter, a slightly modified version of the yin yoga sutras is presented, which we use in our training program.

All forms of yoga aim to increase flexibility and relax muscular tension. Yang yoga also emphasizes strength and endurance. When practicing yang yoga, muscles are contracted, poses are performed repetitively, and are typically held for 10 to 30 s.

Yin yoga emphasizes relaxing fascial contracture, including ligaments, joint capsules and discs. For this reason, yin poses are performed with the muscles relaxed and held for several minutes. Yin poses are primarily floor poses.

Yin yoga sutras

The purpose of yoga asana is to harmonize the flow of chi in the meridians. This is accomplished by stressing 14 skeletal segments and 10 myofascial groups.

The 14 skeletal segments are toes, ankles, knees, hips, pelvis, lumbar, thoracic, cervical, fingers, wrist, radius, ulna, humerus and scavicle. (Note: scapula + clavicle = scavicle.)

The 10 myofascial groups are groin, quads, hip flexors, glutes, hamstrings, rectus abdominis, obliques, thoracolumbar, cervical and scapular.

The two fundamental stresses are tension and compression.

Stress is created by seven asana archetypes. These archetypes are Shoelace, Saddle, Caterpillar, Dragonfly, Twist, Dog and Dragon. The seven archetypes must be adapted to the flexibility and the skeletability of every student. Flexibility refers to the extensibility of soft tissue: myofascia, joint capsules and discs. Skeletability refers to the potential range of motion of a joint segment, the range of motion before bone compression stops the movement. It is not always desirable to develop maximum skeletability. Every bone in every body is different, so what is easy for one skeleton may be impossible for another. Every yogi, therefore, has a unique skeletability. Consequently, there is no such thing as a "perfect pose". If you are effectively stressing the target areas then you are performing the poses correctly. Every hand and foot position either helps or inhibits your ability to stress the target areas. The most effective way to do this varies from person to person.

Feel the rebound. In yin yoga, the rebound is the subjective experience of energy movement within the body. It is accompanied by pleasant feelings of physical ease, mental stillness and

Chapter 38

emotional calm. After practicing a pose for a few minutes, relax in any comfortable position and feel the rebound.

Skeletal joints and skeletal segments

A joint is formed when two bones are in contact. There are approximately 206 bones in the body and their various contacts create over 300 joints. But when considered as functional groups, there are only 14 joint segments, or 24 if you include both arms and both legs.

In yin yoga, the joint segments are labeled with simple mnemonic names and can include more than one joint. For example: the "lumbar segment" includes the 10 facet joints and five intervertebral discs of the five lumbar vertebrae.

When practicing yoga it is not possible to isolate the joints within a segment. For example, it is not possible to twist, bend or stretch just one lumbar vertebra. A yogi must be content to stress all of the lumbar vertebrae. It is sometimes possible to emphasize one particular part of a segment, but all of the joints in the segment will still be affected by a yoga pose.

Muscles and myofascial groups

There are over 600 muscles in the body, but for yoga practitioners it is sufficient to consider the muscles of the body as divided into 10 myofascial groups (or 20 if you include left and right sides). Each group is formed by a shared fascial structure or fascial compartment.

The first eight myofascial groups are involved in the vast majority of yin yoga poses. These eight groups can be schematized as three myofascial groups on each side of the torso and five myofascial groups in each thigh. Each of these groups is clearly delineated by fascial compartments (Grant, 1948; Schuenke et al., 2006).

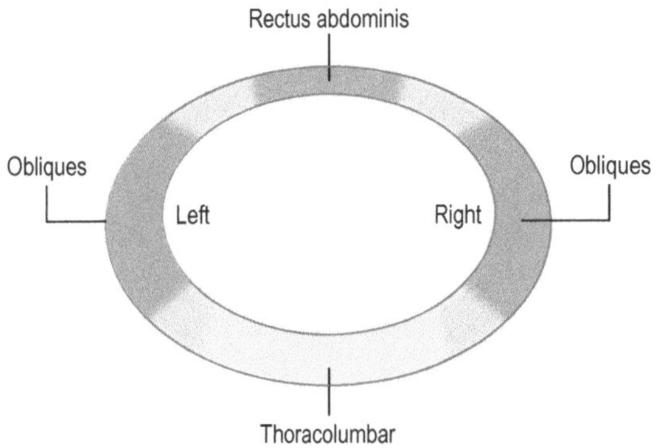

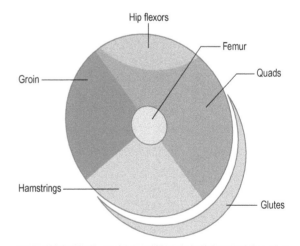

Figure 38.1

The three myofascial groups on each side of the torso can be schematically represented as above. If a yoga practitioner feels the stress of a yoga asana in the specified target area then he or she is performing the asana correctly.

Figure 38.2

The five myofascial groups of the right thigh can be schematically represented as above. If a yoga practitioner feels the stress of a yoga asana in the specified target area then he or she is performing the asana correctly.

Yin yoga as a fascia-oriented practice

Again, it is not possible to isolate just one of the muscles within a group. For example, a yogini cannot do a forward bend and stretch only one of the muscles ensheathed by the thoracolumbar fascia. A yogini is obliged to stretch all the muscles within that group. It is sometimes possible to emphasize one, but all of the muscles in the group will be affected by a yoga pose.

Yoga practice as stressing specific target areas

Presenting yoga as a practice designed to stress joint segments and myofascial groups allows us to sweep aside the various "rules of alignment" floating around in the yoga world and replace them with a system that appears to be simpler, safer and more effective. This simplification is made possible by the fascial compartmentalisation of muscles.

Six-step protocol

This is the protocol for determining how each yoga asana should be developed:

1. Select a target area to be stressed.
2. Select the asana archetype that stresses that area.
3. Select a variation of the archetype that suits your skeletability.
4. Practice the pose for 3–5 min.
5. Be sure not to overstrain the skeletal or myofascial tissues.
6. Rebound for 1 or 2 min.

The first three steps of the protocol are illustrated below.

Stressing the gluteal group: the first three steps

Step 1

Select the target area. The target area in this example will be the gluteal myofascial group, which includes 10 muscles and the iliotibial band. The muscles are gluteus minimus, gluteus medius, gluteus maximus, the six deep rotator muscles, and the tensor fasciae latae. It is not likely that all of these muscles will be affected, but all of them are potential targets. This varies from student to student.

Step 2

Select the asana archetype that stresses the gluteal group. In this instance, it is the Shoelace. All variations of the Shoelace archetype require different degrees of external rotation, abduction and flexion of the femur. The combination of these movements stresses the gluteal group.

Step 3

Select the variation of the archetype that suits your skeletability. For this demonstration both models have selected Sleeping Swan. Skeletability refers to the range of motion that is determined by the shape of your bones. In Sleeping Swan, the relevant bones are the hip socket and the femur.

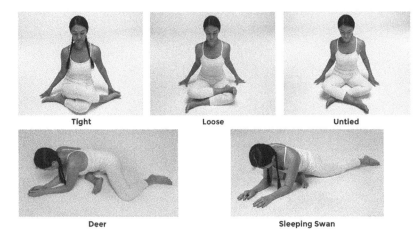

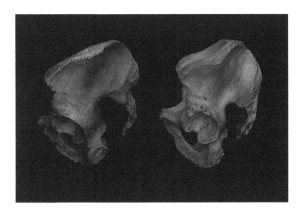

Figure 38.3

Each one of these poses is a variation of the Shoelace. Each variation externally rotates, abducts and flexes the femur. It is the combination of these movements that stresses the gluteal myofascial group. Each variation emphasizes a slightly different combination of these three movements. It is up to the student to carefully test and determine the appropriate variation for her body. For this demonstration, each model will choose the Sleeping Swan.

Figure 38.4

This is an image of two pelvi facing to the reader's left. The hip socket on the left pelvis is oriented forward and down. The hip socket on the right pelvis is oriented towards the camera and nearly horizontal. Without going into detail, I hope that the reader can appreciate that the amount of rotation, abduction and flexion would be dramatically different for these dramatically different hip sockets. Also, keep in mind that the differences in the femur bones are just as dramatic.

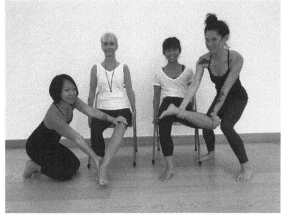

Figure 38.5

The models sitting in the chairs are allowing their left femurs to be passively rotated by a partner. Each of the models is demonstrating the limit of their ability to abduct and externally rotate their femurs. Each of them is experiencing compression of the femur against the lip of the hip socket. This type of compression is not painful, which is why they are smiling.

Yin yoga as a fascia-oriented practice

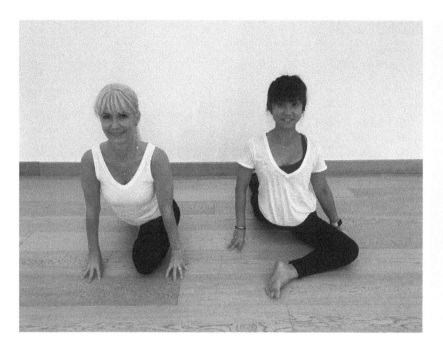

Figure 38.6

The same two models are demonstrating the preferred placement of their left foot and knee. The model on the left has minimized the amount of external rotation and abduction; the model on the right has maximized them. If the model on the left pushed her foot forward and her knee out to the side then she might hurt her knee. If the model on the right brought her foot down and her knee in she would not stress the gluteal group.

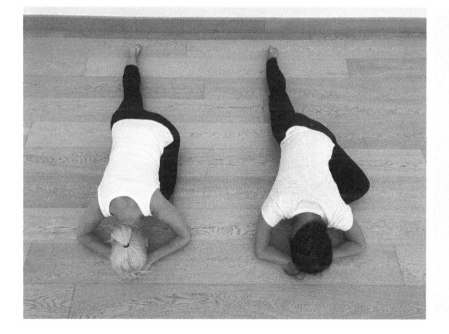

Figure 38.7

Both models are now lying prone over their left leg. Both of these variations of Sleeping Swan are effectively stressing the gluteal myofascial group. There is no perfect or best variation that would be equally effective for both of them.

Chapter 38

Stressing the joint segments of lower body: the first three steps

Step 1

Select the target areas. The target areas in this example will be the skeletal segments of the lower body: toes, ankles, knees, hips, pelvis and the lumbar spine. These joint segments are particularly susceptible to stiffness and degeneration in our modern, chair-bound society.

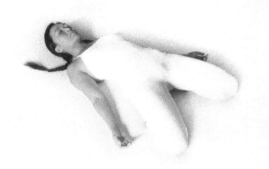

Figure 38.8

This is the Saddle archetype. The student sits on her feet, modestly abducts her femurs, and reclines. All the joints of the lower body are stressed, as well as the quad and hip flexor myofascial groups.

Step 2

Select the asana archetype that stresses these segments. In this instance it is the Saddle. Saddle also stresses two myofascial groups: the quads and hip flexors. But for this analysis, we will focus on the joint segments.

Step 3

Select the variation of the archetype that suits your skeletability. In this example, the variation is foot position. Different foot positions require different degrees of internal rotation of the hip joints and external rotation of the tibia. This analysis will focus on the internal rotation of the hip joint.

Props are frequently used in yin yoga. They are used to reduce tension in the soft tissues or to reduce compression on the bones and discs. Saddle is the epitome of a pose that frequently requires the use of props because so many joint segments are stressed.

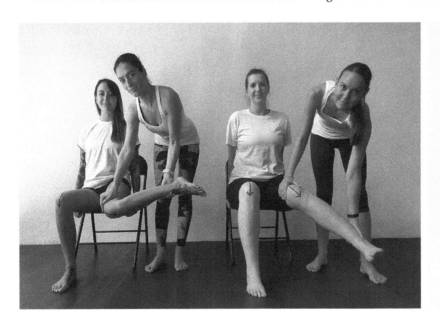

Figure 38.9

The models sitting in the chairs are allowing their left femurs to be passively rotated by a partner. Each of the models is demonstrating the limit of their abilities to internally rotate their femurs. Each of them is experiencing compression of the femur against the lip of the hip socket. This type of compression is not painful, which is why they are smiling.

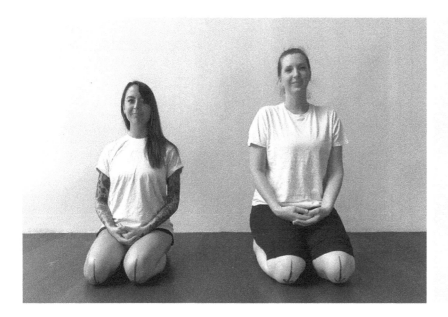

Figure 38.10

The models are sitting on their feet. A line has been drawn to indicate the orientation of the knee. This line approximately divides the condyles of the femur; it is intended only as a reference.

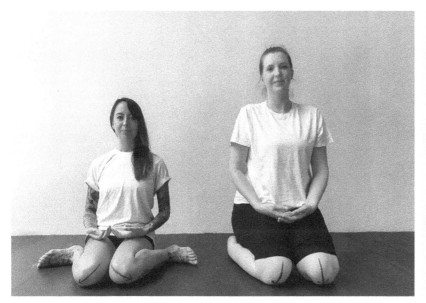

Figure 38.11

In this image both models are attempting to sit between their feet. Sitting between their feet requires more internal rotation than sitting on their feet. The model on the right has very little internal rotation, as is indicated by the very slight change in the vertical lines. And so her feet have moved only slightly apart. The model on the left has a large range of internal rotation, as is indicated by the vertical line becoming nearly horizontal.

Not every student has the props available or the skill to use them as demonstrated in Figure 38.14. In this case there are two possible options:

1: Be content to sit on your feet as in Figure 38.11, or with feet apart and using a cushion as in Figure 38.12. This benefits the toes, ankles, knees and the quads.

2: If practicing at home, kneeling on the floor and leaning back against a couch is stable and effective.

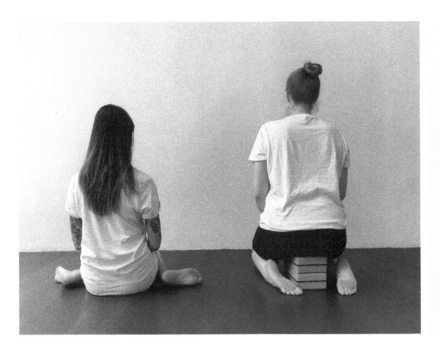

Figure 38.12

The model on the right has minimized femoral rotation by sitting on a cushion and keeping her feet just hip-width. The model on the left has maximized femoral rotation by sitting between her feet and dorsiflexing her ankles. Students with a lot of internal rotation frequently prefer this position as it more effectively stresses the quads and hip flexors.

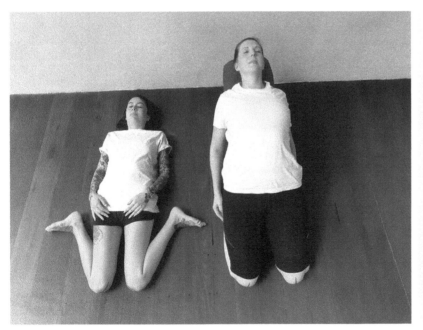

Figure 38.13

Both models are showing their preferred Saddle variation. The model on the right sits on a cushion to prevent knee strain. She also rests her upper body on a cushion to reduce pelvic and lumbar extension.

Yin yoga as a fascia-oriented practice

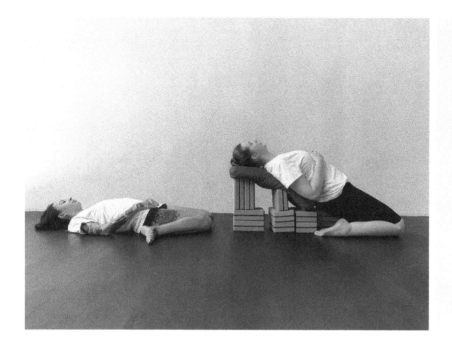

Figure 38.14
Both models are showing their preferred Saddle variation. The model on the right sits on a cushion to prevent knee strain. She also rests her upper body on a cushion to reduce pelvic and lumbar extension.

Remember: it is not always desirable to develop the maximum skeletability of a joint segment.

Stressing the muscles and joints of upper body: the first three steps

Step 1

Select the target areas. The target areas in this example will be the skeletal segments and muscles of the upper body. The skeletal segments include the fingers, wrist, radius, ulna, humerus and scavicle (scapula + clavicle.) The myofascial group is the scapular group. This large group includes the muscles that move and stabilize the scavicle and the humerus. The scavicle muscles include the rhomboids, levator scapulae, pectoralis minor, latissimus dorsi and trapezius. The humeral muscles include the four rotator cuff muscles, deltoid, pectoralis major, biceps, coraco-brachialis, triceps and latissimus dorsi.

Step 2

Select the asana archetype that stresses these target areas. In this instance, it is the Dog. The identifying characteristic of the Dog is bearing weight on the arms.

Step 3

Select the variation of the archetype that suits your skeletability. In this example, the variation will be Chaturanga, a push-up. All the joints of the upper body will have some influence on this pose, but three are most relevant: the scapula, the humerus and the ulna. This analysis will focus on the torsion of the humerus.

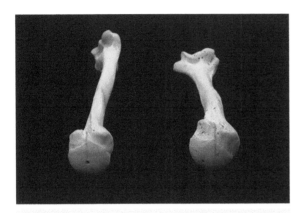

Figure 38.15

This is an image of two right humerus bones. It is the view you would have looking down your right arm. The round, proximal end of the humerus articulates with the scapula to form the shoulder joint. The distal end articulates with the ulna to form the elbow joint. The long bones of the body have torsion, they spiral, but no two long bones are identical. To demonstrate this a line has been drawn through the bicipital grooves of each specimen and these lines are oriented vertically. We could say that the elbow joint of the left specimen is "turned in" relative to the right specimen.

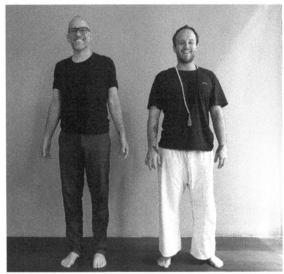

Figure 38.16

These two models are standing relaxed. The inner crease of their elbow joints are turned out on the left model and turned in on the right model. This is indicative of their different humeral torsions.

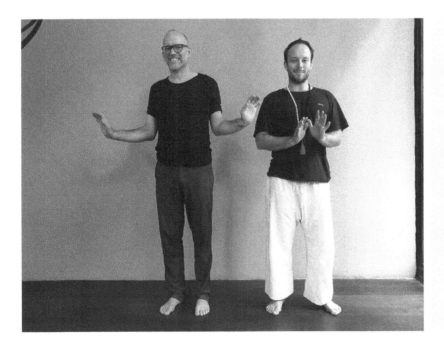

Figure 38.17

Flexing their elbows brings their arms and hands into very different orientations relative to their torsos. When practicing Chaturanga, the model on the left would have to internally rotate his humeri to place his palms on the floor. The model on the right would have to externally rotate his humeri to place his palms on the floor. The stresses on their joint capsules, rotator cuff and deltoid muscles are very different when they practice Chaturanga.

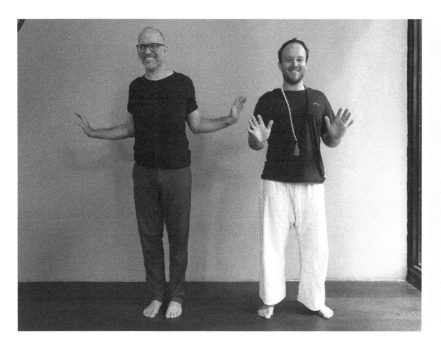

Figure 38.18

A common "alignment cue" in Chaturanga is "squeeze the scapula together". In this image, both models have retracted their scapula. The model on the left has now placed his arms in an even more disadvantageous position. He would have to internally rotate 70 degrees to place his palms on the floor. But the model on the right now has perfect arm position. He would not need to rotate his humeri at all.

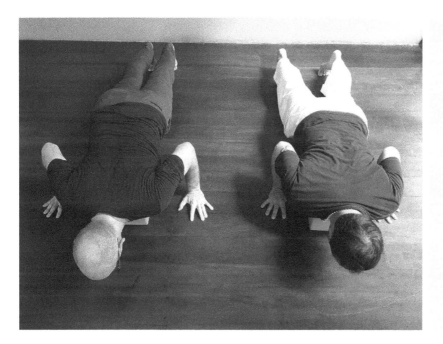

Figure 38.19

Another common "alignment cue" in Chaturanga is "squeeze the elbows into the ribs". The model on the left, because he needs to internally rotate his humeri 70 degrees, feels an uncomfortable strain in his shoulder joints if he holds his elbows to his ribs, so he holds his humeri at an angle away from his body.

Chapter 38

Many variations of an archetype

I do not want to leave the reader with the impression that, for each student, there is one and only one best variation of an archetype. A yogini might practice many variations of an archetype, as long as each variation effectively stresses the target areas.

In our first example, the Sleeping Swan was selected to compare two different skeletons performing the same variation. But each model might also enjoy practicing other variations of the Shoelace. Shoelace stresses the gluteal group. Each variation of Shoelace alters the abduction, rotation and flexion of the femur. These variations will almost certainly emphasize slightly different parts of this large myofascial group. It is important to explore all the variations of an archetype to determine which are effective and which are ineffective stressors of the gluteal group. Every variation that is effective should stay in your repertoire.

In our second example, we saw that the model with excellent internal rotation of the femur was comfortable sitting between her feet. But someone with this skeletability might also enjoy sitting on their feet. Sitting on their feet will elevate their pelvis. This might create a desirable extension of the lumbar spine that one does not experience when sitting between their feet. They might also experience a better stretch on their hip flexors when sitting on their feet.

In our third example, we saw that the model on the right could easily hold his elbows in to his ribs when practicing Chaturanga. But he might choose several different abduction angles of his humerus to emphasize different muscles within the scapular group. Arms abducted emphasizes the pectoral and deltoid muscles. Arms adducted emphasizes the triceps.

Modern meridian theory

The man who initiated my interest in fascia was my teacher Dr. Hiroshi Motoyama, who had PhDs in both Philosophy and Physiological Psychology. He began his scientific investigation of meridians in the 1970s. In 1987, in an address to some of his students, he said:

"Modern Western medicine does not yet understand the meridian system. This is because the meridians lie in a water-rich phase within the connective tissue (fascia). When a person dies, this layer dries out. Since the meridian channels have no walls as the blood vessels do, they cannot be detected by current medical techniques. Actually, however, these water-rich channels crisscross the entire body."

Motoyama (2003).

It is no longer true that practitioners of Western medicine do not understand the meridian system. Indeed, many sides of scientific inquiry appear to be closing in on the meridian system. Two findings of modern fascia research are most relevant to yoga practitioners: fascia's ability to contract and relax, and fascia's ability to absorb, bind and release water.

Rebound and rehydration

It has been demonstrated that slow, compressive massage strokes temporarily force water out of myofascial tissues, and that when the tissues recover the water content is higher than before. It has also been demonstrated that relaxing after long, static stretching can induce a higher hydration in fascia (Schleip et al., 2012).

Yin yoga as a fascia-oriented practice

This super-compensation of the water content aptly describes the subjective experience of the rebound after a yoga pose.

After practicing a pose for several minutes, a yin yogini will rest for a minute or two and focus on what she is feeling in the target area. This period of restful introspection is called "the rebound". During the rebound a yogini typically feels fluid movement and a sense of heat dispersion or vibration. It is innately pleasant and relaxing.

Meridians conduct energy

Dr. Motoyama demonstrated that the water-rich channels in fascia are electrically conductive. He also demonstrated that the currents in these channels propagate at a different velocity than the nervous system, that the pathways of conduction are different from those of the nervous system, and that the local response to electrical stimulus of a meridian is opposite to that of the nervous system (positive vs. negative). He also demonstrated that the pathways of the watery fascial channels correspond very closely to the pathways described in ancient acupuncture texts (Motoyama, 1997).

If and when these findings are confirmed by other researchers, this would have large implications for acupuncture theory, yoga theory and modern medicine. If experiments were to confirm that the interstitial environment has malleable qualities of electrical capacitance and conduction, then the colloquial "I am having a low energy day" would take on a medically testable meaning.

Motoyama noted that a certain electrical response, which he called the "before polarization" current, was higher in healthy people who had good fluid flow in their fascia, and lower in elderly, seriously ill or physically weak people, who had poor fluid flow in their fascia Motoyama, 1997).

One day, I hope that the following statement is a scientifically validated fact:

Some of the mechanical stresses created by yoga postures are converted into greater electrical capacitance and conductance in the meridians. This affects the migration of various cells through the fascia/interstitium, the movement of substances in and out of cells, and alters what cells express. This is why the healing effects of the practice go far beyond flexibility and relaxation.

The rebound is more than physical

During the rebound, yogis also experience emotional contentment and mental calm. A simple theory of fascial rehydration cannot explain the depth of the emotional and mental responses. A yogini would say they are the result of harmonizing the flow of her chi.

Chi is the ancient Chinese term for life force. The theory of a life force was hotly debated and dismissed from modern medicine over 100 years ago but the conception of a life force is central to acupuncture theory and yoga practice. Dr. Motoyama taught that chi is a unique form of energy not reducible to electricity or chemistry.

The ancient theory of chi and the modern theory of meridians are an accurate description of the subjective experience of yoga. I believe there are watery meridian channels penetrating and sustaining all tissues of the body, including bones, joints, viscera and the cerebrospinal fluid. The purpose of yoga asana is to harmonize the flow of chi in these meridians.

References

Grant, J.C.B. (1948) *A Method of Anatomy*, 4th edn. Baltimore, MD: Williams and Wilkins, 386.

Motoyama, H. (1997) *Measurements of Ki Energy: Diagnosis and Treatment*. Tokyo, Japan: Human Sciences Press, 3–5.

Motoyama, H. (2003) *Awakening the Chakras and Emancipation*. Tokyo, Japan: Human Science Press, 194.

Schleip, R., Duerslen, L. & Vleeming, A. et al. (2012) Strain hardening of fascia: static stretching of dense fibrous connective tissues can induce a temporary stiffness increase accompanied by enhanced matrix hydration. *J Bodyw Mov Ther*. 16: 94–100.

Schuenke, M., Schulte, E. & Schumacher, U. (2006) General Anatomy and Musculoskeletal System. In: *THIEME Atlas of Anatomy*. Stuttgart, Germany: Thieme, 128–129.

Other resources

California Institute for Human Science
On the web: CIHS.edu
701 Garden View Court
Encinitas, CA 92024.

Clark, Bernie (2016)

Your Body Your Yoga

Wild Strawberry Productions

Clark, Bernie (2018)

Your Spine Your Yoga

Wild Strawberry Productions

Muscolino.
Youtube: Piriformis Muscle Medially Rotates with Dr. Joe Muscolino.

https://www.youtube.com/watch?v=vGZPw6ARj0s

Acknowledgments

Our thanks to Dr. Tyler Maltman for the term "skeletability".

Our thanks to Jo Phee and Joe Barnett for directing the photo shoots of the various poses.

More thanks to Jo Phee for her images of Sleeping Swan and Saddle.

Our thanks to Annette Pauli and Iris Tan for modeling Sleeping Swan.

Our thanks to Jaclyn Philpott and Hellè Weston for modeling Saddle.

Our thanks to Joe Barnett and Robert John for modeling Chaturanga.

Fascia-focused Pilates training

Elizabeth Larkam

Note Elizabeth Larkam has produced a compilation of short videos to help you gain a deeper understanding. Watch these videos free of charge at **www.pilatesanytime.com/fascia**. To redeem your free access use code **FASCIA**. These short videos were compiled as a companion to her book *Fascia in Motion: Fascia-focused Movement for Pilates* [Handspring, 2017].

Introduction

The movement program created by Joseph Hubertus Pilates (1880–1967) served the bedridden after World War I broke out in 1914, when he taught in a camp for enemy aliens in Lancaster, England. J. H. Pilates took springs from beds, creating his earliest rehabilitation equipment for the internees (Pilates Method Alliance, 2013).

Less than a century later, it was reported that Pilates was the fastest growing activity in the country, with 8.6 million Americans participating in 2009 (Sporting Goods Manufacturers Association, 2010). Participation increased by 456% between 2000 and 2009 (Rovell, 2010). Countless millions have engaged in the practice of Pilates worldwide. In 2015, Statista reported that the number of United States participants aged 6 years and older in Pilates training amounted to ~8.6 million (Statista, 2015).

Pilates programs, informed by principles of fascia-oriented training (Müller & Schleip, 2011) (Chapter 24) have been shown to improve standing balance, seated balance and proximal control of gait for polytrauma members of the military returning from Iraq and Afghanistan with amputations (Moore, 2009), trauma, traumatic stress, brain injury and vestibular dysfunction (Larkam, 2013). Soldiers from Denmark, Israel and the United States demonstrate their fascia-focused Pilates programs, informed by the

organization of the myofascial continuities (Myers, 2020) (Chapter 36) (Pilates Method Alliance Video, 2013).

History of the Pilates method

The Pilates method has been in continuous use in the United States since 1926 when Joseph Pilates and his wife Clara immigrated to New York City from Germany. In 2010 there were 8653000 Pilates participants in the United States (Sporting Goods Manufacturers Association, 2010) and countless millions engaged in the practice of Pilates worldwide. For more than 40 years, J. H. Pilates created and documented a comprehensive movement system that reflected his own physical training and the physical culture of the times. In his youth, he practiced various physical regimens to overcome childhood ailments of rickets, asthma and rheumatic fever. The movement system Joseph Pilates created was influenced by his practice of bodybuilding, gymnastics, skiing, diving, martial arts and boxing. Joseph Pilates did not have any clinical or medical credentials (PMA, 2013). He was self-taught through movement experience, observation and reading. His ideas regarding spinal alignment (Pilates, 1934) were markedly different from the generally accepted view that optimal spine organization requires a cervical and lumbar lordosis and a thoracic kyphosis. In fact, Joseph Pilates designed his entire movement system to straighten spinal curves, reflecting his belief that

Chapter 39

"the normal spine should be straight to successfully function according to the laws of nature in general and the law of gravity, in particular.... Proper carriage of the spine is the only natural preventive against abdominal obesity, shortness of breath, asthma, high and low blood pressure and various forms of heart disease. It is safe to say that none of the ailments here enumerated can be cured until the curvatures of the spine have been corrected" (Pilates, 1934).

Table 39.1 Publications that inform fascia-focused Pilates movement	
Publications (alphabetically by last name)	**Branch of knowledge**
I: Models of movement	
Beach, P. (2010) *Muscles and Meridians: the manipulation of shape*. Edinburgh, UK: Churchill Livingstone.	Osteopathy, Traditional Chinese medicine
Martin, D.-C. (2016) *Living biotensegrity: interplay of tension and compression in the body*. Munich, Germany: Keiner.	Physics, Chinese movement arts
Scarr, G. (2018) *Biotensegrity: the structural basis of life*, 2nd edn. Edinburgh, UK: Handspring. Stephen Levin introduced the term biotensegrity in 1975.	Osteopathy
II: Architecture and anatomy of fascia	
Guimberteau, J.-C. & Armstrong, C. (2015) Architecture of human living fascia: the extracellular matrix and cells revealed through endoscopy. Edinburgh, UK: Handspring.	General medicine, surgery
Stecco, C. (2015) *Functional atlas of the human fascial system*. Edinburgh, UK: Churchill Livingstone.	General medicine, orthopedic surgery, human anatomy
Stecco, A., et al. (2016) *Fascial disorders: implications for treatment. American Academy of Physical Medicine & Rehabilitation Journal* 8(2): 161–168.	General medicine with specialty in physiatry
Van der Wal, J. (2009) The architecture of the connective tissue in the musculoskeletal system—an often overlooked functional parameter as to proprioception in the locomotor apparatus. *International Journal of Therapeutic Massage & Bodywork* 2(4): 9–23.	Fascia research in medical laboratory, general medicine
III: Fascia-informed manual therapies	
Chaitow, L. (2018) *Fascial dysfunction: manual therapy approaches*. Edinburgh, UK: Handspring.	Osteopathy
Myers, T. W. (2020) *Anatomy trains®: myofascial meridians for manual & movement therapists* (3rd ed.). Edinburgh, UK: Elsevier.	Structural integration
Schwind, P. (2006) *Fascial and membrane technique*. Edinburgh, UK: Churchill Livingstone. Schwind studied with Jean-Pierre Barral.	Rolfing®
Stecco, L. & Stecco, C. (2014) *Fascial manipulation® for internal dysfunctions*. Stuttgart, Germany: Schattauer GmbH.	Physiotherapy, general medicine, human anatomy
IV: Fascia-informed theory and movement applications	
Avision, J. S. (2015) *Yoga: fascia anatomy and movement*. Edinburgh, UK: Handspring.	Yoga Structural integration
Schleip, R. (2015) *Fascia in sport and movement*. Edinburgh, UK: Handspring. Robert Schleip and Thomas W. Myers coined the term "Fascial Fitness®"	Fascia research, Rolfing®

Table 39.2 Pilates movement principles correlate with fascia-focused training criteria
The eight movement principles of the Pilates method (Lessen, 2013) correlate substantially with suggested fascia-focused training criteria (Larkam, 2017)

Pilates principles	Fascia-focused movement criteria
Whole-body movement	Whole-body movements simultaneously involving large areas of the neuromyofascial system Whole-body continuity — connect trunk to limbs and limbs to trunk — connect deep structures to superficial ones and superficial structures to deep ones
Centering	Movement initiation — connect proximal structures to distal ones and distal structures to proximal ones
Precision	Kinesthetic acuity — kinesthesia (dynamic proprioception), the aptitude to sense the position and movement of the limbs and trunk
Control	Proprioceptive refinement — proprioceptive sensations are connected with position, tendon and muscle sensations
Concentration	Interoception — interstitial nerves in fascia serve an interoceptive, rather than proprioceptive or nociceptive function. Stimulation of those free nerve endings provides information about the condition of the body in search for homeostasis in relation to physiological needs. Interoceptive signaling is associated with feelings like warmth, nausea, hunger, soreness, effort, heaviness or lightness. Perceptions about internal somatic sensations are associated with emotional preferences and feelings (Schleip, 2015)
Breathing	Flowing movement sequences
Balanced muscle development (optimal activation of the neuromyofascial system)	Multidirectional movements with slight changes of angle
Rhythm	Preparatory countermovement Dynamic stretching — slow and fast tempo variations
These fascia-focused movement criteria do not correlate with specific Pilates principles. However, fascia-focused Pilates movement may involve them	
	Develop glide within the three-dimensional neuromyofascial system
	Force/load transfer — movements that distribute force/load through the neuromyofascial system
	Facilitate tissue hydration
	Develop regular lattice with crimp
	Develop elastic recoil
	Stimulate tissue renewal
	Develop tissue resilience
	Movements are sustainable for motor control refinement and collagen remodeling
	Access all appropriate myofascial continuities in optimal sequence for client profile
	Movements encourage awareness of and embodiment of applied biotensegrity

Chapter 39

Selected mat and reformer exercises provide examples of the Pilates principles

This chapter examines the effectiveness and the limitations of the original Pilates method to fulfill the principles of fascia-focused training.

This photograph suggests that the original Pilates method of unique movement sequences and equipment created a foundation from which contemporary expressions of Pilates can be customized to train fascia. The chapter includes one example of how the J. H. Pilates mat exercise Leg Pull Front provides a foundation for the contemporary Pilates Reformer exercise, Jumping

Table 39.3 Selected mat and Reformer exercises provide examples of the Pilates principles		
Pilates principles	**Pilates mat exercise**	**Reformer exercise**
Rhythm	The One-Leg Stretch with Knees Extended (Pilates Anytime Mat Workout (2016) #2507)	Elastic recoil training with jumpboard
Breathing	The Roll Up (*Figure* **39.2A2**)	Standing side splits
Rhythm	The Saw (*Figure* **39.2E2**)	Knee stretch series Standing/knees off
Rhythm	Fast: The One Leg Kick (*Figure* **39.2C2**) Slow: The Roll Over With Legs Spread (Both Ways) (*Figure* **39.2B1**)	Fast: Stomach Massage Slow: Side Stretch
Whole body movement	Side Bend Twist (*Figure* **39.2F3**)	Long-Stretch
Balanced muscle development (optimal activation of the neuromyofascial system)	The Cork-Screw (*Figure* **39.2E1**)	Feet in straps
Centering	The Teaser (*Figure* **39.2A6**)	Short box advanced abdominals
Concentration control	The Leg-Pull (*Figure* **39.2F2**)	Control back (face ceiling)
Precision	The Hip Twist With Stretched Arms (*Figure* **39.2E4**)	Front splits – hands up
These fascia-oriented training principles do not correlate with specific Pilates principles; however, fascia-focused Pilates movement may fulfill these benefits	The Spine Stretch (*Figure* **39.2A5**) The Spine Twist (*Figure* **39.2E3**) Mat practice 20 min twice per week for between 7 months and 2 years.	Spine-Massage Cleopatra Reformer practice 20 min twice per week for between 7 months and 2 years

"If you will faithfully perform your Contrology exercises regularly only four times a week for just three months as outlined in Return to Life, you will find your body development approaching the ideal, accompanied by renewed mental vigor and spiritual enhancement." Joseph H. Pilates (1945–2010).

Fascia-focused Pilates training

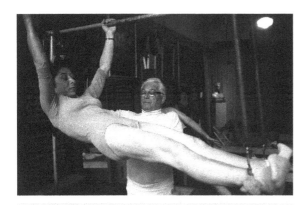

Figure 39.1

Joseph H. Pilates instructing a client in Hanging Pull Up on his trapeze table at Joe's Gymnasium, the 8th Avenue Studio, New York, NY, October 1961. The Universal Reformer is visible in the background.

Copyright I. C. Rapoport.

in Quadruped, which fulfills the principles of fascia-focused training. The Pilates movement principles are explained in *The Pilates Method Alliance Pilates Certification Exam Study Guide* (PMA, 2013), which states: "The body is organised to move by **centering. Balanced muscle development** allows efficient movement and proper joint mechanics. Constant mental **concentration** is required to fully develop the body. **Precision**, meaning exact, defined, specific, intentional movement is necessary for correct form. Only a few repetitions of each exercise are appropriate so that each repetition can be performed with the greatest **control**, using only the necessary muscles and effort necessary for each movement. **Breathing** promotes natural movement and **rhythm** and stimulates muscles to greater activity. Performance of the Pilates exercises is distinguished by always using the **whole body**."

Mat exercises provide the foundation of the Pilates method

Thirty-four mat exercises form the foundation of the movement system that Joseph Pilates called

"Contrology". Joseph Pilates states his philosophy in his 1945 book, *Return to Life*: "Faithfully perform your Contrology exercises only four times a week for just three months...you will find your body development approaching the ideal, accompanied by renewed mental vigor and spiritual enhancement" (Pilates, 1945). Careful study of the mat exercises indicates that, although specific Pilates mat exercises may satisfy the fascia-focused training criteria "Multidirectional Movements with slight changes in angle" (Table 39.2), the majority of exercises will not, given their single plane orientation. Of the mat exercises pictured in *Return to Life Through Contrology*, 15 are organized in flexion in the sagittal plane. Only eight exercises emphasize extension in the sagittal plane. Lateral flexion of the spine is represented by two exercises. Three exercises combine flexion and rotation. Spinal rotation is represented by The Spine Twist. Joseph Pilates intended the remaining five exercises to be performed in a posterior pelvic tilt and lumbar flexion in order to flatten the lumbar lordosis. However, they may be practiced in a neutral pelvis and a neutral lumbar spine.

Given that 29 of the mat exercises are open kinematic chain for the lower extremity, these mat exercises are not optimal for developing elastic recoil in full weight bearing. Only four exercises are closed kinematic chain for both upper and lower extremities. Joseph Pilates performed many of the mat exercises with rather vigorous elastic bounces in the end ranges of available motion (Pilates, 1932–1945) so even his open kinematic chain exercises can be used to develop elastic recoil (Chapter 8).

Joseph Pilates was a prolific inventor of exercise apparatus

Throughout his 4 decades of work in Joe's Gymnasium, Joseph Pilates continued to develop

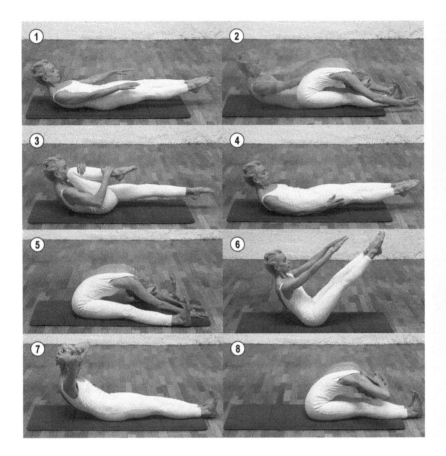

Figure 39.2 A

Seven Pilates mat exercises demonstrate spine flexion in supine and sitting. These movements emphasize activation of the Deep Front (Figure 36.7) and Superficial Front (Figure 36.2) myofascial continuities. From top left to bottom right: **(1)** The Hundred, **(2)** The Roll-Up, **(3)** The One Leg Stretch, **(4)** The Double Leg Stretch, **(5)** The Spine Stretch, **(6)** The Teaser, **(7, 8)** The Neck Pull.

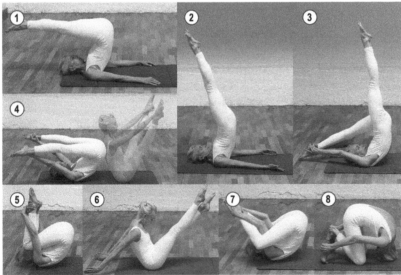

Figure 39.2 B

Eight Pilates mat exercises demonstrate spine flexion with weight bearing on the upper thoracic area. These movements emphasize synergistic activation of the Superficial Front (Figure 36.2) and Superficial Back (Figure 36.1) myofascial continuities. From top left to bottom right: **(1)** The Roll Over, **(2)** Rocker with Open Legs, **(3)** The Jack-Knife, **(4)** The Control Balance, **(5)** Rolling Back, **(6)** The Boomerang, **(7)** The Seal, **(8)** The Crab.

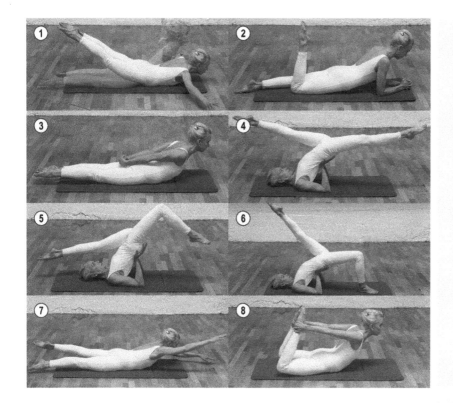

Figure 39.2 C

Eight Pilates mat exercises demonstrate spine extension. These movements emphasize synergistic activation of the Superficial Back (Figure 36.1) myofascial continuity in conjunction with the Deep Front (Figure 36.7) myofascial continuity. From top left to bottom right: **(1)** The Swan-Dive, **(2)** The One Leg Kick, **(3)** The Double Kick, **(4)** The Scissors, **(5)** The Bicycle, **(6)** The Shoulder Bridge, **(7)** Swimming, **(8)** The Rocking.

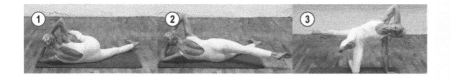

Figure 39.2 D

Two Pilates mat exercises demonstrate lateral flexion of the spine. These movements emphasize activation of the Lateral myofascial continuity (Figure 36.3). Left to right: **(1, 2)** The Side Kick, **(3)** The Side Kick Kneeling.

(Continued)

his movement program, inventing over 14 exercise apparatus that provide assistance, resistance and complexity to the organization required by the mat exercises. The equipment frames provide a number of places to which springs or cords may be attached, creating movement environments that support a variety of vectors, making it possible to satisfy all the criteria of fascia-focused training listed in Table 39.2. Joseph Pilates created a unique movement repertoire for each of his inventions.

Contemporary evolution of the Pilates method serves client and patient diversity

A century has passed since Joseph Pilates began working in a New York City boxer's training gym, teaching a diverse clientele. The proliferation of applications of Pilates techniques has resulted in an expansion of protocols for a

Chapter 39

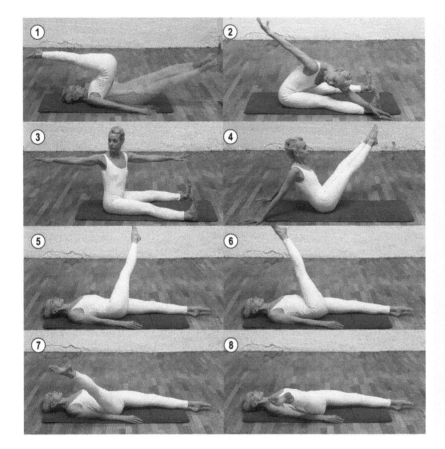

Figure 39.2 E

Five Pilates mat exercises demonstrate spine rotation. These movements emphasize activation of the Spiral myofascial continuity (Figure 36.4). Top left to bottom right: **(1)** The Cork-Screw, **(2)** The Saw, **(3)** The Spine Twist, **(4)** The Hip Twist with Stretched Arms, **(5–8)** The One Leg Circle (Both Ways).

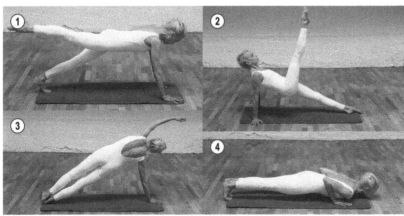

Figure 39.2 F

Four Pilates mat exercises demonstrate closed kinematic chain contact of the hands and feet with the mat. These movements activate the entire neuromyofascial system (Figure 36.1–36.7). From top left to bottom right: **(1)** The Leg-Pull – Front, **(2)** The Leg-Pull, **(3)** The Side Bend, **(4)** The Push Up.

wide range of diagnoses, conditions and performance goals. Research on the properties and function of the neuromyofascial system, as well as the creation of Fascial Fitness (Chapter 24), influences interest in how to train fascia in Pilates.

Fascia-focused Pilates training

Table 39.4 The myofascial continuities[a] and J. H. Pilates mat

Use this Pilates mat fascia-focused training guide to plan your mat classes and individual practice for thorough fascial training. Each exercise cultivates at least one of the fascial-focused movement criteria and activates one primary and several secondary myofascial continuities

Fascia-focused movement criteria

Movement requirements	Biotensegrity model
1. Movements are sustainable for motor control refinement and collagen remodeling 2. Movements encourage awareness of and embodiment of the biotensegrity model[b]	b "A tensegrity structure provides a global response to a local mechanical stress. The result is a degree of independence from the force of gravity. Without a tensegrity model, our fibrillar structure would collapse under gravitational force. With the tensegrity model, our structure absorbs and disperses the compression by spreading the load throughout the entire network, including the structures at the periphery" (Guimberteau and Armstrong, 2015). "The value of the Tensegrity model is *not* that it necessarily changes a particular approach to treatment but that it provides a *better means to visualize the mechanics of the body* in the light of new understandings about functional anatomy" (Scarr, 2018).

The myofascial continuities[a]

Movement intent	Superficial Back	Functional	Lateral	Spiral	Deep Front	Arm	Superficial Front
3. Access all appropriate myofascial continuities in optimal sequence for client profile	The Swan-Dive (*Figure 39.2C1*)	Rocker With Open Legs (*Figure 39.2B2*)	The Side Bend (*Figure 39.2F3*)	The Spine Twist (*Figure 39.2E3*)	Rolling Back (*Figure 39.2B5*)	The Leg-Pull (*Figure 39.2F2*)	The Bicycle (*Figure 39.2C5*)
4. Interoception — Interstitial nerves in fascia serve an interoceptive, rather than proprioceptive or nociceptive function. Stimulation of those free nerve endings provides information about the condition of the body in search for homeostasis in relation to physiological needs. Interoceptive signaling is associated with feelings like warmth, nausea, hunger, soreness, effort, heaviness or lightness. Perceptions about internal somatic sensations are associated with emotional preferences and feelings (Schleip, 2015).							
5. Proprioceptive refinement — Proprioceptive sensations are connected with position, tendon and muscle sensations	The Leg-Pull (*Figure 39.2F2*)	The Jack-Knife (*Figure 39.2B3*)	Rocker With Open Legs (*Figure 39.2B2*)	The Cork-Screw (*Figure 39.2E1*)	The Teaser (*Figure 39.2A6*)	The Leg-Pull – Front (*Figure 39.2F1*)	The Roll Up (*Figure 39.2A2*)
6. Kinesthetic acuity — Kinesthesia (dynamic proprioception), the aptitude to sense the position and movement of the limbs and trunk	Swimming (*Figure 39.2C7*)	Rolling Back (*Figure 39.2B5*)	The Side Kick Kneeling (*Figure 39.2D3*)	The Hip Twist With Stretched Arms (*Figure 39.2E4*)	The Double Leg Stretch (*Figure 39.2A4*)	The Side Bend (*Figure 39.2F3*)	The One Leg Stretch (*Figure 39.2A3*)

(Continued)

Table 39.4 [Continued] The myofascial continuities and J. H. Pilates mat

Use this Pilates mat fascia-focused training guide to plan your mat classes and individual practice for thorough fascial training. Each exercise cultivates at least one of the fascial-focused movement criteria and activates one primary and several secondary myofascial continuities

Fascia-focused movement criteria

Movement attributes

7. Whole-body movements simultaneously involving large areas of the neuromyofascial system	The Shoulder Bridge (Figure 39.2C6)	The One Leg Kick (Figure 39.2C2)	The Side Bend (Figure 39.2F3)	The Cork-Screw (Figure 39.2E1)	The Neck Pull (Figure 39.2A8)	The Push Up (Figure 39.2F4)	The Crab (Figure 39.2B8)
8. Whole-body continuity – Connect trunk to limbs and limbs to trunk – Connect deep structures to superficial ones and superficial structures to deep ones	Swimming (Figure 39.2C7)	The Leg-Pull (Figure 39.2F1)	The Side Kick (Figure 39.2D1, 2)	The Hip Twist With Stretched Arms (Figure 39.2E4)	The Scissors (Figure 39.2C4)	The Side Bend (Figure 39.2F3)	The Double Leg Stretch (Figure 39.2A4)
9. Movement initiation – Connect proximal structures to distal ones and distal structures to proximal ones	The Rocking (Figure 39.2C8)	Swimming (Figure 39.2C7)	The Side Kick (Figure 39.2D1, 2)	The Cork-Screw (Figure 39.2E1)	Rocker With Open Legs (Figure 39.2B2)	The Boomerang (Figure 39.2B6)	The Seal (Figure 39.2B7)
10. Flowing movement sequences	The Swan-Dive (Figure 39.2C1)	The Leg-Pull – Front (Figure 39.2F1)	The Side Kick Kneeling (Figure 39.2D3)	The Saw (Figure 39.2E2)	The Jack-Knife (Figure 39.2B3)	Swimming (Figure 39.2C7)	Rolling Back (Figure 39.2B5)
11. Multidirectional movements with slight changes of angle	The Bicycle (Figure 39.2C5)	The One Leg Circle (Both Ways) (Figure 39.2E5–8)	The Hip Twist With Stretched Arms (Figure 39.2E4)	The Cork-Screw (Figure 39.2E1)	The Hip Twist With Stretched Arms (Figure 39.2E4)	The Hip Twist With Stretched Arms (Figure 39.2E4)	The One Leg Circle (Both Ways) (Figure 39.2E5–8)
12. Force/load transfer – Movements that distribute force/load through the neuromyofascial system	The Rocking (Figure 39.2C8)	The Rocking (Figure 39.2C8)	The Side Kick (Figure 39.2D1, 2)	The Hip Twist With Stretched Arms (Figure 39.2E4)	The Seal (Figure 39.2B7)	The Side Bend (Figure 39.2F3)	The Seal (Figure 39.2B7)
	The Swan-Dive (Figure 39.2C1)	The Leg-Pull – Front (Figure 39.2F1)	Rocker With Open Legs (Figure 39.2B2)	The Cork-Screw (Figure 39.2E1)	The Push Up (Figure 39.2F4)	The Push Up (Figure 39.2F4)	The Crab (Figure 3.3H)

Table 39.4 [Continued] The myofascial continuities[a] and J. H. Pilates mat

Use this Pilates mat fascia-focused training guide to plan your mat classes and individual practice for thorough fascial training. Each exercise cultivates at least one of the fascial-focused movement criteria and activates one primary and several secondary myofascial continuities

Fascia-focused movement criteria	The Double Kick (Figure 39.2C3)	The Side Kick Kneeling (Figure 39.2D3)	The Side Kick (Figure 39.2D1,2)	The Spine Twist (Figure 39.2E3)	The Shoulder Bridge (Figure 39.2C6)	The Spine Twist (Figure 39.2E3)	The Bicycle (Figure 39.2C5)
13. Preparatory counter movement							
14. Facilitate tissue hydration	Approximately two-thirds of the volume of fascial tissues is made up of water. During application of mechanical load, whether by stretching or via local compression, a significant amount of water is pushed out of the more stressed zones. Application of external loading of fascial tissues can result in a refreshed hydration with improvement in the viscoelastic tissue properties (Schleip and Baker, 2015, p. 8).						
15. Develop glide within the three-dimensional neuromyofascial system	The normal glide of the collagen layers over one another may be hampered by loose connective tissue that has accumulated a variety of waste products. Failure of loose connective tissue gliding occurs in cases of overuse syndrome, trauma and surgery. Increase of local temperature contributes to fascial gliding. When the temperature is increased to over 40°C, the three-dimensional superstructure of hyaluronan chains break down progressively. This decreases hyaluronan viscosity of the loose connective tissue that is present within and beneath deep fasciae and muscles. The temporary increase in temperature can be provided by massage, movement or a warm shower. It is possible that during sleep, immobilization may cause increased hyaluronan viscosity and consequently a stiffness of the deep fasciae and muscles (Stecco, 2015, p. 60, p. 64).						
16. Develop regular lattice with crimp	The microstructure of collagen fibers shows undulations called crimp, which is reminiscent of elastic springs. When people age or when fascial fibers are immobilized, the structure of the fiber appears to loose crimp and springiness. Regular proper exercise loading of the fascial fibers may induce a more youthful collagen architecture with wavy fibers and increased elastic storage capacity (Schleip and Baker, 2015, p. 7).						
17. Develop elastic recoil							
18. Stimulate tissue renewal	The renewal speed of the body-wide fascial network is quite slow, with a half-life between months and years rather than days or weeks. During the first 3 hours after appropriate exercise loading, collagen synthesis is increased. However, collagen degradation is also increased. During the first one and a half days following exercise loading, collagen degradation outweighs collagen synthesis. Forty-eight hours after exercise, net synthesis of collagen production becomes positive (Schleip and Baker, 2015, pp. 8–9). The mobile, adaptable, fibrillar network with its intersecting fibers develops a mechanical harmony that is lost when healthy tissue is damaged. The body's repair mechanisms are unable to restore the fibrillar network in the damaged area to its original condition. The replacement tissue is of poor quality but can be improved by early mobilization of the injured area by manual therapy to enhance the flexibility of the scar tissue (Guimberteau and Armstrong, 2015, p. 162).						
19. Develop tissue resilience	According to the biotensegrity model, the neuromyofascial system accommodates movement as a self-adjusting whole. The myofascial meridians map out a set of connective tissues that form the outer tensional network that pulls in on the skeleton. The "isolated muscle theory" that has predominated our thinking has limited our perception of this body-wide "give" that is essential to resilience (Myers, p. 46; Ch. 6 in Schleip and Baker, 2015).						

[a] *Anatomy Trains* by Thomas W. Myers (2015) introduces the term myofascial meridians. In this chapter I replace "meridians" with "continuities".

Table 39.5 The myofascial continuities[a] and J. H. Pilates Reformer

Use this Pilates Reformer fascia-focused training guide to plan your Reformer classes and individual practice for thorough fascial training. Each exercise cultivates at least one of the fascia-focused movement criteria and activates one primary and several secondary myofascial continuities

Fascia-focused movement criteria	The myofascial continuities[a]						
Movement requirements	Biotensegrity model						
1. Movements are sustainable for motor control refinement and collagen remodeling	[b] "A tensegrity structure provides a global response to a local mechanical stress. The result is a degree of independence from the force of gravity. Without a tensegrity model, our fibrillar structure would collapse under gravitational force. With the tensegrity model, our structure absorbs and disperses the compression by spreading the load throughout the entire network, including the structures at the periphery" (Guimberteau and Armstrong, 2015).						
2. Movements encourage awareness of and embodiment of the biotensegrity model[b]	"The value of the Tensegrity model is not that it necessarily changes a particular approach to treatment but that it provides a better means to visualize the mechanics of the body in the light of new understandings about functional anatomy" (Scarr, 2014).						
	Superficial Back	Functional	Lateral	Spiral	Deep Front	Arm	Superficial Front
3. Access all appropriate myofascial continuities in optimal sequence for client profile	Thigh-Stretch	Balance-Control 3	Swimming – Backstroke	Horseback 2	Control Stretch	Long-Stretch	Balance-Control 4
Movement intent							
4. Interoception — Interstitial nerves in fascia serve an interoceptive, rather than proprioceptive or nociceptive, function. Stimulation of those free nerve endings provides information about the condition of the body in search for homeostasis in relation to physiological needs. Interoceptive signaling is associated with feelings like warmth, nausea, hunger, soreness, effort, heaviness or lightness. Perceptions about internal somatic sensations are associated with emotional preferences and feelings (Schleip, 2015).							
5. Proprioceptive refinement — Proprioceptive sensations are connected with position, tendon and muscle sensations	Breaststroke	Horseback 1	Control Stretch – Lifting	Horseback 1	Long-Stretch	Rowing – Back	Spine-Massage
6. Kinesthetic acuity — Kinesthesia (dynamic proprioception), the aptitude to sense the position and movement of the limbs and trunk	Long-Backstretch	Back-Bending 3	Control Stretch – Bending	Chest-Expansion	Horseback 2 & 3	Rowing – Front	Semicircles Up & Down

Table 39.5 [Continued] The myofascial continuities[a] and J. H. Pilates Reformer

Use this Pilates Reformer fascia-focused training guide to plan your Reformer classes and individual practice for thorough fascial training. Each exercise cultivates at least one of the fascia-focused movement criteria and activates one primary and several secondary myofascial continuities

Fascia-focused movement criteria							
Movement attributes							
7. Whole-body movements simultaneously involving large areas of the neuro-myofascial system	Swan-Dive	Russian-Stretch 2	Side Stretch & Control Stretch	Twist	Twist	Long-Backstretch	Russian-Stretch 1
8. Whole-body continuity — Connect trunk to limbs and limbs to trunk — Connect deep structures to superficial ones and superficial structures to deep ones	Rocking	Russian-Stretch 1	Long Spine Stretch	Corkscrew	Back-Bending 2	Tendon-Stretch	Swimming – Backstroke
9. Movement initiation — Connect proximal structures to distal ones and distal structures to proximal ones	Rocking & Pull	Balance-Control 1	Side Stretch & Control Stretch	Chest-Expansion	Stomach Massage	Balance-Control 1	Rowing – Front
10. Flowing movement sequences	Back-Bending 1	Russian-Stretch 1 & 2	Swimming – Backstroke	Twist	Back-Bending 3	Triceps	Triceps
11. Multidirectional movements with slight changes of angle	Swimming	Corkscrew	Side Stretch & Control Stretch	Corkscrew	Corkscrew	Twist	Corkscrew
12. Force/load transfer — Movements that distribute force/load through the neuromyo-fascial system	Lifting	Balance-Control 1	Long Spine Stretch	Horseback 3	Overhead	Side Stretch & Control Stretch	Arches (Footwork)
	Down-Stretch	Twist	Side Stretch & Control Stretch	Russian-Stretch 2	Tendon-Stretch	Balance-Control 3	Spine-Massage

(Continued)

Table 39.5 [Continued] The myofascial continuities' and J. H. Pilates Reformer

Use this Pilates Reformer fascia-focused training guide to plan your Reformer classes and individual practice for thorough fascial training. Each exercise cultivates at least one of the fascia-focused movement criteria and activates one primary and several secondary myofascial continuities

Fascia-focused movement criteria	Swan-Dive	Swimming	Control Stretch – Bending	Horseback 2	Feet & Knees (Footwork)	Swan-Dive	Tiger-Stretch
13. Preparatory counter movement	Swan-Dive	Swimming	Control Stretch – Bending	Horseback 2	Feet & Knees (Footwork)	Swan-Dive	Tiger-Stretch
14. Dynamic stretching — Slow and fast tempo variations	Down-Stretch	Side Stretch & Control Stretch	Side Stretch & Control Stretch	Corkscrew	Tiger-Stretch	Horseback 3	Semicircles Up & Down
Movement outcomes							
15. Facilitate tissue hydration	Approximately two-thirds of the volume of fascial tissues is made up of water. During application of mechanical load, whether by stretching or via local compression, a significant amount of water is pushed out of the more stressed zones. Application of external loading of fascial tissues can result in a refreshed hydration with improvement in the viscoelastic tissue properties (Schleip and Baker, 2015, p. 8).						
16. Develop glide within the three-dimensional neuro-myofascial system	The normal glide of the collagen layers over one another may be hampered by loose connective tissue that has accumulated a variety of waste products. Failure of loose connective tissue gliding occurs in cases of overuse syndrome, trauma and surgery. Increase of local temperature contributes to fascial gliding. When the temperature is increased to over 40°C, the three-dimensional superstructure of hyaluronan chains break down progressively. This decreases hyaluronan viscosity of the loose connective tissue that is present within and beneath deep fasciae and muscles. The temporary increase in temperature can be provided by massage, movement or a warm shower. It is possible that during sleep, immobilization may cause increased hyaluronan viscosity and consequently a stiffness of the deep fasciae and muscles (Stecco, 2015, p. 60, p. 64).						
17. Develop regular lattice with crimp	The microstructure of collagen fibers shows undulations called crimp, which is reminiscent of elastic springs. When people age or when fascial fibers are immobilized, the structure of the fiber appears to loose crimp and springiness. Regular proper exercise loading of the fascial fibers may induce a more youthful collagen architecture with wavy fibers and increased elastic storage capacity (Schleip & Baker, 2015, p. 7).						

Table 39.5 [Continued] The myofascial continuities[a] and J. H. Pilates Reformer

Use this Pilates Reformer fascia-focused training guide to plan your Reformer classes and individual practice for thorough fascial training. Each exercise cultivates at least one of the fascia-focused movement criteria and activates one primary and several secondary myofascial continuities

Fascia-focused movement criteria	
18. Develop elastic recoil	
19. Stimulate tissue renewal	The renewal speed of the body-wide fascial network is quite slow, with a half-life between months and years rather than days or weeks. During the first 3 hours after appropriate exercise loading, collagen synthesis is increased. However, collagen degradation is also increased. During the first one and a half days following exercise loading collagen degradation outweighs collagen synthesis. Forty-eight hours after exercise, net synthesis of collagen production becomes positive (Schleip and Baker, 2015, pp. 8–9). The mobile, adaptable, fibrillar network with its intersecting fibers develops a mechanical harmony that is lost when healthy tissue is damaged. The body's repair mechanisms are unable to restore the fibrillar network in the damaged area to its original condition. The replacement tissue is of poor quality but can be improved by early mobilization of the injured area by manual therapy to enhance the flexibility of the scar tissue (Guimberteau and Armstrong, 2015, p. 162).
20. Develop tissue resilience	According to the biotensegrity model, the neuromyofascial system accommodates movement as a self-adjusting whole. The myofascial meridians map out a set of connective tissues that form the outer tensional network that pulls in on the skeleton. The "isolated muscle theory" that has predominated our thinking has limited our perception of this body-wide "give" that is essential to resilience (Myers, p. 46; Ch. 6 in Schleip & Baker, 2015).

[a] *Anatomy Trains* by Thomas W. Myers (2020) introduces the term myofascial meridians. In this chapter I replace "meridians" with "continuities".

Table 39.6 The myofascial continuities[a] and fascia-focused Reformer exercises
Use this Pilates Reformer fascia-focused training guide to plan your Reformer classes and individual practice for thorough fascial training. Each exercise cultivates at least one of the fascia-focused movement criteria and activates one primary and several secondary myofascial continuities

Fascia-focused movement criteria							
Movement requirements	Biotensegrity model						
1. Movements are sustainable for motor control refinement and collagen remodeling 2. Movements encourage awareness of and embodiment of the biotensegrity model[b]	b "A tensegrity structure provides a global response to a local mechanical stress. The result is a degree of independence from the force of gravity. Without a tensegrity model, our fibrillar structure would collapse under gravitational force. With the tensegrity model, our structure absorbs and disperses the compression by spreading the load throughout the entire network, including the structures at the periphery" (Guimberteau and Armstrong, 2015). "The value of the Tensegrity model is not that it necessarily changes a particular approach to treatment but that it provides a better means to visualize the mechanics of the body in the light of new understandings about functional anatomy" (Scarr, 2014).						

The myofascial continuities[a]

	Superficial Back	Functional	Lateral	Spiral	Deep Front	Arm	Superficial Front
3. Access all appropriate myofascial continuities in optimal sequence for client profile	Semicircles up & down with hip external and internal rotation	Hip joint mobility, supine leg abduction/adduction	Seated thoracic lateral flexion and rotation (Advanced Mermaid)	Hip joint mobility, standing lunge hip external/internal rotation	Quadruped hip flexion, emphasize Anterior Oblique Sling System	Seated thoracic lateral flexion and rotation (Advanced Mermaid)	Quadruped hip extension with lateral translation on the Rocker Reformer

Movement intent

4. Interoception — Interstitial nerves in fascia serve an interoceptive, rather than proprioceptive or nociceptive, function. Stimulation of those free nerve endings provides information about the condition of the body in search for homeostasis in relation to physiological needs. Interoceptive signaling is associated with feelings like warmth, nausea, hunger, soreness, effort, heaviness or lightness. Perceptions about internal somatic sensations are associated with emotional preferences and feelings (Schleip, 2015).

| 5. Proprioceptive refinement

— Proprioceptive sensations are connected with position, tendon and muscle sensations | Thoracic rotation with lateral translation, hands on shoulder rests, standing | Supine lateral translation (all three variations) | Quadruped lateral translation | Bridging with rotation | Long-stretch with lateral translation on Rocker Reformer | Thoracic rotation with lateral translation, hands on shoulder rests in quadruped and standing | Hip joint mobility, supine femur circles |

Table 39.6 [Continued] The myofascial continuities' and fascia-focused Reformer exercises

Use this Pilates Reformer fascia-focused training guide to plan your Reformer classes and individual practice for thorough fascial training. Each exercise cultivates at least one of the fascia-focused movement criteria and activates one primary and several secondary myofascial continuities

Fascia-focused movement criteria							
6. Kinesthetic acuity — Kinesthesia (dynamic proprioception), the aptitude to sense the position and movement of the limbs and trunk	Quadruped hip extension with foot on foot bar, emphasize Anterior Oblique Sling System	Quadruped lateral translation	Thoracic rotation with lateral translation, hands on shoulder rests in quadruped and standing	Seated thoracic lateral flexion and rotation (Advanced Mermaid)	Elastic recoil arm jumps in quadruped	Elastic recoil arm jumps in quadruped	Hip joint mobility, standing medial hip glide
Movement attributes							
7. Whole-body movements simultaneously involving large areas of the neuromyofascial system	Standing assisted squats standing on carriage on diagonal axis with respect to springs, thoracic and cervical rotation	Hip joint mobility, standing medial hip glide	The side kick kneeling position with foot on foot bar	Standing assisted squats standing on carriage on diagonal axis with respect to springs, thoracic rotation	Elastic recoil leg jumps, quadruped single leg jumps in hip extension	Semicircle Up & Down with rotation of pelvis and lumbar spine and hip external and internal rotation	Spine-massage with single cord to opposite foot
8. Whole-body continuity — Connect trunk to limbs and limbs to trunk — Connect deep structures to superficial ones and superficial structures to deep ones	Prone on long box, feet on foot bar, hip and knee extension with thoracic extension	Semicircles up & down with hip external and internal rotation	Standing side splits on a diagonal with respect to the springs, thoracic lateral flexion	Differentiated spine rotation standing on diagonal axis facing away from the foot bar holding a Magic Circle	Elastic recoil leg jumps, supine ankle jumps with knees extended	Standing assisted squats standing on carriage on diagonal axis with respect to springs, thoracic and cervical rotation	Quadruped lateral translation

(Continued)

Table 39.6 [Continued] The myofascial continuities' and fascia-focused Reformer exercises

Use this Pilates Reformer fascia-focused training guide to plan your Reformer classes and individual practice for thorough fascial training. Each exercise cultivates at least one of the fascia-focused movement criteria and activates one primary and several secondary myofascial continuities

Fascia-focused movement criteria							
9. Movement initiation — Connect proximal structures to distal ones and distal structures to proximal ones	Elastic recoil leg jumps, quadruped single leg jumps in hip extension	Supine lateral translation (all three variations)	Elastic recoil arm jumps seated single arm	Bridging with rotation	Hip joint mobility, supine femur circles	Elastic recoil arm jumps in quadruped	Elastic recoil leg jumps, quadruped lower leg jumps
10. Flowing movement sequences	Bridging with rotation	Long-stretch with lateral translation on Rocker Reformer	The side kick kneeling position with foot on foot bar, hip extension with thoracic rotation	Semicircles up & down with rotation of pelvis and lumbar spine	Semicircles up & down with hip external and internal rotation	Seated thoracic lateral flexion and rotation (Advanced Mermaid)	Spine-massage with single cord to opposite foot
11. Multidirectional movements with slight changes of angle	Elastic recoil leg jumps, quadruped single leg jumps in hip extension (all landing variations)	Quadruped hip extension with foot on foot bar (all variations)	Elastic recoil leg jumps, side lying single leg jumps (all landing variations)	The side kick kneeling position with foot on foot bar, hip extension with thoracic rotation	Elastic recoil leg jumps, supine ankle jumps with knees extended	Elastic recoil arm jumps in quadruped	Quadruped hip extension with lateral translation on the Rocker Reformer
12. Force/load transfer — Movements that distribute force/load through the neuromyofascial system	Standing assisted squats, stand on floor on diagonal axis with respect to springs	The side kick kneeling position with foot on foot bar (all variations)	Elastic recoil arm jumps seated single arm	Thoracic rotation with lateral translation, hands on shoulder rests in quadruped and standing	Elastic recoil leg jumps, quadruped single leg jumps in hip extension	Differentiated spine rotation Standing on the diagonal axis facing toward the foot bar without Magic Circle	Spine-massage with single cord to opposite foot

Table 39.6 [Continued] The myofascial continuities[a] and fascia-focused Reformer exercises

Use this Pilates Reformer fascia-focused training guide to plan your Reformer classes and individual practice for thorough fascial training. Each exercise cultivates at least one of the fascia-focused movement criteria and activates one primary and several secondary myofascial continuities

Fascia-focused movement criteria							
	Elastic recoil arm jumps in quadruped	Standing assisted squats standing on carriage on diagonal axis with respect to springs, thoracic and cervical rotation	Thoracic rotation with lateral translation, hands on shoulder rests, standing	Standing assisted squats standing on carriage on diagonal axis with respect to springs, thoracic and cervical rotation	Spine-massage with single cord to opposite foot	Elastic recoil arm jumps seated single arm	Elastic recoil leg jumps, quadruped lower leg jumps
13. Preparatory counter movement	Spine-massage with single cord to opposite foot	Elastic recoil leg jumps, quadruped single leg jumps in hip extension	Elastic recoil leg jumps, side lying single leg jumps	Elastic recoil arm jumps seated with trunk rotation	Elastic recoil arm jumps in quadruped	Elastic recoil arm jumps seated with trunk rotation	Elastic recoil leg jumps, supine ankle jumps with knees extended
14. Dynamic stretching — Slow and fast tempo variations	Standing side splits on a diagonal with respect to the springs	Standing side splits on a diagonal with respect to the springs, thoracic rotation	Standing side splits on a diagonal with respect to the springs	Standing side splits on a diagonal with respect to the springs	Hip joint mobility, standing lunge hip external/internal rotation	Seated thoracic lateral flexion and rotation (Advanced Mermaid)	Hip joint mobility, standing lunge hip external/internal rotation
Movement outcomes							
15. Facilitate tissue hydration	Approximately two-thirds of the volume of fascial tissues is made up of water. During application of mechanical load, whether by stretching or via local compression, a significant amount of water is pushed out of the more stressed zones. Application of external loading of fascial tissues can result in a refreshed hydration with improvement in the viscoelastic tissue properties (Schleip and Baker, 2015, p. 8).						

(Continued)

Table 39.6 [Continued] The myofascial continuities* and fascia-focused Reformer exercises
Use this Pilates Reformer fascia-focused training guide to plan your Reformer classes and individual practice for thorough fascial training. Each exercise cultivates at least one of the fascia-focused movement criteria and activates one primary and several secondary myofascial continuities

Fascia-focused movement criteria

Criteria	Exercises
16. Develop glide within the three-dimensional neuromyofascial system	The normal glide of the collagen layers over one another may be hampered by loose connective tissue that has accumulated a variety of waste products. Failure of loose connective tissue gliding occurs in cases of overuse syndrome, trauma and surgery. Increase of local temperature contributes to fascial gliding. When the temperature is increased to over 40°C, the three-dimensional superstructure of hyaluronan chains break down progressively. This decreases hyaluronan viscosity of the loose connective tissue that is present within and beneath deep fasciae and muscles. The temporary increase in temperature can be provided by massage, movement or a warm shower. It is possible that during sleep, immobilization may cause increased hyaluronan viscosity and consequently a stiffness of the deep fasciae and muscles (Stecco, 2015, p. 60, p. 64).
17. Develop regular lattice with crimp	The microstructure of collagen fibers shows undulations called crimp, which is reminiscent of elastic springs. When people age or when fascial fibers are immobilized, the structure of the fiber appears to loose crimp and springiness. Regular proper exercise loading of the fascial fibers may induce a more youthful collagen architecture with wavy fibers and increased elastic storage capacity (Schleip and Baker, 2015, p. 7).
18. Develop elastic recoil	Elastic recoil leg jumps, quadruped lower leg jumps / Elastic recoil arm jumps in quadruped / The side kick kneeling position with foot on foot bar in hip flexion—jumping with foot on jump board / Elastic recoil arm jumps seated with trunk rotation / Elastic recoil leg jumps, supine ankle jumps with knees extended / Elastic recoil arm jumps in quadruped / Elastic recoil leg jumps, quadruped lower leg jumps
19. Stimulate tissue renewal	The renewal speed of the body-wide fascial network is quite slow, with a half-life between months and years rather than days or weeks. During the first three hours after appropriate exercise loading, collagen synthesis is increased. However, collagen degradation is also increased. During the first one and a half days following exercise loading, collagen degradation outweighs collagen synthesis. Forty-eight hours after exercise, net synthesis of collagen production becomes positive (Schleip and Baker, 2015, pp. 8–9). The mobile, adaptable, fibrillar network with its intersecting fibers develops a mechanical harmony that is lost when healthy tissue is damaged. The body's repair mechanisms are unable to restore the fibrillar network in the damaged area to its original condition. The replacement tissue is of poor quality but can be improved by early mobilization of the injured area by manual therapy to enhance the flexibility of the scar tissue (Guimberteau and Armstrong, 2015, p. 162).
20. Develop tissue resilience	According to the biotensegrity model, the neuromyofascial system accommodates movement as a self-adjusting whole. The myofascial meridians map out a set of connective tissues that form the outer tensional network that pulls in on the skeleton. The "isolated muscle theory" that has predominated our thinking has limited our perception of this body-wide "give" that is essential to resilience (Myers, p 46; Ch. 6 in Schleip and Baker, 2015).

* *Anatomy Trains* by Thomas W. Myers (2020) introduces the term "myofascial meridians". In this chapter I replace "meridians" with "continuities".

Fascia-focused Pilates training

Fascial training inspires development of Pilates teaching techniques

Although the Pilates movement principles correlate with fascia-focused training criteria, the design of fascia training programs in the contemporary Pilates environment requires new consideration of all elements of Pilates program design. Research on the neuromyofascial system suggests new criteria for exercise sequencing, new choices of movement tempo and rhythm and different language for verbal cueing, as well as clarification of the quality and direction of touch for tactile cues.

The practice of training fascia in Pilates has been inspired by the publication of Thomas W. Myers' book (Myers, 2020) (Chapter 36). Pilates teachers seeking to augment their movement education with interdisciplinary study applied the 11 myofascial chains described by Myers (for an evidence-based review, see Chapter 36) to the Pilates mat and apparatus repertoire and began the paradigm shift from "isolated muscle theory" to the "longitudinal anatomy" (Myers, 2020). Figure 39.3 shows the 11 myofascial chains drawn on Pilates mat and apparatus exercises,

illustrating the effectiveness of this movement program for fascia-focused training. Table 39.7 provides the key to Figure 39.3, naming each myofascial chain according to the model detailed by Myers in *Anatomy Trains*.

Phillip Beach proposed the Contractile Field model of movement (Beach, 2010). "Seeing movement as whole organism fields of contractility that have evolved along functional pathways offers us fresh approaches to assessment and treatment of the moving body...Core patterns of contractility, allied to field-like behaviour, suggest new ways to understand human movement" (Beach, 2010). The Contractile Field theory has not yet exerted a significant influence on fascia-focused training in Pilates. This may be due, in part, to the complexity of his theories and the fact that *Muscles and Meridians* is less richly illustrated than *Anatomy Trains*. The publication in 2012 of *Fascia: The Tensional Network of The Human Body* (Schleip et al., 2012) inspired the author to pursue interdisciplinary study of the properties and function of the neuromyofascial system and apply this research to movement education in the contemporary Pilates environment.

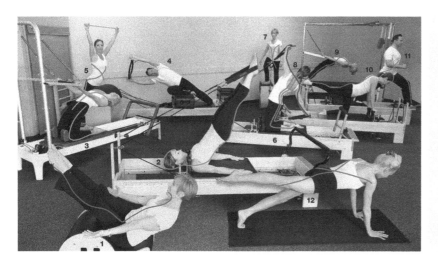

Figure 39.3

Myofascial continuities drawn on Pilates mat and apparatus exercises illustrate the effectiveness of this movement system for fascia-focused training. Table 39.7 names each myofascial meridian, each exercise, and the equipment based on the original designs of J. H. Pilates.

Copyright 2013, Elizabeth Larkam

Chapter 39

Table 39.7 Key to Figure 39.3. Each model in Figure 39.3 performs a Pilates exercise that activates several myofascial continuities. The primary myofascial continuity is identified here together with the exercise name and equipment evolved from the inventions of J. H. Pilates		
Myofascial continuity* drawn on Pilates mat and apparatus exercise	**Pilates exercise**	**Pilates equipment**
1. The Deep Front myofascial continuity	Teaser reverse	Clara step barrel
2. The Superficial Back myofascial continuity	Long spine massage — advanced version	Reformer with long straps
3. The Superficial Front myofascial continuity	Thigh-Stretch with spine extension and left rotation	Reformer with tower push through bar
4. The Lateral myofascial continuity	Mermaid — advanced version	Reformer and short box
5. The Spiral myofascial continuity front section	Swan-Dive rotations	Ladder Barrel and dowel in hands
6. The Spiral myofascial continuity back section	Thigh-Stretch — advanced version with spine extension and right rotation	Reformer with short straps
7. The Front Functional myofascial continuity	Side lunge with weight shift — advanced version	Combo chair and rotator disc under right foot
8. The Arm myofascial continuity Left – Deep Front Arm myofascial continuity Right – Superficial Back Arm myofascial continuity	Kneeling arm work and thigh stretch — advanced version with spine extension and right rotation	Reformer with short straps
9. The Deep Front myofascial continuity	Bridging — advanced version	Trapeze table with push through bar
10. The Superficial Back myofascial continuity	Jumping on footplate in quadruped	Reformer with footplate (footplate is hidden behind model #6)
11. The Spiral myofascial continuity front section	Standing/side splits with diagonal orientation	Reformer with standing platform
12. The Back Functional myofascial continuity	Leg-Pull – Front	Mat
*Continuity is used here as a synonym for the term "myofascial meridian", used by Myers (2020). In this chapter I replace "meridians" with "continuities".		

The Pilates movement principles of Precision, Control, Centering, Flow and Whole Body Movement all correlate with the fascia-focused training principle of Proprioceptive Refinement and Kinesthetic Acuity. Jaap van der Wal's (2009) writing on proprioception (Schleip et al., 2012) may guide Pilates teachers who seek clarity on the perception of movement. "To understand the mechanical and functional circumstances of the fascial role in connecting and in conveying stresses and in proprioception, it is therefore more important to know the architecture of the connective and muscle tissue than the regular anatomical order or topography" (Schleip et al., 2012).

Fascia-focused Pilates training

Table 39.8 Fascia-focused movement criteria and J. H. Pilates high back chair and Wunda chair examples

Fascia-focused movement criteria		
Movement requirements	Biotensegrity model	
1. Movements are sustainable for motor control refinement and collagen remodeling 2. Movements encourage awareness of and embodiment of the biotensegrity model*	* "A tensegrity structure provides a global response to a local mechanical stress. The result is a degree of independence from the force of gravity. Without a tensegrity model, our fibrillar structure would collapse under gravitational force. With the tensegrity model, our structure absorbs and disperses the compression by spreading the load throughout the entire network, including the structures at the periphery" (Guimberteau and Armstrong, 2015). "The value of the Tensegrity model is not that it necessarily changes a particular approach to treatment but that it provides a better means to visualize the mechanics of the body in the light of new understandings about functional anatomy" (Scarr, 2014).	
	Pilates principles	**J. H. Pilates high back chair and Wunda chair examples**
3. Access all appropriate myofascial continuities in optimal sequence for client profile	Whole-body movement	Reverse Swan/Torso Press Sit (Supine atop Chair)
Movement intent		
4. Interoception — interstitial nerves in fascia serve an interoceptive, rather than proprioceptive or nociceptive function. Stimulation of those free nerve endings provides information about the condition of the body in search for homeostasis in relation to physiological needs. Interoceptive signaling is associated with feelings like warmth, nausea, hunger, soreness, effort, heaviness or lightness. Perceptions about internal somatic sensations are associated with emotional preferences and feelings (Schleip, 2015)	Breathing	Interoceptive sensations are unique to each individual
5. Proprioceptive refinement — proprioceptive sensations are connected with position, tendon and muscle sensations	Concentration Control	Seated Leg Pumps
6. Kinesthetic acuity — kinesthesia (dynamic proprioception), the aptitude to sense the position and movement of the limbs and trunk	Precision	Piano Lesson Back (Squat in external rotation back to Chair)
Movement attributes		
7. Whole-body movements simultaneously involving large areas of the neuromyofascial system	Whole-body movement Breathing	Side Arm Twist (Seated atop Chair)
8. Whole-body continuity — connect trunk to limbs and limbs to trunk while connecting deep structures to superficial ones and superficial structures to deep ones	Whole-body movement	Cat (Kneeling atop Chair)
9. Movement initiation — connect proximal structures to distal ones and distal structures to proximal ones	Centering Breathing	Pike/Teaser on Floor (Seated on floor in front of Chair)
10. Flowing movement sequences	Breathing	Tendon Stretch One Leg

(Continued)

Chapter 39

Table 39.8 (Continued) Fascia-focused movement criteria and J. H. Pilates high back chair and Wunda chair examples		
Fascia-focused movement criteria		
11. Multidirectional movements with slight changes of angle	Balanced muscle development (optimal activation of the neuromyofascial system)	Jack-Knife from Floor and Corkscrew
12. Force/load transfer — movements that distribute force/load through the neuromyofascial system		Washer Woman Over the Chair (Standing behind Chair) Press Up with Handles Facing In
13. Preparatory counter movement	Rhythm	Swan Front/Chest Press (Prone atop Chair)
14. Dynamic stretching — slow and fast tempo variations	Rhythm	Seated Mermaid/Side Arm Sit
Movement outcomes		
15. Facilitate tissue hydration		
16. Develop glide within the three dimensional neuromyofascial system		
17. Develop regular lattice with crimp		
18. Develop elastic recoil	*J. H. Pilates high back chair and wunda chair exercises do not develop elastic recoil of the neuromyofascial system*	
19. Stimulate tissue renewal		
20. Develop tissue resilience		

Reframe Pilates concepts with new understanding of the structure and function of the neuromyofascial system

In fascia-oriented training one practices body movements that engage the longest possible myofascial chains (Müller and Schleip, 2011). This is in harmony with the Pilates principle of whole body movement. In our second week of development, the fascial network is a unified whole and remains a single, unifying and communicating network from birth until death (Earls and Myers, 2010). Fascia-focused training shaped by research on the properties and function of fascia reinforces the Pilates practice of whole body movement. The "Powerhouse" of J. H. Pilates (Pilates, 1945) and the inner unit of core control (Lee, 2012) may be understood in the context of whole-body continuity by an understanding of the Deep Front Line myofascial chain (Myers, 2020) (Chapter 36).

The concept of lumbopelvic stability and the Pilates principle of balanced muscle development may be informed by biotensegrity, derived from "biology", "tension" and "integrity" (Scarr, 2018). The internal balance of tension and compression supports structural integrity. Any deformation

Table 39.9 Fascia-focused movement criteria and fascia-focused combo chair examples

Fascia-focused movement criteria	Pilates principles	J. H. Pilates high back chair and Wunda chair examples	Fascia-focused combo chair examples
Movement requirements			
Biotensegrity model			
*"A tensegrity structure provides a global response to a local mechanical stress. The result is a degree of independence from the force of gravity. Without a tensegrity model, our fibrillar structure would collapse under gravitational force. With the tensegrity model, our structure absorbs and disperses the compression by spreading the load throughout the entire network, including the structures at the periphery" (Guimberteau and Armstrong, 2015). "The value of the Tensegrity model is not that it necessarily changes a particular approach to treatment but that it provides a better means to visualize the mechanics of the body in the light of new understandings about functional anatomy" (Scarr, 2014).			
1. Movements are sustainable for motor control refinement and collagen remodeling			
2. Movements encourage awareness of and embodiment of the biotensegrity model*			
3. Access all appropriate myofascial continuities in optimal sequence for client profile	Whole-body movement	Reverse Swan/Torso Press Sit (Supine atop Chair)	Stand on rotator discs, one hand per pedal, thoracic and cervical rotation
Movement intent			
4. Interoception — Interstitial nerves in fascia serve an interoceptive, rather than proprioceptive or nociceptive function. Stimulation of those free nerve endings provides information about the condition of the body in search for homeostasis in relation to physiological needs. Interoceptive signaling is associated with feelings like warmth, nausea, hunger, soreness, effort, heaviness or lightness. Perceptions about internal somatic sensations are associated with emotional preferences and feelings (Schleip, 2015)	Breathing	Interoceptive sensations are unique to each individual	
5. Proprioceptive refinement — proprioceptive sensations are connected with position, tendon and muscle sensations	Concentration Control	Seated Leg Pumps	Standing ankle plantar/dorsi flexion hip neutral, external/internal rotation
6. Kinesthetic acuity — kinesthesia (dynamic proprioception), the aptitude to sense the position and movement of the limbs and trunk	Precision	Piano Lesson Back (Squat in external rotation back to Chair)	Side to chair, one foot per pedal, inside foot in front, hands on top of chair in seven different positions
Movement attributes			
7. Whole-body movements simultaneously involving large areas of the neuromyofascial system	Whole-body movement Breathing	Side Arm Twist (Seated atop Chair)	Standing pelvic unleveling with ankle plantar flexion and thoracic lateral flexion and rotation

(Continued)

Table 39.9 [Continued] Fascia-focused movement criteria and fascia-focused combo chair examples

Fascia-focused movement criteria

8. Whole-body continuity — connect trunk to limbs and limbs to trunk while connecting deep structures to superficial ones and superficial structures to deep ones	Whole-body movement	Cat (Kneeling atop Chair)	Side to chair, one foot per pedal, outside foot in front, hands on top of chair in seven different positions
9. Movement initiation — connect proximal structures to distal ones and distal structures to proximal ones	Centering Breathing	Pike/Teaser on Floor (Seated on floor in front of Chair)	Seated spine extension with rotation
10. Flowing movement sequences	Breathing	Tendon Stretch One Leg	Seated lateral spine flexion with rotation
11. Multidirectional movements with slight changes of angle	Balanced muscle development (optimal activation of the neuromyofascial system)	Jack-Knife from Floor and Corkscrew	Facing chair, one foot per pedal, hands on wobble board, variation one—turn towards leg with knee flexion, variation two—turn away from leg with knee flexion
12. Force/load transfer — movements that distribute force/load through the neuromyofascial system		Washer Woman Over the Chair (Standing behind Chair) Press Up with Handles Facing In	One hand on rotator disc, one hand on chair pedal, single leg plank / Facing chair, one foot per pedal, hands on top of chair in seven different positions
13. Preparatory counter movement	Rhythm	Swan Front/Chest Press (Prone atop Chair)	Seated lateral spine flexion with rotation (side bend away from pedal before side bending toward the pedal)
14. Dynamic stretching — slow and fast tempo variations	Rhythm	Seated Mermaid/Side Arm Sit	Seated spine extension with rotation
Movement outcomes			
15. Facilitate tissue hydration			
16. Develop glide within the three dimensional neuromyo-fascial system			
17. Develop regular lattice with crimp			
18. Develop elastic recoil		*The high back chair and Wunda chair do not support elastic recoil training*	*The combo chair does not support elastic recoil training*
19. Stimulate tissue renewal			
20. Develop tissue resilience			

Fascia-focused Pilates training

Table 39.10 Fascia-focused movement criteria and J. H. Pilates trapeze table examples

Fascia-focused movement criteria

	Pilates principles	J. H. Pilates trapeze table examples
Movement requirements	Biotensegrity model	
1. Movements are sustainable for motor control refinement and collagen remodeling		* "A tensegrity structure provides a global response to a local mechanical stress. The result is a degree of independence from the force of gravity. Without a tensegrity model, our fibrilar structure would
2. Movements encourage awareness of and embodiment of the biotensegrity model*		collapse under gravitational force. With the tensegrity model, our structure absorbs and disperses the compression by spreading the load throughout the entire network, including the structures at the periphery" (Guimberteau and Armstrong, 2015).
		"The value of the Tensegrity model is not that it necessarily changes a particular approach to treatment but that it provides a better means to visualize the mechanics of the body in the light of new understandings about functional anatomy" (Scarr, 2014).
3. Access all appropriate myofascial continuities in optimal sequence for client profile	Whole-body movement	Rolling In and Out
Movement intent		
4. Interoception — Interstitial nerves in fascia serve an interoceptive, rather than proprioceptive or nociceptive function. Stimulation of those free nerve endings provides information about the condition of the body in search for homeostasis in relation to physiological needs. Interoceptive signaling is associated with feelings like warmth, nausea, hunger, soreness, effort, heaviness or lightness. Perceptions about internal somatic sensations are associated with emotional preferences and feelings (Schleip, 2015)	Breathing	Interoceptive sensations are unique to each individual
5. Proprioceptive refinement — proprioceptive sensations are connected with position, tendon and muscle sensations	Concentration Control	Thigh Stretch
6. Kinesthetic acuity — kinesthesia (dynamic proprioception), the aptitude to sense the position and movement of the limbs and trunk	Precision	Magician
Movement attributes		
7. Whole-body movements simultaneously involving large areas of the neuromyofascial system	Whole-body movement Breathing	Hanging Down
8. Whole-body continuity — connect trunk to limbs and limbs to trunk while connecting deep structures to superficial ones and superficial structures to deep ones	Whole-body movement	Parakeet

(Continued)

Table 39.10 [Continued] Fascia-focused movement criteria and J. H. Pilates trapeze table examples

Fascia-focused movement criteria		
9. Movement initiation — connect proximal structures to distal ones and distal structures to proximal ones	Centering Breathing	Push-Through Seated Back
10. Flowing movement sequences	Breathing	Spread Eagle
11. Multidirectional movements with slight changes of angle	Balanced muscle development (optimal activation of the neuromyofascial system)	Butterfly
12. Force/load transfer — movements that distribute force/load through the neuromyofascial system		Tower Hanging Up
13. Preparatory counter movement	Rhythm	Side-Lying Bicycle
14. Dynamic stretching — slow and fast tempo variations	Rhythm	Mermaid
Movement outcomes		
15. Facilitate tissue hydration		
16. Develop glide within the three dimensional neuromyofascial system		
17. Develop regular lattice with crimp		
18. Develop elastic recoil		J. H. Pilates trapeze table exercises do not develop elastic recoil of the neuromyofascial system
19. Stimulate tissue renewal		
20. Develop tissue resilience		

Table 39.11 Fascia-focused movement criteria and fascia-focused trapeze table examples

Fascia-focused movement criteria	Biotensegrity model		
Movement requirements			
1. Movements are sustainable for motor control refinement and collagen remodeling	*"A tensegrity structure provides a global response to a local mechanical stress. The result is a degree of independence from the force of gravity. Without a tensegrity model, our fibrillar structure would collapse under gravitational force. With the tensegrity model, our structure absorbs and disperses the compression by spreading the load throughout the entire network, including the structures at the periphery" (Guimberteau and Armstrong, 2015).		
2. Movements encourage awareness of and embodiment of the biotensegrity model*	"The value of the Tensegrity model is not that it necessarily changes a particular approach to treatment but that it provides a better means to visualize the mechanics of the body in the light of new understandings about functional anatomy" (Scarr, 2014).		
	Pilates principles	**J. H. Pilates trapeze table examples**	**Fascia-focused trapeze table examples**
3. Access all appropriate myofascial continuities in optimal sequence for client profile	Whole-body movement	Rolling In and Out	Prone scapula patterning
Movement intent			
5. Interoception — Interstitial nerves in fascia serve an interoceptive, rather than proprioceptive or nociceptive function. Stimulation of those free nerve endings provides information about the condition of the body in search for homeostasis in relation to physiological needs. Interoceptive signaling is associated with feelings like warmth, nausea, hunger, soreness, effort, heaviness or lightness. Perceptions about internal somatic sensations are associated with emotional preferences and feelings (Schleip, 2015)	Breathing	Interoceptive sensations are unique to each individual	
6. Proprioceptive refinement — proprioceptive sensations are connected with position, tendon and muscle sensations	Concentration Control	Thigh Stretch	Seated on rotator disc scapular depression, elbow flexion, arm external rotation
7. Kinesthetic acuity — kinesthesia (dynamic proprioception), the aptitude to sense the position and movement of the limbs and trunk	Precision	Magician	Supine to side lying assisted trunk rotation with arm internal and external rotation
Movement attributes			
9. Whole-body movements simultaneously involving large areas of the neuromyofascial system	Whole-body movement Breathing	Hanging Down	Seated "circle-saw"

(Continued)

Table 39.11 [Continued] Fascia-focused movement criteria and fascia-focused trapeze table examples

Fascia-focused movement criteria			
10. Whole-body continuity — connect trunk to limbs and limbs to trunk while connecting deep structures to superficial ones and superficial structures to deep ones	Whole-body movement	Parakeet	Parakeet with single hip flexion
11. Movement initiation — connect proximal structures to distal ones and distal structures to proximal ones	Centering Breathing	Push-Through Seated Back	Supine assisted spine extension with arms crossed in external rotation
12. Flowing movement sequences	Breathing	Spread Eagle	Bridge with knees extended
13. Multidirectional movements with slight changes of angle	Balanced muscle development (optimal activation of the neuromyofascial system)	Butterfly	Seated on rotator disc scapular depression, elbow flexion, arm external rotation
14. Force/load transfer — movements that distribute force/load through the neuromyofascial system		Tower Hanging Up	Prone scapula patterning Parakeet with double knee flexion and extension
15. Preparatory counter movement	Rhythm	Side-Lying Bicycle	Supine to side lying assisted trunk rotation with arm internal and external rotation
16. Dynamic stretching — slow and fast tempo variations	Rhythm	Mermaid	Seated "circle-saw"
17. Movement outcomes			
18. Facilitate tissue hydration			
19. Develop glide within the three dimensional neuromyofascial system			
20. Develop regular lattice with crimp			
21. Develop elastic recoil			*The trapeze table does not support elastic recoil training.*
22. Stimulate tissue renewal			
23. Develop tissue resilience			

Fascia-focused Pilates training

Table 39.12 Fascia-focused movement criteria and J. H. Pilates spine-corrector examples

Fascia-focused movement criteria		
Fascia-focused movement criteria		
Movement requirements	Biotensegrity model	
1. Movements are sustainable for motor control refinement and collagen remodeling	* "A tensegrity structure provides a global response to a local mechanical stress. The result is a degree of independence from the force of gravity. Without a tensegrity model, our fibrillar structure would collapse under gravitational force. With the tensegrity model, our structure absorbs and disperses the compression by spreading the load throughout the entire network, including the structures at the periphery" (Guimberteau and Armstrong, 2015).	
2. Movements encourage awareness of and embodiment of the biotensegrity model*	"The value of the Tensegrity model is not that it necessarily changes a particular approach to treatment but that it provides a better means to visualize the mechanics of the body in the light of new understandings about functional anatomy" (Scarr, 2014).	

	Pilates principles	**J. H. Pilates spine-corrector examples**
3. Access all appropriate myofascial continuities in optimal sequence for client profile	Whole-body movement	Back Arch and Bridge
Movement intent		
4. Interoception — Interstitial nerves in fascia serve an interoceptive, rather than proprioceptive or nociceptive function. Stimulation of those free nerve endings provides information about the condition of the body in search for homeostasis in relation to physiological needs. Interoceptive signaling is associated with feelings like warmth, nausea, hunger, soreness, effort, heaviness or lightness. Perceptions about internal somatic sensations are associated with emotional preferences and feelings (Schleip, 2015).	Breathing	Interoceptive sensations are unique to each individual
5. Proprioceptive refinement — proprioceptive sensations are connected with position, tendon and muscle sensations	Concentration Control	Balance
6. Kinesthetic acuity — kinesthesia (dynamic proprioception), the aptitude to sense the position and movement of the limbs and trunk	Precision	Swimming
Movement attributes		
7. Whole-body movements simultaneously involving large areas of the neuromyofascial system	Whole-body movement Breathing	Teaser
8. Whole-body continuity — connect trunk to limbs and limbs to trunk while connecting deep structures to superficial ones and superficial structures to deep ones	Whole-body movement	Helicopter

(Continued)

Table 39.12 [Continued] Fascia-focused movement criteria and J. H. Pilates spine-corrector examples

Fascia-focused movement criteria		
9. Movement initiation — connect proximal structures to distal ones and distal structures to proximal ones	Centering Breathing	Swan
10. Flowing movement sequences	Breathing	Rolling In and Out
11. Multidirectional movements with slight changes of angle	Balanced muscle development (optimal activation of the neuromyofascial system)	Corkscrew
12. Force/load transfer — movements that distribute force/load through the neuromyofascial system		The Rollover with Legs Spread (Both Ways) Grasshopper
13. Preparatory counter movement	Rhythm	Low Bridge
14. Dynamic stretching — slow and fast tempo variations	Rhythm	Scissors
Movement outcomes		
15. Facilitate tissue hydration		
16. Develop glide within the three dimensional neuromyofascial system		
17. Develop regular lattice with crimp		
18. Develop elastic recoil	*J. H. Pilates spine-corrector exercises do not develop elastic recoil of the neuromyofascial system*	
19. Stimulate tissue renewal		
20. Develop tissue resilience		

Table 39.13 Fascia-focused movement criteria and J. H. Pilates ladder barrel examples

Fascia-focused movement criteria	Pilates principles	J. H. Pilates ladder barrel examples
Movement requirements		
	Biotensegrity model	
1. Movements are sustainable for motor control refinement and collagen remodeling	*"A tensegrity structure provides a global response to a local mechanical stress. The result is a degree of independence from the force of gravity. Without a tensegrity model, our fibrillar structure would collapse under gravitational force. With the tensegrity model, our structure absorbs and disperses the compression by spreading the load throughout the entire network, including the structures at the periphery" (Guimberteau and Armstrong, 2015).	
2. Movements encourage awareness of and embodiment of the biotensegrity model*	"The value of the Tensegrity model is not that it necessarily changes a particular approach to treatment but that it provides a better means to visualize the mechanics of the body in the light of new understandings about functional anatomy" (Scarr, 2014).	
3. Access all appropriate myofascial continuities in optimal sequence for client profile	Whole-body movement	Horseback
Movement intent		
4. Interoception — Interstitial nerves in fascia serve an interoceptive, rather than proprioceptive or nociceptive function. Stimulation of those free nerve endings provides information about the condition of the body in search for homeostasis in relation to physiological needs. Interoceptive signaling is associated with feelings like warmth, nausea, hunger, soreness, effort, heaviness or lightness. Perceptions about internal somatic sensations are associated with emotional preferences and feelings (Schleip, 2015).	Breathing	Interoceptive sensations are unique to each individual
5. Proprioceptive refinement — proprioceptive sensations are connected with position, tendon and muscle sensations	Concentration Control	Side Sit-Ups
6. Kinesthetic acuity — kinesthesia (dynamic proprioception), the aptitude to sense the position and movement of the limbs and trunk	Precision	Twist
Movement attributes		
7. Whole-body movements simultaneously involving large areas of the neuromyofascial system	Whole-body movement Breathing	Swan Dive
8. Whole-body continuity — connect trunk to limbs and limbs to trunk while connecting deep structures to superficial ones and superficial structures to deep ones	Whole-body movement	Grasshopper

(Continued)

Table 39.13 [Continued] Fascia-focused movement criteria and J. H. Pilates ladder barrel examples

Fascia-focused movement criteria			
9. Movement initiation — connect proximal structures to distal ones and distal structures to proximal ones	Centering Breathing	Bicycle	
10. Flowing movement sequences	Breathing	Climb-a-Tree	
11. Multidirectional movements with slight changes of angle	Balanced muscle development (optimal activation of the neuromyofascial system)	Helicopter	
12. Force/load transfer — movements that distribute force/load through the neuromyofascial system		Horseback Stomach Jumps	
13. Preparatory counter movement	Rhythm	Scissors	
14. Dynamic stretching — slow and fast tempo variations	Rhythm	Back Bend to Forward Bend	
Movement outcomes			
15. Facilitate tissue hydration			
16. Develop glide within the three dimensional neuromyofascial system			
17. Develop regular lattice with crimp			
18. Develop elastic recoil		*J. H. Pilates barrel exercises do not develop elastic recoil of the neuromyofascial system*	
19. Stimulate tissue renewal			
20. Develop tissue resilience			

will create strain that is distributed throughout the body. Any injury rapidly becomes a strain distribution patterned into the whole body that requires a whole-body assessment and whole-body treatment. Pilates teachers are challenged to see the whole body in terms of biotensegrity, in order to develop coherent movement program designs that address the neuromyofascial system and develop motor control in support of functional movement.

Fascia-focused training has the criteria of Proximal Initiation. This correlates with the Pilates principle of Centering. J. H. Pilates used the term "Powerhouse" to refer to the girdle of strength between the top of the pelvis and the bottom of the ribcage responsible for Centering or Proximal Initiation. Contemporary Pilates teacher education, influenced by Diane Lee (2011), explains that the inner unit of core control is the key to efficient, graceful, balanced movement (St. John, 2013).

The thoracolumbar fascia is essential for lumbar spine stability and force closure of the sacroiliac joint

The thoracolumbar fascia (TLF) is a three-dimensional girdling structure consisting of several aponeurotic and fascial layers that separates the paraspinal muscles from the muscles of the posterior abdominal wall. Several muscles attach to the TLF and its thick composite, which attaches to the posterior superior iliac spine and the sacrotuberous ligament. The thoracolumbar composite assists in maintaining the integrity of the lower lumbar spine and the sacroiliac joint. The latissimus dorsi, gluteus maximus and abdominal muscles, primarily the transversus

abdominis, attach to the TLF. Tension applied by these muscles, especially the transversus abdominis, can be transmitted through the TLF to beneficially stiffen the lumbar spine, creating stability, and increase the force closure of the sacroiliac joint. Flexion of the spine stretches the TLF, diminishing its lateral dimensions. Resistance to lateral retraction of the TLF by the abdominal muscles will stiffen this tissue and increase resistance to flexion of the lumbar region. Contraction of the paraspinal muscles increases intracompartmental pressure and contributes to the hydraulic amplifier effect supporting the lumbar spine. Increased tone in the lumbar multifidus muscle should increase the tension created by the thoracolumbar composite between the two posterior superior iliac spines. This increased, medially directed tension leads to force closure of the sacroiliac joint, thus stabilizing the pelvis (Willard et al., 2012).

As Pilates teachers advance their interdisciplinary education, aligning Pilates movement principles and practices with recent findings in motor learning, neuroscience and fascia-focused movement, it is likely that the movement form founded by J. H. Pilates will continue to attract practitioners worldwide (Larkam, 2017).

Augment fascia-focused Pilates training with fascial release for structural balance

Fascia-focused Pilates training may be integrated with manual therapy or fascial release for structural balance. When one practitioner has acquired both skill sets, the client will be fortunate enough to receive fascia-focused training for motor control and movement education together

Chapter 39

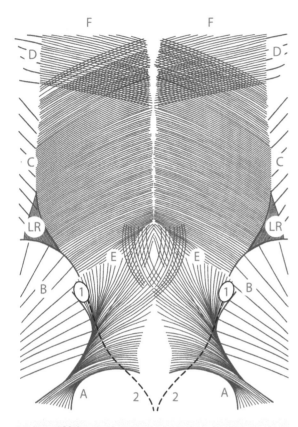

Figure 39.4

The deep layer of the thoracolumbar fascia and different fiber directions of attachments to: **(A)** sacrotuberous ligament connecting to hamstrings, **(B)** fascia of gluteus medius, **(C)** fascia of internal oblique, **(D)** serratus posterior inferior, **(E)** erector spinae muscles, **(1)** posterior superior iliac spine, **(2)** sacrum, **(LR)** lateral raphe.

Reproduced with permission from Schleip, R. & Baker, A. (Eds) (2015). Fascia in Sport and Movement. © Handspring Publishing.

with fascia release for structural balancing. If the practitioner has only one skill set, the client may seek two practitioners who can provide complementary sessions. Precise, whole body movement is necessary for training the fascia but may not be sufficient to facilitate efficient movement. The body as a biotensegrity system responds to trauma, contracting and retracting around all axes (Earls and Myers, 2010). When fascial release for structural balance opens the body in one dimension, it seems to respond in all dimensions.

Design tactile cues to reinforce fascia-focused Pilates training

The tactile cues modeled by Joseph Pilates in his films (Pilates, 1932–1945) indicate a strong touch, sometimes forcefully pushing the client into the intended position. Fascia-focused training encourages a perceptual refinement of shear, gliding and tensioning motions in superficial fascial membranes (Müller & Schleip, 2011) (Chapter 24). This is inspired by the finding that the superficial fascia layers are more densely populated with mechanoreceptive nerve endings than the tissue situated more internally (Stecco et al., 2014) (Chapter 15). Although this perceptual refinement is recommended in terms of movement, it seems reasonable to apply this discovery to shaping tactile cues for fascia-focused Pilates training. By applying precise vectors at the depth of the superficial fascia layer, conveying myofascial continuity to a bony landmark or organ, a clear direction in space can be given. For example, in Figure 39.3, in Exercise no. 12, the desired thoracic kyphosis has been lost. Accurate spinal organization may be reinforced by placing the pads of the four fingers of the teacher's hand on the posterior spinous processes of the thoracic vertebrae between the scapulae. Instruct the client to increase pressure from the little finger side of the heel of the hand into the mat as she brings the sternum up, in the direction of the vertebrae, bringing the spinous processes convex toward the ceiling.

Another example of a tactile cue harmonious with fascia-focused training involves exercise no. 10 in Figure 39.3. Support of the thoracolumbar junction has been lost, resulting in compression in the area of T11, T12 and L1. The palm surface of the instructor's fingers are placed on the anterior lateral surfaces of the lower ribs, guiding the ribs towards the back of the thorax, asking the client to draw the lower ribs in and up toward the ceiling. Tactile cues are to be used judiciously, to inform or encourage rather than to force or overwhelm. In fascia-focused Pilates training, the client is the active agent who has the responsibility of shaping the movement rather than the role of a passive recipient of instructor actions.

Fascia-focused Pilates training is a young field undergoing rapid development

The intentional practice of fascia-focused Pilates training has only been in development since 2001. It has not been scientifically evaluated. The principles of fascia-focused training may inform all elements of Pilates program design, including utilization of all planes of motion, movement sequencing, tempo, duration, frequency, selection of resistance, verbal cues and tactile cues.

The work of the international community of Pilates teachers, who are evolving the field of fascia-focused Pilates training, occurs in Pilates studios throughout the world. In these movement laboratories, Pilates teachers engage in interdisciplinary enquiry and collaborate with clients to facilitate functional, elegant movement in activities of daily living, athletics and performance.

Practical application

Transform a J. H. Pilates mat exercise, that addresses muscular function, into a Pilates reformer sequence that stimulates fascial tissues, satisfying the principles of fascia-focused training. In Figure 39.3, exercise no. 12, a Leg Pull Front is demonstrated. This J. H. Pilates mat exercise requires integration of all the Myofascial chains (Myers, 2020) (Chapter 36). However, Leg Pull Front does not satisfy the Fascia-focused training criteria (Table 39.2) (Chapter 24). This demanding mat exercise provides limited opportunities for Preparatory Counter-Movement, Flowing Movement Sequences, Tempo Variation and Multidirectional Movements, with slight changes in angle that lead to Tissue Hydration and Renewal. Leg Pull Front does not involve elastic recoil (Chapter 8). Contrast Leg Pull Front to the Fascia-focused Pilates Reformer exercise shown in Figure 39.3, exercise no. 10. Jumping on the Footplate in Quadruped requires integrated action of all the Myofascial chains utilized in Leg Pull Front. (The Footplate, or Jump Board, is hidden by the person doing Exercise 6.) One blue spring connects the reformer carriage to the frame. In addition to fulfilling the myofascial chain requirements of Fascia-focused training, exercise no. 10 satisfies a number of Fascia-focused criteria. The dancer's demi plié or knee bend prepares for the ankle plantar flexion and knee extension required for each jump. This is Preparatory Counter-Movement (Chapter 24). Landing from each jump involves deceleration through the entire lower kinematic chain together with enhanced tensioning of the long fascial chains that connect the feet with the pelvic girdle, spine, thorax, shoulder girdle, arms and hands. This creates a flowing movement sequence. The jumps may be quick and small or slow and large. This is Tempo Variation. The jumping leg may be oriented in neutral hip rotation, external rotation or internal rotation. This fulfills Multidirectional Movements with slight changes in angle. The elastic recoil property of Reformer Jumping in quadruped makes additional demands on proprioceptive refinement and kinesthetic acuity, resulting in tissue hydration and tissue renewal.

Chapter 39

References

Avision, J (2015) *Yoga: fascia anatomy and movement.* Edinburgh, UK: Handspring.

Beach, P. (2018) *Muscles and Meridians.* Churchill Livingstone Elsevier.

Chaitow, L (2018) *Fascial dysfunction: manual therapy approaches.* Edinburgh, UK: Handspring.

Earls, J. (2014) *Born to Walk: Myofascial Efficiency and the Body in Movement.* Lotus Publishing.

Earls, J. & Myers, T. (2010) *Fascial Release for Structural Balance.* Chichester, UK: Lotus Publishing.

Guimberteau, J.-C. & Armstrong, C. (2015) *Architecture of human living fascia: the extracellular matrix and cells revealed through endoscopy.* Edinburgh, UK: Handspring.

Larkam, E. (2013) *Heroes in Motion.* 9 minutes 31 seconds. Available through: Pilates Method Alliance: https://www. heroesinmotion.org; https://www.youtube.com/watch?v=YdsTMB61dBo.

Larkam, E. (2017) *Fascia in Motion: Fascia-focused movement* for Pilates. Edinburgh, UK: Handspring.

Lee, D. (2011) *The Pelvic Girdle.* 4th ed. Churchill Livingstone Elsevier.

Lessen, D. (2013) *The PMA Pilates Certification Exam Study Guide*, 3rd edn. Miami, FL: Pilates Method Alliance Inc.

Martin, D.-C. (2016) *Living biotensegrity: interplay of tension and compression in the body.* Munich, Germany: Keiner.

Moore, J. (2009) MPT, OCS, ATC, CSCS *Physical Therapist.* Lower Extremity Amputation: Early Management Considerations. Naval Medical Center San Diego Military Amputees Advanced Skills Training (MAAST) Workshop July 28–30. Comprehensive Combat and Complex Casualty Care Naval Medical Center, San Diego.

Muller, M.G. & Schleip, R. (2011) Fascial Fitness: Fascia oriented training for bodywork and movement therapies. *IASI Yearbook* 2011: 68–76.

Myers, T.W. (2020) *Anatomy Trains Myofascial Meridians for Manual and Movement Therapists.* Elsevier.

Myers, T. (2011) *Fascial Fitness: Training in the Neuromyofascial Web.* Available through: IDEA http://www.ideafit.com/fitness-library/fascial-fitness.

Pilates, J.H. (1932–1945) *Joe and Clara Historic Video.* DVD 70 minutes. Available through Mary Bowen at www.pilatesmarybowen.com/videos/video.html.

Pilates, J.H. & Miller, W.R. (1945) *Return to Life Through Contrology.* Reprinted 2003. Presentation Dynamics Inc.

Pilates, J.H. (1934) *Your Health.* Reprinted 1998. Presentation Dynamics Inc.

Scarr, G. (2018) *Biotensegrity: the structural basis of life*, 2nd ed. Edinburgh, UK: Handspring.

Schleip, R. (2015) *Fascia in sport and movement.* Edinburgh, UK: Handspring.

Schleip, R., Findley, T.W., Chaitow, L. & Huijing, P.A. (2012) *Fascia: The Tensional Network of the Human Body.* Churchill Livingstone Elsevier.

Schwind, P. (2006) *Fascial and membrane technique.* Edinburgh, UK: Churchill Livingstone.

Sporting Goods Manufacturers Association (2010) *Single Sport Report – 2010 Pilates.* sgmaresearch@sgma.com; www.sgma.com.

St. John, N. (2013) *Pilates Instructor Training Manual Reformer 1.* Balanced Body University.

Stecco, A., et al. (2016) Fascial disorders: implications for treatment. *American Academy of Physical Medicine & Rehabilitation Journal.* 8: 161–168.

Stecco, C. (2015) *Functional atlas of the human fascial system.* Edinburgh, UK: Churchill Livingstone.

Stecco, L. & Stecco, C. (2014) *Fascial Manipulation for Internal Dysfunction.* Piccin Nuova Libraria S.p.A.

Turvey, M.T. & Fonseca, S.T. (2014) The medium of haptic perception: a tensegrity hypothesis. *J Mot Behav.* 46: 143–187.

van der Wal, J. (2009) The architecture of the connective tissue in the musculoskeletal system—an often overlooked functional parameter as to proprioception in the locomotor apparatus. *Int J Ther Massage Bodywork.* 2: 9–23.

Further reading

Note: Elizabeth Larkam has produced a compilation of short videos to help you gain a deeper understanding. Watch these videos free of charge at www.pilatesanytime.com/fascia. To redeem your free access use code FASCIA

These short videos were compiled as a companion to her book *Fascia in Motion: Fascia-focused Movement for Pilates* (Handspring, 2017).

Blom, M.-J. (2012) Pilates and Fascia: The art of 'working in'. *Fascia: The Tensional Network of The Human Body.* 7 (22): 451–456. Churchill Livingstone Elsevier.

These five contemporary Pilates classes reflect the influence of Fascia-focused training and the myofascial continuities discussed in the chapter. Viewers have a 30-day free trial on the Pilates Anytime website with the Code: LARKAM.

Larkam, E. (2012) *#1014: Reformer Workout Level 2 90 minutes.* http://www.pilatesanytime.com/class-view/1014/video/Elizabeth-Larkam-Pilates-Pilates-Class-by-Elizabeth-Larkam

Larkam, E. (2012) *#889: Reformer Workout Level 2/3 75 minutes.* http://www.pilatesanytime.com/class-view889/video/Elizabeth-Larkam-Pilates-Pilates-Class-by-Elizabeth-Larkam

Larkam, E. (2012) *#866: Wunda Chair Workout Level 2/3 60 minutes.* http://www.pilatesanytime.com/class-view/866/video/Elizabeth-Larkam-Pilates-Pilates-Class-by-Elizabeth-Larkam

Larkam, E. (2012) *#863: Mat Workout Level 2 50 minutes.* http://www.pilatesanytime.com/class-view/863/video/Elizabeth-Larkam-Pilates-Pilates-Class-by-Elizabeth-Larkam

Larkam, E. (2012) *#829: Pilates Arc Workout Level 2 60 minutes.* http://www.pilatesanytime.com/class-view829/video/Elizabeth-Larkam-Pilates-Pilates-Class-by-Elizabeth-Larkam

St. John, N. (2013) *Pilates Instructor Training Manual Mat 1.* 2nd ed. Balanced Body University.

St. John, N. (2013) *Pilates Instructor Training Manual Mat 2.* 2nd ed. Balanced Body University.

St. John, N. (2013) *Pilates Instructor Training Reformer 2.* 2nd ed. Balanced Body University.

St. John, N. (2013) *Pilates Instructor Training Reformer 3.* 2nd ed. Balanced Body University.

St. John, N. (2013) *Pilates Instructor Training Pilates Chair.* 2nd ed. Balanced Body University.

St. John, N. (2013) *Pilates Instructor Training Trapeze Table.* 2nd ed. Balanced Body University.

St. John, N. (2013) *Pilates Instructor Training Barrels.* 2nd ed. Balanced Body University.

Three-dimensional fascia-oriented training

Stefan Dennenmoser

Introduction

Fascia is a ubiquitous, three-dimensionally networked structure, which takes on different forms depending on the nature of the load present (Stecco et al., 2007; Schleip et al., 2012). This varying structure is certainly not "in-born", rather it is formed by the individual strains on the body, according to the motor development of a person (Blasi et al., 2015; Wilke et al., 2016). The developmental steps one can observe usually occur in a pattern: from gross movement towards a target action, from experimental movement to movement pattern, and from repeated prevention of falling to locomotion. On confronting gravity, the exclusively kyphotic curve that is characteristic of the spine of a newborn baby is transformed, taking on a S-shaped curve that extends along the sagittal plane. The baby's crawling motion first produces lateral flexion and then spinal rotation as a function of that side-to-side movement. During this time, the movements are driven entirely by neuromuscular activity as the myofascial reinforcement present in an adult body is as yet undeveloped (Schultz et al., 1996). Only through repeated use and the related tensile loading does the tissue become more dense and stronger over months and years and, depending on the level of physical activity and movement habits, integrated into the individual's movement dynamics.

Strong differences can arise, for example, between people who suffer with paralysis from birth and those who are exposed to a very high level of repetitive or one-sided strain: for the person in a wheelchair, the fascia lata is not palpable as a reinforced structure whereas in athletes it is well-defined; for cowboys who spend hours every day on the back of a horse, a corresponding reinforcement of tissue can be found on the insides of the upper legs (Otsuka et al., 2018).

Myofascial coordination and fascial trigger mechanisms

Fascial reinforcement can serve to lessen strain on the musculature because it takes on a large portion of the load in eccentric (Chapter 26) as well as slow or almost static movements. It, furthermore, shapes the posture of the body via its base level of tension. The harmonic interplay between fascia and the involved musculature is thus a characteristic of a properly functioning system (Holleran et al., 1995). If the body perceives pain, then this interplay can be impaired. This leads to an increase in persistent tension of the musculature, which contributes to acidosis, fibrosis and fascial adhesions, and if not resolved the pathology could become chronic (Pavan et al., 2014).

It would be sensible here to keep the concept of myofascial coordination in mind because the muscular system and the fascial system are obviously inseparably linked, and each is dependent on the functionality of the other.

Chapter 40

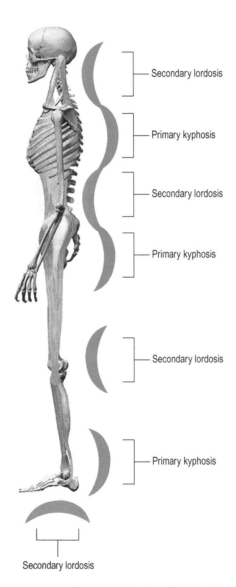

Secondary lordosis

Primary kyphosis

Secondary lordosis

Primary kyphosis

Secondary lordosis

Primary kyphosis

Secondary lordosis

Figure 40.1

The lordotic curves of the body result first from muscle tension. Then they become reinforced by fascial structures.

© www.faszienfit.de

This connection becomes particularly obvious for quick or elastic movements. Here, it is not about a gradual transfer of tension, rather the fascial regaining force is employed; the Achilles tendon is one example. For repeated two-legged hopping with brief ground contact, it appears that a large amount of the energy for the jump can be gained by the stretching of the Achilles tendon (Kawakami et al., 2002). During that movement the calf musculature only has an isometric function: it has to bring the Achilles tendon to the right level tension in anticipation for jumping, so as to generate its "catapult effect" (Sugisaki et al., 2011) Repeated studies in athletes have shown that the interplay between the fascia and muscular pre-tensioning is trainable (Fouré et al., 2012; Hirayama et al., 2017) and apparently this is also the case for the increasingly elastic movement quality of athletes in most sports.

Aside from these parallel and serial mechanisms of muscular and fascial tension, a spatial deformation of the muscle can be observed as it increases in thickness with contraction, and this then deforms the epimysium which transmits power to adjacent structures (Findley et al., 2015).

Tensegrity

Fascia training is thus also always muscle training, and muscle training also always affects—in varying amounts—the fascial system. The more naturally, gracefully or explosively a movement is executed, the more the fascial tissue becomes involved and trained. If one accepts the tensegrity model as the basis for human posture and movement, two factors emerge: the joint-stabilizing function of the myofascial base tension, and long-chain impulse transmission along the myofascial lines of tension.

According to the model of tensegrity, human bones function like distance pieces, kept in place by tension within the long lines of myofascial

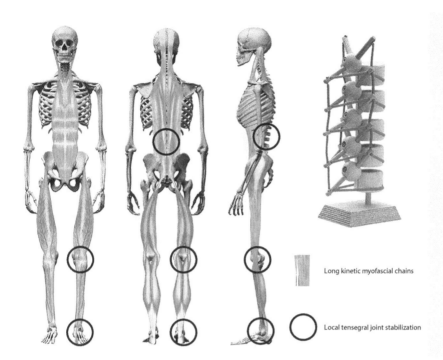

Long kinetic myofascial chains

Local tensegral joint stabilization

connections. The position of the bones is dictated by means of the tensile elements, and the bones somehow "float" in a fascial frame of tension (Dischiavi et al., 2018). This is why a harmonic balance in tension guarantees functional posture and movement.

An interesting side effect of this model is that, given these conditions, compressive stress does not exist in the joint because the joints are actually not needed as contact surfaces. By contrast, the positive tension surrounding the joint, i.e. tensegrity, even leads to less strain on the joint. While in the traditional and common model of linear-functioning muscle tension, where each increase in tension leads to an increase in load on the joint, targeted tensioning allows for and delivers relief for the joint surfaces through a three-dimensional, spiral and oblique arrangement of tension around the joint (Hashizume et al., 2014; Dischiavi et al., 2018).

Training of the tensional integrity system is markedly more difficult than common strength training, as it requires more attentiveness, acuity and body awareness. Such exercises can be found in existing body and movement schools, even if their principles are not explicitly formulated as being fascial in nature. These include approaches to the resolution of existing dysfunctional tension with Eutony (Alexander, 1983), the Feldenkrais Method and the Alexander Technique. Here, the training mostly takes place through inductive movement imagery (ideokinesis), which serves to coordinate the structure of individual tension elements. To this end, some movement schools use movements that are primitive in origin, for example, Continuum Movement or Animal Moves, which elaborate on and imitate the movements of various animals. Others, like Crawling Fitness, seek to trace human movement development by creating a

Chapter 40

modern and improved form of Klapp's Crawling. Still others look to kinematic concepts of strength and tensions centers (Pilates) or lines of tension (Spiraldynamik, Gyrokinesis). The orientation of movement in space represents a further element, which can be found in Laban Movement Analysis or the Gyrotonic Method.

Fundamentals: the three-dimensional architecture of the foot

If one adheres to the model of Spiraldynamik then the arch of the human foot is not determined by the shape of bones of the feet or the linear tension of the foot musculature, rather it

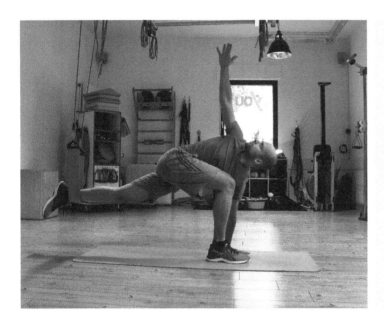

Figure 40.3

Three-dimensional training in Functional Fitness.

© www.you-personaltraining.de

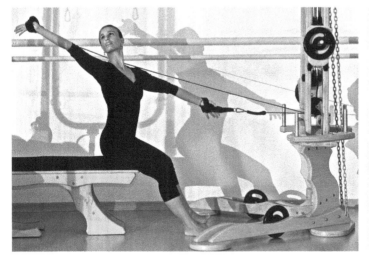

Figure 40.4

Three-dimensional training with a special apparatus: Gyrotonic Method©.

© Fabiana Bernardes, www.gyrotonic-sjcampos. com.br

Three-dimensional fascia-oriented training

results from the spiral screw-like connection of the intricate forefoot in relation to the solid form of the heel. While great apes possess a similar boney foot structure, this spiral screwing action is missing; rather, they primarily put weight through the outside edge of the foot, which is why they run stiffly on their back legs (Gray, 2016). Whenever people attempt to simulate a foot arch in this way, exactly the same precarious and unstable gorilla-like gait is the result.

In order to achieve a healthy arch in the structure of the foot, a number of things need to be done:

- Structural work on the fixations and thickening of the connective tissue of the foot, particularly the soles of the feel, the most painful point under the tarsal bones (navicular), the forefoot bones (metatarsals) and the area around the ankles (retinaculi). This can be done manually, or possibly using tennis or foam balls. Furthermore, initiation of the spiral screwing can be achieved through manual work (Figure 40.5).
- Bring awareness to the three contact surfaces when standing: the heel, the ball of the foot proximal to the little toe, and the ball of the big toe. When actively loading the ball of the big toe, the heel must remain stable. Neither the foot nor the knee should give way or fold inwards for this action.
- While maintaining an emphasis on the loading of the ball of the big toe, the stable heels can be a raised a bit and, if a step is available, the heels can also be lowered.
- If a sufficient level of coordination is present, the loading of the big toe can be practiced in movement: first simply by shifting weight forward and backward, then in walking backwards, and finally in forward locomotion.

Stabilization: three-dimensional body tensioning

Almost without exception, the joint partners in human anatomy are comprised of surfaces that fit more or less well on top of one another, which must be held in their functional position through appropriate muscular, ligamentous and capsular tension. As mentioned above, the oblique

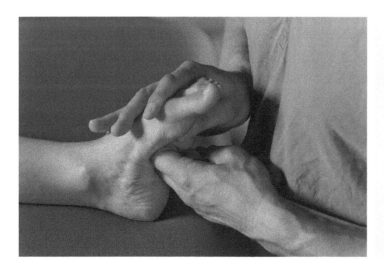

Figure 40.5

Structural work.

© Dennenmoser, Faszien – Therapie und Training, 1. Auflage 2016 © Elsevier GmbH, Urban & Fischer, München.

Chapter 40

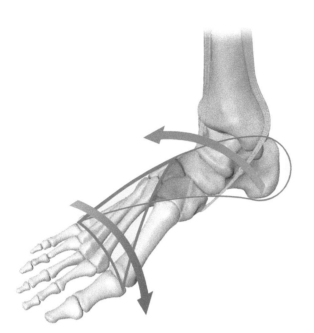

Figure 40.6

Spiraling model of the foot.

© www.spiraldynamik.com.

and spiral arrangement of the tension elements makes such stabilization possible. Again we find this model in Spiraldynamik, in the Franklin® Method known as "bone rhythms", in the Gyrotonic Method as "narrowing" (in dance), as "expanding", or also as "powerhouse" in the Pilates method. In all cases, the body seems to become taller or longer, and at the same time well-balanced and more stable.

An absence of such tension can be observed in people who are standing a lot every day, and shifting their body weight primarily to one side. In doing this, the loaded leg seems to screw inwards, the arch of the foot collapses, the lower leg rotates to the outside, the upper leg rotates to the inside and the knee is in turn locked in place.

This position does indeed require a minimum of muscle tension, but puts a considerable strain on the joints. In order to reverse this sinking

inwards, the muscles that move the joint must be active and the joint partners have to de-rotate against gravity. The forefoot must push against the ground via the ball of foot behind the big toe and the heels have to remain stable; while the lower legs rotate internally, the upper legs rotate externally and the ilia again rotate inwards. One can imagine pushing with the feet and legs against a floor that yields to the force, or similarly the lengthening action of the legs as a downward moving elevator comes to a stop and gravity is thus enhanced.

This image of enhanced gravity or tension-induced lengthening is then transferred to the torso and the upper extremities. While the arms function in a similar way to the legs, the torso has at its disposal a number of additional oblique and spiral connections, and moreover additional horizontal tension through the transverse abdominal muscles, pelvic floor and diaphragm.

Three-dimensional fascia-oriented training

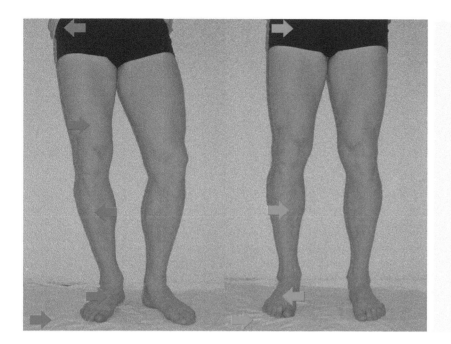

Figure 40.7
Compressed and decompressed joints via active de-rotation. www.faszienfit.de.

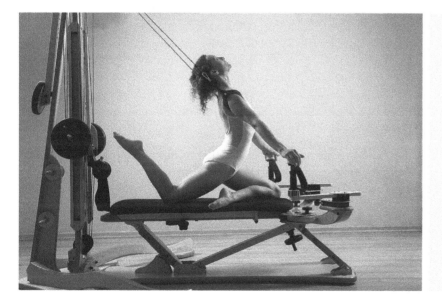

Figure 40.8
Gyrotonic® an Gyrokinesis® as an example of elongation/expansion).

© www.ronnyperry.com.

The most graceful combination of simultaneous three-dimensional stabilizing and expansive movement is clear to see in the Gyrotonic Method.

Training required: expansion in motion

A striking characteristic of the pre-tensioning mentioned above is that the amplitude of

Chapter 40

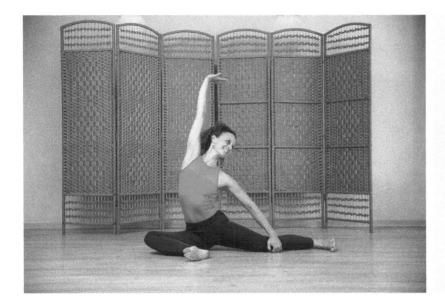

Figure 40.9

Gyrotonic® an Gyrokinesis® as an example of elongation/expansion).

© www.ronnyperry.com.

movement seems to be reduced in the first moment. This is obvious, because a movement using maximum range of motion requires "long", i.e. relaxed, muscles. But through the initiation of pre-tensioning, the elastic forces around the joint become active earlier. In this respect, two advantages of pre-tensioning come together: on the one hand, the joint is kept safe and the joint surfaces are relieved of strain, and on the other hand, elastic power is available for rapid movement.

Since the pull of muscles does not only act in a linear way on the skeleton, but its forces are distributed to the capsular and ligamentous structures around the joint, the linear power available for a movement is reduced by 20–30% (Maas et al., 2001). In order to develop a movement that is more refined and easier on the joints, the focus should be shifted an even greater amount in favor of the capsule tension so that the person performing the movement might be only making 50% or less power available for the target movement. For practice, to whatever extent is possible, the main portion of the power should contribute to the positioning of the joint. For all practical purposes this is achieved through kinetic images of great resistance (e.g. weight, pull, water), against which a movement is made. Further useful ideas include the imaginary extension of a part of the body that participates in the movement or a yawning quality of movement (pandiculation). The base tension is always at least as important as the target movement. Narrowing, expanding or the stable powerhouse are movements done with this in mind.

The initial over-tensioning on the joint capsule certainly can (and must!) be increasingly reduced in advanced practitioners until the movement is made in a truly elastically way, although the body does not lose length and the movement does not lose amplitude. A well-coordinated body, in this sense, anticipates the coming load and establishes just the right amount of pre-tension.

Long connections: myofascial functional chains

One of the most well-known myofascial functional chains is the long superficial backlines.

Three-dimensional fascia-oriented training

The fascial connections are really three-dimensional, but with spiral and spirally functional lines. These have been amply established in research (Wilke et al., 2016) and connect the torso with the respective contralateral extremities. Any locomotion, jumping or throwing motion requires this crossing-over connection. Whether in soccer, golf or javelin throwing, as soon as an object needs to be moved, the respective movement of the extremities is not only supported by the torso. An optimal movement impulse is also carried out through the spiral pre-stretching and successive shortening of the myofascial tracts.

Comparing the throwing abilities of gorillas and people, the apparent lack of this spiral-screwing motion is striking in the great apes, a characteristic limitation in contrast to the human thrower (Goldman, 2014). Great apes accelerate an object like a person who is just learning to throw, and moreover has not practiced very much. It is solely an arm movement: the monkey has anatomical limits to movement and the human beginner who has not yet learned to coordinate the movement are thus

similar throwers. In order to really utilize the elastic energy of the contralateral-oblique myofascial tracts, differentiated timing is required in terms of the muscular tensioning in the eccentric lengthening phase, isometric support during the maximal stretch and the elastic power of the fascia in the acceleration phase.

In order to train this quality of movement, the "reaching back" aspect has to be clearly emphasized. This involves keeping both the amplitude and also the source of the movement impulse in mind. In the field of strength training, this is described as dynamic eccentric or plyometric training. At the turnaround point of the movement, when the "reaching back" is transferred into the concentric target movement, maximal tensile forces are realized. If this movement coupling happens quickly enough, the body can utilize the elasticity of the tendons and fascia and maximally accelerate the body or object, often called the "catapult effect" (Kawakami et al., 2002) The timespan for this is dependent on things like the length of the myofascial chain: the longer the elastic chain, the longer the reversal

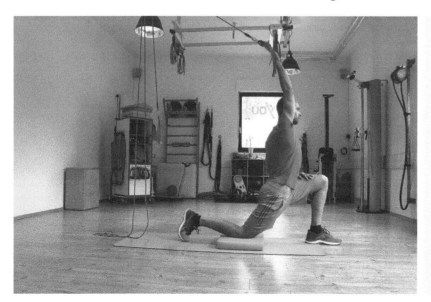

Figure 40.10

Throwing movement/
stretching.

© www.you-personaltraining.de.

Chapter 40

of motion can last. For example, while skipping rope with a low jump height, the ground contact time is under 0.1 s; it amounts to about 0.15 s for a long jump and, for a high jump, for which the entire body is elastically involved, about 0.2 s. The optimal value of the duration of this elastic movement reversal is different among individuals and depends on the environment, but it decreases in general as progress is made in athletic training, which reflects the increasing role of the fascial elasticity (Fouré et al., 2012; Hirayama et al., 2017).

Three-dimensional equipment training

The most ineffective forms of movement, from a functional as well as a fascial standpoint, involve isolated, limited, single-joint loading, like those that are dictated by some strength training equipment. A knee curl machine only offers a movement that is neither present in any sports nor any everyday activity. Such training only makes sense for countering muscular imbalance, or if one is working with people who are absolute beginners when it comes to physical activity. With increasing athletic experience, the equipment training must become more complex,

as fascia connects structures in multiple directions, involving more joints, i.e. closer to natural everyday movements, because of its elastic storage function. Newer trends, like Functional Training, Animal Moves or Paleo Training shift the person training into a natural wilderness, to work against these conditions. The delight of self-experience through proprioception (which derives from fascial tissue) in these archaic forms of movement has a balancing effect, making them restorative and enhancing creativity to compensate for a lack of everyday movement.

Concepts like Pilates or the Gyrotonic Method place emphasis on improving the control of movement, and thus position fascia-related whole-body coordination in the foreground. The devices of both of these disciplines are expressions of this attempt to support the manifold human movement possibilities with appropriate equipment.

Nonetheless, classic equipment like steel cables, free weights or other systems also allow for functional application: it is possible to use bodyweight training, and in so doing attempt to maximally train the possibility for differentiated movement.

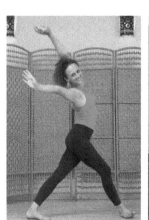 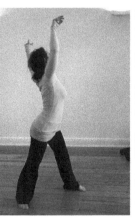 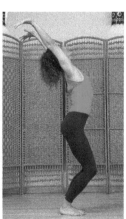

Figure 40.11

Dancing workout with expansion in all dimensions. www.LinkinMotion.eu / www.ronnyperry.com.

© Diana van Zon, www.LinkinMotion. eu / www.ronnyperry.com

Conclusion

The modern world of everyday movement is becoming increasingly two-dimensional. Many people sit in front of screens for a long time, and as a result fall into a more and more hunched posture. This tendency towards imbalance leads first to habitual postural adaptations and then to structural adaptations of the soft tissue, which in turn cause imbalances, overloading syndromes and degenerative processes (Bishop et al., 2014; Pavan et al., 2014). In the past, advice included "sit up straight", which fortunately has been replaced with "sit movable". Workplaces are being designed to be more adaptable and more "movement friendly". Nevertheless, the crucial and decisive factor is the movement experience of the individual themselves. In athletic activity as well as in therapy and everyday movements, there is a need to carry out complex and three-dimensional movement tasks, resulting first in the enhancement of neuromuscular coordination and subsequently the improvement myofascial structures.

References

Alexander, G. (1983) Eutony means balance of tensions. Psychophysical education, re-education and therapy. *Panminerva Med.* 25: 61–65.

Bishop, J.H., Fox, J.R., Maple, R., Loretan, C., Badger G.J., Henry, S.M., Vizzard, M.A. & Langevin, H.M. (2016) Ultrasound evaluation of the combined effects of thoracolumbar fascia injury and movement restriction in a porcine model. *PLoS One.* 11: e0147393.

Blasi, M., Blasi, J., Domingo, T., Pérez-Bellmunt, A. & Miguel-Pérez, M. (2015) Anatomical and histological study of human deep fasciae development. *Surg Radiol Anat.* 37: 571.

Dischiavi, S.L., Wright, A.A., Hegedus, E.J. & Bleakley, C.M. (2018) Biotensegrity and myofascial chains: a global approach to an integrated kinetic chain. *Med Hypotheses.* 110: 90–96.

Findley, T., Chaudhry, H. & Dhar, S. (2015) Transmission of muscle force to fascia during exercise. *J Bodyw Mov Ther.* 19: 119–123.

Fouré, A., Nordez, A. & Cornu, C. (2012) Effects of plyometric training on passive stiffness of gastrocnemii muscles and Achilles tendon. *Eur J Appl Physiol.* 112: 2849–2857.

Goldman, J.G. (2014) http://www.bbc.com/future/story/20140225-human-vs-animal-who-throws-best.

Gray, R. (2016) http://www.bbc.com/earth/story/20161209-the-real-reasons-why-we-walk-on-two-legs-and-not-four.

Hashizume, S., Iwanuma, S., Akagi, R., Kanehisa, H., Kawakami, Y. & Yanai, T. (2014) The contraction-induced increase in Achilles tendon moment arm: a three-dimensional study. *J Biomech.* 47: 3226–3231.

Hirayama, K., Iwanuma, S., Ikeda, N., Yoshikawa, A., Ema, R. & Kawakami, Y. (2017) Plyometric training favors optimizing muscle-tendon behavior during depth jumping. *Front Physiol.* 8: 16.

Holleran, K., Pope, M., Haugh, L. & Absher, R. (1995) The response of the flexion-relaxation phenomenon in the low back to loading. *Iowa Orthop J.* 15: 24–28.

Kawakami, Y., Muraoka, T., Ito, S., Kanehisa, H. & Fukunaga, T. (2002) In vivo muscle fibre behaviour during counter-movement exercise in humans reveals a significant role for tendon elasticity. *J Physiol.* 540: 635–646.

Maas, H., Baan, G.C. & Huijing, P.A. (2001) Intermuscular interaction via myofascial force transmission: effects of tibialis anterior and extensor hallucis longus length on force transmission from rat extensor digitorum longus muscle. *J Biomech.* 34: 927–940.

Otsuka, S., Yakura, T., Ohmichi, Y., Ohmichi, M., Naito, M., Nakano, T. & Kawakami, Y. (2018) Site specificity of mechanical and structural properties of human fascia lata and their gender differences: a cadaveric study. *J Biomech.* 77: 69–75.

Pavan, P.G., Stecco, A., Stern, R. & Stecco, C. (2014) Painful connections: densification versus fibrosis of fascia. *Curr Pain Headache Rep.* 18: 441.

Sugisaki, N., Kawakami, Y., Kanehisa, H. & Fukunaga, T. (2011) Effect of muscle contraction levels on the force-length relationship of the human Achilles tendon during lengthening of the triceps surae muscle-tendon unit. *J Biomech.* 44: 2168–2171.

Wilke, J., Krause, F., Vogt L. & Banzer, W. (2016) What is evidence-based about myofascial chains: a systematic review. *Arch Phys Med Rehabil.* 97: 454–461.

Dance

Liane Simmel

Introduction

Dancers are easily spotted on the street, as their bodies seem to show a special "connectivity" that allows for harmonious, continuous and elegant movement. There are many different factors contributing to this impression, one of which might be the state of the fascial system. Dance in its variety of different styles offers a great source of body and movement expertise, gained through physical experience. By teaching it, the expertise of generations of dancers and dance teachers is passed on in the studios being adapted anew by each individual dancer and thus practically tested over a wide range of different body types. However, big sections of this knowledge have not yet been proven scientifically.

Since the 1980s, there has been an increasing interest in dance from a medical perspective. In its early years, the new field of dance medicine focused mainly on the dancer's health, his/her working conditions, typical dance injuries and injury prevention (Laws et al., 2005; Hincapié et al., 2008; Simmel, 2014). Analogous to the development in sports medicine, where the focus has changed from the management of sports injuries to a broader definition of a medicine of exercise, dance medicine is widening its horizons towards the dancer's body expertise, motor learning abilities and specific training methods (Wyon et al., 2016). It is the expanded knowledge from medical research, sports medicine and exercise science that allows for a deeper scientific understanding of many traditional dance training methods.

Dancers train to combine a high degree of flexibility, exceptional balance (Bläsing et al., 2018) and remarkable coordination of whole-body movements (Bronner, 2012) with suppleness and elegance. The flow of multidimensional movements and the constant variation of exercise patterns may play an important role in stimulating the fascial system.

Dancers often describe their dance training as an outstanding training for body connectivity. As a dancer in transition to her second profession states: "Searching in all varieties of sports, I could not find any other athletic training which provides the same feeling of a whole-body training as dance training does. After a ballet class my body feels trained from head to toe". The ongoing research on fascial tissue might help to find a scientific explanation for this body experience. Meanwhile, looking at dance training from a fascial training perspective can expand today's training recommendations by highlighting ideas which might increase the effectiveness of a fascial-orientated fitness training.

Dance training

In contrast to many sports, where the attention is focused on achieving measurable external goals, dance emphasizes not only the outer shape and the outcome of the movement but also the perception and awareness of the sensations within the dancer's body (De Lima, 2013). It is the ability to perceive, classify and react to one's individual inner body perspective that creates a

Chapter 41

sophisticated dancer. Dance seems to be a special combination between strong athletic performance ability and high body perception and awareness.

When speaking of dance and dance training, one has to keep in mind the enormous variety of different dance techniques. From classical ballet, modern and contemporary dance to urban, break dance or tap, many different dance styles are shown on stage and might be part of a choreography. This great diversity in dance styles places high demands on the dancer's body. Obviously, there is not one specific training method that can provide everything dancers need for their fitness (Angioi et al., 2009). However, even today, for many dancers the classical ballet technique seems to be the basis of their dance career as well as their daily training routine. Even dance companies who mainly perform contemporary dance or dance theatre tend to offer daily ballet classes to their dancers. Enriched with somatic principles and contemporary dance elements, these classes seem to offer helpful training methods, most of them being developed practically through trial and error, yet still do not have scientific proof.

"Somatic movement education" (Hanna, 2004) describes the process of a sensory motor training creating improved muscle function, enhanced sensory awareness and adaptation of muscle patterns. With its integration, listening to the body and responding to perceived sensations by consciously questioning movement habits and altering movement patterns became an important tool in teaching and learning dance. Dance and somatic approach influenced each other mutually with the dancer's experience supporting somatic investigation and the somatic approach being applied to the dance technique (Bartenieff and Lewis, 1980). By addressing the inner body perspective, dance stimulates both the proprioception and interoception of the body. The highest density of proprioceptive and interoceptive receptors are found within the fascial tissue (Schleip et al., 2012B), so it seems to play an important role in the perception of inner sensations. It can, hence, be assumed that training body awareness is deeply associated with the fascial system.

Adaptation of fascial tissue

"Form follows function". This statement by the American sculptor, Horatio Greenough, which addressed the organic principles in architecture, is quoted in many bodywork methodologies to refer to the impressive adaptability of the body. How the body is used and the way the individual tissues are put under strain influences its formation and architecture. It is this principle that, for example, explains the tightening of the iliotibial band at the outside of the thigh in many classical trained dancers as the turnout position of the leg increases the tension on this structure.

Research has shown that fascial tissue is particularly adaptable to regular strain. When put under increasing physiological stress, it reacts to the loading patterns by remodeling the architecture of its collagenous fiber network, resulting in a change in length, strength, elasticity, and an increasing ability to withstand shearing forces (Schleip and Müller, 2013). By contrast, aging processes and lack of movement—at least in animals—lead to a more haphazard and disoriented arrangement of the collagenous fibers, diminishing the elasticity of the fascial tissue (Järvinen et al., 2002). Thus the local architecture of the fasciae reflects the individual history of previous strain and movement demands.

To achieve adaptation in human fasciae, applied strains need to exceed the degree of normal daily life activities. This requires a specific training that stimulates the fibroblasts to build

Dance

up an elastic fiber architecture. Movements that load the fascial tissues over diverse whole-body extensions using their elastic springiness for fast form and position changes seem to be especially efficient. There are many examples in dance, like high jumps starting from a deep squat position or leg extensions that proceed in contra directional upper body and arm movement with fast direction changes. As many dance exercises require a great range of motion and a variety of movement angles, dance offers a large repertoire of exercises potentially helping to maintain and train the strength, elasticity and shearing ability of the fascial tissue.

Dance offers both training and challenge to the fascial network. Dance sequences are, in general, practiced on both sides, right and left, as well as forwards and backwards. By using these multidirectional whole-body movements, dance trains a wide variety of motions, which calls for a high shearing ability of the different fascial layers. Additionally, by putting specific focus on alignment and placement, dance supports to counteract potential harmful asymmetries within the body, for example, like a hyperlordosis of the lumbar spine, which could lead to a tightening of the thoracolumbar fascia. With targeted flexibility training being an integral part of most dance classes, dance seems to keep the soft tissue compliant and extensible. Counter-movements, dynamic muscle loading and springy motions are part of many dance steps, challenging the elastic storage capacity of the fascial tissue. Furthermore, by focusing on inner body awareness while performing exercises, dance stimulates proprioception.

In summary, dance engages the fascial system through:

- Multidirectional whole-body movements
- Specific focus on alignment and placement to counteract body asymmetries

- Targeted flexibility training
- Counter-movements, dynamic muscle loading and springy motions
- proprioceptive stimulation.

Dance as fascial training

Although results from fascia research are only beginning to be included specifically, many dance elements, exercises and corrections address the fascial connective tissue and correspond with the principles of fascial fitness training (Schleip and Müller, 2013).

Aspects of dance as fascial training:
- Myofascial release
- Stretching
- Preloading – counter-movements
- Cyclic training
- Body awareness.

Myofascial release

Findings from animal studies suggest that immobility quickly fosters the development of additional cross-links, which render the fascial tissue less flexible (Järvinen et al., 2002). It seems a natural conclusion that whole-body mobility is an important prerequisite for the elasticity and shearing ability of the fascial system. In our daily movement habits, we are a long way away from using the full range of motion our joints would permit. Instead, we tend to stick to familiar movement patterns which, over time, might limit our general range of motion and reduce mobility. This is where the targeted mobilization exercises of dance come to the fore.

Exercise: Release of the dorsal fascia

This exercise is thought to gradually release the dorsal fasciae, starting from the cervical area all

Chapter 41

the way down over the heels to the plantar side of the toes. Start by standing upright, feet parallel and hip-width apart, with the hands crossing at the back of the head. Slowly roll down, vertebra by vertebra, flexing the spine, starting from the top of the head. When an initial stretch can be felt at the back of the spine, stop and gently increase the pressure on the head, resisting by performing an isometric contraction of the back muscles. Hold the contraction for 8 s, then release the tension and slowly continue rolling down, stopping at any newly felt stretch. Slowly proceed in this manner until reaching the deepest possible stretching position (Figure 41.1).

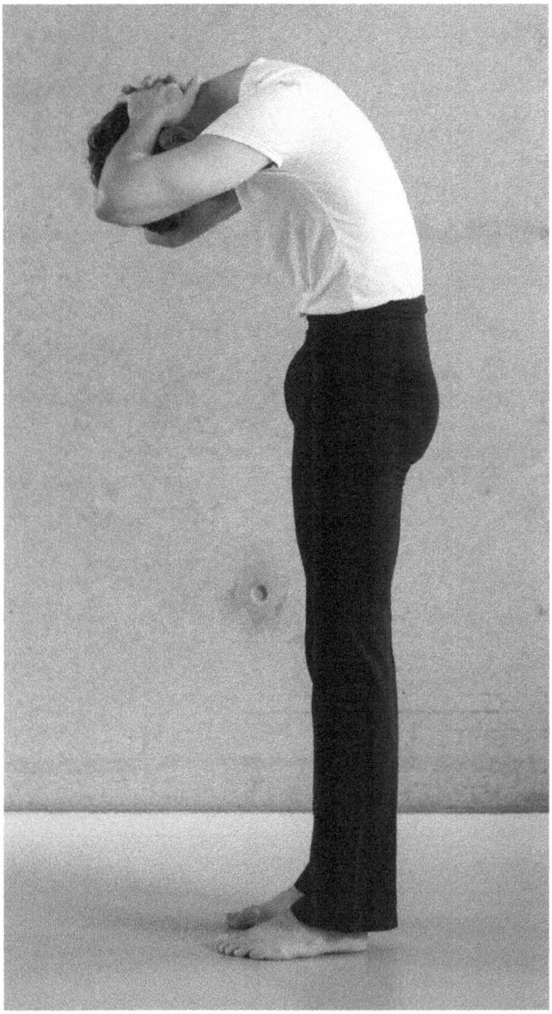

Exercise: Release of the plantar fascia

This exercise focuses on releasing the plantar fascia of the feet while preloading the dorsal fasciae. Start by standing in the yoga downward-facing-dog position, feet parallel and hip-width apart. Feel the connection between the soles of the feet and the hands flat on the floor, focusing on the stretch of the dorsal fasciae by lifting up the sit bones high in the air. Shift the weight onto the hands and slowly walk step-by-step towards the hands using the mobility of the foot and the elasticity of the sole to deepen the stretch on the dorsal fascia (Figure 41.2).

Stretching

The collagen fibers of the fascial system are primarily shaped by tensional strain rather than by

Figure 41.1

Release of the dorsal fasciae

With permission from Andreas Siegel.

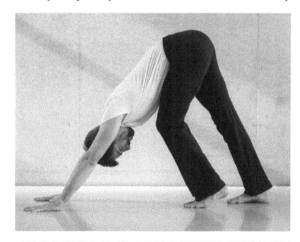

Figure 41.2

Release of the plantar fascia

With permission from Andreas Siegel.

compression (Schleip and Müller, 2013). This fact, and the decrease in range of motion that usually accompanies aging, reducing the shearing ability between distinct fascial layers, leads to a strong recommendation for regular stretching in order to remodel and train the fascial tissue. Using variations of different stretching styles seems to be more effective than sticking to only one method. Thus, alternating between slow passive stretches at different angles and dynamic and bouncing stretches has been recommended. Research suggests that fast dynamic stretching is even more effective as a fascial training when combined with a preparatory counter-movement (Fukashiro et al., 2006).

Dance uses a wide variety of stretching and flexibility methods throughout its training. Passive stretching methods are common to increase general flexibility. The typical multidirectional movements, with slight changes in angle while deepening the stretch, are beneficial for the fascial system. Active and dynamic stretching are naturally integrated into most dance steps. Each controlled high extension of the leg and each leg-kick elongates the muscular and fascial tissue, placing tensional strain on the collagenous fibers. The dynamic swinging used in leg swings, whether lying on the floor or standing, stimulates many epimysial tissues in the leg and pelvis, which are extended beyond their habitual conditions. In dance, all these stretches engage myofascial chains extending over multiple joints.

Exercise: Dynamic stretching of the back of the leg

This exercise uses a dynamic muscular loading pattern in which the muscle is briefly activated while in its lengthened position. For this purpose, Schleip and Müller (2013) propose soft elastic bounces at the end ranges of available motion. Start by standing upright, feet parallel and hip-width apart, with the balls of the feet standing on a stair. Be aware of the connection between heel and head letting the head easily "float" on the cervical spine, and slowly lower the heel. At the end of the available movement, perform soft elastic bounces, lowering the heel even further. Finish the exercise with a short isometric contraction of the calf muscles while still in the deepest stretching position (Figure 41.3).

Preloading – counter-movements

The elasticity of the fascial tissue is key to its high capacity to store kinetic energy. Using the dynamic catapult effect of the collagen fibers allows for an energetic and elastic movement, not only when jumping and running, but also in daily activities, i.e. walking. The higher the demands on velocity and momentum, the more the elasticity

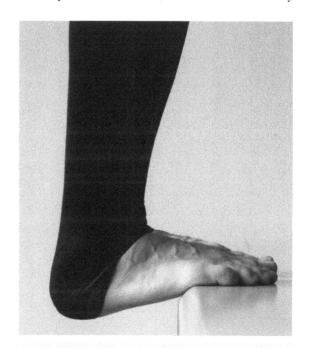

Figure 41.3

Dynamic stretching of the back of the leg

With permission from Andreas Siegel.

Chapter 41

of the fascial system comes into account. In a healthy fascial system, actively preloading the fascial tissue before an action facilitates the dynamic impulse. This can be used by starting a movement with a slight counter-movement in the opposite direction. While performing the actual movement, the stored energy will dynamically release in a passive recoil action, thereby using the catapult effect of the connective tissue.

Preparatory counter-movements are common in dance. Many dance exercises implement the energy-loading momentum as preparation for a dance step. Using a deep demi-plié (bending the knees without lifting the heels off the floor) before jumping or in preparation for a pirouette, loads the soft tissue and allows for a dynamic passive recoil to start the actual movement. The principles of fall, rebound and recovery, as used in many contemporary dance techniques (Diehl and Lampert, 2011), seem an ideal training for the preloading and recoil capacity of the fascial tissue. Breathing in before bending backwards increases the elastic tension in the upper body and thus elongates the spine, diminishing the pressure on the discs as well as on the intervertebral joints.

Exercise: Leg swings

The focus of this exercise is on the preloading of the posterior fascial chain. Start by lying supine, both knees bent, feet parallel and aligned with the sit bones. The right knee drops to the left side. The momentum of the movement allows the lower right leg to swing along the floor to the left, thereby also rotating the pelvis to the left. The entire right posterior fascial chain from the shoulder to the foot becomes preloaded, supporting the right leg, at the end of its loading capacity, to swing back along the floor to the starting position. The left side takes over the momentum, starting to swing to the right, preloading the left posterior fascial chain. Repetitive alternation between right and left swing preloads the fascial chains and facilitates the passive recoil action at the end of the preloading capacity (Figure 41.4).

Cyclic training

Experimental research shows that fluid is pressed out of the fascial tissue when subjected to strain, similar to a sponge being squeezed. When releasing the strain, this area will refill with fluid, which comes from the surrounding tissue, the lymphatic network and the vascular system (Schleip et al., 2012A). Although the optimal durations for the loading and unloading phases have yet to be elucidated, their proper timing is important to facilitate optimal rehydration, as the short pause gives the tissues the chance to absorb nourishing fluid, thereby boosting the fascial metabolism. A cyclic training character that alternates periods of intense strain with targeted breaks is therefore recommended.

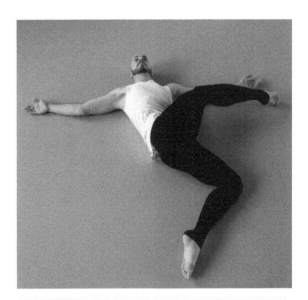

Figure 41.4

Leg swings

With permission from Andreas Siegel.

Dance

In general, rhythm plays a vital role in dance: be it using music as an external "pacemaker", focusing on one's individual breath pattern or engaging with the "inner rhythm" of the movement itself. Rhythmically loading and unloading the fascial tissue comes naturally in dance, alternating between stretching and releasing, between elongating and contracting. Thus many dance exercises implement a cyclic fascial training and hence support fascial health.

Body awareness

Good coordination and awareness of one's whole-body connectivity are essential keystones for dance. Allowing movements to fluently continue through the body, focusing on maintaining the alignment and expanding the body in space, brings attention to the fascial network. Dance, especially contemporary dance, implements a large repertoire of fascial awareness exercises, which focus on the body's inner communication network and the stretching of the connecting tissue.

Exercise: Rocking the dorsal fasciae on the floor

Focus on the dorsal fasciae to facilitate their mobility. Start by lying supine, both legs parallel with the feet in dorsal flexion, anchoring the heels into the floor. Rhythmically point and flex the feet allowing the momentum to continue up to the head, gently flexing and extending in the most upper cervical joint. Feel the connectivity from the toes up to the head and register the impulses of the feet as they induce the motion of the head.

Exercise: Awareness of whole-body connectivity

Elongate and mobilize the lateral myofascial chain: lying supine with legs stretched, and arms opened out to the side with palms facing towards the ceiling, start with the impulse of the right foot slowly pulling the right leg across to the left side, allowing the pelvis and spine to follow. Feel the resistance by holding the right arm and shoulder on the floor. To perform the stretch dynamically, alternate the pulling impulse between right leg and right arm. Roll back to the starting position, taking time to compare both sides of the body, then continue the exercise on the left side (Figure 41.5).

Supplementary fascial training through dance

In addition to offering a large selection of exercises, dance also provides helpful supplementary ideas to support fascial training. Although these practices have been inspired by physical feedback and are not yet proven scientifically, they have been applied practically by generations of dancers and have helped dancers to gain their specific "whole body connectivity" for which they are renowned. By performing most of the exercises on both sides, dance provides an "equilibrium" for the body. Regarding fascial training, there are four movement

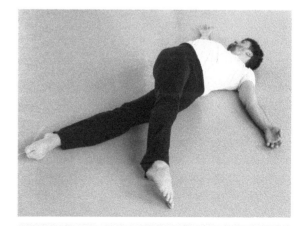

Figure 41.5

Awareness of whole-body connectivity

With permission from Andreas Siegel.

Chapter 41

principles, which are fundamental to almost every dance training and which, in application to the specific fascial training, could increase its effectiveness.

> ### Increase fascia-oriented training training by the use of dance-specific movement principles:
> - Awareness of oppositions
> - Elongation
> - Counter-movements
> - Momentum and rebound.

The awareness of opposition is key for body connectivity. As a preparation for the exercise, the dancer is focusing on the specific body parts affected by the movement to follow, their connection and their separation. This allows for the feeling of space and elongation, yet connection between the opponents. For example, when bending the upper body to the right side, the left foot firmly keeps its contact to the floor. The two opponents, head to the right side and left foot, stay connected, thus allowing elongation and stretching of the fascial tissue on the left side of the body.

When lifting one leg off the floor or using the arms for expressive dance movements, dancers tend to focus on the elongation of their extremities. With the image of widening the movement into space, filling out the surrounding area, the dancer increases their bodily borders. From the perspective of fascial training, this elongation of the extremities allows for further loading and prestretching of the fascial tissue.

Keeping one's balance is crucial in dance. To achieve a natural equilibrium, regardless of the performed dance movement, the dancer makes use of small counter-movements that allow for

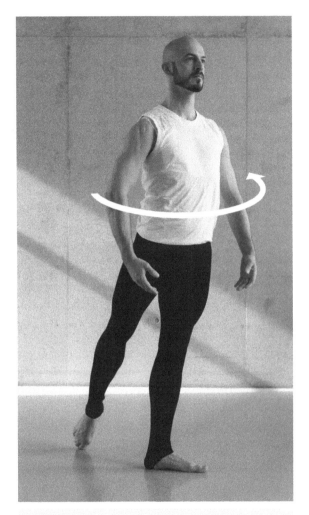

Figure 41.6

In order to achieve an economic equilibrium, the dancer performs a small rotation of the spine to the left when lifting the right leg to the back.

With permission from Andreas Siegel.

stability and counter-strain. For example, to achieve economic equilibrium, a small rotation of the spine to the left may be used when lifting the right leg to the back (Figure 41.6). Fascially speaking, this small counter-movement allows loading of the corresponding fascial tissue.

Dance

Jumping, rolling on the floor, or lifting, each of these dance movements demands perfect timing of the impulse, momentum and rebound: the optimal timing in releasing the preloaded muscular and connective tissues. A cat-like jump with a noiseless landing requires a high level of elasticity within the fascial tissue, using the body like a spring, preloading its fibers in preparation for the movement. Applying this momentum and rebound to daily life activities, for example, by using the elastic rebound while walking fast or jumping up stairs, allow for an implemented fascial fitness training.

Although these dance movement principles still require further research regarding their effect on the fascial tissue, applying them into fascial training might add helpful aspects and increase its effectiveness.

Dance uses a wide variety of fascial training techniques and principles, which are nowadays recommended and supported by an increasing body of evidence. In its practical application, dance provides ideas for further research in fascial fitness training. However, with its highly complex movement patterns and its whole-body integration, dance remains challenging for scientific research. Yet further investigation on the dancer's body expertise might help to deepen the understanding of fascial structures and their trainability.

References

Angioi, M., Metsios, G., Koutedakis, Y. & Wyon, M.A. (2009) Fitness in contemporary dance: a systematic review. *Int J Sports Med*. 30: 475–484.

Bartenieff, I. & Lewis, D. (1980) *Body Movement: Coping with the Environment*. Oxon, New York: Routledge.

Bläsing, B., Puttke M. & Schack, T. (Eds) (2018) *The Neurocognition of Dance*. 2nd ed. Oxon, New York: Routledge.

Bronner, S. (2012) Differences in segmental coordination and postural control in a multi-joint dance movement: Développé arabesque. *J Dance Med Sci*. 16: 26–35.

De Lima, C. (2013) Trans-meaning – Dance as an embodied technology of perception. *J Dance Somat Pract*. 5: 17–30.

Diehl, I. & Lampert, F. (Eds) (2011) *Dance Techniques 2010: Tanzplan, Germany*. Leipzig, Germany: Seemann Henschel.

Fukashiro, S., Hay, D. & Nagano, A. (2006) Biomechanical behavior of muscle-tendon complex during dynamic human movements. *J Appl Biomech*. 22: 131–147.

Hanna, T. (2004) *Somatics: Reawakening the Mind's Control of Movement, Flexibility, and Health*. Cambridge: Da Capo Press.

Hincapié, C.A., Morton, E.J. & Cassidy, J.D. (2008) Musculoskeletal injuries and pain in dancers: a systematic review. *Arch Phys Med Rehabil*. 89: 1819–1829.

Järvinen, T.A.H., Józsa, L., Kannus, P., Järvinen, T.L.N. & Järvinen, M. (2002) Organization and distribution of intramuscular connective tissue in normal and immobilized skeletal muscles. An immunohistochemical, polarization and scanning electron microscopic study. *J Muscle Res Cell M*. 23: 245–254.

Laws, H., Apps, J., Bramley, I. & Parker, D. (2005) *Fit to Dance 2: Report of the Second National Inquiry Into Dancers' Health and Injury in the UK*. Regina Saskatchewan, Canada: Newgate Press.

Schleip, R., Duerselen, L., Vleeming, A., Naylor, I., Lehmann-Horn, F., Zorn, A. & Klingler, W. (2012a) Strain hardening of fascia: static stretching of dense fibrous connective tissues can induce a temporary stiffness increase accompanied by enhanced matrix hydration. *J Bodyw Mov Ther*. 16: 94–100.

Schleip, R., Findley, T.W., Chaitow, L. & Huijing, W.A. (Eds) (2012b) *Fascia: The Tensional Network of the Human Body: The Science and Clinical Applications in Manual and Movement Therapy*. Churchill Livingstone, Elsevier.

Schleip, R. & Müller, D.G. (2013) Training principles for fascial connective tissues: scientific foundation and suggested practical applications. *J Bodyw Mov Ther*. 17: 103–115.

Simmel, L. (2014) *Dance Medicine in Practice*. Oxon, New York: Routledge.

Chapter 41

Wyon, M.A., Allen, N., Cloak, R., Beck, S., Davies P. & Clarke, F. (2016) Assessment of maximum aerobic capacity and anaerobic threshold of elite ballet dancers. *Med Probl Perform Art*. 31: 145–150.

Further reading

Quin, E., Rafferty S. & Tomlinson, C. (2015) *Safe Dance Practice*. Champaign, IL: Human Kinetics.

Todd, M. (2008) *The Thinking Body*. Gouldsboro: Gestalt Journal Press.

Wilmerding, M.V. & Krasnow, D.H. (Eds) (2017) *Dancers Wellness*. Champaign: Human Kinetics.

Kettlebell training

Frieder Krause

Introduction

The kettlebell (KB) is a cast-iron or cast-steel weight shaped like a cannonball with a handle on top (Figure 42.1). The name kettlebell stems from its distinctive form resembling an old water kettle. Originally developed in the 1700s as a counterweight for market scales in Russia, KBs have been used as training tools in eastern Europe since then (Tsatsouline, 2006). In the past decade, training with KBs has become increasingly popular in the worldwide functional training and fitness community. Since the 1960s, there have been competitive events, where athletes compete in different lifting forms. However, the competitive nature of KB sport will not be the focus of this chapter.

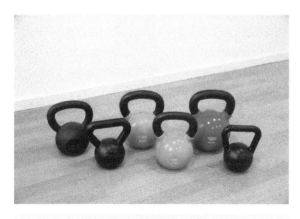

Figure 42.1 A selection of kettlebells with different weights and forms

What makes KB training unique and different from other forms of weight training? Unlike traditional dumbbells, the center of mass in a KB lies outside the hand, which predisposes KBs for ballistic and swinging movements involving the whole body (Jay et al., 2011). That being said, KB training usually consists of multi-joint movements and exercises focusing on functional or myofascial chains rather than on isolated muscles or body parts. Of course, this holistic approach to exercise and physical training is not necessarily limited to KB training alone. Other training forms such as Olympic lifting, powerlifting or so-called functional training also focus on complex movements rather than isolating muscles as in traditional bodybuilding. However, the swinging component of most KB exercises is indeed a unique feature that has potential benefits for the connective tissue network.

Traditionally, training with KBs has been popular in policemen, special forces and military personnel because it is thought to improve explosive power, strength endurance as well a mental toughness (Tsatsouline, 2006; Sukopp, 2016; Kwella, 2017). Today, its use has spread to fitness clubs and rehabilitation clinics around the world. Research has shown that KB training leads to acute responses in hormones triggering muscle adaptation (Budnar et al., 2014), reduced neck and lower back pain (Jay et al., 2011), improved postural stability (Jay et al., 2013), increased aerobic fitness (Thomas et al., 2014;

Chapter 42

Falatic et al., 2015) as well as enhanced maximal and explosive strength (Lake and Lauder, 2012A). Therefore, it serves as a good addition to any regular health and fitness training regimen. The aim of this chapter is to elaborate how KB training may affect the fascial system and how it can be integrated into a training program tailored to improve connective tissue properties. One of the most commonly used KB exercises, the KB swing, as well as other exercises that can be utilized to impact the myofascial system, will be introduced and thoroughly described. After practicing the described examples, the reader will be able to apply the underlying principles to other KB exercises or similar forms of training.

Potential effects of KB training on the fascial system

To date, there is no scientific evidence on the impact of KB training on the fascial system. However, the swinging movements in many KB exercises could affect connective tissue renewal as well as its energy storage capacity. Mechanical loading, especially eccentric muscle work, has been shown to induce increased collagen remodeling in tendons (Kjær et al., 2009). As swinging the KB often requires an eccentric deceleration at the point of movement reversal, such an effect may also occur in KB training. In this context, it has to be underlined that the three-dimensional nature of the exercises may stimulate the fibers of the fascial system more effectively than movements occurring in one plane only. The storage and release of elastic energy is one of the main tasks of our connective tissue during functional tasks such as walking (Ishikawa et al., 2005). The KB might be an ideal tool to train and improve this energy storage capacity, because smooth movement execution and swinging exercises as the ones used in KB training have generally been proposed as positive training stimuli for the fascial system (Schleip and Müller, 2013).

The KB swing

The KB swing unarguably represents one of the most commonly used KB exercises. It is an exercise with relatively low technical demands that can be executed with relatively light loads. Both features make it an exercise than can easily be integrated into a training program for both novices and experienced lifters (Lake and Lauder, 2012B). Furthermore, its complex and ballistic nature involves most muscles of the posterior body (the hamstrings, glutes, erector spinae and latissimus dorsi) (Budnar et al., 2014) and the corresponding connective tissue, in particular the thoracolumbar fascia (TLF).

In the starting position, the feet are placed about a shoulder width apart, with the toes facing slightly outward. The arms should remain extended during the whole exercise, allowing the entire energy created by the hip, knee and core muscles to be fully transferred into the KB. The KB is placed on the floor, 5 cm in front of the feet. The movement is initiated by actively flexing, or "hinging" the hip joint with little to no flexion of the knee and a neutral spine. The KB is then actively pulled backwards between the knees and behind the pelvis (the "backswing"). The end position is governed by hamstring flexibility and the ability to maintain a neutral spine.

From this position, the hip is explosively extended to accelerate the KB forward and upwards. The forearms should remain in contact with the body during the swinging phase until the KB passes the hip, ensuring that the energy is fully transferred from the feet through the torso and arms into the KB. The knees, hips and upper body should all be fully extended while swinging the KB to about shoulder height. In the next

Kettlebell training

step, either actively pull the KB back down or let gravity take over and wait until the KB is accelerated downwards. When the forearms touch the body, actively flex the hip. In this portion of the movement, the hamstrings, the glutes and the lumbar extensors work eccentrically, and the momentum and energy are absorbed in the connective tissue, like in an elastic spring. When the KB reaches the end position, the hips are again explosively extended to accelerate the KB forward and upward in a fluid movement. During the entire exercise, the movement should be led by the hip joint, not the arms and shoulders. Beginners tend to pull the KB cranially with their shoulders instead of using the momentum generated by the hip to swing the KB. One consequence is that they reduce weight because their shoulders fatigue rapidly. Also, the amount of force generated during hip extension will determine the height of the KB. If you cannot swing the KB high enough, do not use your arms but try to extend the hip faster after the backswing. See Figure 40.2 for a detailed illustration of the KB swing.

Key points for the KB swing:

- Actively pull the KB back to start the exercise
- Explosively extend hip and knees while keeping arms straight
- Swing KB to shoulder height, keeping the entire body extended
- Do not pull the KB upwards with your shoulders
- Keep the hips extended until the forearm touches your torso
- Flex hips (and knees slightly) to slow down the KB, absorbing the energy
- The movement should look smooth and easy

As mentioned, the KB swing mostly works on the muscles of the posterior body, especially the hamstrings, gluteal muscles and the latissimus dorsi, all of which are linked by connective tissue that has the ability to transfer force (Krause et al., 2016; Wilke et al., 2016) (Chapter 13). In both end positions, elastic energy can be stored during the eccentric movement phase in the myofascial system and released in the subsequent

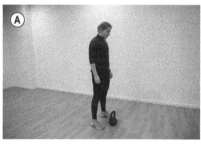
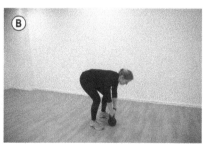
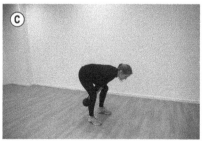
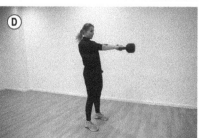
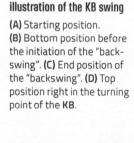

Figure 42.2 Detailed illustration of the KB swing

(A) Starting position. **(B)** Bottom position before the initiation of the "backswing". **(C)** End position of the "backswing". **(D)** Top position right in the turning point of the **KB**.

Chapter 42

concentric movement: in the flexed low position, the TLF as well as the fascia of the anterior shoulder and arm act like a spring, being stretched and releasing kinetic energy as the KB is accelerated in the anterior direction. In the extended high position, energy is stored and released in the myofascial tissue of the anterior body, as well as in the posterior shoulder and arm.

Alterations in TLF morphology (Langevin et al., 2009) and sliding properties (Langevin et al., 2011) have been shown in patients with low back pain. Similarly, changes in fascial thickness of the sternocleidomastoid muscle seem to manifest in patients with neck pain (Stecco et al., 2014). KB swing training might impact connective tissue remodeling and elastic properties of the TLF and the entire myofascial tissue of the shoulder-arm complex. These alterations may, in turn, explain the positive effect of KB exercises for patients with low back and neck pain (Jay et al., 2011). In sum, the KB swing seems to be a good exercise for preventing non-specific myofascial pain, as well as for treating patients with low back or neck pain, as long as the weight is chosen according to the functional abilities and the physical status of the patient.

One-handed KB swing

If one is able to perform a KB swing with proper form and good technique, progression can be achieved via the one-handed swing. Due to the unilateral character of the exercise, the core muscles are engaged in an anti-rotational manner, increasing complexity and effectiveness (Kwella, 2017). The stress on the muscles and the connective tissue on the KB swinging arm is also greater than in the two-handed swing. Additionally, one-handed swings are the foundation for more complex KB lifts like the KB clean or the KB snatch, and should therefore be mastered before further progressing the training routine.

The movement itself, as well as the general recommendations, are the same as for the two-handed swing. With regard to the grip, there are essentially three different ways to hold the KB, each of which has an impact upon muscle activation in the forearm and shoulder. The neutral grip is the most commonly used, although internal or external rotation of the shoulder and rotation of the KB by 90° to grab the corner of the KB in the starting position are also possible.

The "backswing" is again initiated by actively pulling the KB between the legs, backwards. Then the hip and knees are explosively extended while keeping the arm straight, swinging the KB to about shoulder height. On the return, ensure the weight and the momentum of the KB do not "twist" the body by actively engaging the muscles of the core (especially the external and internal obliques), to counteract the rotational forces which the KB creates while gravity accelerates it downwards. Keeping the forearm as close to the inside of the ipsilateral leg as possible, flex the hip when the KB reaches the midline, absorbing the energy of the KB and transferring it to the next hip extension movement to accelerate the KB back upwards (see Figure 42.3 for a detailed illustration of the one-handed KB swing.)

Key points for the one-handed swing:

- Actively pull the KB back with one hand to start the exercise
- Explosively extend hip and knees while keeping the arm straight
- Swing KB to shoulder height, ensuring the torso does not twist
- While the KB is accelerated downwards, make sure that the body stays straight
- The movement should look smooth and easy

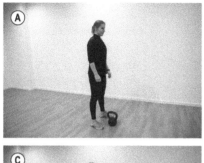
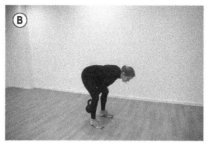
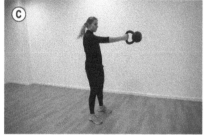
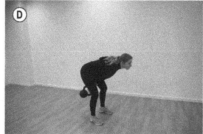

Figure 42.3 Detailed illustration of the one-handed KB swing

(A) Starting position. **(B)** End position of the "backswing". **(C)** Top position right in the turning point of the KB. **(D)** End position of the subsequent "backswing" phase.

Rotational outside swing

To focus even more on the three-dimensional structure of the connective tissue network of the body, a rotational component can be added to the conventional KB swing. The rotational outside swing creates the opportunity to play with the amplitude of both swinging height as well as rotation, thus targeting even more of the connective tissue's fibers and muscles. In the starting position, the KB lies on the floor next to the right or left foot (depending on which side the exercise is started). To grab the KB, internally rotate the contralateral femur and flex the hip, lift the KB of the floor with both hands, slightly swinging it forward as the hips are extended. While swinging the KB, rotate the hip back into a neutral position (facing forward) to create a straight standing position when the KB reaches shoulder height. While the KB swings to the contralateral side, internally rotate the other hip and slightly flex the hips and knees to decelerate the KB. Repeat the procedure to first decelerate and then accelerate the KB back to the starting position

(see Figure 42.4 for a detailed illustration of the rotational outside swing).

Key points for the rotational outside swing:

- Start with the KB on the floor next to one foot
- Internally rotate the contralateral hip to grab the KB
- Swing the KB forward and then to the opposite side while internally rotating the other hip
- Extend the hips back to neutral to accelerate the KB back forward and to the opposite side
- The movement should look smooth and easy

The rotational component of the exercise means the elastic energy in the bottom position is stored more in the glutes, the latissimus and the connecting TLF in a three-dimensional manner. When adjusting the amount of rotation, the exercise gives the perfect opportunity to reach more connective tissue fibers than with the normal two-handed KB swing. It is also possible to switch between the rotational out-

Chapter 42

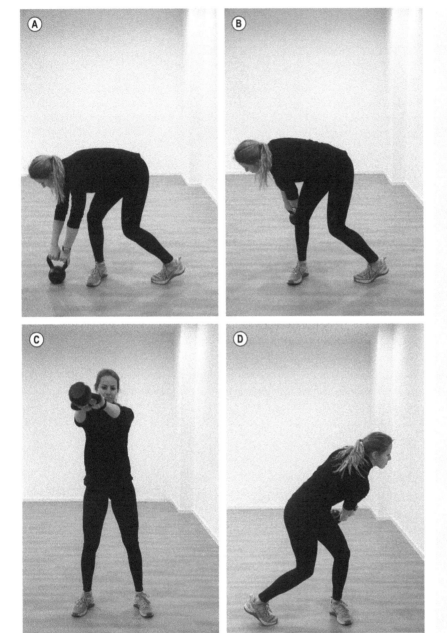

Figure 42.4 Detailed illustration of the rotational outside swing

(A) Bottom position before the initiation of the "backswing" (notice the internal rotation in the left hip joint). **(B)** End position of the "backswing". **(C)** Top position right in the turning point of the KB (notice the neutral position in both hip joints). **(D)** End position of the backswing at the contralateral side (notice the internal rotation in the right hip joint).

Kettlebell training

side swing, the conventional KB swing and the one-handed KB swing, making this a complex workout that involves several functional and myofascial chains in one exercise.

Practical tips

What is the correct weight to start KB training as a novice?

Although it is not easy to give general recommendations, there is no need to start with less than 8 to 12 kg if you are healthy, depending on the exercise. For a woman, consider beginning with 12 kg, although a trained woman could start with 16–20 kg. For a man, start with 16–20 or 20–24 kg if a more experienced lifter (Kwella, 2017). If unsure, start with a lighter KB and then progressively increase the weight. Loading can be increased without increasing the weight by swinging the KB faster.

How many repetitions and sets should I start with?

As a beginner, it is important that you learn the exercise with proper form and technique. In KB training, the loading is usually determined using work and rest time in an interval training manner rather than counting repetitions as in traditional weight training. In the studies by Jay et al. (2011, 2013), a total of 10 sets with a ratio of 30 s of work and 60 s of rest was used in the first 4 weeks, which might be a good starting point for a beginner. In the last 4 weeks of their studies, the rest period was reduced to 30 s. Lake and Lauder (2012A) used 12 sets of 30 s with 30 s of rest during their 6-week study. However, you will find a plethora of interval training methods for KB training, each of which can be used effectively, depending on your training goal.

How should I warm up prior to KB training?

It is generally advised that a warm-up consists of a period of aerobic exercise, followed by dynamic stretching, and ending with a period of movement similar to the upcoming activity (McGowan et al., 2015). As you use almost the entire body during KB training, the dynamic stretching portion of the warm-up should also incorporate multi-joint exercises. As an even more specific warm-up, you can do the KB swing without weights, or with lower weights than you use during the actual workout. This approach has also been used in research (Jay et al., 2011, 2013) and seems an appropriate choice.

What other equipment is required to start KB training?

Besides a set of KBs with different weights, there is no need for additional equipment. Shoes with a hard sole are recommended; also, exercises can be performed barefoot, although there is the danger of dropping a KB and causing injury.

Conclusion

Although there is no scientific evidence for the impact of KB training on the fascial system, the swinging nature of KB exercises can potentially have a positive effect on connective tissue remodeling and energy storage capacity. Training with KBs has been shown to reduce back and neck pain. Although this is more of a speculative nature, it might partly be explained by normalization of connective tissue morphology and sliding properties due to KB swing training. Training with KBs focuses on entire myofascial chains and complex movements rather than on isolated muscles, which makes it a valuable addition to any exercise program. There are many more KB exercises than those described in this chapter, which is intended as a starting point to discover the benefits of KB as a training tool.

Chapter 42

References

Budnar, R.G. Jr, Duplanty, A.A., Hill, D.W., McFarlin, B.K., & Vingren, J.L. (2014) The acute hormonal response to the kettlebell swing exercise. *J Strength Con Res*. 28: 2793–2800.

Falatic, J.A., Plato, P.A., Holder, C., Finch, D., Han, K. & Cisar, C.J. (2015) Effects of kettlebell training on aerobic capacity. *J Strength Con Res*. 29: 1943–1947.

IIshikawa, M., Komi, P.V., Grey, M.J, Lepola, V. & Bruggemann, G. (2005) Muscle-tendon interaction and elastic energy usage in human walking. *J Appl Physiol*. 99: 603–608.

Jay, K., Frisch, D., Hansen, K., Zebis, M.K., Andersen, C.H., Mortensen, O.S., & Andersen, L.L. (2011) Kettlebell training for musculoskeletal and cardiovascular health: a randomized controlled trial. *Scand J Work Env Hea*. 37: 196–203.

Jay, K., Jakobsen, M.D., Sundstrup, E., Skotte, J.H., Jørgensen, M.B., Andersen, C.H., Pedersen, M.T. & Andersen, L.L. (2013) Effects of kettlebell training on postural coordination and jump performance: a randomized controlled trial. *J Strength Con Res*. 27: 1202–1209.

Kjær, M., Langberg, H., Heinemeier, K., Bayer, M.L., Hansen, M., Holm, L., Doessing, S., Kongsgaard, M., Krogsgaard, M.R., Magnusson, S.P. (2009) From mechanical loading to collagen synthesis, structural changes and function in human tendon. *Scand J Med Sci Sports*. 19: 500–510.

Krause, F., Wilke, J., Vogt, L. & Banzer, W. (2016) Intermuscular force transmission along myofascial chains: a systematic review. *J Anat*. 228: 910–918.

Kwella, J. (2017) *Die Kraft der Kettlebell: Übungsausführung. Fehlerbehebung. Trainingsplanung.* Berlin, Germany: Strength Academy UG.

Lake, J.P. & Lauder, M.A. (2012a) Kettlebell swing training improves maximal and explosive strength. *J Strength Con Res*. 26: 2228–2233.

Lake, J.P. & Lauder, M.A. (2012b) Mechanical demands of kettlebell swing exercise. *J Strength Con Res*. 26: 3209–3216.

Langevin, H.M., Fox, J.R., Koptiuch, C., Badger, G.J., Greenan-Naumann, A.C., Bouffard, N.A., Konofagou, E.E., Lee, W., Triano, J.J. & Henry S.M. (2011) Reduced thoracolumbar fascia shear strain in human chronic low back pain. *BMC Musculoskel Disord*. 12: 203.

Langevin, H.M., Stevens-Tuttle, D., Fox, J.R., Badger, G.J., Bouffard, N.A., Krag, M.H., Wu, J. & Henry, S.M. (2009) Ultrasound evidence of altered lumbar connective tissue structure in human subjects with chronic low back pain. *BMC Musculoskel Disord*. 10: 151.

McGowan, C.J., Pyne, D.B., Thompson, K.G. & Rattray, B. (2015) Warm-up strategies for sport and exercise: mechanisms and applications. *Sports Med*. 45: 1523–1546.

Schleip, R. & Müller, D.G. (2013) Training principles for fascial connective tissues: scientific foundation and suggested practical applications. *J Bodyw Mov Ther*. 17: 103–115.

Stecco, A., Meneghini, A., Stern, R., Stecco, C. & Imamura, M. (2014) Ultrasonography in myofascial neck pain: randomized clinical trial for diagnosis and follow-up. *Surg Radiol Anat*. 36: 243–253.

Sukopp, T. (2016) *Das große Kettlebell-Trainingsbuch*. München, Germany: Riva.

Thomas, J.F., Larson, K.L., Hollander, D.B & Kraemer, R.R. (2014) Comparison of two-hand kettlebell exercise and graded treadmill walking: effectiveness as a stimulus for cardiorespiratory fitness. *J Strength Con Res*. 28: 998–1006.

Tsatsouline, P. (2006) *Enter the Kettlebell! Strength Secret of the Soviet Supermen*. New York, NY: Dragon Door Publications.

Wilke, J., Krause, F., Vogt, L. & Banzer, W. (2016) What is evidence-based about myofascial chains: a systematic review. *Arch Phys Med Rehabil*. 97: 454–461.

Fascia-oriented strength training in a conventional gym environment

Robert Schleip

Introduction

Previous chapters described fascia-oriented training concepts, which do not use any external tools, or they use mobile tools such as small weights, or take advantage of stationary equipment—like the Pilates reformer—which is specially designed to allow for a rich variety of joint motions. However, for many of our clients, modern fitness gyms, with their stationary muscle-strengthening machines, have become a regular or at least easily accessible part of their lifestyles.

Muscle strength-oriented training offers indeed many health benefits that cannot be equally replaced by cardiovascular training or by fascia-oriented training. For example, several myokines—cellular messenger substances produced by muscle cells—have been described, which are upregulated after muscular strength training and exert beneficial anti-aging effects, not only on the trained muscles themselves, but also on most other organs and tissues in the human body, including our brains (Pedersen, 2019). Fascia training should therefore not be recommended as an alternative but rather as a useful complement to muscular strength training. This chapter describes how fascia-oriented training can be conducted in a conventional gym environment.

Panther versus bull

A shift in attitude is recommended when switching to a fascia-oriented movement style in a gym.

This can be nicely illustrated by the movement style of a panther, versus that of a bull (Schleip and Buschmann, 2016). A bull often increases its power by making the body more condensed—i.e. shorter, more compressed and more rounded—to increase the power behind its pushing force. This is also how some people push the resistance handles away in a conventional gym exercise, and it seems to work well for that purpose. What we advocate for a fascia-oriented workout style is to work with less resistance than in the bull style, but to emphasize a more graceful and elongated orchestration, maybe similar to the movements of an elegant panther. As a basic orientation we recommend starting with 50–60% of the usual resistance load, compared with a bull-type application style, although that percentage may need to be adjusted to a significant degree downwards or upwards for a given individual and situation.

Unless a more specific application purpose is chosen (as described later), we recommend working in two to three exercise sets per machine, with the following steps per set:

- Concentric phase 2–3 s
- Three to five mini-bounces around end point
- Eccentric phase 2–3 s
- Three to five mini-bounces around end point.

These should be performed with 90-s breaks between sets. The resistance should allow 10 to 15 cycles over the full range. If it allows more or

Chapter 43

only less than that then it should be adjusted. A specific myofascial tissue region should not be trained in this manner more than once or twice per week (with gaps of at least 2–3 days in between) to allow for sufficient recovery and adaptation. A time of 3 months can be expected before a visible and palpable tissue improvement can be noticed with this training style, based on the relatively slow remodeling times of dense collagenous tissues (see Chapter 1).

Principles of Panther training

The principles of Panther training are outlined below. In a basic application, the exercise starts with a preparatory counter-movement in the opposite direction to that anticipated for the main resistance movement. For example, in the example shown in Figure 43.1, the individual starts by extending their hands away from the chest and slightly backwards.

Panther training

Basic principles:

1. Preparatory counter movement
2. Proximal initiation
3. Directional variations
4. Mini bounces.

Advanced principles:

1. Tensegral pre-tension
2. Final exhaustion at end range
3. Embodiment.

Next, the main movement, against the resistance of the machine, is not initiated at the distal contact point with the equipment (e.g. the hands holding a bar), but rather at a much more proximal body part. In the example shown in Figure 43.1, this means that a small reaching-forward motion of the lower chest region precedes the subsequent forward motion of the arms. The combination of

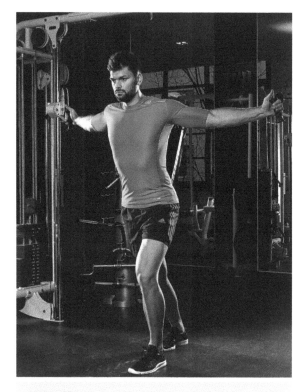

Figure 43.1

For better loading of the fascial tissues, it is recommended to start the exercise by a preparatory counter-movement (extending the hands away from the chest and slightly backwards) before the main forward motion is initiated with a proximal body part, in this example with the lower chest.

From Schleip, R. et al.: Faszien Krafttraining. Riva Verlag, Muenchen, 2016, with permission.

these first two principles tends to increase the tensile load on the fascial components during the subsequent main motion. For the main motion, the inclusion of different directional variations is recommended, such as shown in Figure 43.2. In addition, the inclusion of three to five quick elastic mini-bounces at both the long-range as well as the short-range end positions is recommended. A brief pause of a few split seconds after the last bounce ensures that the subsequent slow resistance motion includes the end point position at which the mini bounces occurred.

Fascia-oriented strength training in a conventional gym environment

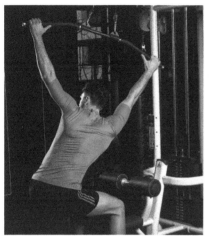 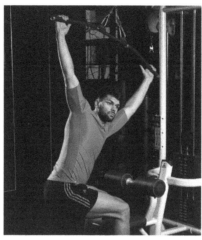

Figure 43.2

For conventional muscle fiber training, exact repetitions along the same loading vector are usually recommended for optimal training effectiveness. By contrast, the fascia-oriented Panther training suggests exploring different loading vectors. This way many different tissue areas within larger myofascial sheets can be reached within the same exercise set.

From Schleip, R. et al.: Faszien Kraft-training. Riva Verlag, Muenchen, 2016, with permission.

When familiar with these basic principles, an inclusion of the following advanced principles can be explored. Before starting an exercise, a brief moment (like one breathing cycle) should be devoted to slightly increasing the fascial pre-tension via a multidirectional expansion of the whole body in an integrated manner, which is described as "tensegral movement" by Dr. Daniele-Claude Martin (2016). In the example shown in Figure 43.1, this could mean a slight simultaneous extension of the whole body upwards and downwards together with subtle widening of the chest and arms.

Another added principle includes continuing the resistance movement at the final long-range position (in case this is possible) over shorter distances, until even that is no longer possible. In conventional muscle strength workouts, one is advised to repeat the basic movement as long as possible but to stop once a "clean" movement over the full range of motion is no longer possible. By contrast, in our fascia-oriented workout style, the trainee then continues the resistance motion over a much smaller distance ("squeezing the last drop out") until the body exhaustion prevents

even this small motion. This serves to enhance an increasing range-of-motion remodeling effect, as will be shown later. It should not be included for individuals who have been classified as hypermobile after undertaking the Beighton test (see Chapters 7 and 19).

Finally, each set can be finished with a brief moment of open attention, in which the trainee pays curious attention with a mindful attitude towards any positive or interesting proprioceptive, interoceptive or emotional after-effects in themselves. While in a conventional muscle gym exercise it is not uncommon to see the trainee fall into a "slump position" for a brief moment when being exhausted at their last repetition, an individual engaged in a Panther workout will sit (or stand) quietly for a brief moment in a continued tensegral posture, and may feel tiny expansional body changes or increased vitality perceptions in the body, similar to listening to the after-effects of a stone thrown into a quite pond (Figure 43.3). Only after such a brief "embodiment moment" does the trainee then continue with the next set or with the next exercise.

Chapter 43

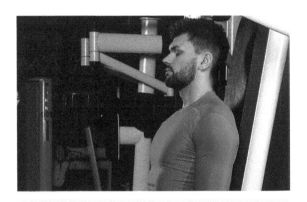

Figure 43.3

In the advanced version of our recommended Panther training, the trainee completes each set with a brief "embodiment" moment, in which any immediate after-effects in terms of altered body sensations or emotional changes are greeted with an attitude of open-minded curious attention.

From Schleip, R. et al.: Faszien Krafttraining. Riva Verlag, Muenchen, 2016, with permission.

Specific guidelines for different purposes

Hypomobile type

If you have been classified as a general hypomobile type in the respective Viking Test (Chapter 16) then it is suggested that you perform only the first move of each set over the full available range of motion, and that you continue to conduct all subsequent moves over the last quarter of the available range of motion in the long stretched position for the primarily loaded muscles. It is also recommended that you conduct the mini-bounces in the long stretched position only (and not in the opposite position, in which the loaded muscle fibers are shortened), and that you apply the principle "Final exhaustion at end range" with enhanced emphasis. And, as an additional booster, we recommend conducting the eccentric phase—i.e. when the machine lengthens your muscle fibers against your resistance—twice as slowly compared with the concentric phases.

These recommendations are based on the research of Aquino et al. (2009), who showed that muscular resistance training in a stretched position induced a more powerful long-term increase in hip flexion mobility than a conventional stretching application. In addition, new insights about the role of the intramuscular titin fiber showed that this unique fiber plays a key role as a "third contractile element" (in addition to actin and myosin), and also as a very important mechanosensor, the signaling of which takes priority over the signaling from other mechanoreceptors. In particular, titin signaling tends to induce a long-term increase in muscle fiber length. Such titin signaling only happens when muscle fibers are either contracting at long lengths (independent of the type of contraction) or undergoing eccentric contraction (then it can occur at any length condition) (Herzog, 2018).

Hypermobile type

If you have been tested as positive for generalized hypermobility (see Chapters 7 and 19), then we recommend that you perform only the first move of each set over the full available range of motion, and that you continue to conduct all subsequent moves over a shorter range of motion only, close to the shortest length position of the primarily working muscle fibers. For example, in the exercise shown in Figure 43.4, this means loading the knee in a more extended position only. It is also recommended that you do not perform mini-bounces and that you also do not apply the principle "Final exhaustion at end range" with enhanced emphasis. And finally, it is suggested that you conduct the concentric phase—i.e. when the primarily working muscle fibers are actively shortening against resistance—two to three times as slowly compared to the eccentric phases.

Fascia-oriented strength training in a conventional gym environment

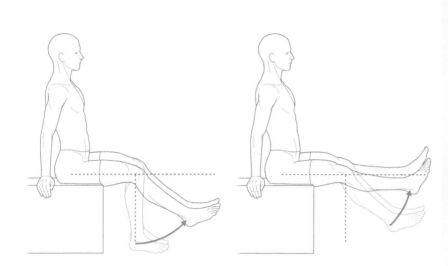

Figure 43.4
Two (of many) different options for conducting knee extension resistance training. In the example on the left, the knee extensors are only loaded in a position at which they are at a longer muscle fiber length. This training style is generally recommended if a long-term increase in knee flexion ability is desired. By contrast, the example on the right shows a resistance training style in which the loaded muscle fibers tend to be at a shorter length. This style is recommended for hypomobile individuals as well as for cancer fighters.

These recommendations are based partly on the new insights about titin signaling, and also on increasing evidence of a long-term shortening effect on muscle fiber length when repeatedly challenging the muscle in a short position against resistance (Gajdosik, 2001). While titin signaling, which we suggest utilizing for hypomobile (Viking) body types, tends to increase muscle fiber length by an increase in the number of the sarcomeres (i.e. the functional contractile units within one fiber), it is assumed that the opposite happens, i.e. a decrease in the number of sarcomeres, when the maximal loading of the muscle tends to happen within its shortest length condition.

Nevertheless, research on hypermobility seems to indicate a tendency for decreased proprioception (Smith et al., 2013), particularly close to the end position of the available range of motion, at which the muscle fibers are at long length. For this purpose, it is essential that the first cycle of movement is conducted over the full available range of motion and is performed more slowly and with an even higher proprioceptive attention than the subsequent movements within the same set.

Cross-over type

If you were classified as a cross-over type (Chapter 19) and/or if you happen to search for more flexibility in some areas of your body and for more joint stability in other areas, then a mixture of the above recommendations is suggested. For those joints to which you wish to increase your flexibility, then you apply the training style for a Viking-type individual, and for those joints to which you wish to increase joint stability (rather than mobility), we suggest applying the training style described for the hypermobile condition. If you are not certain about a particular body area or exercise regarding your desired preference, then just follow the general Panther training recommendations.

Chapter 43

Tendon training for athletes

If you are an athlete who is doing regular sports not just for fun or health purposes, but rather for a performance orientation within a competition environment, then we suggest applying the Berlin Method of tendon training (Bohm et al., 2014). This method has been shown to induce an increase in both collagen synthesis and tendon resistance over a period of several months, and was larger via this specific training protocol compared with other training types, which involved either more rapid loading or longer lasting tendon stimulations. An increase in tendon resistance is generally regarded as evoking an increased injury protection within an athletic loading environment (Mersmann et al., 2017).

In this protocol, high loads should be applied in five sets of four repetitions with a stress and relaxation duration of ~3 s. Breaks between sets should be 1–2 min (see Figure 43.5). The muscular contraction should be at very high force (≥85% of isometric voluntary force maximum). Due to the length-force relationship of muscle fiber contractions, such high forces are usually only possible around the mid-range position of the available range of motion. For the Achilles tendon contractions, an angle of ~90° at the foot joint is recommended, and for the patellar tendon contractions, a knee joint angle of ~70°.

Cancer fighters

Resistance training has been shown to reduce mortality in cancer survivors (Hardee et al., 2014). Fascia researcher Thomas Findley advocates a gym-based resistance training, in which the loading happens primarily in the short length position (Findley, 2015). Oriented on a 10-repetition maximum (10RM), patients perform sets of training by performing the first set of 10 at 50% 10RM, the second at 75% 10RM, and the third and final set at 100% of the 10RM. He showed that if the muscles are loaded close to their short length position then the longitudinal stress is less than at mid-range or long positions. However, the lateral stress—forces passing via the epimysium to structures parallel to the working muscle fibers—is much higher (Findley et al., 2015). Findley cites preliminary results which indicate that such a force distribution results in a lowering of TGF- 1 expression, a substance which is usually regarded as having a having an aggravating effect on tissue stiffness and cancer progression (Findley, 2015). Figure 43.6 illustrates an example of a preferred loading position in this protocol.

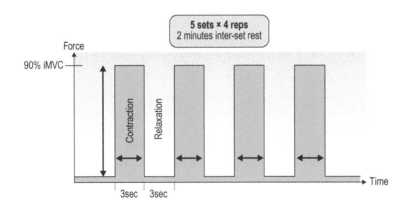

Figure 43.5

Training protocol of the Berlin Method of tendon training for the purpose of enhanced injury (and overload pathology) protection in competitive athletes. High intensity loading to the tendon should be applied in five sets of four repetitions with a contraction and relaxation duration of 3 s each, and an inter-set rest of 2 min.

Illustration from Mersmann et al. (2017).

Fascia-oriented strength training in a conventional gym environment

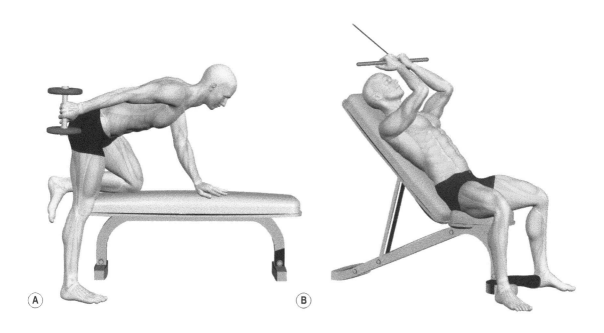

Figure 43.6

Examples of different triceps curls. **(A)** With the muscle fibers at short length, and **(B)** with the muscle fibers at long length. The suggested training protocol for cancer fighters recommends resistance training around the short length position **(A)**.

Clinical summary

Fascia-oriented training does not need to stop at the gym door. Several training recommendations have been developed by different authors for using conventional muscle training machines in a modified manner with the aim of influencing fascial tissue remodeling. Different protocols have been presented for specific mobility body types as well as for other purposes. Fascia-oriented exercises in a gym environment should be regarded not as an alternative but rather as complementing muscle strength-oriented training. We recommend practicing fascia-oriented training and conventional muscle training on different days with sufficient resting time in between to allow for adequate recovery and adaptation.

References

Aquino, C.F., Fonseca, S.T., Gonçalves, G.G., Silva, P.L., Ocarino, J.M. & Mancini, M.C. (2009) Stretching versus strength training in lengthened position in subjects with tight hamstring muscles: a randomized controlled trial. *Man Ther.* 15: 26–31.

Bohm, S., Mersmann, F., Tettke, M., Kraft, M. & Arampatzis, A. (2014) Human Achilles tendon plasticity in response to cyclic strain: effect of rate and duration. *J Exp Biol.* 217: 4010–4017.

Chaudhry, H., Bukiet, B., Anderson, E.Z., Burch, J. & Findley, T. (2017) Muscle strength and stiffness in resistance exercise: Force transmission in tissues. *J Bodyw Mov Ther.* 21: 517–522.

Findley, T.W. (2015) Link between Manual Therapy, Movement, Fascia and Cancer. Video presentation from the 2015 Joint Conference on Acupuncture, Oncology and Fascia, November 14, 2015, Boston. https://

oshercenter.org/joint-conference-2015-video-presentations/.

Findley, T., Chaudhry, H. & Dhar, S. (2015) Transmission of muscle force to fascia during exercise. *J Bodyw Mov Ther.* 19: 119–123.

Gajdosik, R.L. (2001) Passive extensibility of skeletal muscle: review of the literature with clinical implications. *Clin Biomech.* 16: 87–101.

Hardee, J.P., Porter, R.R., Sui, X., Archer, E., Lee, I.M., Lavie, C.J. & Blair, S.N. (2014) The effect of resistance exercise on all-cause mortality in cancer survivors. *Mayo Clinic Proceedings.* 89: 1108–1115.

Herzog, W. (2018) The multiple roles of titin in muscle contraction and force production. *Biophys Rev.* 10: 1187–1199.

Martin, D.-C. (2016) *Living Biotensegrity – Interplay of tension and compression in the body*. München, Germany: Kiener Press.

McMahon, G.E., Morse, C.I., Burden, A., Winwood, K. & Onambele-Pearson, G.L. (2013) The manipulation of strain, when stress is controlled, modulates in vivo tendon mechanical properties but not systemic TGF-b1 levels. *Physiol Rep.* 1: e00091.

Mersmann, F., Bohm, S. & Arampatzis, A. (2017) Imbalances in the development of muscle and tendon as risk factor for tendinopathies in youth athletes: a review of current evidence and concepts of prevention. *Front Physiol.* 8: 987.

Pedersen, B.K. (2019) Physical activity and muscle-brain crosstalk. *Nat Rev Endocrinol.* 15: 383–392.

Schleip, R. & Buschmann, B. (2016) *Faszien Krafttraining*. München, Germany: Riva Verlag.

Smith, T.O., Jerman, E., Easton, V., Bacon, H., Armon, K., Poland, F. & Macgregor, A.J. (2013) Do people with benign joint hypermobility syndrome (BJHS) have reduced joint proprioception? A systematic review and meta-analysis. *Rheumatol Int.* 33: 2709–2716.

Rehabilitation in sport medicine

Raúl Martínez Rodríguez and Fernando Galán del Río

Introduction

Physical activity is associated with improved quality of life. However, being physically active carries the risk of injury and re-injury. At the present time, the incidence and recurrence of overuse injuries are high. Recent longitudinal studies in professional soccer players have shown that muscle injury rates and their recurrence rates increased during 11 consecutive seasons by 4% annually from 2001 to 2014, despite ongoing scientific investigation as well as improved educational background and knowledge of the different professionals involved in the rehabilitation process (Ekstrand et al., 2013). Therefore, there is a substantial interest in sports medicine to improve the prevention, treatment and rehabilitation of sports-related injuries.

The specific training of fascial tissues is suggested to lead the augmentation of the mechanical efficiency of the musculoskeletal system. However, the rise of external loads required to increase sport performance does also represent an additional stress factor in the medium term, which may eventually be associated with an increase of the risk of sport-related injury due to mechanical overuse. Even in the short term, tissue repair processes following a traumatic acute injury modify the mechanical properties of soft tissue around the scar area in a more direct and precise way. As a consequence, the involvement of fascial tissue in human movement, as regards its capacity to absorb and transmit mechanical forces via different musculoskeletal structures, may be distorted and, hence, be the origin in the development of local and remote dysfunctions. From a therapeutic standpoint, skillful application of manual forces to the fascial system may help to condition and reverse collagen overproduction, thus improving tissue functionality and optimizing rehabilitation of musculoskeletal injuries.

Against this background, the boom in scientific knowledge on myofascial tissues and its potential clinical implications in the physiopathology of sport-related injuries invites us to continue exploring and developing new ways to detect, treat and control the mechanical properties of connective tissue.

Tissue adaptation following overuse

Mechanotransduction is the means by which external mechanical loads across the fascial network (shearing, tension and/or torsion) are transduced into biochemical responses at an effector cell level, generating structural and functional modifications on different musculoskeletal system components (Kjaer, 2004). Optimization of sport performance necessarily entails an increase of training loading and a decrease of rest periods, which drive a process of physiological adaptation associated with progressive and steady changes in the muscle, the muscle fascia and the tendon (Kjaer, 2004; Miller

Chapter 44

et al., 2005). Nonetheless, different papers suggest that the mechano-adaptation of the connective tissue after frequent high-intensity loadings includes a persistent and low-grade inflammatory reaction around the extracellular matrix, even in the absence of structural alterations on the macro-level (Barbe et al., 2013; Zügel et al., 2018). Such micro-inflammation is linked to an extended release of several proinflammatory and nociceptive substances, which, in the case of some cytokines (interleukin 1 , tumour necrosis factor and, mainly, TGF -1), cause tissue stiffness through distinction and proliferation of fibroblasts as well as excessive collagen synthesis (Barbe et al., 2013; Zügel et al., 2018).

Mechanical tissue behavior following overuse

Structural changes in muscle fascia micro-architecture, and especially in the configuration of joints and intramuscular septa connecting adjacent muscles, are crucial in force distribution since they increase pre-tension in the deep fascia and optimize longitudinal force transmission to the tendon (Huijing, 2009; Bernabei et al., 2017). When no discomfort or pain appears, and when it is associated with high sports performance, the decrease of viscoelasticity and force absorption capacity must be considered as a physiological adaptation helping to optimize force transmission between muscles and tendons. However, in the medium term, the ensuing restructuring process could give rise to a stiffer fascial network, hence decisively modifying the soft tissue's viscoelastic behavior. In this context, decreases of local elasticity limit the fascial system's capacity for deformation and force absorption, which, in turn, magnifies the risk of musculoskeletal injury (Purslow, 2010). In sum, continuous high-intensity loading, reduced rest periods and an inadequate monitoring of the

mechanical connective tissue properties, may result in a lower tolerance threshold to musculoskeletal system loading, particularly during eccentric movements. Therefore, it is necessary to understand the association between tissues of the fascial system and the origin of muscular, tendinous and joint injuries related to sport practice.

Relevance of fascial stiffness in selected overuse injuries

Myofascial (muscle) injury

Different modifiable factors in the prevention and treatment of muscle injury have been suggested, including, but not limited to, muscle fatigue, muscle strength imbalance, neuromuscular inhibition, poor motor control of the pelvic and trunk muscles, limited flexibility or premature return to play (Silder et al., 2010). In addition, considering that the susceptibility for sustaining a muscle strain injury is greater in high-force eccentric contractions from a lengthened position, adequate viscoelastic behavior of soft tissues would be essential to dissipate and absorb the kinetic energy required during eccentric terminal movements, as well as during external loading via foot-ground contact (Chumanov et al., 2011) (Chapter 16).

Tendon injury

The increase of fascial stiffness may directly influence the development of tendinous disorders, since the tendon is directly connected to the deep fascia (Dalmau-Pastor et al., 2014; Grob et al., 2016). Indeed, new research shows tendon architecture as a specialized structure made of terminal layers of connective tissue arranged in the shape of a spiral with disruption between a profound muscle fascia (paratendon) and intra- and intermuscular connective tissue, as well as intermuscular septa and other collagen-reinforced structures. The connective tissue provides important stiff connections between agonist and antagonist muscles, from which force is transmitted to the tendon (Grob et al., 2016). Thus, the force generated by the muscle that is transferred to bones via tendons to produce movement is not only transmitted by each myofibril, made up of sarcomeres arranged in series and equipped with a myotendinous junction (myotendinous force transmission), but also by the existing fascial continuity between muscle fascia and tendon. This important functional continuity hence enables force transmission via the muscular supporting connective tissue (myofascial force transmission) (Huijing et al., 2009). As stated above, mechanical loading at physiological levels is beneficial to tendons, which directly respond to physical activity by increased metabolic activity and collagen synthesis. However, the mechanical properties of tendons, including their Young's modulus (a measure of the stiffness of an elastic material), may undergo modifications in response to excessive loading, modifying the adequate stress-strain balance (Järvinen et al., 2005 A).

Joint injury

Contraction and activation of the different muscle groups lead (1) to an increase of joint compressive forces through muscle shortening, and (2) to the augmentation of stiffness in peri-articular tissues (Barker et al., 2014). Also, higher pre-tension of the fascial system and reduced deformability of peripheral structures, transmitting mechanical tension to the articulation, could be related to an increase of the physiological compression forces at joint level as well as to a reduction in the quality of accessory movements (gliding, bearing, translation and/or rotation). Indeed, an article showed a higher level of stiffness and thickness of external peripatellar structures in patients with patellar chondropathy

when compared with asymptomatic controls. This finding has been related to the increase of pain in joints due to stronger compression forces in patellofemoral joint level (Schoots et al., 2013).

Relevance of fascial stiffness in sports injuries related to muscle healing

Once injured, muscle tissue undergoes a slow and spontaneous healing process that results in the formation of connective (scar) tissue, which is usually fibrotic and stiff. Thus, during the initial phases of the healing process, due to structural damage and/or surgery (iatrogenesis) within the area of ruptured and necrotized fibers, there is a proliferation of inflammatory cells stimulating fibroblast activity and collagen production around the scar (Järvinen et al., 2005 B). Initially, the scar tissue is characterized by a disorganized and random arrangement of the new collagen fibers. The absence of parallel fiber orientation relative to their original force transmission axis is a feature common to scars missing mechanical stimuli. In the long term, it can frequently be observed that presumed healed sport injuries are, in fact, highly scarred, increasing the overall mechanical stiffness of the myofibrous tissue it replaces (Järvinen et al., 2005). In addition, proliferation of scar tissue leads to greater strain in the affected structures during eccentric contractions, which could contribute to discomfort and pain, as well an increased re-injury risk during high speed and high amplitude movements (Silder et al., 2010).

Relevance of fascial stiffness in sensory motor alterations

Histological studies have demonstrated the presence of free nerve endings of A-δ and C fibers in fascia, which are polimodal receptors acting as unspecific mechanoreceptors and potential nociceptors when facing pressure and/or excessive mechanical tension (Taguchi et al., 2013; Schilder et al., 2014). Interestingly, the density of such receptors is three times higher in the lumbar fascia than in the deep spinal muscles (Barry et al., 2015). In addition to the muscular fascia, free nerve endings are also located in the continuous network of connective tissue found in joints (joint capsule, ligaments and subchondral bone), tendons (paratendon), bones (periosteum) and the nervous system (epineurium). Their concentration is higher than the number of specialized mechanoreceptors (Cabuk and Cabuk, 2016).

Significantly, various experimental studies prove the existence of a functional connection between changes in mechanical properties of the connective tissue and the nociceptive processes resulting from repetitive strains. The release of proinflammatory and pronociceptive substances not only leads to an increase of fibroblastic activity and tissue stiffness, but is also related to different stages of sensorimotor alterations, such as peripheral sensitization and force decreases (Barbe et al., 2013; Zugel et al., 2018).

Essentially, the mechanical forces generated by the musculoskeletal system are decisive for tissue remodeling. Thus, a correct control of loadings will improve mechanical efficiency and the tolerance threshold for mechanical stress. However, pathological adaptations related to stiffening or scarring may result in changes in joint range of motion and muscle-tendon force transmission, as well as an activation of nociceptive mechanisms. At this point, the following question arises: Could a stage of excessive fascial pre-tension (fascial stiffness) be modified by a focused manual treatment? And, from a global perspective, how could this treatment be integrated into classical models for prevention, treatment and rehabilitation of musculoskeletal injuries?

Optimization of the rehabilitation process from a fascia-oriented perspective

It seems apparent that there is a need to apply skillful manual forces over the more rigid areas to restore and improve the fascial system's capacity to absorb and dissipate repetitive mechanical loads. At the same time and following a structural injury, it will be necessary to control the effects of arthrofibrosis, a well-known sequela of structural injuries after sports trauma, when treatment choice has involved immobilization and protection of the injured area for primary treatment or post-operative management (Figure 44.1).

Rehabilitation in myofascial (muscle) injury

The mechanisms of mechanical loading and mechanotransduction are well recognized in the treatment of muscle injuries as they can accelerate the recovery process due to activation/production of satellite cells and growth factors (Järvinen et al., 2005 B). Nonetheless, the healing process may be conditioned by an inadequate regeneration-repair equilibrium. Considering the high mechanosensitivity of fibroblasts, the early use of external loads may also cause an increase in collagen synthesis in the mechanical area of the scar as well as in adjacent associated tissues, leading to incomplete or unfunctional healing with decreased extensibility and eccentric force (Opar et al., 2012). Indeed, some specialists have proved a decrease of eccentric hamstring muscle force in athletes with reasonably high functional

Rehabilitation in sport medicine

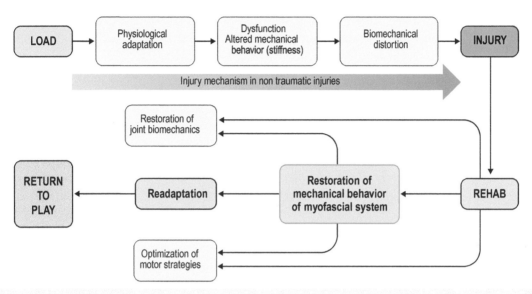

Figure 44.1 Injury mechanism in overuse injuries. Relevance of mechanical properties of fascial system during sports rehabilitation (rehab) physical and manual therapy

Mechanical loading and decrease of rest intervals renders the musculoskeletal system more load-resistant but at the same time it also considerably decreases its stress-susceptibility. In the medium term it can be related to biomechanical distortion and, consecutively, an increase in the risk of structural injury. We propose the need to optimize the process of sports rehabilitation, not only through the use of exercise-based programs, but also through the use of manual matrix remodeling techniques to optimize the mechanical behavior of the fascial system and the movement efficiency.

level (Sole et al., 2011). That study suggested the relevance, not only of neurophysiological factors (neuromuscular inhibition associated with pain or fear of recurrence), but also of mechanical factors of myofascial tissue in high eccentric movements. For this reason, beyond the fear-avoidance model and in line with the content of this chapter, we suggest the need to focus attention on both structural changes observed on echography or MRI and, most importantly, on the optimization of viscoelastic properties of scars, which would be essential to dissipate and absorb the kinetic energy needed for deceleration and high amplitude and high velocity movements (Martínez-Rodríguez and Galán del Río, 2013). This is why the optimization of tensile capacity of scars using the manual techniques described in this chapter may be a

way to lessen the excessive fascial stiffness of intermuscular septa and, more locally, the area around the scar.

Rehabilitation in tendon injury

With regard to the treatment of chronic tendon disorders, a variety of studies show the benefits of eccentric training programs (Murtaugh and Ihm, 2013). These include an increased loading tolerance, a higher rate of force development associated with a decrease in the traction supported by the tendon in the terminal eccentric movements, as well as an improved ability to store elastic energy. Even so, understanding the tendon as a collagenous terminal structure linked to the intramuscular connective tissue, and knowing the role of said connective tissue in the transmission of forces towards the tendon

Chapter 44

(Huijing, 2009), it must be remembered that tendon deformation not only depends on its own internal characteristics but also on the mechanical behavior of the deep fascia and intermuscular septa (Bernabei et al., 2017). Concurrently, the fascial system has been equipped with the capacity to dissipate and distribute force through the continuity of the fascial network. Thus, repetitive overuse initially causes cell matrix changes that thicken and harden the tendon (reactive tendinopathy). This becomes especially obvious in actions that combine high articular amplitude movements and eccentric contractions, during which a stiff fascial network is continually tensed by external forces (distancing of bone levers) and internal forces (muscular contraction). In the medium term, once micro-injured, the tendon undergoes a slow and spontaneous healing process (tendon disrepair) that results in the formation of scar tissue and a loss of normal collagen fiber organization. In this way, from the authors' clinical experience, prior to the execution of the eccentric and/or stretching exercises' protocols, the introduction of different manual techniques, as described below, is proposed to normalize the fascial network's tensional homeostasis and reduce the previously mentioned interfaces' stiffness.

Rehabilitation of bone and joint injuries

Historically, conventional rehabilitation programs base their treatment of decreased range of articular motion after an arthrofibrosis on the application of stretching as well as passive and active articular glide mobilization. However, within this context, the connective tissue intimately related to the joint (capsule, ligaments, periarticular myofascia) dehydrates, loses its elastic capacity, and presents considerable disorganization (intercrossing collagen fibers and capsule shrinkage). As a result, deformation and sliding capacity between fascial layers are limited and, consequently, the movement capacity between articular surfaces is also reduced (gliding, bearing, translation and/or rotation). Recent research introduces the limitations of static stretching techniques for the optimization of the range of motion and the capacity of displacement within layers in lumbar fascia when restriction and fibrosis are detected (Langevin et al., 2018). Early and progressive exercise programs, together with structural techniques specifically designed to treat stiffer areas, are strongly recommended in this case. This said, and considering the anatomy of periarticular connective tissue and the direct relation of mechanical behavior and joint pain, a previous introduction to fascial tissue manipulation directly addressed to the fascial periarticular system should be proposed. This therapy would comprise different alternatives, such as matrix remodeling techniques, deep massage, deep friction and neuromuscular techniques, as well as several options of instrumental proceedings on restrictive and fibrosic areas. Such methodology, on the one hand, intends to induce the rehydration of the ground substance, enabling collagen fibers to move friction-free against each other, and, on the other, encourages the rupture of pathological collagen cross-links (Bove et al., 2016). Subsequently, the execution of progressive active loading exercises is suggested to improve the organization and arrangement of collagen fibers parallel to the main axes of mechanical tension.

It is important to highlight that stiffness within the periarticular myofascial tissue may alter muscle tone regulation and negatively influence protocols designed for muscle strengthening, proprioceptive re-education and training for restoration of sport-based movements. All three are required during the treatment process involving these types of injuries. This is intimately related to the role of the fascial tissue as a substrate of proprioception (mechanosensitive signaling system) and to the function of mechanoreceptors (Stecco et al., 2007; Van der Wal, 2009), specifically of muscle spindles, which are specialized structures of connective tissue within the muscle (endomysium and perimysium). They are characterized as being highly sensitive to even small tension variations. Therefore, considering that the main stimulus for these receptors is deformation, it can be inferred that an increase in stiffness and disorganization within the fascial system after immobilization protocols may decisively alter the capacity of adaptation in such a system. As a conclusion, the authors emphasize the importance of applying manual structural techniques so as to model the periarticular fascial tissue, to normalize the stimulatory mechanism of mechanoreceptors, thereby enabling effective efferent motor responses during muscle strengthening and proprioceptive protocols.

Manual matrix remodeling and control of fascial stiffness

To restore the tissue's normal viscoelastic behavior and allow the release of the elastic energy accumulated (not dissipated) within the surrounding area, thereby stimulating the extracellular matrix muscle to return from a high-tension to a low-tension state, the authors suggest the implementation of manual matrix remodeling techniques. These are based on the use of various mechanical stimuli to apply force through skin and superficial fascia until a deep

steady or progressive deformation of fascial tissue occurs by mixing torsion, shearing, traction, axial and/or compressive manual vectors. However, some fascial structures are of such thickness, fiber composition and resistance (iliotibial band, plantar fascia and other tendons of lower limb) that an immediate deformation may not be possible (Chaudhry et al., 2014). Due to this, and to modify the dynamic behavior of fascial tissue, we propose an approach over all fascia layers, connections, connective tissues, retinacula, septa and/or intramuscular trabecular systems. Although these have been traditionally disregarded by descriptive anatomy given their suggested low structural relevance, they directly intervene in mechanical tension transmission and force balance (Figure 44.2) (Huijing, 2009; Cruz-Montecinos et al., 2016; Bernabei et al., 2017). Principles of application in the use of matrix remodeling techniques can also be extended to stiff scar caused by excessive healing after a traumatic accident and/or surgical history (Martínez-Rodríguez and Galán del Río, 2013).

The following is a detailed description of the different phases of remodeling techniques for application in septa and scars (Figure 44.3):

- Contact phase: an initial compressive vector is provided with the second, third and fourth finger. Pressure must be applied progressively and should be enough to achieve a primary withstand level.
- Stimulation phase: at this stage, an axial, spiral and/or circular input is added to initial vector compression. The physiotherapist's fingers proceed to a deformation of tissue, slowly and continuously creating tension until a tensile barrier more resistant than the first is reached. The time that

Chapter 44

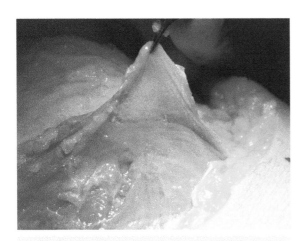

Figure 44.2 Image corresponding to the dissection of the crural fascia at the level of the vastus medialis

There is no solution of real continuity between fascia and muscle fibers, but there is continuity of fascial tissue to the inside of the muscle cells themselves. The separation muscle fascia is created by the analytical mind of the anatomist, determining in this way the understanding of the lesion mechanism, and consequently the manner in which we design the rehabilitation programs.

Image owned by Martínez y Galán, Faculty of Medicine and Health Sciences of Barcelona.

compression and torsion are applied simultaneously may vary (30–90 s).

- Release phase: in this phase, a release of elastic energy in the shape of "local unwind" may appear, depending on the response of the tissue after the initial stimulus. This is followed by a progressive decrease of original tension while there is still contact and reorganization of tissues in the restriction area, which leads to a natural repositioning of fingers as the barrier changes.

This process must be repeated as many times as necessary (usually from three to five times) until, eventually, an ease of "first tension feeling" is detected.

Re-adaptation and return to play

The processes of re-adaptation and retraining before return to play are usually based on progressive loading exercise programs adapted to the individual requirement of each athlete (core training, eccentric exercise and/or dynamic stabilization/muscle activation) and management of pain-avoidance behavior. However, this progressive loading model needs to be optimized since high-load training is required to increase sports performance. For that reason, we propose the use of manual matrix remodeling techniques to optimize the tissue tolerance and increase the fascial system's capacity for deformation and force absorption before and after return to play.

In regard to this, some specific examples are presented in this subsection.

With regard to return to play in muscle injuries, more specifically calf muscle injuries, it should be remembered that the dynamic adaptation of fibrotic scar tissue and nearby areas may influence muscle tissue lengthening and, consequently, strength performance at longer muscle lengths (Järvinen et al., 2005 B; Opar et al., 2012). For that reason, the authors emphasize the importance of using manual structural techniques applied to the intermuscular connective tissue between soleus and gastrocnemius muscles, as well as between the intermuscular septa of the medial and lateral gastrocnemius muscles to improve the soft tissue's viscoelastic behavior (Figure 44.3). In this way, the tolerance of the tissue may be increased to load during the lengthening phase of the eccentric contraction, when the susceptibility to sustain muscle distension is higher (Figure 44.4). To show the benefits of these therapeutic techniques, ultrasound elastography has been used to evaluate (in real time) the stiffness and elasticity

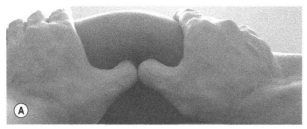
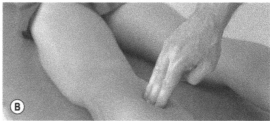

Figure 44.3 Manual matrix remodeling technique

These techniques are based on axial and compressive vectors over the intermuscular septa and/or fibrotic scars to release elastic energy and decrease the excessive stiffness and the pre-tension state of the fascial tissue.

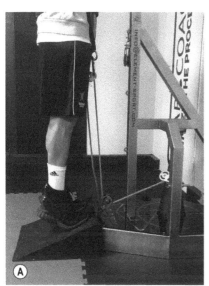
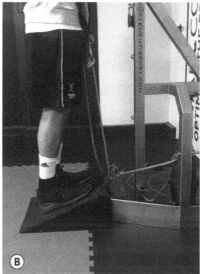

Figure 44.4 High-force eccentric contractions from a lengthened position

Mechanical factors can decrease muscle activity in the lengthened range of eccentric contraction when the susceptibility to sustain a muscle distension is higher. For this reason, we suggest the need to optimize the viscoelastic properties of septa and intermuscular scars using the manual techniques described in the corresponding section before progressive loading exercise programs (i.e. isoinertial training with inclinated wedge to increase eccentric muscle strengthening in calf muscles).

of the tissue. Figure 44.5 reveals the elasticity curve registering the myofascial tissue pre-tension during muscle repair and fibrosis (sonoelastographic evolution control). This information is then used to apply the proper treatment, according to the response of the myofascial tissue, after the fascial therapy is performed (Martínez-Rodríguez and Galán del Río, 2013).

In the rehabilitation of chronic tendon injuries, more specifically Achilles tendinopathy, different authors have studied the multiple benefits derived from the use of eccentric work programs using a progressive overload sequence adapted to the tendon's deformation capacity (Malliaras et al., 2013). However, beyond the protocols of eccentric work and the need to individualize the processes of re-adaptation, it is important to observe the following: in order to increase sports performance, increased loads (stresses) are required. However, at the same time, we also know that

Chapter 44

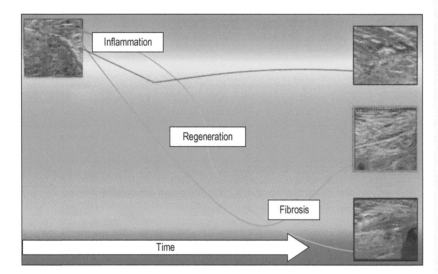

Inflammation

Regeneration

Fibrosis

Time

Figure 44.5 Schematic relationship between the physiological scarring process and the elastography chromatic scale

An elasticity curve shows the ideal moment for implementation of manual matrix remodeling techniques to prevent fibrosis. The lines represent the wound-healing process (inflammation, skeletal muscle regeneration and remodeling), which may lead to fibrosis. The green line represents wound healing with restitution of local elasticity after manual modeling of the scar and the blue line shows the wound-healing process with elasticity loss and a high risk of relapse.

From Martínez and Galán del Río (2013) with permission.

the Achilles tendon has a limited deformation capacity (Järvinen et al., 2005 A). In this context, is it possible to increase training and competition loads without conditioning the proper stress-strain relationship? In other words, is it possible to increase the force-absorbing capacity of the Achilles tendon and plantar fascia while taking into account the composition and resistance of these rigid structures (as indicated above)? Understanding the anatomical and functional continuity of the Achilles-calcaneus-plantar system with the triceps surae (Chapter 12), we propose a manual approach of the gastrocnemius-soleus complex (Figure 44.3). Using this approach, it is possible to improve sliding between the fascial layers of the medial head and lateral heads of the gastrocnemius, as well as between gastrocnemius muscles and soleus muscle in the medial and lateral septa

of the lower limb. In other words, by optimizing the mechanical behavior of intermuscular septa, it is possible to improve the adaptability of the Achilles-calcaneus-plantar system and increase the training loads and mechanical efficiency of the tendon.

Finally, core training exercises are usually incorporated in multiple rehabilitation and return to play programs, as core stability is related to an increase of athletic performance and a decrease in re-injury risk (Huxel Bliven and Anderson, 2013). However, a recent study showed that the effectiveness of core training programs, based on the adequate transmission of force between the transverse musculature and the lumbar fascia, may be limited in those cases where there is an increased thickening of the posterior musculofascial junction of the lumbar

Rehabilitation in sport medicine

fascia via interfascial lumbar triangle. This interface integrates the aponeurosis of the transversus abdominis with lumbar fascia that bifurcates at this level into the middle and posterior layer of the thoracolumbar fascia (Schuenke et al., 2012; Chen et al., 2016). For that reason, prior to performing core training exercises, we suggest the use of manual techniques in the interfascial lumbar triangle to increase sliding of transverse abdominis during contraction and, subsequently, to increase the functional efficiency of the lumbopelvic region during movements that require eccentric strength and efficient deceleration, as well as fast and explosive changes of direction.

Summary

If fibroblast behavior depends on surrounding mechanical processes, it is relevant to try to fully understand these processes, not only during prevention and treatment of myofascial and tendon injury, but also in soft tissue, bone and joint injuries after sports-related traumata.

Many of the existing rehabilitation protocols offer programs involving progressive loading exercises. However, based on the authors' clinical experience, this widely used approach would not consider the pre-existing state of collapse and restriction in the fascial network associated with a repetitive overuse pattern, which is common in most sports. Therefore, the authors would like to stress the benefits of initiating any rehabilitation process by using manual therapy on the restricted and fibrotic areas, aimed at encouraging the rearrangement and remodeling of fascial architecture.

In addition, to optimize sports rehabilitation modification of the mechanical properties of the fascial system, alongside mechanical load control, motor strategies should be considered before and after return to play.

References

Barbe, M.F., Gallagher, S., Massicotte, V.S., Tytell, M., Popoff, S.N. & Barr-Gillespie, A.E. (2013) The interaction of force and repetition on musculoskeletal and neural tissue responses and sensorimotor behavior in a rat model of work-related musculoskeletal disorders. *BMC Musculoskel Disord.* 25,14: 303.

Barry, C.M., Kestell, G., Gillan, M., Haberberger, R.V. & Gibbins, I.L. (2015) Sensory nerve fibres containing calcitonin gene related peptide in gastrocnemius, latissimus dorsi and erector spinae muscles and thoracolumbar fascia in mice. *Neuroscience.* 16: 106–117.

Barker, P.J., Hapuarachchi, K.S., Ross, J.A., Sambaiew, E., Ranger, T.A. & Briggs, C.A. (2014) Anatomy and biomechanics of gluteus maximus and the thoracolumbar fascia at the sacroiliac joint. *Clin Anat.* 27: 234–240.

Bernabei, M., Van Dieën, J.H. & Maas, H. (2017) Longitudinal and transversal displacements between triceps surae muscles during locomotion of the rat. *J Exp Biol.* 220: 537–550.

Bove, G.M., Harris, M.Y., Zhao, H. & Barbe, M.F. (2016) Manual therapy as an effective treatment for fibrosis in a rat model of upper extremity overuse injury. *J Neurol Sci.* 15: 161–180.

Cabuk, H. & Cabuk F. (2016) Mechanoreceptors of the ligaments and tendons around the knee. *Clin Anat.* 29: 789–795.

Chaudhry, H., Schleip, R., Ji, Z., Bukiet, B., Maney, M. & Findley, T. (2008) Three-dimensional mathematical model for deformation of human fasciae in manual therapy. *J Am Osteopath Assoc.* 108: 379–390.

Chen, Y.H., Chai, H.M., Shau, Y.W., Wang, C.L. & Wang, S. F. (2016) Increased sliding of transverse abdominis during contraction after myofascial release in patients with chronic low back pain. *Man Ther.* 23: 69–75.

Chumanov, E., Heiderscheit, B.C. & Thelen, D.G. (2011) Hamstring musculotendon dynamics during stance and swing phases of high-speed running. *Med Sci Sports Exer.* 43: 525–532.

Cruz-Montecinos, C., Cerda, M., Sanzana-Cuche, R., Martín-Martín, J. & Cuesta-Vargas, A. (2016) Ultrasound assessment of fascial connectivity in the lower limb during maximal cervical flexion: technical aspects and practical application of automatic tracking. *BMC Sports Sci Med Rehabil*. 11: 18.

Dalmau-Pastor, M., Farques-Polo, B. Jr., Casanova-Martínez, D. Jr., Vega, J. & Golano, P. (2014) Anatomy of the triceps surae: a pictorial essay. *Foot Ankle Clin*. 19: 603–635.

Ekstrand, J., Häglund, M., Kristenson, K., Magnusson, H. & Waldén, M. (2013) Fewer ligament injuries but no preventive effect on muscle injuries and severe injuries: an 11-year follow-up of the UEFA Champions League injury study. *Br J Sports Med*. 47: 32–37.

Grob, K., Manestar, M., Filgueira, L., Ackland, T., Gilbey, H. & Kuster, M.S. (2016) New insight in the architecture of the quadriceps tendon. *J Exp Orthop*. 3: 32.

Huijing, P.A. (2009) Epimuscular myofascial force transmission: a historical review and implications for new research. *J Biomech*. 42: 9–21.

Huxel Bliven, K.C. & Anderson, B.E. (2013) Core stability for injury prevention. *Sports Health*. 5: 514–522.

Järvinen, T.A., Kannus, P., Maffulli, N. & Khan, K.M. (2005a) Achilles tendon disorders: etiology and epidemiology. *Foot Ankle Clin*. 10: 255–266.

Järvinen, T.A., Järvinen, T.L., Kääriäinen, M., Kalimo, H. & Järvinen, M. (2005b) Muscle injuries: biology and treatment. *Am J Sports Med*. 33: 745–764.

Kjaer, M. (2004) Role of extracellular matrix in adaptation of tendon and skeletal muscle to mechanical loading. *Physiol Rev*. 84: 649–698.

Langevin, H.M., Bishop, J., Maple, R., Badge, G.J. & Fox, J.R. (2018) Effect of stretching on thoracolumbar fascia

injury and movement restriction in a porcine model. *Am J Phys Med Rehabil*. 97: 187–191.

Malliaras, P., Barton, C.J., Reeves, N.D. & Langberg, H. (2013) Achilles and patellar tendinopathy loading programmes: a systematic review comparing clinical outcomes and identifying potential mechanisms for effectiveness. *Sports Med*. 43: 267–286.

Martínez-Rodríguez, R. & Galán del Río, F. (2013) Mechanistic basis of manual therapy in myofascial injuries. Sonoelastographic evolution control. *J Bodyw Mov Ther*. 17: 221–234.

Miller, B.F., Olesen, J., Hansen, M., Døssing, S., Crameri, R., Welling R, et al. (2005) Coordinated collagen and muscle protein synthesis in human patella tendon and quadriceps muscle after exercise. *J Physiol*. 567: 1021–1033.

Murtaugh, B. & Ihm, J.M. (2013) Eccentric training for the treatment of tendinopathies. *Curr Sports Med Rep*. 12: 175–182.

Opar, D.A., Williams, M.D. & Shield, A.J. (2012) Hamstring strain injuries: factors that lead to injury and re-injury. *Sports Med*. 42: 209–226.

Purslow, P. (2010) Muscle fascia and force transmission. *J Bodyw Mov Ther*. 14: 411–417.

Schilder, A., Hoheisel, U., Magerl, W., Benrath, J., Klein, T. & Treede, R.D. (2014) Sensory findings after stimulation of the thoracolumbar fascia with hypertonic saline suggest its contribution to low back pain. *Pain*. 155: 222–231.

Schoots, E.J., Tak, I.J., Veenstra, B.J., Drebbers, Y.M. & Bax, J.G. (2013) Ultrasound characteristics of the lateral

retinaculum in 10 patients with patellofemoral pain syndrome compared to healthy controls. *J Bodyw Mov Ther*. 17: 523–529.

Schuenke, M.D., Vleeming, A., Van Hoof, T. & Willard, F.H. (2012) A description of the lumbar interfascial triangle and its relation with the lateral raphe: anatomical constituents of load transfer through the lateral margin of the thoracolumbar fascia. *J Anat*. 221: 568–576.

Silder, A., Reeder, S.B. & Thelen, D.G. (2010) The influence of prior hamstring injury on lengthening muscle tissue mechanics. *J Biomech*. 43: 2254–2260.

Sole, G., Milosavljevic, S., Nicholson, H.D. & Sullivan, S.J. (2011) Selective strength loss and decreased muscle activity in hamstring injury. *J Orthop Sports Phys Ther*. 41: 354–363.

Stecco, C., Gagey, O., Belloni, A., Pozzuoli, A., Porzionato, A., Macchi, V., et al. (2007) Anatomy of the deep fascia of the upper limb. Second part: study of innervation. *Morphologie*. 91: 38–43.

Taguchi, T., Yasui, M., Kubo, A., Abe, M., Kiyama H., Yamanaka, A., et al. (2013) Nociception originating from the crural fascia in rats. *Pain*. 154: 1103–1114.

van der Wal, J. (2009) The architecture of the connective tissue in the musculoskeletal system—an often over-looked functional parameter as to proprioception in the locomotor apparatus. *Int J Ther Mass Bodyw*. 2: 9–23.

Zügel, M., Maganaris, C.N., Wilke, J., Jurkat-Rott, K., Klingler, W., Wearing, S. C., et al. (2018) Fascial tissue research in sports medicine: from molecules to tissue adaptation, injury and diagnostics. *Br J Sports Med*. 1–9.

How to train fascia in soccer

Klaus Eder and Helmut Hoffmann

Positive and negative influences on the myofascial system in soccer

Excellence in any sport demands a sport-specific level of physical conditioning, combined with corresponding technical skill, to ensure mastery of sport-specific patterns of movement, as well as the tactical insights needed to engage in competitive play.

Soccer, in particular, is characterized by a wide range of stereotypical patterns of movement that are sport- or discipline- specific. Related sports like American Football or Australian Rules Football show comparable stereotypical kicking movements. If these patterns of movement are performed cumulatively in sufficient number, over a prolonged period of time, it is reasonable to expect that these football-specific movement stimuli will provoke reactions that manifest themselves as adaptations of the particular biological structures involved (joints, ligaments, neuromeningeal and myofascial structures) to permit adequate "processing" of the incident stresses and loads (Chapters 4 and 5). Over the past 20 years, in the course of delivering medical care to soccer players at virtually every performance level from amateurs to professionals who represent their countries internationally, we have empirically identified a wide diversity of changes to which soccer players are prone. In this context, because it involves the side-specific dominance of a kicking leg and a support leg,

soccer is also characterized by corresponding asymmetries in adaptations and changes, particularly with regard to the myofascial system.

These adaptations maximize the quality of the sport-specific patterns of movement and thus serve to enhance the individual's performance in their particular sport. However, they are also often the cause of changes in muscular stress patterns within the sport and may, in certain circumstances, lead to abnormal loading or overloading of the body structures involved. Knowledge of the soccer-specific changes affecting the musculoskeletal, neuromuscular and myofascial systems enables coaches and the medical team to assess any structural and functional implications more easily, and lays the groundwork so that athletes can engage in structure-specific preparation and recovery routines. The information below is intended to raise awareness among coaches and the medical team concerning the existence of soccer-specific adaptations and to ensure these phenomena receive proper attention.

Soccer-specific changes and adaptations involving the musculoskeletal system

The following sections outline typical soccer-specific adaptations, with a special focus on myofascial changes which are encountered repeatedly in practice, even in the absence of

Chapter 45

injuries. A correspondingly high probable incidence of such changes must be anticipated in the active soccer player (that may also persist for years afterwards), and it is important to bear this in mind when preparing for both training and competitive matches. The following categories of change figure prominently in soccer and deserve attention.

Changes in the kicking leg due to ball contact

By definition, soccer entails a varying number of contacts with the ball.

In this process, the mechanical stresses associated with ball contact, if generated in sufficient number and magnitude, provoke changes in the biological structures. During the course of evolution, nature has developed our musculoskeletal system, and especially our lower limbs as components of the pelvic-leg axis, specifically for locomotion, walking and running (Chapters 29 and 30). Our feet, with their longitudinal and transverse arches, are ingeniously designed to cushion the impact of our body mass with each step, and to propel our bodies forward in the terminal phase of the gait cycle. Upon contact with the ball, a force is generated over a short period of time that is precisely opposed to the arched construction of the foot, giving rise to corresponding mechanical forces and stresses. With each individual kicking action, the mechanical reaction forces released by the ball mass are of a magnitude that remains well within the physiological range and generally does not exceed the stress tolerance of the structures involved. However, if this action is repeated a sufficient number of times over a prolonged period, possibly many years, the resultant stimuli then act as a form of micro-trauma, eventually leading to changes in the musculoskeletal system. Such changes have

been postulated and discussed since the mid-1980s, for example, by Hess (1985), and by Lees and Nolan (1998).

To ensure appropriate preparation for the sudden and brief tensile stresses generated by ball contact, strengthening occurs at the insertion sites of the talonavicular ligament, which is placed under tensile stress by the action of kicking. The increased numbers of more strongly developed Sharpey's fibers take up an increased amount of space and may then frequently be visible radiologically as a talar beak and/or tibial peak, a phenomenon that results in reduced dorsiflexion mobility at the ankle joint. Furthermore, the majority of soccer players have a flatter medial longitudinal arch (1–3 mm) in the kicking leg compared with the support leg, which consequently provokes an ascending chain of causes and effects with a subtly enhanced tibial internal rotation onto the navicular bone, with corresponding effects on the knee joint in the form of an increased "dynamic genu valgum" during the standing phase.

Alongside this and as a result of these direct changes to the ankle joint in response to kicking movements, soccer players are also likely to develop muscle changes that are characterized by varying degrees of right-left asymmetry (support leg vs. kicking leg). The kicking movement of the leg axis in question represents an "open kinetic chain" type of load in which the foot is moved with maximum forward velocity (moving point) and the hip remains relatively stationary (fixed point). At the same time, every kicking movement necessarily imposes a "closed kinetic chain" type of load on the non-kicking side. In this case, the non-kicking foot is planted on the ground (fixed point), while the structures above it throughout the pelvic-leg axis and torso are in motion (moving point) and need to be adequately stabilized against gravity by a complex set of coordination mechanisms. Similarly varied neuromuscular control actions then create the basis for long-term muscular adaptations to these soccer-specific movement patterns. In the long term, the active musculoskeletal system, as well as the myofascial system, may be assumed to adapt progressively to the characteristic movements that they are called upon to perform, and to the loads associated with those movements as they develop an optimized muscular response.

Reports describe muscle differences between the support leg in relation to the kicking leg (Ekstrand et al., 1983; Knebel et al., 1988). Kicking the ball is a multiple-joint movement, in which an obviously explosive extension movement at the knee is combined with active flexion of the hip and extension (plantar flexion) of the foot at the ankle joint. In general, these authors describe both an increased maximum strength capacity and an increased striking force during quadriceps extension on the kicking-leg side, accompanied by increased maximum strength and striking force of the knee flexors on the support-leg side (Figure 45.1).

Our own empirical observations on the degree of quadriceps muscle development in soccer players suggest additional neurophysiological aspects and considerations relating to long-term functional adaptations. Although soccer players have greater quadriceps strength on the kicking-leg side than on the support-leg side, examination of the thighs in most players shows that the thigh circumference tends to be slightly reduced in the area where the vastus medialis muscle is most fully developed. Evidently the variable "muscular configuration" of the quadriceps is an adaptive response of the musculoskeletal system to years of locally varying, stereotypical functional demands (the kicking leg with its

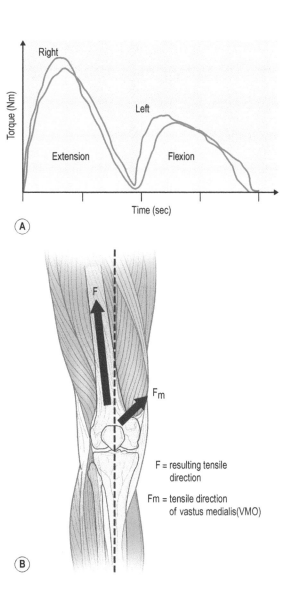

Figure 45.1 Agonist-antagonist relationship in the muscles of the knee joint

numerous open kinetic-chain loads, in contrast to the support leg with its closed kinetic-chain loads). It is not uncommon for there to be clearly identifiable volume deficiencies in the territory of the vastus medialis muscle of the kicking leg in some players.

Chapter 45

From a neurophysiological standpoint, a "chronic" vastus medialis deficiency in the kicking leg can be explained by the absence of any need during open kinetic-chain activity to stabilize the knee joint in terms of tibial rotation relative to the femur in response to gravitational effects. The long-term change in the innervation pattern gradually results in adaptation that is optimized for kicking the ball. The other side of the coin is that this process alters the relative contributions of the individual quadriceps muscles to the resultant quadriceps force. Deficiency of the vastus medialis tends to lateralize the quadriceps pull on the patella, thereby altering the kinematics of the femoropatellar joint. By contrast, the loads on the support leg during running and sprinting tend not to alter the physiological pattern of intra-articular kinematics. Consequently, degenerative changes in the femoropatellar joint are detected far more commonly on the kicking-leg side than on the support-leg side.

Support leg changes due to kicking technique

The changes in the kicking leg, described above, suggest that the contralateral support leg is obviously exposed to different loads during the kicking of a soccer ball. It is interesting that all soccer players, virtually irrespective of their performance level, tend to place their support leg in a very precise position when kicking the ball, with the instep or with the inside/outside of the foot. This results in a highly consistent pattern of stereotypical mechanical loads acting on the musculoskeletal structures. To ensure successful ball acceleration by following through with the kicking leg to transfer momentum effectively to the ball, the support leg must be planted correctly next to the ball on the ground. The following

initial observations are important in this regard (Hoffmann, 1984):

- As far as possible, soccer players plant their support leg next to the ball with remarkable consistency and precision. Tests have shown that intra-individual differences from one ball contact to the next are less than 1 cm (Hoffmann, 1984).
- Soccer players plant their support leg level with the ball (relative to the frontal plane).
- As the foot is planted on the ground, the body's center of gravity shifts outward towards the support leg, usually moving beyond the left knee or even further laterally.
- The lateral distance of the support leg from the ball can vary markedly from one player to the next. Despite these pronounced differences, however, the individual solutions and movement patterns are performed with great precision (intra-individual consistency). However, the further the support leg is placed away from the ball, the greater the lateral shift in the body's center of gravity. The joints along the pelvic-leg axis of the support leg have to stabilize and compensate for this position and this will then culminate in corresponding adaptive changes over time. These side-specific changes are most clearly identified in the ankle joint. The greater the lateralization of the pelvic-leg axis, the greater the lateral and shear forces acting on the joints of the foot. Even in the absence of injuries and/or trauma, these forces have the potential to induce long-term adaptations.

Adaptations of the lumbopelvic-hip region

The muscular adaptations, described above, which occur on the support-leg and kicking-leg sides in response to the demands of soccer also bring in their wake long-term changes in the entire lumbopelvic-hip complex. Our own gait analyses (kinematic, dynamic and palpatory findings) together with manual therapy assessments have highlighted the following aspects: the dominance of the powerful quadriceps and hip flexors (especially the iliopsoas muscle) on the kicking-leg side causes the pelvis to tilt posteriorly on that side (posterior pelvic tilt with inflare component). This, in turn, may cause an anterior pelvic tilt (relatively upright ilium with outflare component) to develop on the contralateral support-leg side in an attempt to stabilize the body's center of gravity in the long term. Additionally, these changes are often accompanied by a decreased range of motion in the sacroiliac joint on the kicking-leg side. This asymmetrical range of motion, combined with torsion of the hips, seems to produce apparent lengthening of the support-leg axis and leads to functional pelvic obliquity. Furthermore, the new stress patterns are transmitted to the structures of the lumbar spine. As a result of the posterior pelvic tilt on the kicking-leg side, physical examination of soccer players often reveals that the lumbar spine is rotated posteriorly to the right due to increased tension on the iliolumbar ligaments.

Implications for the myofascial system

To summarize, soccer players can be expected to exhibit changes and side-specific adaptations affecting all the joints and ligaments of the lower limb, and hence the associated musculoskeletal structures together with the entire functional unit of the pelvic-leg axis with its associated myofascial chains. Varying in degree between different players, and depending on individual predisposition and the duration (years of training) and quantity (scope of training) of the loads and stereotypical movement patterns, these changes may become a source of problems.

Table 45.1 Muscles of the myofascial inflare and outflare chains Adapted from Meert, 2003	
Myofascial inflare chain **Torsion + flexion (e.g. left-sided chain)**	**Myofascial outflare chain** **(Torsion + extension (e.g. left-sided chain))**
Rectus capitis lateralis muscle, left	Obliquus capitis muscles, left longissimus capitis muscle, left trapezius muscle (descending part), left
Scalene muscles, left sternocleidomastoid muscle, left	Levator scapulae muscle, left
Major and minor pectoralis muscles, left	External rotators, left shoulder superior posterior serratus muscle, left
Intercostal muscles, left	Inferior posterior serratus muscle, left
External oblique abdominal muscle, left internal oblique abdominal muscle, right	Diaphragm (transverse separating structure) thoracolumbar fascia, quadratus lumborum muscle, left
Diaphragm (transverse separating structure)	Psoas muscle, right
Iliopsoas muscle, right	Gluteal musculature, right; tensor fasciae latae muscle, right
Obturator muscles, right adductor muscles, right vastus medialis muscle, right	Vastus lateralis muscle, right
Peroneal musculature, right	Sartorius muscle, right mediocrural musculature, right
Plantar fascia	Plantar fascia

Chapter 45

In consequence, some rethinking of priorities will be necessary, both when preparing for training/competitive matches and during the recovery (cool down) phase to optimize regeneration processes. Furthermore, alongside the classic and now conventional strategies (with their focus on joints, ligaments and the musculoskeletal system), consideration should also be given to the myofascia and to relevant exercises that will enable such considerations to be translated into practice. In this context, side-specific connective-tissue properties may also manifest themselves as a result of adaptation to the stereotypical stresses of training/competitive matches. Both connective tissue properties are often found to be reduced on the kicking-leg side. Both the long anterior myofascial chain (components still missing here) and the diagonal anterior myofascial chain (like m. adductor longus and m. rectus abdominis) are found to be less taut and, because of this reduced firmness, paradoxically less elastic. The three-dimensional architecture of collagen "network structures" could therefore be altered in terms of firmness and elasticity (Chapter 8).

The lateral fascia (fascia lata and tractus iliotibialis) of the thigh is also more clearly pronounced with increased firmness. A dominant straight posterior myofascial chain and crossed posterior myofascial chain are found on the support-leg side (Figure 45.2).

Building up optimized fascial structures/networks in the medium and long term

On the basis of the anatomical, biomechanical and physiological principles previously outlined, we can formulate the following general pragmatic "fascial training principles" for the medium and long-term:

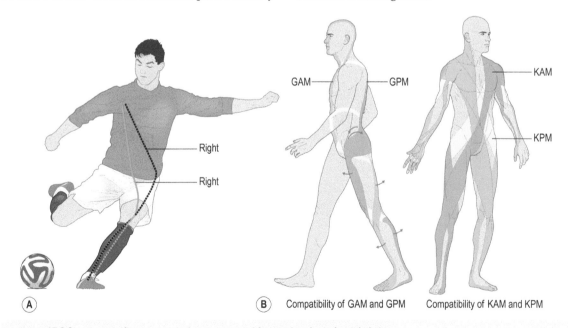

(A)   Right   Right

(B)   GAM   GPM   KAM   KPM

Compatibility of GAM and GPM   Compatibility of KAM and KPM

Figure 45.2 Soccer-specific stereotypical movements with associated myofascial chains

How to train fascia in soccer

Table 45.2 Fascial training principles			
	Fascial tissue stretch	**Fascial tissue elasticity**	**Fascial tissue tension**
Training objective	• Increased synthetic activities of fibroblasts • Alignment of collagen fiber structure • Optimized nourishment of collagen fibers	• Optimization of strength development specifically related to the type of sport • Development of jumping power specific to the type of sport • Economization of energy metabolism	• Improvement of 3D-musculoskeletal stability work in the tensegral system • Formation of myofibroblasts in musculoskeletal transition
Training method	• Multidirectional stretches of myofascial chains across several joints • Self-myofascial release/foam rolling • Plyometric exercises (focus tendon energy storage via stretch-shortening cycles)	• Plyometric exercises (focus muscle-tendon connection via muscular force training effects) • Exercise variants with activation of the stretch-shortening cycle	• Whole-body exercises with high tension of the musculoskeletal system • Exercises with >65% of current maximum strength rating

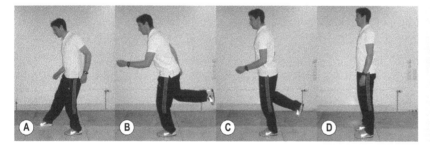

Figure 45.3 Soccer-specific complex stabilization exercise with contralateral trunk rotation and reversal of support/kicking leg function

Exercises and forms of movement, which by and large are focused on the turning points of movement that are specific to the type of sport (such as the kicking movements in soccer), where the agonists operating in synergy and the stretched antagonists meet, demand a virtually isometric tension of the contractile elements. This enables further small movements with directional change via the fascial (elastic) elements, as well as a developmental and directional stimulus. Preparatory counter-movements of this type, close to the turnaround points of movements, may be combined with a variety of rotational components (3D arrangement of the fascial network) (Chapter 40).

Taking account of the myofascial system when preparing for training and competition

Physiotherapeutic modalities

The soccer-specific profile of requirements and adaptations of the locomotor system should be taken into consideration in all preparation for training/competition. Although no reliable scientific evidence exists for the protective effectiveness of most of the following specific training recommendations, these recommendations reflect the current thinking and observations of our group and associated colleagues based on

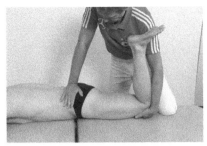

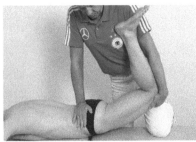

Figure 45.4 Mobilization of the iliopsoas muscle

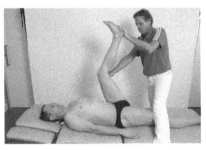

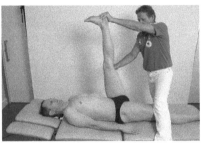

Figure 45.5 Mobilization of the hamstrings

our extensive work with professional soccer players. The following two mobilizations may be performed for the prevention of dysfunctions and/or dysbalances.

The iliopsoas muscle
- is connected to the respiratory diaphragm (Prometheus, 2005) and therefore, its proper function is important for breathingis
- is "connected" with all of the discs in the lumbar spine
- surrounds the lumbar plexus of the motor and, among others, sensory of the quadriceps muscle and the knee joint
- contributes to the determination of stride length.

The hamstrings
- connect the pelvis to the lower extremity
- "interact" with the menisci (Barral and Croibier, 2013)
- "surround" the ischiatic nerve and its end-branches, the tibial and peroneal nerves

- in the case of certain restrictions, irritate the structures of the affected pelvis-leg axis to a major extent and may thereby increase the risk of injury.

Preparing for training and competition

Passive modalities: Elastic taping and kinesiotaping

In preparing for training/competitive matches, elastic tapes and kinesiotapes may be used to stabilize joints. Functional tapes replace and supplement ligamentous and osseous joint-stabilizing factors and produce tensile and relaxing effects on the skin and subcutaneous receptors, thus selectively facilitating or inhibiting muscle tone/activity (neurophysiological and myotensive/myofascial improvement of joint stability via muscular joint stabilization factors). See Eder and Mommsen (2007), and Mommsen et al. (2007), for further information on these techniques.

How to train fascia in soccer

Active modalities

The purpose of all preparatory modalities/activities in this context can be subsumed under the following definition: optimal psychological and physical preparation for subsequent soccer-specific psychological and physical demands to achieve the current best possible level of performance.

In line with ideas originally outlined by Schlumberger (Eder and Hoffmann, 2006), these active modalities comprise, in general, the following key areas:

- Boosting physiological metabolic activities using moderate running with varying intensity to raise core body temperature, increase general metabolic activities, and optimize neuromuscular control processes.
- Structure-specific preparation of the musculoskeletal system for soccer-specific movement sequences utilizing dynamic stretching and taking account of myofascial structures (Chapter 40).
- Preparation for soccer-specific stereotypical movement patterns with progressively increasing complexity and intensity. In particular, soccer-specific cutting movements with directional changes of varying intensity should be integrated in this process, as well as phases of acceleration and deceleration, initially without the ball, and then as preparation advances, receiving the ball and running with it, as well as situation-specific movement sequences (corners, free kick variations, etc.).

In terms of structure-specific preparation of the musculoskeletal system, in particular, the widespread practice of static stretching immediately prior to the stresses of training/competitive matches should be discarded

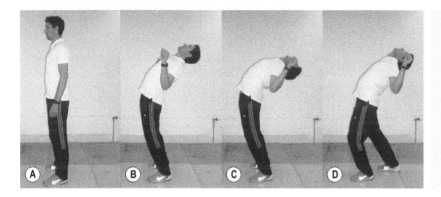

Figure 45.6 Stretching the straight anterior myofascial chain to prevent entrapment

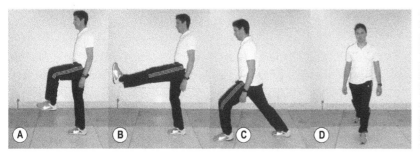

Figure 45.7 Example to illustrate dynamic stretching: hurdle walk

Chapter 45

(Chapter 10). Similarly, we propose that the exercise forms involving preparatory counter-movement and rapid bouncing as a type of "dynamic stretching" to shape and develop the fascial network are less suitable (if not actually unsuitable) as immediate preparation for the stresses of training/competitive matches. Instead, the suitable approach involves "dynamic stretching" that, as well as catering for the myotensive (muscular contractile) and neuromuscular (proprioceptive) movement prerequisites, also prepares the myofascial structures for the stresses and loads that are to follow.

In our experience, plyometric exercises (Chapter 25), initially with a unidirectional character and then building up with a multidirectional three-dimensional character (linear and lateral as well as rotatory), have proved themselves useful for activating joint-specific capsular receptors to round off structure-specific preparation, and can then transition into soccer-specific stereotypical movement patterns with and without the ball (Chapter 24).

Taking account of the myofascial system during recovery after the stresses of training/competitive matches

Generally recognized measures, after the stresses of training and competitive matches, for the timely restoration and recovery of physical performance, have the following objectives:

- Replenishment of exercise-induced fluid and energy deficits (for example, muscle glycogen stores).

- Optimization of physiological metabolic status (supply and removal in the context of biochemical regeneration processes) by promoting the circulation using moderate, low-intensity aerobic (alactic) movement types incorporating exercises that are not soccer-specific, such as cycling or aqua-jogging (characterized by reduced intra-articular load stresses on the joints).

- Possibly, physiotherapy to monitor the status of the joints and ligaments of the lower limb and spinal column.

These activities should be supplemented with special reference to the fascial network. To release fascial adhesions and resolve swellings that have developed following the stresses of training/competitive matches, self-myofascial techniques can be integrated into the regeneration strategy, thereby promoting dynamic hydration of the collagenous ground substance (although these effects have not been confirmed by research so far) (Chapter 27). Notwithstanding, foam rollers may be suitable for this purpose. The locally limited contact surface of these rollers permits a slow gradual rolling movement via the gravitational application of the athlete's bodyweight and so encourages a continuous further rolling movement along the course of the affected fascia. Here, too, in the specific context of soccer, it is important to direct such efforts preferentially to the most commonly affected fascia. In our experience these are the lateral structures of the kicking leg due to soccer-specific adaptations.

Conclusion

More recent scientific insights have brought about a paradigm shift in our understanding and appreciation of the function and importance of the fascial network. Alongside the classic targets of training, such as musculoskeletal function and performance, cardiopulmonary function and performance, and neuromuscular coordination and control, this radical change of perspective highlights the imperative to revise and re-orient training objectives, and their

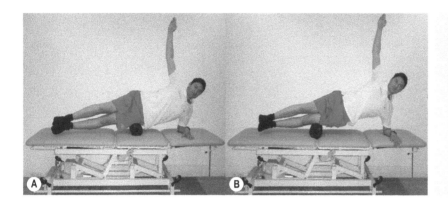

Figure 45.8 Myofascial auto-release techniques for the dorsolateral fascia of the kicking-leg thigh

implementation and achievement, by adopting appropriate training modalities. In terms of fascial training, this requires measures and methods to develop and optimize a fascial network, as well as strategies to integrate fascial aspects into direct preparation for and recovery from the stresses of training/competitive matches, thus ensuring that the fruits of modern fascia research are incorporated into the soccer-specific training process.

References

Barral, J.-P. and Croibier, A. (2013) *Gelenke-ein neuer osteopathischer Behandlungsansatz-untere Extremitäten*. Munich, Germany: Urban & Fischer-Verlag.

Eder, K. & Hoffmann, H. (2006) *Verletzungen im Fußball –vermeiden – behandeln – therapieren*. Munich, Germany: Elsevier Verlag.

Eder, K. & Mommsen, H. (2007) *Richtig Tapen – Funktionelle Verbände am Bewegungsapparat optimal anlegen*. Balingen, Germany: Spitta Verlag GmbH & Co. KG.

Ekstrand, J., Gillquist, J. & Liljedahl, S.O. (1983) Prevention of soccer injuries. Supervision by doctor and physiotherapist. *Am J Sports Med*. 11: 116–120.

Hess, H. (1985) Fussball. In: Pförringer (Ed.), *W. Sport – Trauma und Belastung*. Erlangen, Germany: Perimed Fachbuch-Verlagsgesellschaft mbH.

Hoffmann, H. (1984) *Biomechanik von Fußballspannstößen*. Frankfurt/Main: unpublished thesis, University of Frankfurt/M.

Knebel, K.P., Herbeck, B. & Hamsen, G. (1988) *FußballFunktionsgymnastik. Dehnen, Kräftigen, Entspannen*. Reinbeck, Germany: Rowohlt Verlag.

Lees, A. & Nolan, I. (1998) The biomechanics of soccer: a review. *J Sports Sci*. 16: 211–234.

Meert, G.F. (2003) *Das Becken aus osteopathischer Sicht*. Munich/Jena, Germany: Urban & Fischer Verlag.

Mommsen, H., Eder, K. & Brandenburg, U. (2007) *Leukotape K – Schmerztherapie und Lymphtherapie nach japanischer Tradition*. Balingen, Germany: Spitta Verlag GmbH & Co. KG.

Mueller-Wohlfahrt, H.-W., Ueblacker, P., Haensel, L. & Garrett, W.E. Jr. (2013) *Muscle Injuries in Sports*. Stuttgart/New York: Georg Thieme Verlag.

Prometheus (2005) *LernAtlas der Atomie*. Stuttgart-New York: Georg Thieme Verlag.

Movement therapy for breast cancer survivors

P. J. O'Clair

Introduction

Breast cancer is the second most common type of cancer in the world and by far the most prevalent in women, with over two million new cases reported each year. It is estimated that 627,000 women died from breast cancer in 2018, that is, ~15% of all cancer deaths among women (World Health Organization, 2018). Fortunately, due to early detection and advancements in screening, many patients diagnosed will survive and go on to live out their normal life expectancy. Despite this good news, cancer treatments take an enormous toll: in just 1 year of treatment, the body can age a decade. Between the inherent weight gain, muscle atrophy and premature bone loss, women are left emotionally frail and physically weak, often challenged by normal day-to-day activities (Helms et al., 2008).

Treatments and side effects

Breast cancer treatments aim both to rid the body of disease and to minimize the possibility of the cancer returning. They are either local or systemic, with patients receiving either one form or a combination, based on individual needs. Local treatments are used to remove or destroy damaged tissue at and around the cancer site; they include surgery such as lumpectomy, mastectomy, breast-conserving surgery and axillary (underarm) lymph node removal. Systemic treatments are used to destroy or control cancer cells throughout the entire body rather than at a specific site; these methods include chemotherapy,

hormone therapy and biological therapy. Side effects to breast cancer treatments—such as pain, temporary swelling, tenderness, infection, increased stiffness in joints, "hardness" due to scar tissue that forms at the surgical site (Fourie, 2008), and very high levels of fatigue from surgery, radiation and chemotherapy—impact a patient's ability and/or desire to exercise. Weight gain and low self-esteem are also common challenges.

Movement therapy for breast cancer survivors

There is a growing body of exercise-oncology research that strongly suggests exercise can greatly reduce the risk of breast cancer recurrence as well as enhance functionality and quality of life (Kaelin et al., 2006; Mutrie et al., 2007; Sprague et al., 2007). It has recently been suggested that physical activity above all other possible lifestyle modifications, including weight management, diet, cessation of tobacco and reduction in alcohol consumption, may have the most robust effect on reducing breast cancer recurrence (Dieli-Conwright & Orozco, 2015). The challenge for the newly diagnosed patient is in selecting which exercise is most appropriate for them, especially if they are not currently engaged in regular physical activity. Often they look to their medical teams for advice and direction. Those who work with breast cancer, or any types of cancer patients, should be well versed in the type of cancer, the treatments administered and their associated side effects. Treatments for

Chapter 46

breast cancer patients differ from individual to individual due to many factors: age, extent of disease, co-morbid state and current physical condition. These factors, along with the current stage of treatment, type of medication(s) and potential side effects with exercise, should be taken into account and help guide the movement practitioner. Appropriately directed movement therapy is a critical component in the breast cancer patient's journey to recovery.

Movement therapy aims to strengthen the body-mind connection, which is essential through all phases of healing. It can provide a gentle restorative approach to exercise and is perfectly suited for women as they recover and work to rebuild their bodies both pre- and post-treatment (the benefits, most likely, also extend to the very small minority of breast cancer patients who are men). The goal of this therapeutic program is to restore the health of the damaged or compromised myofascial continuities, facilitate the slide and glide of tissues between adjacent structures, decrease excessive scar tissue build-up, build strength of the entire kinematic chain, address postural dysfunctions, help to regain sensory awareness, and teach or restore proper breathing techniques.

Many of the breast cancer patients my team and I have worked with report feeling better post-exercise and believe that movement is the key to tolerating the side effects and symptoms from cancer-related treatments, such as chemotherapy and radiation. Cancer-related fatigue (CRF) is one of the most widespread side effects and often begins immediately upon diagnosis. Studies report a prevalence of CRF in patients of up to 96% (Stasi et al., 2003). One study investigating the effects of supervised exercise training on both cardiopulmonary function and CRF in breast cancer survivors suggests that individualized exercise at a moderate intensity maintains or improves cardiopulmonary function with associated reductions in CRF. In addition, breast cancer survivors receiving a combination of chemotherapy and radiation following surgery appear to benefit to a greater extent as a result of an individualized exercise intervention (Hsieh et al., 2008). Along with the intense bouts of CRF, breast cancer patients experience minor to often severe postural effects from cancer-related treatments (Haddad et al., 2013). Patients who undergo multiple surgical procedures including the various types of reconstructive procedures are the most compromised physiologically.

One patient came to me complaining of hip pain. She was looking for exercises to help her with her condition. While completing a comprehensive health history screen, she revealed that she had had breast cancer years before and had had a mastectomy with a transverse rectus abdominis muscle (TRAM) flap reconstruction. Her TRAM flap reconstructive surgery involved making an incision along the lower abdomen and taking an oval section of skin, fat, blood vessels, and the rectus abdominis muscle from the lower half of the belly, and rerouting it to the chest to form a breast. The rectus abdominis muscle mobilizes the trunk into flexion by pulling the ribs and pelvis inward, but it also serves as a facilitator in upright posture and, along with the deeper abdominal muscles, acts as a shield and protects the viscera. The absence of this muscle could result in movement compensation. During evaluation we found that she had overactive hip flexors with a resulting tightness of the ipsilateral (same side) lumbar erector spinae and quadratus lumborum muscles. We concluded that her hip pain was likely due to her years of movement compensation post-breast cancer surgery and not necessarily an isolated hip joint problem. The good news is that after following a protocol similar to the one outlined in this chapter, within 3 months she was pain-free, and within 9 months her audible hip clicking with basic everyday movements was gone. She was able to resume her passion for long walks and hiking without discomfort or pain.

Postural dysfunctions resulting from multiple life-saving surgical procedures and treatments require careful attention and specifically designed exercise regimens to help re-establish proper neuromuscular patterns and restore optimal posture.

Potential movement therapy benefits for breast cancer survivors

(N.B. The benefits listed below have not been proven and are hypothetical; more research is needed before they can be stated as absolutes).

Movement therapy
- improves shoulder girdle mechanics, specifically scapula-humeral rhythm, to aid in the breakdown of scar tissue and frozen shoulder
- improves lympathic drainage through breathing
- restores overall range of motion, flexibility
- re-establishes proper muscular firing patterns
- increases the strength of local and global stabilizing muscles
- enhances core muscular strength and endurance
- restores upright postural alignment and balance
- improves overall sensory awareness
- assists with weight management
- increases self-confidence and overall well-being
- reduces both physiological and emotional stress
- improves appearance.

The key to the success of any exercise and movement-based therapy program is to proceed slowly and to consistently monitor how the patient feels. Developing a continual dialogue will ensure that they are not taking on more than they can handle. Just as crucial is the practitioner's bedside manner; there is a strong emotional element when working with breast cancer survivors, and positive reinforcement from the wellness professional is vital in all phases.

Movement therapy program design: five key concerns

It is imperative that movement professionals understand that patients recovering from breast cancer differ from those healing from injury and address the physiological conditions resulting from treatment (Kaelin et al., 2006). Movement therapy practitioners should take these conditions into account when implementing exercise programs for breast cancer survivors.

Lymphedema

This condition relates specifically to axillary lymph node dissection, axillary radiation or surgical infection (swelling of the arm). The swelling occurs when the lymph channels are altered and no longer able to properly drain lymph fluid from the arm back into the body's general circulation. Patients who have developed lymphedema should follow the guidelines outlined by their medical team and may be advised to wear compression garments when exercising. Lymphedema is managed by compression garment wear, exercise and elevation (APTA, 2020).

Rotator cuff

Breast cancer surgeries affect the rotator cuff muscles, resulting in "faulty" shoulder girdle mechanics, poor posture, increased stiffness, decreased mobility and pain (Ebaugh et al., 2011). Restoring the function of these muscles will help with daily life activities that involve pulling and pushing actions.

Chapter 46

Sarcopenia

This condition results in a simultaneous loss of muscle and gain in fat tissue. Inactivity during treatment, chemotherapy, premature menopause and other hormonal changes brought on by breast cancer treatments may lead to sarcopenia. Sarcopenia is associated with an increased risk of overall mortality in breast cancer survivors and may be associated with breast cancer-specific mortality (Villaseñor et al., 2012).

Premature osteoporosis

As a result of both local and systemic treatment, many breast cancer survivors experience a loss of ovarian function and, consequently, a drop in estrogen levels. This can increase bone loss and lead to osteoporosis. Women who were pre-menopausal before their cancer treatment may go through menopause earlier than those who have not had breast cancer (National Institutes of Health Osteoporosis and Related Bone Diseases National Resource Center, 2016).

Physiological muscular imbalances

After a mastectomy, a woman may opt to have surgery to reconstruct her breast(s) using an artificial implant or her own tissue, referred to as an autologous tissue flap. Flap surgery takes tissue from the abdomen, back or buttocks and uses it to reconstruct the breast. The effect of this procedure varies significantly from patient to patient. Flap surgeries often create muscular imbalances, and compensation patterns. Most patients have no difficulty in day-to-day life activities (Cyriac et al., 2010). However, there is insufficient long-term research detailing the effects on the long-term function of the associated prime movers, such as the rectus abdominis gluteus and latissimus dorsi. It can be assumed that loss of prime mover function may result in a greater demand on synergistic muscles, such as the obliques, rhomboids, and mid and lower trapezius.

The relationship between cancer and fascia

While the relationship between cancer and fascia has been a relatively unexplored topic in the scientific and therapeutic worlds, researchers are starting to recognize the potential importance of fascia in cancer, especially when it comes to integrative medicine, not just drugs and pharmacology (Langevin et al., 2016). Therapeutic work to rebuild the body may involve rehabilitation of the fascia, which could have been damaged in treatment.

Reports have shown that individuals with dense breast tissue have a 4- to 6-fold increased risk of developing breast carcinomas and that a third of all breast cancer cases are attributed to breast density, making it one of the greatest risk factors for carcinoma (Provenzano et al., 2008). When the tissue underlying the tumor is stiffer, it encourages the cancer to not only grow but to spread. In addition, the cancer secretes factors that increase the stiffness of the tissue creating a vicious cycle of disease (Provenzano et al., 2008). The stiffness and architecture of the collagen in the connective tissue plays a role in cancer progression. Collagen fiber bundles with a specific structured organization around tumors, as opposed to unstructured wavy collage fibers, have been shown to be more evident in cancer that has spread, as in metastatic breast cancer. These structured collagen fibers contribute to cancer progression and facilitate invasion out from primary tumors (Provenzano et al., 2008). While there is not much we can do to change ones predisposed breast tissue density, the knowledge of how tissue density impacts the disease can help direct our therapeutic approach with patients both during and post-cancer treatments. We will want to minimize the build-up of scar tissue and restore tissue mobility as quickly and as safely as possible. Recommendations in programming should include diaphragmatic breathing techniques and stretching or release methods to enhance the range of motion and improve movement quality.

Survivorship is a complex road in a breast cancer patient's journey. In addition to the enormous physical challenges, many patients experience psychological trauma resulting in depression, anxiety and fear. Dealing with a life-threatening disease and living with extended periods of stress can often lead to an increase in sympathetic nervous system activity (Won and Kim, 2016). Findings have shown that sympathetic activation may cause fascial contractions and potentially lead to an increase in fascial stiffness (Staubesand and Li, 1996; Bhowmick et al., 2009). The combination of moderate to low intensity movement therapy with integrative, contemplative practices such as yoga, meditation, Pilates and tai chi has shown improvements in sleep, anxiety, depression and quality of life for cancer patients (Buettner et al., 2006; Stan et al., 2012). Given that contemplative practices help decrease sympathetic tone, it could be speculated that it may, in turn, help decrease fascial stiffness.

Inflammation is another exercise-oncology research topic of interest. Inflammation is an extremely problematic human condition and is related to chronic musculoskeletal pain, different types of inflammatory diseases and cancer. Utilizing physically based treatments, known as mechano-therapeutics, as opposed to drugs

may play a positive role in the development and progression of cancer cells/tumors. Factors such as tissue stiffness, architecture of the tissue, and tissue forces in the matrix have a profound effect on the sustainability and progressive nature of cancers. When it comes to forces, there many unanswered questions: How much force? How should it be applied and for how long? (Berrueta et al., 2018).

For much of the 20th century, the vast majority of scientific efforts to understand and destroy cancer have focused on the cells, but not on the environment in which they live: the microenvironment. Cells in the human body, when operating under normal conditions, have specific jobs to do. They receive instructions from their genetic material and from signals in their environment and respond by obeying these commands. Langevin (2018) states that "cancer cells are cell that have gone rogue: they march to the beat of their own drum." Under normal circumstances there is a dynamic yet stable interaction between cells and their surrounding extra cellular matrix (ECM). Cancer development results when there are alterations to those normal interactions. Cancer cells appear to behave as masters of division, multiplying out of control and not stopping when it is appropriate, gradually invading the body.

Cellular response to both chronically inflamed tissue and cancer-associated tissues is to become contractile, increasing stiffness in the ECM by generating sustained and continued tension on the ECM. Increased stiffness in the ECM is accompanied by greater interstitial pressure and lymphatic flow, which may predispose an individual to fibrosis, cancer invasion and metastasis. Mechanical factors, i.e. physical force, can be a potential target for

Chapter 46

therapeutic intervention. As observed in animal models, just 10 min per day of simple stretching can potentially slow down the advancement of cancer (Langevin, 2018).

Movement therapy: phases of recovery

The movement therapy exercises outlined in this chapter are a sample of movements that may prove helpful with the various phases of breast cancer healing and recovery:

(1) Pre-habilitation (prehab) is a preparatory phase that begins as early as the day of diagnosis and continues until medical treatments commence. In this phase you are able to provide movement education and to prepare the patient for surgery and cancer treatment.

(2) Post-rehabilitation – phases I and II. The rehabilitation process is broken down into two segments that begins after preliminary tissue rehabilitation has occurred and/or the medical team has cleared the patient to perform a gentle range of motion and low-load strengthening. These phases are designed to re-educate the body-mind connection and to develop a strong physical foundation. The exercises can be used throughout the course of the patient's cancer journey to restore and rebuild their bodies.

Diagnosis and prehab

Upon diagnosis, patients undergo a continuum of defensive and protective behaviors, both emotional and physical. This is the time to begin preparing the mind and body for what is to come. Because this is pre-treatment, there are not many exercise restrictions. However, there should be a significant focus on muscular strength and endurance, especially of the upper body and core. Daily movement is key to keep both the mind stimulated and all systems of the body functioning.

For almost a decade, Hubert Godard and a team of researchers from the National Cancer Institute in Milan observed the physical and psychological damage of women with breast cancer. They conducted experiments with different groups of patients while walking and performing movements of daily life. One group was in the pre-operative phase and the other was in the post-surgical phase. In the pre-operative group, the researchers observed that as many as 50% of women had already begun to lose pendulousness or rhythmic swing quality in their affected limbs (arms) with just the news of the diagnosis, and also that the pendulousness would further decrease after surgery, in some cases as a complete arrest of the arm. In the post-surgical group, the researchers found unusual post-surgical limitations of the shoulder girdle, which could not be explained through traditional examinations. When walking, 65% of women demonstrated a loss of pendular motion in the arm on the affected side. The arm appeared anchored to the trunk, almost lifeless. Yet, when prompted to swing their arms symmetrically, they did so with no difficulty (Godard and Martino, 2001).

As witnessed in these experiments, patients diagnosed with breast cancer will begin to guard their body, subconsciously protecting the arm on the affected side, keeping it close to their side, not allowing it to hang loosely, or even swing naturally with gait. The early onset of this protective behavior may result in a physical manifestation, and greatly impact the health and function of the muscles and connective tissue, making them more rigid and stiff. Within as little as 2 to 3 weeks, immobilized rat limbs become rigid, lose elasticity and the connective tissue fibers become adhesive (Jarvinen, 2002). In my experience, the patients who enter the treatment process more aware of their bodies

Movement therapy for breast cancer survivors

and physically stronger have an easier time dealing with the physical limitations post-surgery. And as evidenced by Godard and Martino (2001), the patients were not aware they had developed this protective mechanism. The overall body posture in women who undergo mastectomies may be negatively affected, especially for those with large, heavy breasts (Haddad et al., 2013). Restrictions in the upper limbs and difficulty with upper-body tasks leave many women feeling physically and psychologically drained: the dysfunctions may remind them of their illness and lack of potential or full capacity in life (Collins et al., 2004). For the breast cancer patient, movement awareness and education is critical in the recovery process and may help with some of the painful and dehabilitating postural side effects from surgical and systemic treatments (Hojan et al., 2013).

Potential benefits of prehab movement therapy

- Maintain energy
- Remain emotionally grounded
- Build stamina
- Increase circulation and overall blood flow
- Foster mind-body connection
- Strengthen areas likely compromised by local and systemic treatments

Post-rehab phase I: movement therapy for breast cancer

At the first session, ensure you review the client's overall health history as well as the types of treatments and surgeries which they may have undergone. This information is instrumental in developing an effective and safe movement therapy program. Remember that you are not here to diagnose but to help with rehabilitation. Therefore, it is imperative that you prepare by gathering all of the facts before you begin. Keep in mind that the usual stages for tissue healing and exercise progression for a client who has had cancer differ greatly from a client who has an acute or chronic injury. Symptoms like muscle tightness and joint stiffness are present in both instances. However, while the symptomology may appear similar, you cannot treat a mastectomy or a lumpectomy as you would a rotator cuff or joint injury. Treatments such as chemotherapy and radiation coupled with surgery greatly affect the time it takes to heal and fully recover. Also, keep in mind that there are ongoing side effects that this client may experience which are unlike those an injured client may have.

Phase I exercises focus on developing the client's kinesthetic awareness and teach very basic biomechanical movement principles. These principles are foundational and can be part of the client's daily exercise regimen forever. After the initial screening, introduce simple biomechanical movement principles. The basic principles selected here are essential to both dynamic stability and mobility. These include:

- Breathing
- Pelvic placement
- Ribcage placement
- Scapula movement and stabilization
- Head and cervical placement

(Further information is available at https://www.merrithew.com/stott-pilates-basic-principles.)

In addition to the previously mentioned principles, listed below are five additional exercises which are appropriate for phase I.

Chapter 46

Focused breathing with mini-stability balls

Benefits: regulate the lymphatic system and rid the body of toxins. In addition to gravity and muscular contractions, the breath serves as the primary pump for the lymphatic system. The breath also encourages engagement of the deep core musculature: transversus abdominis, internal obliques, pelvic floor and multifidus, all of which are important for restoring posture and functional strength.

Start position: seated, kneeling or standing, holding the ball at chest or underarm. Choose ball size according to comfort level and range of motion.

Exercise and breath pattern: inhale deeply into the ball, exhale allow the ball to gently press against body. Stay for 3–5 full breaths in each position.

Beneficial cues: use the ball as a focal point to send the breath, expand the breath into the ball.

Limb bouncing – arms

Benefits: bouncing fosters rhythmic movement, spring-like, non-muscular, almost effortless action, and is intended to calm and restore.

Start position: lying supine on mat, knees bent.

(A) Arm by side with blue ball

(B) Arm in flexion with orange ball

Pre-tension arm before bouncing to feel tensional integrity in limb and to spark and sustain rhythmic bouncing.

Exercise and breath pattern: breathing is not dictated, it is natural. Stay for 20–30 s or until the movement feels like an effort.

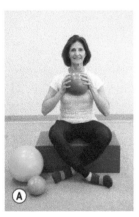 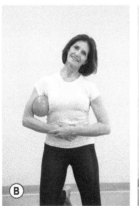 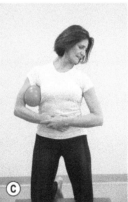

Figure 46.1 Focused Breathing with mini stability balls

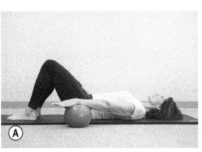 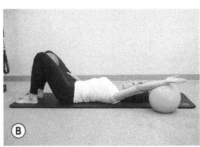

Figure 46.2 A&B Limb Bouncing – Arms

Movement therapy for breast cancer survivors

Beneficial cues: music is beneficial to foster one's rhythmic quality. Music at ~130 beats per min is optimal with arm bouncing.

Limb bouncing – legs

Benefits: bouncing fosters rhythmic movement, spring-like, non-muscular, almost effortless action, and is intended to calm and restore.

Start position: lying supine on mat with knees bent. Pre-tension leg before bouncing to feel tensional integrity in limb and to spark and sustain rhythmic bouncing.

Exercise and breath pattern: breathing is not dictated, it is natural. Stay for 20–30 s or until the movement feels like an effort.

Beneficial cues: music is beneficial to foster one's rhythmic quality when bouncing. Music at ~120–130 beats per min is optimal with leg bouncing.

Hamstring curls with sliders

Benefits: works the posterior chain, which is critical in regaining verticality and good posture. The slider provides proprioceptive stimulus to enhance stability of core musculature

and enable an ease of glide and facilitate smooth movement.

Start position: lying supine on mat with entire spine neutral, knees bent, feet dorsiflexed with heels on the sliders.

Exercise and breath pattern: inhale, slide both feet out as far as a neutral spine can be maintained exhale. Slide both feet back in to start position. Repeat 8–12 times.

Beneficial cues: apply just enough pressure to feel the muscles activate, use the breath to help control the movement. Keep upper body relaxed and focus on keeping trunk stable.

Standing hinge and low row with resistance loop

Benefits: hinging is a primary foundational movement pattern, necessary in many functional moves of daily living. Rows strengthen the shoulder girdle and posterior chain.

Start position: standing on resistance loop, holding ends of loop, palms facing in.

Exercise and breath pattern: inhale to hinge at hip maintaining neutral spine (Figure 46.5B),

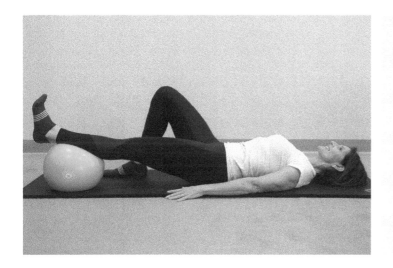

Figure 46.3 Limb Bouncing – Legs

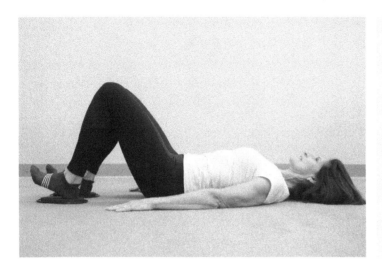

Figure 46.4 Hamstring Curls with Sliders

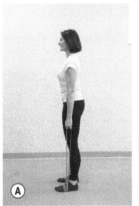
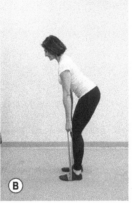
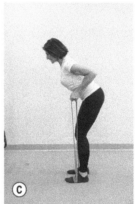

Figure 46.5 A-C Standing Hinge & Low Row with Resistance Loop

exhale, squeeze shoulder blades together and slightly down, and pull band in close to the body (Figure 46.5C). Repeat row pattern 8–12 times.

Beneficial cues: keep body from shifting back when hinging at hips, keep spine neutral throughout.

Movement therapists should remember that it is critical in phase I to avoid taxing or overworking any one area of the body. Select one or two exercises for the upper body and then one or two for the lower body. Follow the recommended repetitions but pay close attention to the ability of the client and let the weaker side determine the amount of resistance and number of repetitions.

Always support the affected limbs with pillows or cushions when necessary, and only work in a comfortable range of motion. Never work through pain.

Post-rehab phase II – movement therapy for breast cancer

The goal of the phase II exercises is to continue building upon the foundations set in the previous phase. These foundations focus on restoring joint mobility with a range of gentle motion exercises designed to break down residual scar tissue, both from surgery and various treatments. We continue our work to increase

Movement therapy for breast cancer survivors

overall body awareness with slow, controlled and concentrated movements. Introduce the following low-load exercises to strengthen the local stabilizers, promote joint stability and enhance neuromuscular control. Use a layering effect as you add each new exercise, and keep a record of what you have added. This will help you to determine which exercises the client can withstand and which may be overly challenging. If you add too many new exercises at once then you will not know which move could be problematic.

Limb bouncing – arms

Benefits: bouncing fosters rhythmic movement, spring-like, non-muscular, almost effortless action, and is intended to calm and restore.

Start position: supine on mat, arm in flexion overhead resting on ball, palm up or in any comfortable position. Pre-tension arm before bouncing to feel tensional integrity in limb and to spark and sustain rhythmic bouncing.

Exercise and breath pattern: breathing is not dictated, it is natural. Stay for 20–30 s or until the movement feels like an effort.

Beneficial cues: music is beneficial to foster one's rhythmic quality when bouncing. Music at ~130 beats per min is optimal with arm bouncing.

Hamstring curl bridge combo

Benefits: this version adds the bridge, which will increase the workload of the posterior chain and place additional emphasis on the core.

Start position: lying supine with hips extended to a lower hover over mat, knees bent, feet dorsiflexed with heels on the sliders.

Exercise and breath pattern: inhale, slide one foot out as far as a neutral spine can be maintained. Exhale, return to start position. Repeat, alternating legs 5–8 times.

Note: to progress this exercise slide both feet out.

Beneficial cues: apply just enough pressure to feel the muscles activate, use the breath to help control the movement, keep the upper body relaxed and focus on keeping trunk stable.

Standing flexion and abduction

Benefits: increase strength in abductors of hip, improves posture and balance.

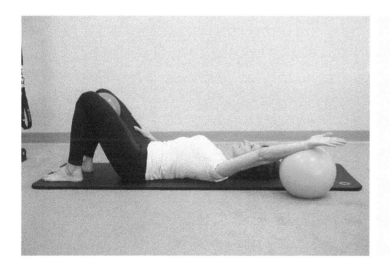

Figure 46.6 Limb Bouncing – Arms

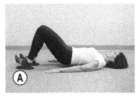 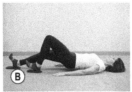 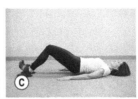

Figure 46.7 A–C Hamstring Curl Bridge Combo

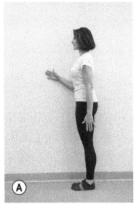 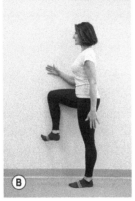 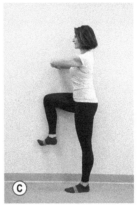

Figure 46.8 A–C Standing Flexion & Abduction

Start position: standing sideways about one foots distance from wall. Place inside arm against wall for balance.

Exercise and breath pattern: inhale to lift inside knee to hip height, exhale press knee against wall (Figure 46.8B) and if possible bring arms to the genie position in front of body for balance (Figure 46.8C). Stay and breath for 2–3 full breaths and return to start position. Repeat three times on each side of the body.

Beneficial cues: keep tension on lateral aspect of outside leg but maintain neutral foot and knee alignment, stay tall.

Standing low row with resistance loop

Benefits: enhances slide and glide of scapula, increases strength in shoulder girdle muscles, excellent for posture. The loop anchored high will strengthen the lower trapezius muscles.

Start position: standing facing anchor of resistance loop (loop anchored high), hold loop with hands, palms facing in, arms extended long in front of body.

Exercise and breath pattern: inhale, prepare. Exhale, squeeze shoulder blades together and slightly down, and pull band in close to body. Repeat row pattern 8–12 times.

Beneficial cues: think of the scapula sliding in and down the back.

Forearm plank scapula isolations

Benefits: the plank is the gold standard in core stability, using the ball supports the trunk and provides a good assist until strength to hold full plank is achieved.

Start position: prone with forearms on mat, orange ball placed under the pelvis and lower trunk, knees bent, toes curled under.

Exercise and breath pattern: inhale to prepare. Exhale to lift knees off mat to full plank position. Remain in plank for 3–5 full breaths breathing normally.

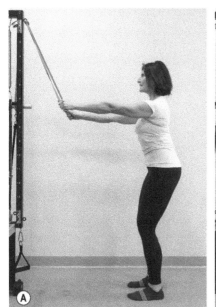

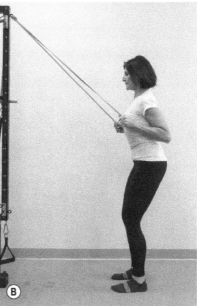

Figure 46.9 A&B Standing Low Row with resistance loop

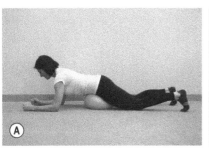

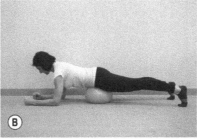

Figure 46.10 A&B Forearm Plank Scapula Isolations

Beneficial cues: keep the body taut to avoid sagging or collapse. Use the breath to maintain posture. Avoid sinking into the ball.

Be mindful of these phase II contraindications:

- Progressing too quickly
- Using too heavy a load and potentially stressing the joints
- Not adhering to a client's needs and physician recommendations
- Overworking the limbs, especially in the affected areas
- Not allowing for adequate rest and recovery between sessions

A strong component of body-mind exercise is empowering the client by increasing their kinesthetic awareness. As this happens, the client becomes more familiar with her own body from one day to the next and can recognize when things are not quite right.

By arming our clients with simple, effective exercises, we provide them with the tools they need to become self-reliant, to enjoy a higher quality of life and be more functional in everyday activities.

Chapter 46

References

APTA (2020) Lymphedema Fact Sheet for Consumers https://oncologypt.org/wp-content/uploads/2020/02/Lymphedema-Fact-Sheet-for-Consumers.pdf [last accessed September 2020]

Berrueta, L., Bergholz, J., Munoz, D., Muskag, I., Badger, G.J., Zhao, J.J. & Langevin, H.M. (2018) Stretching reduces tumor growth in a mouse breast cancer model. *Sci Rep*. 8: 1–7.

Bhowmick, S., Singh, A., Flavell, R.A., Clark, R.B., O'Rourke, J. & Cone, R. (2009) The sympathetic nervous system modulates CD4 FoxP3 regulatory T cells via a TGF-β-dependent mechanism. *J Leukoc Biol*. 86(6): 1275–1283.

Buettner, C., Kroenke, C.H., Phillips, R.S., Davis, R.B., Eisenberg, D.M. & Holmes, M.D. (2006) Correlates of use of different types of complementary and alternative medicine by breast cancer survivors in the nurses' health study. *Breast Cancer Res Treat*. 100: 219–227.

Collins, L.G., Nash, R., Roud, T. & Neuman, B. (2004) Perceptions of upper-body problems during recovery from breast cancer treatment. *Support Care Cancer*. 12: 106–113.

Cyriac, C., Sharma, R.K. & Singh, G. (2010) Assessment of the abdominal wall function after pedicled TRAM flap surgery for breast reconstruction: use of modified mesh repair for the donor defect. *Indian J Plast Surg*. 43: 166–172.

Dieli-Conwright, C.M. & Orozco, B.Z. (2015) Exercise after breast cancer treatment: current perspectives. *Breast Cancer (Dove Med Press)*. 7: 353–362.

Ebaugh, D., Spinelli, B. & Schmitz, K.H. (2011) Shoulder impairments and their association with symptomatic rotator cuff disease in breast cancer survivors. *Med Hypotheses*. 77: 481–487.

Fourie, W. (2008) Considering wider myofascial involvement as a possible contributor to upper extremity dysfunction following treatment for primary breast cancer. *J Bodyw Mov Ther*. 12: 349–355.

Godard, H. & Martino, G. (2001) Motioned e-motion. In: Biondi, M., Costantini, A. & Grassi, L. (Eds), *Manuale di oncologia in psicooncologia*. Milan, Italy: Masson, 875–881.

Haddad, C.A., Saad, M., Perez, M. & Miranda Júnior, F. (2013) Assessment of posture and joint movements of the upper limbs of patients after mastectomy and lymphadenectomy. *Einstein (Sao Paulo)*. 11: 426–434.

Helms, R.L., O'Hea, E.L. & Corso, M. (2008) Body image issues in women with breast cancer. *Psychol Health Med*. 13: 313–125.

Hojan, K. & Milecki, P. (2013) Opportunities for rehabilitation of patients with radiation fibrosis syndrome. *Rep Pract Oncol Radiother*. 19: 1–6.

Hsieh, C.C., Sprod, L.K., Hydock, D.S., Carter, S.D., Hayward, R. & Schneider, C.M. (2008) Effects of a supervised exercise intervention on recovery from treatment regimens in breast cancer survivors. *Oncol Nurs Forum*. 35: 909–915.

Jarvinen, T.A., Jozsa, L., Kannus, P., Jarvinen, T.L. & Jarvinen M. (2002) Organization and distribution of intramuscular connective tissue in normal and immobilized skeletal muscles: An immunohistochemical polarization and scanning electron microscopic study. *J Musc Res Cell Mot*, 23: 245–54.

Kaelin, C.M., Coltrera, F., Gardiner, J. & Prouty, J. (2006) *The breast cancer survivor's fitness plan: a doctor-approved workout plan for a strong body and lifesaving results*. New York, NY: McGraw-Hill Education.

Langevin, H.M., Keely, P., Mao, J., Hodge, L.M., Schleip, R., Deng, G., Hinz, B., Swartz, M.A., deValois, B.A., Zick, S. & Findley, T. (2016) Connecting (t)issues: how research in fascia biology can impact integrative oncology. *Cancer Res*. 76: 6159–6162.

Langevin, H. (2018) Connective tissue, inflammation and cancer. Lecture presented June 5, 2018 at Grand Rounds at Osher Center for Integrative Medicine, Harvard Medical School, Boston, MA.

Mutrie, N., Campbell, A.M., Whyte, F., McConnachie, A., Emslie, C., Lee, L., Kearney, N., Walker, A. & Ritchie, D. (2007) Benefits of supervised group exercise programme for women being treated for early stage breast cancer: pragmatic randomized controlled trial. *BMJ*. 334: 517.

National Institutes of Health Osteoporosis and Related Bone Diseases National Resource Center (2016) What breast cancer survivors need to know about osteoporosis. NIH Publication No. 16–7898.

Provenzano, P.P., Inman, D.R., Eliceiri, K.W., Knittel, J.G., Yan, L., Rueden, C.T., White, J.G. & Keely, P.J. (2008) Collagen density promotes mammary tumor initiation and progression. *BMC Med.* 6: 11.

Sprague, B.L., Trentham-Dietz, A., Newcomb, P.A., Titus-Ernstoff, L., Hampton, J.M. & Egan, K.M. (2007) Lifetime recreational and occupational physical activity and risk of in situ and invasive breast cancer. *Cancer Epidemiol Biomarkers Prev.* 16: 236–243.

Stan, D.L., Collins, N.M., Olsen, M.M., Croghan, I. & Pruthi, S. (2012) The evolution of mindfulness-based physical interventions in breast cancer survivors. *Evid Based Complement Alternat Med.* 2012: 1–15.

Stasi, R., Abriani, L., Beccaglia, P., Terzoli, E. & Amadori, S. (2003) Cancer-related fatigue: evolving concepts in evaluation and treatment. *Cancer.* 98: 1786–1801.

Staubesand, J. & Li, Y. (1996) On the fine structure of the crural fascia, with particular reference to the epi- and intrafascial nerves. *Manuelle Medizin.* 34: 196–200.

Villasenor, A., Ballard-Barbash, R., Baumgartner, K., Baumgartner, R., Bernstein, L., McTiernan, A. & Neuhausen, M.L. (2012) Prevalence and prognostic effect of sarcopenia in breast cancer survivors: the HEAL Study. *J Cancer Surviv.* 6(4): 398–406.

Won, E. & Kim, Y.K. (2016) Stress, the autonomic nervous system, and the immune-kynurenine pathway in the etiology of depression. *Curr Neuropharmacol.* 14: 665–673.

World Health Organization (2018) Breast cancer. https://www.who.int/cancer/prevention/diagnosis-screening/breast-cancer/en/.

Additional resources

Courneya, K.S., Mackey, J.R., Bell, G.J., Jones, L.W., Field, C.J. & Fairey, A.S. (2003) Randomized controlled trial of exercise training in postmenopausal breast cancer survivors: cardiopulmonary and quality of life outcomes. *J Clin Oncol.* 21: 1660–1668.

Dubashi, B., Vidhubala, E., Cyriac, S. & Sagar, T.G. (2010) Quality of life among young women with breast cancer: study from a tertiary cancer institute in south India. *Indian J Cancer.* 47: 142–147.

Eyigor, S. & Kanyilmaz, S. (2014) Exercise in patients coping with breast cancer: an overview. *World J Clin Oncol.* 5: 406–411.

Eyigor, S., Karapolat, H., Yesil, H., Uslu, R. & Durmaz, B. (2010) Effects of pilates exercises on functional capacity, flexibility, fatigue, depression and quality of life in female breast cancer patients: a randomized controlled study. *Eur J Phys Rehabil Med.* 46: 481–487.

Hamer, J. & Warner, E. (2017) Lifestyle modifications for patients with breast cancer to improve prognosis and optimize overall health. *CMAG.* 189: E268–E74.

Holmes, M.D., Chen, W.Y., Feskanich, D., Kroenke, C.H., & Colditz, G.A. (2005) Physical activity and survival after breast cancer diagnosis. *JAMA.* 20: 2479–2486.

Irwin, M.L., Smith, A.W., McTiernan, A., Ballard-Barbash, R., Cronin, K., Gilliland, F.D., Baumgartner, R.N., Baumgartner, K.B. & Bernstein, L. (2008) Influence of pre- and postdiagnosis physical activity on mortality in breast cancer survivors: the health, eating, activity, and lifestyle study. *J Clin Oncol.* 26: 3958–3964.

Kummer, F., Catuogno, S., Perseus, J.M., Bloch, W. & Baumann, F.T. (2013) Relationship between cancer-related fatigue and physical activity in inpatient cancer rehabilitation. *Anticancer Res.* 33: 3415–3422.

Lahart, I.M., Metsios, G.S., Nevill, A.M. & Carmichael, A.R. (2015) Physical activity, risk of death and recurrence in breast cancer survivors: a systematic review and meta-analysis of epidemiological studies. *Acta Oncologica.* 54: 635–654.

McNeely, M.L., Campbell, K.L., Rowe, B.H., Klassen, T. P., Mackey, J. R. & Courneya, K. S. (2006) Effects of exercise on breast cancer patients and survivors: a systematic review and meta-analysis. *Oncol Nurs Forum.* 25: 107–113.

Schwartz, A.L., Mori, M., Gao, R., Nail, L.M. & King, M.E. (2001) Exercise reduces daily fatigue in women with breast cancer receiving chemotherapy. *Med Sci Sports Exerc.* 33: 718–723.

Mental imagery, fascia and movement

Amit Abraham and Eric Franklin

Introduction

Cognition (the neural processes involved in perceiving, interpreting and using sensory information) is an integral component of movement. Cognitive elements of awareness, consciousness, somatics and mindfulness have traditionally referred to an individual's power to strategically use the mind to influence physical and emotional spheres. Cognition is important to daily functioning, mind-body and movement practices, sports and rehabilitation. As sensory stimuli from the environment often require split-second motor responses, the body and mind work together to make predictions and take appropriate actions. Cognitive tools of mentally envisioning and rehearsing scenes or outcomes are known as mental imagery (MI) (Guillot and Collet, 2010). Such tools are particularly relevant in sport and movement, for which a combination of mental and physical elements is fundamental. Research into the potential associations between cognition, including MI, and fascia, is in its infancy. However, based on research to date, there are at least three possible avenues in which a pairing of MI with fascia can be identified to support movement and well-being: (1) Fascia can serve as an attentional focus, including during MI; (2) MI positively affects muscle tissue (Slimani et al., 2016) and, given the cellular, physiological and functional similarities existing between muscle and fascia tissue, MI likely also affects fascia; and (3) fascia can respond to

chemical and mechanical stimuli (Schleip et al., 2019), so its responsiveness to cognitive stimuli such as MI cannot be ruled out.

This chapter presents a rationale for possible interactions between MI and fascia, and discusses ways in which the two can communicate to support mental and physical well-being. Specifically, examples are provided of traditional and novel ways in which fascia-related MI can assist the mind-body synergy within a context of movement, sports and rehabilitation.

What is mental imagery?

MI is the self-generated cognitive process of creating any picture, experience (visual, kinesthetic, auditory, gustatory, etc.) or scene in the mind, typically with the goal of influencing a physical or psychological outcome (Guillot and Collet, 2010). The closer the mental image is to creating a multisensory experience of realism, the better and more effective MI is. For example, sitting in an armchair at home, one can image being at the beach with feet resting on warn sand (kinesthetic), watching the sun dipping below the horizon (visual), hearing the sound of the waves breaking on the shore (auditory), and tasting the salt air (gustatory), all in order to bring the imaged experience closer and closer to that of actually being there.

As a fundamentally trainable human skill, the ability to easily and clearly create a mental image gets better with practice, even in cases where cognition is negatively impacted, such as in sport-related concussions or neurodegenerative diseases (Abraham et al., 2018). When associated with movement, MI is called motor imagery, which can be used solely or in conjunction with actual physical execution of the movement. For example, while imaging bending and extending the elbow, a person can focus on the feeling (kinesthetic) and/or visual experience, with or without actually moving it. The details of a real and/or an imaged experience can arise as the performer notices his or her internal kinesthetic experiences of the body, movement, sensations and thoughts, as well as details of the imaged environment's scenes and objects. Visual MI can take the perspective of an internal (first-person) imaging of the scene through one's own eyes or an external (third-person) view of oneself in a scene from some distance away.

Mental images can include both real (anatomical or biomechanical) or fictional (metaphorical) contents about the body itself, including its tissues, cells, organs and body parts. Metaphorical images are those that adapt a borrowed quality/ idea from one object and apply it to another. For example, if while landing from a jump one can image the foot to be an elastic arched rubber band that is being slightly flattened on impact, the quality and characteristics of the metaphor (the rubber band s elasticity and energy absorption and storage capabilities) may facilitate the foot's normal biomechanics and thus possibly enhance the mobility and flexibility required for maximum performance and injury prevention.

Beneficial effects of MI include increased muscle power, range of motion and movement efficiency; improved memory and dual tasking; and increased self-confidence and reduced anxiety and pain (motor, cognitive and psychological

outcomes, respectively). Such diverse beneficial effects explain why MI is used as a training method to enhance performance in sports, movement and rehabilitation (Dickstein and Deutsch, 2007; Abraham et al., 2016, 2017). As a training method, MI can be used in isolation or in conjunction with other physical training approaches, including physical and occupational therapy, Feldenkrais, yoga and Pilates. Furthermore, MI has assisted with movement outcomes in a variety of populations, from athletes and dancers to older adults and people with neurodegenerative conditions, such as Parkinson s disease and multiple sclerosis. Indeed, MI is available even when pain, paralysis or physical confinement limits or prohibits physical training, such as after an injury or surgery.

MI assists beginners and elite experts at all stages of learning a task by cueing attention to the body, for example, by saying, "As you move, image your entire body filled with balloons" (Figure 47.1) or by offering a reassuring image to overcome fear or other limitations in range of motion. MI s advantages include its ready availability, low cost and safety of use.

How does mental imagery work?

How and why MI positively affects physiological and psychological aspects of movement is not yet fully understood. It is known that mentally imaging a motor task (e.g. lifting a leg) activates the same brain regions as those responsible for actually performing the task, albeit to a somewhat more limited degree (Guillot and Collet, 2010). Such brain activation provides a training effect without physical execution. Furthermore, mentally replicating a motor task, along with other task-related sensory and cognitive information, allows for further improvements in the performance of the task.

Mental imagery, fascia and movement

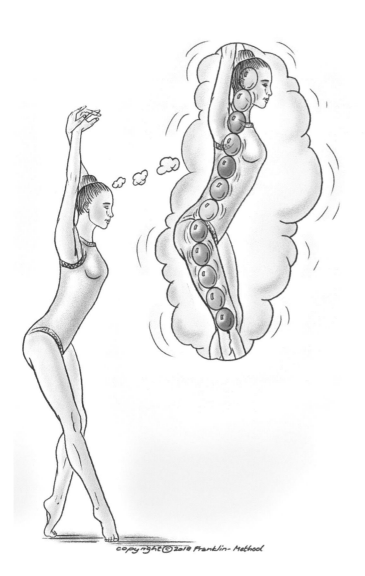

Figure 47.1 Cueing attention to the body through MI's metaphor of moving while imaging one's entire body filled with balloons
Original drawing by Mr. Eric Franklin, all rights reserved.

MI s contribution to neural changes in the central nervous system results in greater relaxation and improved programming of the motor system (Yue and Cole, 1992; Yue et al., 1996). Given the close anatomical and functional association between muscle and fascia tissues, neural processes within the myofascial system can contribute to MI s physiological and psychological mechanisms of effect. For example, by addressing both muscle sarcomeres and their surrounding fascia, MI could intensify the recruitment of motor units (Helm et al., 2015). Insofar as MI addresses the autonomic nervous system, blood flow and other physiological variables, such as heart rate and stress levels, are impacted (Collet et al., 2013).

Potential psychological mechanisms of MI include facilitation of the cognitive elements

Chapter 47

associated with skill execution and motor learning, including attentional focus, self-awareness and various movement patterns. As MI directs attentional focus to the engaged fascial tissue throughout movement preparation and execution, fascia's role in skill execution and motor learning can interact with, and potentially be enhanced by, the cognitive tool of MI for mutual benefit. As MI supports healthy functional fascial tissue, movement and performance are improved. In return, as the body feels and functions better, one more easily imagines positive outcomes and so is able to use MI more effectively. Details of the ways in which this beneficial interaction could happen are included below.

The role of sensory information in mental imagery

Previous experiences play a part in perceiving, interpreting and responding to subsequent ones, as in conscious perception where memories or experiences become integrated with the ongoing sensory information. Similarly, personal experiences and sensory information can affect MI. That is, having a previous experience with a motor task, scene or sensation often promotes a more vivid, accurate and complete mental image created by the brain more quickly and easily. A previous experience that entails wrong or negative information and memories about the task tends to hamper both physical performance and MI. For example, people experiencing pain are often limited in their physical capabilities and so are prone to generate more negative mental images. Individuals with chronic pain experience greater difficulties engaging in MI when compared with asymptomatic individuals, including more time being required to complete MI tasks and less clarity of the mental images being formed (Bowering et al., 2013). It is logical to assume that pain originating from fascial tissue (such as in low back pain or fascia-related syndromes) will also impede MI. Interestingly, MI can reduce, or increase, pain depending on the imaged contents (Fardo et al., 2015). Facilitating more positive mental images about the fascial tissue could, therefore, offer a therapeutic tool for sufferers of fascia-related pain.

Another way in which sensory information from fascia can affect MI is through its effects on body schema. Body schema is the mental representation of one s body and its parts in space and in relation to each other. Body schema is formed from sensory information derived from the different body parts and tissues (often referred to as proprioception). Body schema deficits, as seen in brain damage or neuro-degenerative diseases, degrades MI. Insofar as the sensory and mechanical capabilities of fascial tissue involved in biomechanics, posture and movement contribute to body schema, sensory-proprioceptive information from fascia can affect MI, including that of body schema. In a study of people with Parkinson's disease, participants were able to improve their pelvic schema (assessed by self-drawings) following a 2-week MI training intervention (Abraham et al., 2019b). An improvement in body schema due to MI training can be, at least in part, attributed to clearer and intensified fascia-related sensory-proprioceptive information leading to increased fascial awareness. More ways in which MI can affect sensory and motor experiences are discussed below.

Can mental imagery modulate actual motor and sensory experiences?

As MI uses, and is affected by, sensory and motor experiences and information that includes those from the fascia, the path from MI to fascia-related sensory-motor experiences opens the door to fascia-related cognitive-motor integration. MI's facilitation of correct body biomechanics and schema enhances motor and non-motor aspects of performance. By directing attentional focus and facilitating the many components associated with a task, MI helps shape the mental experience of that motor task. Adding movement to MI further promotes better and safer movement as increased brain activity facilitates a direct, immediate and concrete connection between the mental image and its desired effect on movement, posture, body schema and emotional well-being. In a study in dancers, MI ability and MI "positive" contents were positively correlated with increased confidence and decreased anxiety levels, suggesting that MI plays a role in psychological aspects of performance (Monsma and Overby, 2004).

In summary, MI is affected by motor and sensory experiences and information from the body and the environment. MI is also capable of facilitating and modulating sensory and motor actual experiences and information.

Mental imagery of fascia

Mental imagery of fascia (aka fascial MI) specifically addresses the dynamic structure, range of function, and applicable metaphors of fascial tissue, given that the latter is often not easily felt, palpated, or recognized. One fascial MI approach currently practiced is a division of Dynamic Neuro-Cognitive Imagery (DNI®; also known as "The Franklin Method"®). DNI is an evidence- and science-based (Heiland et al., 2012, 2013; Franklin, 2014; Abraham et al., 2019a) MI approach to movement, postural retraining and rehabilitation that combines MI components (e.g. metaphorical imagery, anatomical imagery, and visual and kinesthetic imagery) with anatomical and biomechanical embodiment and mindful movement. DNI's tools of self-talk and self-touch increase fascial understanding and awareness through experiential embodiment. DNI's fascial MI combines anatomical, biomechanical and metaphorical cues with visual and kinesthetic MI of the dynamic, three-dimensional nature of the movement's fascial actions. For example, the thoraco-lumbar fascia can be imaged as a slippery web changing its shape as the arm reaches forward and up (Figure 47.2). Given the dynamic nature of fascia and its contribution to biomechanics and movement, fascial MI used alongside actual movement in training and rehabilitative settings can later be used by the performer and the trainer/therapist to communicate the desired aspects of the movement. For example, the expression "thoracolumbar fascia as a web" (Figure 2) could serve as a means of communication between the performer and their trainer/therapist to provide a clear and efficient cue in subsequent interactions.

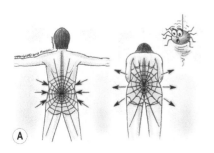

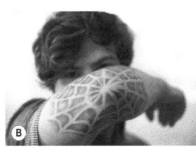

Figure 47.2

(A) Metaphorical DNI of the thoracolumbar fascia as a moveable web (drawn by Mr. Eric Franklin, all rights reserved). **(B)** A tattoo of a web on a skin illustrates the dynamic nature of the web (photographer: Karina Glikin-Yaari, all rights reserved).

Chapter 47

Using mental imagery as a cueing and instructional strategy

Integrating MI within an exercise and training regimen involving fascia is a process of combining art and science from the fields of cognition, communication and psychology. Communicating MI with cues and instructions in movement practice requires concentration, self-awareness and attentional focus. It also requires that the cues be tailored to the knowledge, skills and experiences of the performer. Anatomical and biomechanical MI especially require a knowledge and vocabulary of the field. Metaphorical MI is personal and subjective, so such cues need to be adjusted and tailored to the specific individual. For example, cueing a client to relax the shoulders with the DNI image of "the fascia of your upper trapezius melting like honey" may unexpectedly lead to tense shoulders in an individual who is allergic to honey. Therefore, creating efficient and effective MI requires ongoing mutual feedback between the instructor/therapist and the performer. It is important to regularly ask the performer to notice and report any thoughts about the experiences with different mental images. Doing so allows the brain to register and record the novel mental image and the experience associated with it. Additionally, asking for feedback from the performer allows for a clear and common MI language to be built with the goal of optimizing motor performance. With this caveat in mind, we invite you to "try on, like trying on different outfits" the DNI images below. Notice for yourself any changes in your physical and cognitive experiences of movement.

Dynamic neuro-cognitive imagery exercises for mental imagery and fascia

Below are three examples that specifically address fascial tissue with fascial DNI. Each consists of anatomical, biomechanical and metaphorical MI, although to different degrees, and all three are performed while moving.

Exercise 1. Reciprocal motion of the fascia of the arm (Figure 47.3)

1. Focus on the muscles of the right upper arm and image the fascia located there surrounding, separating and connecting the muscles (brachialis, biceps, triceps).

2. Image the fascia to be a stocking, with a color and a texture of your choosing.

3. Flex your elbow, and as the biceps contracts, image the stocking around it shortening and widening.

4. Image the biceps muscle bulging and filling the fascial stocking, as the fascial stocking is expanding and creating space for the biceps muscle (Figure 47. 3B).

5. Image the triceps stocking stretching, lengthening and narrowing as the elbow flexes.

6. Image the fascia "squishing the triceps into length, like squishing toothpaste down its tube".

7. As you extend the elbow, image the opposite: the triceps muscle is bulging and filling the fascial stocking and the fascial stocking expanding and pushing back against the triceps muscle.

8. At the same time, image the biceps stocking stretching, lengthening and narrowing as the elbow extends. Image the fascia squishing the biceps into length, like squishing toothpaste down its tube (Figure 47. 3A).

9. Repeat 5–6 times while focusing on this mental image during the movement.

10. Let go of the hands and compare the right and the left side. Do you feel any

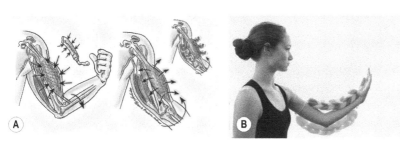

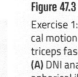

Figure 47.3

Exercise 1: Imaging reciprocal motion of the biceps and triceps fascia of the arm. **(A)** DNI anatomical and metaphorical illustration (drawn by Mr. Eric Franklin, all rights reserved), and **(B)** visual and kinesthetic modeling with sponges (photographer: Karina Glikin-Yaari, all rights reserved).

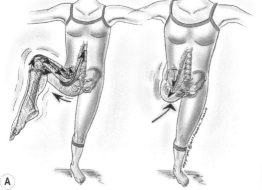

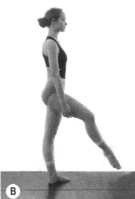

Figure 47.4

Exercise 2: Fascial mobility during a leg motion. **(A)** DNI illustration of fascial movement during a leg swing (drawn by Mr. Eric Franklin, all rights reserved), and **(B)** a model demonstrating a leg swinging forward (photographer: Karina Glikin-Yaari, all rights reserved).

differences? Do you feel the right arm more relaxed, elongated and energetic?

11. Repeat the exercise on the left arm.

Exercise 2. Fascial envelope during a leg swing (Figure 47.4)

1. Stand on one leg and swing the other leg backwards and forwards with the thigh lifted and the knee bent.

2. As the leg swings to the front, image the fascia of the posterior aspect of the lower extremity (all the way to the toes) lengthening. Try to image its dynamic connections with the thoraco-lumbar fascia. Image the hip flexors and specifically the iliopsoas muscles shortening and bulging against its fascia (Figure 47.4A).

3. When swinging the leg backward, image the pushing and bulging of the gluteus muscle and erector spinae muscles against their fasciae. Image also the fascia of the anterior aspect of the leg (all the way to the toes) lengthening. Focus specifically on the fascia of the iliopsoas muscle lengthening (Figure 47.4B).

4. You can also image the fascial envelope around the whole body and notice how it changes during the movement. As the leg swings forward, image the posterior fascia with a metaphor of a big net stretching across the wall of your whole back and leg. As the leg swings backward, image the metaphorical net of the anterior fascia lengthening across the front of the body, particularly on the side of the extending leg.

Chapter 47

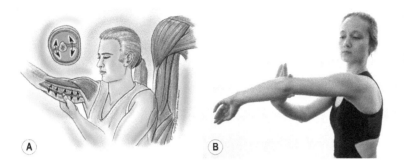

5. Pause and compare sides. Do you feel any difference? Do you feel one leg is more vivid and elastic?

6. Now perform the same exercise on the other leg.

Exercise 3. Anatomical and metaphorical imagery of the inter-muscular septa of the arm (Figure 47.5)

1. Place your left hand on top of the right biceps muscle with your thumb on the medial intermuscular septum and your fingers on the lateral intermuscular septum, so that your hand is on top of the biceps.

2. Image the space between the biceps and the triceps muscles; this is where the septum is located and the humerus bone can be felt. Now try to palpate it with your fingers, carefully as these areas contain nerves and vessels, and the area may be tender.

3. Rotate your arm medially and laterally, and use your other hand to pull the biceps muscle in the opposite direction. Mobilize both medial and lateral septa, and image them being stretchy like rubber.

4. Now switch to holding the triceps muscle with fingers and thumb on both septa and rotate your arm counter to your gentle pull on the triceps. Image stretchy septa (Figure 47.5A).

5. Move your left fingers down the arm along the septa to the medial and lateral epicondyles of the humerus. As you rub and mobilize the area, image the fascial tissue of the septa below. Also, image the anatomical fascial boundary between the biceps muscle on top of the humerus and the triceps muscle beneath it.

6. Gently rub both septa just proximal to the medial and lateral epicondyles. Then push outward on both epicondyles of humerus. Image the septa lengthening as if you were pulling on a rubber band in a variety of directions (Figure 47.5B).

7. Let go of both hands and notice any differences between the right and left arms. Does the right arm feel more relaxed or energetic? Flex both elbows and notice any differences between them in power and ease of movement.

8. Now switch hands and repeat the process on the other arm. Notice any differences between the two sides.

Conclusion

MI is a dynamic, complex phenomenon affected by and interacting with various elements, including sensory stimuli from within the body as well as from the environment. The relationship suggested in this chapter between MI and fascia relies on mutual and interactive cognitive and anatomical-physiological mechanisms. As MI of fascial tissue holds potential for enhancing fascial awareness and perception, including it in therapy (e.g., bodywork, physical and occupational therapy, osteopathy, structural integration, etc.), may result in positive outcomes in movement, body schema and pain reduction. Complementary to that, by potentially modulating sensory information from and about the fascia, MI may affect actual fascia-related sensory and motor experiences. These mechanisms of effect are currently only science-driven hypotheses, but ones which open a window to new research paths. If confirmed, proven connections between MI and fascia could enhance collective knowledge about fascial movement, awareness and perception.

Insofar as MI is a creative process of self-discovery and given the effect of movement on it, the more one moves, the more it is possible for the brain to form and offer mental images and metaphors. Respecting individual differences among movers as well as trial and error is encouraged when it comes to MI. If one image does not work, try a different one. You may be surprised by the results.

References

Abraham, A., Dunsky, A. & Dickstein, R. (2016) Motor imagery practice for enhancing elevé performance among professional dancers: a pilot study. *Med Probl Perform Art.* 31: 132–139.

Abraham, A., Dunsky, A. & Dickstein, R. (2017) The effect of motor imagery practice on elevé performance in adolescent female dance students: a randomized controlled trial. *J Imagery Res Sport Phys Activ.* 12: 20160006.

Abraham, A., Gose, R., Schindler, R., Nelson, B.H. & Hackney, M.E. (2019a) Dynamic neuro-cognitive imagery (DNITM) improves developpé performance, kinematics, and mental imagery ability in university-level dance students. *Front Psychol.* 10: 382.

Abraham, A., Hart, A., Dickstein, R., Hackney, M.E. (2019b) "Will you draw me a pelvis?" Dynamic neuro-cognitive imagery improves pelvic schema and graphic-metric representation in people with Parkinson's disease: a randomized controlled trial. *Complement Ther Med.* 43: 28–35.

Abraham, A., Hart, A., Andrade, I. & Hackney, M.E. (2018) Dynamic neuro-cognitive imagery (DNI™) improves mental imagery ability, disease severity, and motor and cognitive functions in people with Parkinson's disease. *Neural Plast.* 2018: 6168507.

Bowering, K.J., O'Connell, N.E., Tabor, A., Catley, M.J., Leake, H.B., Moseley, G.L. & Stanton, T. R. (2013) The effects of graded motor imagery and its components on chronic pain: a systematic review and meta-analysis. *J Pain.* 14: 3–13.

Collet, C., Di Rienzo, F., El Hoyek, N. & Guillot, A. (2013) Autonomic nervous system correlates in movement observation and motor imagery. *Front Hum Neurosci.* 7: 415.

Dickstein, R. & Deutsch, J.E. (2007) Motor imagery in physical therapist practice. *Phys Ther.* 87: 942–953.

Fardo, F., Allen, M., Jegindo, E.M., Angrilli, A. & Roepstorff, A. (2015) Neurocognitive evidence for mental imagery-driven hypoalgesic and hyperalgesic pain regulation. *Neuroimage.* 120: 350–361.

Franklin, E. (2014) Fascia Release and Balance: Franklin Method Ball and Imagery Exercises, OPTP.

Guillot, A. & Collet, C. (2010) *The neurophysiological foundations of mental and motor imagery.* USA: Oxford University Press.

Heiland, T. & Rovetti, R. (2013) Examining effects of Franklin method metaphorical and anatomical mental images on college dancers' jumping height. *Res Dance Educ.* 14: 141–161.

Heiland, T.L., Rovetti, R., Dunn, J. (2012) Effects of visual, auditory, and kinesthetic imagery interventions on dancers' plié arabesques. *J Imagery Res Sport Phys Activ.* 7: article 5.

Helm, F., Marinovic, W., Kruger, B., Munzert, J. & Riek, S. (2015) Corticospinal excitability during imagined and observed dynamic force production tasks: effortfulness matters. *Neuroscience.* 290: 398–405.

Monsma, E.V. & Overby, L.Y. (2004) The relationship between imagery and competitive anxiety in ballet auditions. *J Dance Med Sci.* 8: 11–18.

Schleip, R., Gabbiani, G., Wilke, J., Naylor, J., Hinz, B., Zorn, A., Jäger, H., Breul, R., Schreiner, S. & Klingler, W. (2019) Fascia is able to actively contract and may thereby influence musculoskeletal dynamics: a histochemical and mechanographic investigation. *Front Physiol.* 10: 336.

Slimani, M., Tod, D., Chaabene, H., Miarka, B. & Chamari, K. (2016) Effects of mental imagery on muscular strength in healthy and patient participants: a systematic review. *J Sports Sci Med.* 15: 434–450.

Yue, G. & Cole, K.J. (1992) Strength increases from the motor program: comparison of training with maximal voluntary and imagined muscle contractions. *J Neurophysiol.* 67: 1114–1123.

Yue, G., Wilson, S.L., Cole, K J., Daring, W.G. & Yuh, W.T.C. (1996) Imagined muscle contraction training increases voluntary neural drive to muscle. *J Psychophysiol.* 10: 198–208.

Further reading suggestions

Franklin, E. (2012) *Dynamic Alignment through Imagery*, 2nd edn. Champaign, IL: Human Kinetics.

Franklin, E. (2014) *Dance Imagery for Technique and Performance*, 2nd edn. Champaign, IL: Human Kinetics.

Periodized fascia training for speed, power, and injury resilience

Bill Parisi and Johnathon Allen

In the 1990s, the common assumption was that speed was not something you could dramatically improve through training. It was a genetic gift. You were either born to be fast or you weren't. It was believed that if you had more fast-twitch type II muscle fibers and a leaner frame, you were inevitably going to be faster. While there's obviously some inherent truth to that, it turns out that this is not the end of the story. Our understanding of speed has evolved significantly over the past few decades to give us new insights. Not only have we proven that human speed can be significantly enhanced through targeted training, we have a much better understanding of how and why (Clark and Weyand, 2014). In addition to demonstrating that the fascial system is both adaptable and trainable, modern research and imaging technology suggest it may play a significant role in the body's ability to generate speed in all of its many forms (Schleip and Müller, 2012) – from running a sub-10-second 100-meter dash, to throwing a 100-mph fast ball, and delivering a lightning-fast knockout punch. In all these examples, speed comes from multiple anatomical systems working together in a highly coordinated unison, enabled by the body's integrated myofascial web. When I was in high school, I went to Finland to train with the top javelin throwers and coaches in the world. While I was there, I was exposed to advanced functional training and medicine ball techniques not previously seen in the US. My belief is that those techniques optimize the adaptive remodeling and elastic energy-storage properties of the body's tendons and fascial system. This functional approach to three-dimensional, fascia-focused training allowed me to learn that throwing things is one of the most complete forms of athleticism. To be a great thrower, you need powerful legs and a stiff, super-strong core. Tremendous amounts of force are channeled from the lower body through your trunk, torso, shoulder, arm, elbow, wrist, and fingers. It's a whole-body experience (Naito et al, 2011) (see Chapter 33).

Fascia loves variability – variability in load, variability in movement, and variability of vectors (Zügel et al, 2018). And the sport of basketball is a three-dimensional game with constantly changing variables happening on multiple planes with submaximal loads and explosive movements that engage the entire body from foot to finger in a bullet-fast chain reaction of proprioception and elasticity. Spend three-plus hours a day playing basketball from a very young age (and avoid injury) and you will likely develop thicker Achilles' tendons with powerful dynamic recoil properties that give you kangaroo-like abilities for jumping, accelerating, and rapidly changing direction (Wiesinger, 2017). So, with this in mind, the question I ask is: How do we create a fascia-aware curriculum backed by research that any athlete or coach can use to improve athletic performance and injury resilience?

Fascia training 101

According to Davis's Law, fascial tissue continuously remodels itself in triple-helix strands of collagen produced by thousands of tiny fibro-blast cells that organize along the lines of load and stress in the body's extra-cellular matrix using a biological process called mechanotrans-duction (Ingber, 1998). Essentially, the net of your body-wide fascia system is constantly remodeling itself based on movements, loading patterns, diet, and lifestyle. If you sit hunched over at a desk all day, you will probably develop densely matted concentrations of collagen in the myofascial layers of your shoulders and your upper and lower back where the stress and load are concentrated. Although this process has not yet been proven to occur, animal studies show substantial disorganization of the muscular con-nective tissue (perimysium, epimysium) after sustained immobilization (Järvinen and Lehto, 1993). Therefore, it may be argued that without a regular program of variable movements moving those fibers and pumping viscous fluid into those matted tissues, they will eventually harden into dense adhesions that limit your mobility. On the other hand, if you spend your days working on a farm or an Alaskan tuna boat struggling against gravity under constantly variable loads happen-ing on multiple planes of motion that challenge your body's kinetic chain in frequently awkward positions (and avoid injury), it seems probable that you will develop a resilient three-dimen-sional fascia system that in conjunction with thick, powerful tendons – can give you the ability to generate tremendous amounts of force despite having a leaner/smaller frame than someone who bulks up at the gym. Science is showing us that this enhanced capability for power genera-tion comes from the elastic amplification prop-erties of tendons and fascia tissue and a pulsing neurological chain reaction of co-contractions happening across multiple myofascial structures that combine to create a finely-tuned balance of stability and mobility (Maas and Sandercock,

2010). If you doubt this assertion, challenge a farm kid or deep-sea fisherman to a wrestling match and see how it goes. But this takes us back to the million-dollar question: How do we har-ness this biological dynamic to create functional athletic training programs that improve speed, power, and injury resilience?

Fascial tissue and its behavior are based on its biological structure. If we understand the basic structure of fascia and how it behaves, we will understand how to train it. Observed simply, fascia is made up of cells, fibers, the extra cellular matrix, and water (see Fig.1.3). When it comes to the cells within fascia, we've got fibroblasts, mast cells, adipose cells, and macrophages. And all of them do very specific things. During the tissue remodeling phase of healing, macrophage activ-ity and collagenase enzymes clean up the old tissue so we can lay down the new. Fibroblasts are the cells that lay down the new. Fibroblasts build fascia just like osteoblasts build bone. They line up along the lines of stress – or 'load paths' – and produce the protein fibers of collagen, elastin, and reticulin. Since farm kids and deep sea fish-ermen stress their bodies in all sorts of different lengths, angles, and positions, they end up laying down an omnidirectional latticework of protein fibers throughout their bodies that is driven by the wide variety of loading patterns happening along the many different lines of stress they are subjected to.

Importantly, though, fascia tissue remodeling is rate/load specific (Bohm et al., 2014). Elastic energy is stored and released by tendons and fascia tissue very quickly – in less than 1.2 seconds (Kawakami et al., 2002). If a force lasts longer than that, the plasticity properties of fascia will adjust to accommodate to the load. This means that training tendons and fascia tissue for more elastic explosiveness requires short, cyclic, quickly repeated motions, like bouncing, jumping rope, or running on the balls of your feet (as opposed to slower-contraction cycles, like bicycling or rowing). Another key aspect in this dynamic is that the Type I collagen fibers that store and release elastic energy need to be connected and glued down in the extracellular matrix. They're glued down by a fluid called ground substance, which contains soluble carbohydrate polymers. These polymers take these protein fibers and glue them together omnidirectionally. The other key element in fascia tissue is water. We have either bound water or unbound water in our tissues. Unbound water consists of free-floating H_2O molecules that are not bonded with each other. Bound water is where H_2O molecules are bonded with each other and a hydrophilic surface in their vicinity. When that happens there is strong evidence to suggest that fascia becomes stiffer and more dynamic because it is more resistant to compression (Pollack, 2001). If you're an athlete, and you've got stiffer, more dynamic fascia tissue, that means you're wearing a kind of internal weightlifting compression suit that is tighter and stretchier. This means we want the water in fascia to be bound. This can be achieved through specific movement techniques, stretching, foam rolling, mechanical manipulation, eating fresh food, drinking plenty of water, alongside other strategies.

Vector variability

One of the first things to explore when designing a periodized training program is anatomical adaptation and the importance of vector variability in preparing the body for increased levels of exertion. The basic periodization premise is that the preparation phase of anatomical adaptation leads to strength, which leads to power (i.e. the expression of strength), which leads to speed, agility, and quickness. Traditionally,

weight, rep schemes, tempos, and rest periods were the only variables in the anatomical adaptation phase of a periodized training program. Typically, weights would be used to do mostly linear, sagittal-plane movements in the gym with higher reps for anatomical adaptation, lower reps with heavier weights for strength, and even lower reps using lighter weights and faster bar movements for power. However, in a fascia-aware approach to periodization, the process of anatomical adaptation is not just a matter of repeating the same movement patterns over and over with the same tempos along the same lines of stress. If it's true that fascia likes variability, then a fascia-aware approach to anatomical adaptation should include a variety of loads, vectors, and angles that stimulate omnidirectional tissue remodeling from the outset. This is because fibroblasts will lay down collagen in a more balanced latticework of fibers that provides increased shape stability, greater elastic recoil capability, and resistance to deformation which helps improve injury resilience. If tissues in the ankles, knees, hip, trunk, arms, and shoulders are exposed to different loads at different angles during the anatomical adaptation phase, the power of mechanotransduction for omnidirectional tissue remodeling across the entire body can be harnessed. This makes vector variability a key ingredient in anatomical adaptation. It is important to understand that both linear track athletes and multidirectional field and court sport athletes will benefit from a more dynamic multidirectional stretch/recoil capacity of the fascia system. An important part of linear sprinting is the ability to maintain joint and core stiffness in the transverse plane. And it is likely that inexperienced sprinters often over-rotate or leak energy from their core and joint systems because they do not have a well-balanced fascia system and strong core.

Chapter 48

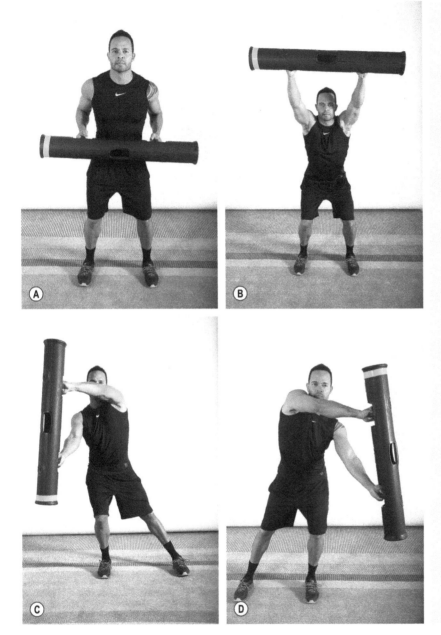

Figure 48.1 A–D Box Pattern

The box pattern drill provides vector variability. It activates the core and fascia connections in a whole-body chain reaction along the frontal plane. Work with any loaded movement tool such as a ViPR PRO (pictured), medicine ball, or kettlebell to achieve vector variability using the external load and gravity as drivers. **1.** Start by holding the load in an athletic stance. **2.** Raise the load overhead. **3.** Rotate the load vertically while lunging to the right. **4.** Return to the overhead position. **5.** Rotate the load vertically while lunging to the left. **6.** Repeat an equal number of reps on each side (**6–8**).

Odd position strength

For the strength training phase of a fascia-aware periodization program, our focus is on working with submaximal loads in odd positions at length. The idea is to load odd positions at length so we can engage tissue paths across the entire body on all three planes. To be clear, we're not saying that shortening muscles under load is

Periodized fascia training for speed, power, and injury resilience

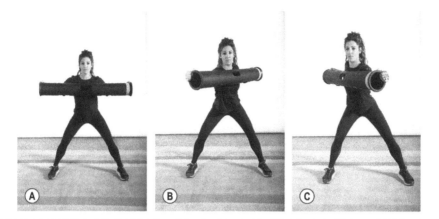

Figure 48.2 A–C Alternate Interior Reach

The alternate interior reach drill is another example of vector variability. It activates the core and engages fascia connections in a chain reaction along the transverse plane. **1.** Start by holding the load by the outside edges in an athletic stance. **2.** Rotate torso while reaching across the frontal plane as far as possible with each hand. **4.** Repeat an equal number of reps on each side (**6–8**).

bad and lengthening under load is good. They are both good, but they are different inputs that produce different results. From a fascia training perspective, the body needs to be subjected to a variety of different load paths on all three planes involving multiple joints, tissues, and structures. By lengthening muscles under load, shape stability and strength can be developed across the entire fabric of the body, not just over a local joint or segment.

Power and speed

In the world of athletic training, power is considered an expression of strength. If strength is being expressed at speed, it is often described in the industry as either speed-strength or strength-speed. While these terms are sometimes used interchangeably, they involve different training approaches and outcomes. Speed-strength refers to moving a load at a high rate of speed (e.g. a lineman in football pushing his opponent), while strength-speed is moving a relatively heavy load with the intention of moving it as fast as possible (e.g. Olympic lifting). In the power development phase of periodized training, the focus is on movements that involve rapid oscillating speeds and rebound motions where the contact times are under 1.2 seconds (Kawakami et al., 2002). This means doing things like bouncing a medicine ball against a wall, jumping a rope, running on the balls of the feet, or quickly moving a submaximal load overhead from one shoulder to the other. When these inputs are done at a faster athletic pace, they will stimulate cell signaling to lay down new collagen in the fascia tissue. The elastic recoil power of collagen fiber is best exemplified by a kangaroo's astounding ability to jump 40-feet at a time in rapid succession and achieve speeds of up to 40-mph. Studies show that this impressive ability doesn't come from kangaroos having more fast twitch muscle fibers than other animals, as was originally thought (in fact, they have roughly the same amount of type II muscle fibers as koala bears). It comes from the stored potential energy in

Chapter 48

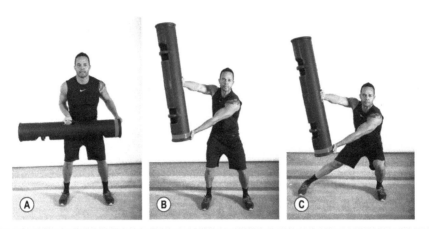

Figure 48.3 A–C Flag Lunge

The flag lunge helps develop odd-position strength by activating whole-body load paths and co-contractions in three dimensions on all three planes. Work with any loaded movement tool such as a ViPR PRO (pictured), medicine ball, or kettle bell to develop odd-position strength using the external load and gravity as drivers. **1.** Start by holding a load at midline with a shovel grip in an athletic stance. **2.** Raise the load laterally to one side, like a flag. **3.** Lunge across the frontal plane in the opposite direction of the load while exhaling forcefully. **4.** Return to the starting position. **5.** Repeat an equal number of repetitions on each side (**6–8**).

the collagen rich fascia tissue of their massive hindleg tendons and a pulsing elastic recoil dynamic called the "catapult effect" (Kram and Dawson, 1998). Humans are the only primates who have this same biological ability. The catapult effect is enabled by the surrounding muscles, which pre-contract isometrically to stretch the attached connective tissues—loading them like a stretched rubber band—and then relax to quickly release the stored elastic energy in an explosive pulse of force (Kawakami et al., 2002). The key to harnessing this powerful dynamic is the ability to create "super-stiffness" across the body's integrated myofascial system. Studies conducted by Stuart McGill and Stephen Brown revealed that super-stiffness comes from multiple structures co-contracting simultaneously to create a "mechanical composite" of tissues that provide a pulse of rock-solid stability (Brown and McGill, 2009). These pulses of super-stiffness create the anchor points a kangaroo (or human) needs to rapidly store and release elastic energy relative to the density of

collagen fibers in their tendons. Therefore, a well-structured fascia-aware training program should start by developing a solid foundation of odd position strength with omnidirectional shape stability first. Power and speed can then be stacked on top.

When it comes to speed training, regardless of whether you're training for linear speed or the rapid change of direction speeds experienced in field and court sports, it turns out that maximum velocity sprinting is unequaled as a training stimulus when prescribed in the right amounts. In fact, there is a growing body of evidence showing that maximum velocity sprinting not only improves overall speed and agility in short distances, it helps reduce soft tissue injuries in the groin and hamstring (Edouard et al., 2019).

Speed, agility, and quickness

As a running back in American football, the first line of defense is passed by cutting, darting, and

Periodized fascia training for speed, power, and injury resilience

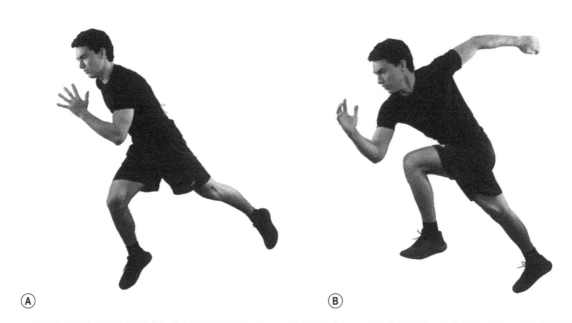

Ⓐ　　　　　　　　　　　Ⓑ

Figure 48.4 A–B Power Bounds

Power bounds develop the ability to use the "catapult effect" of the tendons and fascia system. Powerful extension and flexion from the ankle, knee, hip, core and shoulder are needed to maximize force generation. This exercise forces the tendons and fascia system to engage in the high-intensity movement of loaded single-leg bounding. Step **1**: Begin in a sprinter's stance and start by exploding backward off one leg while driving the opposite knee forward and the opposite arm backward. Step **2**: Let the ground come to you on each stride. Upon landing, immediately explode off the ground again into the next stride driving the opposite arm and leg backward. Step **3**: Repeat the power bounds continuously while striving to cover more horizontal distance on each side. Step **4**: Perform for 20–40 yards for 4–8 sets.

quickly changing directions. This rapid darting ability comes from the capacity to convert power into braking, accelerating, and rapidly reaccelerating in different directions. It requires the ability to instantly read visual and audio cues and quickly respond with appropriate countermovements while controlling your momentum and body mass. It is a responsive motor skill that is reactive and unplanned. It therefore has a significant neurological component that is facilitated in part by the proprioceptive properties of the fascia system (Schleip, 2017). This means power-conversion drills that combine timing, balance, and posterior chain strength—like the speed-skater bound—are a crucial component in periodized speed training. Because they require refined movement literacy, neurological tuning,

and core strength. Rapid, whole-body compound movements prompt the body to utilize multiple fascial sling systems to absorb force, stabilize momentum, decelerate body mass, and produce explosive power using the catapult effect of the tendons working in conjunction with the myofascial system.

Rest and recovery

When it comes to rest and recovery, the traditional focus is on neural and metabolic recovery periods between workout sessions or circuits. However, there is a strong reason to monitor work-to-rest ratios over the course of each workout: this concerns the extra cellular matrix. For example, in a metabolically-intense CrossFit

Chapter 48

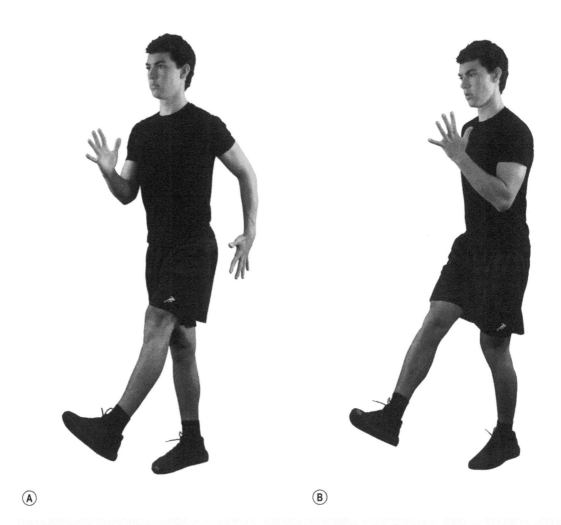

Figure 48.5 A–B Straight-Leg Bounding

Straight leg bounding is designed to activate the hamstrings and generate horizontal and vertical driving force off the ground. By keeping the leg straight and knees locked it forces the hamstrings to do more of the work as opposed to the quad and glut muscles. Since the hamstrings are a complex, two-jointed muscle responsible for hip extension and knee flexion it is commonly injured. Step **1**: Start by standing tall with both legs firmly locked at the knee joint. Step **2**: Flex and extend the hip in a shuffle like action while moving forward and slowly increase the intensity of the force production off the ground on each stride. Step **3**: Stay leaning slightly forward with a strong active anterior core while syncing the arms with the legs to maximize force production into the ground. Step **4**: Do two sets of 20–30 yards.

style workouts, injury rates tend to increase after about 30 minutes of exercise (Weisenthal et al., 2014). This is due to repetitive, aggressive muscle contractions that push blood and water away from localized areas of the body via muscle pumping and osmotic fluid pressure. When water is pushed out of localized areas, the composition of the ECM is changed, and the fascia tissue becomes less dynamic and stiffness is reduced (Schleip and Müller, 2012). However, when water binds to a sugar receptor within fascia (i.e. it becomes bound water), the tissue

Periodized fascia training for speed, power, and injury resilience

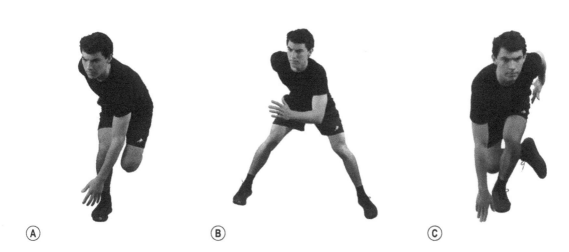

(A) (A)

(B)

(C)

Figure 48.6 A–C Speed-Skater Bounds

The speed skater bound is an example of speed-strength conversion. It is a total body movement with a focus on the gluteus maximus and posterior fascia chain. Due to the extreme hip flexion and stretch put on the glute complex while in this bent over position, the initial dynamic contraction challenges the body's fascia slings more than traditional exercises. It is an expression of power and control that relies on neural activity, proprioception, and timing. Step **1**: Start standing on one leg flexed at the hip and knee with the opposite hand down in front of the grounded leg. Step **2**: Dynamically and explosively jump laterally as fast as possible landing and balancing on the opposite leg. Focus on full extension of the hip and knee of the jumping leg while engaging in the lateral movement. Step **3**: Immediately upon landing, jump back laterally as fast as possible. Step **4**: Repeat continuous jumps for 12–16 total reps, 6–8 reps on each leg for 2–3 sets

becomes stiffer and more resistant to compression. Therefore, it is important to include strategic recovery sessions within workout routines, as opposed to purely between sessions. During an intense session, we recommend 10 minutes of rest for every 30 minutes of exhaustive exercise, using restorative pumping actions that return water and blood to the challenged tissues. This may enable water to bind to the fascia cells and sugar receptors, arguably creating a more robust, dynamic, and supportive fascial network throughout the workout.

In conclusion, the goal of periodized training is to engineer structural and functional adaptations in the body's tissues over time that improve athletic performance and resiliency. These adaptations are shown to be directly proportional to the mechanical stress inputs created by the intensity (load), volume (quantity), tempo (rate), and frequency, of the training. With increasing challenge along omni-directional paths using varying loads at varying tempos—and enough time to recover and remodel—the tissues will adapt by becoming three-dimensionally stronger and more elastic along the lines of stress. Therefore, a fascia training periodization program should progress through a series of whole-body exercise routines that emphasize vector variability, then odd-position strength, then power, then speed, agility, and quickness—utilizing different loads, angles, and speeds throughout. By using this structure for a periodized program, the fascia system's natural biological behavior can potentially be utilized to make athletes stronger, faster, and bouncier, with less injury risk—which is the ultimate win.

Chapter 48

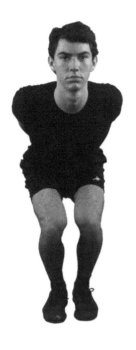

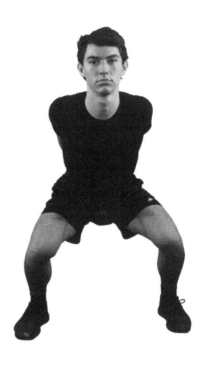

(A)   (B)

Figure 48.7 A-B Wide Outs

Wide-outs dynamically activate the gluteus medius/maximus and adductor group. By staying low and abducting then, immediately upon ground contact, adducting the legs in a jumping fashion while maintaining balance and a low athletic position, this exercise is a great lateral quickness drill. **Step 1:** Start in a wide stance squat position with knees in-line with your toes and hands behind your back.

Step 2: Without increasing your jump height, bring your feet close together by adducting the legs in a synchronized jump; then land softly maintaining a strong core without increasing the height of your head or hips. **Step 3:** Immediately upon landing, jump again abducting both legs and separating them back to the starting position. **Step 4:** Repeat the jumps continuously for two sets of 8–12 reps.

References

Bohm, S., Mersmann, F., Tettke, M., Kraft, M. & Arampatzis, A. (2014) Human achilles tendon plasticity in response to cyclic strain: Effect of rate and duration. *Journal of Experimental Biology.* 217: 4010–4017

Brown, S. & McGill, S. (2009) Transmission of muscularly generated force and stiffness between layers of the rat abdominal wall. *SPINE.* 34 (2).

Clark, K.P. & Weyand, P.G. (2014) Are running speeds maximized with simple-spring stance mechanics? *Journal of Applied Physiology.* 117 (6).

Edouard P., Mendiguchia, J., Guex, K., et al. (2019) Sprinting: a potential vaccine for hamstring injury? *Science Performance and Science Reports.*

Ingber, D. (1998) The Architecture of Life. *Scientific American.*

Järvinen, M.J. & Lehto, M.U.K. (1993) The effects of early mobilisation and immobilisation on the healing process following muscle injuries. *Sports Med.* 15(2): 78–89.

Kawakami, Y., Muraoka, T., Ito, S., Kanehisa, H. & Fukunaga, T. (2002) In vivo muscle fiber behavior during counter-movement exercise in humans reveals a significant role for tendon elasticity. *Journal of Physiology.* 540 (pt2): 635–646.

Maas, M. & Sandercock, T.G. (2010) Force transmission between synergistic skeletal muscles through connective tissue. *Journal of Biomedicine and Biotechnology.* April 12.

Kram, R. & Dawson, T. (1998) Energetics and biomechanics of locomotion by red kangaroos *(Macropus rufus). Comp Biochem Physiol.* 120 (1).

Naito, K., Takagi, H. & Maruyama, T. (2011) Mechanical work, efficiency and energy redistribution mechanisms in baseball pitching. *Journal of Sports Technology.* 4 (1–2).

Pollack, G.H. (2001) *Cells, Gels, and the Engines of Life. A New, Unifying Approach to Cell Function.* Seattle, Washington: Ebner and Sons Publishers.

Sawicki, G. (2009) *It Pays to Have a Spring in Your Step.* Department of Ecology and Evolutionary Biology, Brown University.

Schleip, R. & Müller, D.G. (2012) Training principles for fascial connective tissues: Scientific foundation and suggested practical applications. *Journal of Bodywork and Movement Therapies* 17 (1).

Schleip, R. (2017) Fascia as a sensory organ: clinical applications. *Terra Rosa.* 20.

Weisenthal, B.M., Beck, C.A., Maloney, M.D. et al. (2014) Injury Rate and Patterns Among CrossFit Athletes. *Orthop J Sports Med.* 2(4).

Wiesinger, H.P, Rieder, F. et. al. (2017) Sport-specific capacity to use elastic energy in the patellar and achilles tendons of elite athletes. *Frontiers in Physiology.* 8 (132).

Zügel, M. et al. (2018) Fascial tissue research in sports medicine: From molecules to tissue adaptation, injury and diagnostics. *British Journal of Sports Medicine.* 52 (23).

PERMISSIONS

Fig 1.2 Illustration courtesy of fascialnet.com

Fig 1.3 Illustration courtesy of fascialnet.com

Fig 1.4 Illustration courtesy of fascialnet.com, modified after Reeves et al., 2006.

Fig 1.5 Illustration courtesy of fascialnet.com

Fig 1.6 © 2015 fascialnet.com

Fig 1.7 Illustration courtesy of fascialnet.com, modified after Magnusson et al. (2010).

Fig 3.1 Reprinted from Leblanc et al. (2017). Copyright © 2017 John Wiley and Sons. Used with permission.

Fig 3.2 Reprinted from Magnusson et al. (2007). Copyright © 2007 John Wiley and Sons. Used with permission.

Fig 3.3 Lower part reprinted from Laver et al. (2018). Copyright © 2018 Springer-Verlag GmbH, DE part of Springer Nature. Used with permission.

Fig 3.4 Copyright © 2009 The American Physiological Society. Used with permission.

Fig 4.2 Modified from Nishimura et al. (1994) with permission.

Fig 4.3 Illustration from Svensson et al. (2016) with permission.

Fig 4.4 Illustration from Mikkelsen et al. (2017) with permission.

Fig 5.3 Mersmann et al. (2017a) used with permission by Frontiers Media SA.

Fig 9.1 Illustration: U.S. National Cancer Institute's Surveillance, Epidemiology and End Results (SEER) Program.

Fig 9.2 Photograph with the permission of James Heilman.

Fig 9.3A © Mfigueiredo, wikicommons, CCBY-SA 3.0.

Fig 9.3B Illustration based on data from Fede et al., 2018.

Fig 9.4A © JC Guimberteau, www.endovivo.com

Fig 9.5 Illustration modified after Sommer and Zhu (2008).

Fig 11.1 Model by Graham Scarr.

Fig 11.3 Artist: Amanda Williams.

Fig 11.4 Credit: Thomas Stephan Photography.

Fig 11.6 Thanks to 3D Life Prints, NTC, Ireland, and the Fascia Research Society

Fig 15.1 Illustration courtesy offascialnet.com

Fig 15.2 Images from Department of Neuroscience, Institute of Human Anatomy, University of Padova.

Fig 17.2 © iStock.com/nirat

Fig 17.3 Adapted from Mueller-Wohlfahrt et al.,2013, with permission.

PERMISSIONS

Fig 17.4 © iStock.com/fizkes

Table 17.1 Adapted from Mueller-Wohlfahrt et al., 2013. Reproduced with permission.

Fig 18.3 Adapted from Idorn & Hojman (2016) with permission from Elsevier Science & Technology Journals.

Fig 18.4 Adapted from: Hojman, J., Gehl, J., Christensen, J. F., et al. (2018). Molecular mechanisms linking exercise to cancer prevention and treatment. *Cell Metabolism* 27(1): 10-21, with permission from Elsevier Science & Technology Journals.

Fig 19.1 © fascialnet.com

Fig 21.3 Photo: fascialnet.com

Fig 21.6 Photo: Philips Health System.

Fig 24.3 Photograph reprints with permission from www.blackroll.com.

Fig 25.1 Reproduced with permission from Pullsh, Germany.

Fig 25.2 Reproduced with permission from Omegawave, Finland.

Fig 25.3 Reproduced with permission from Exxentric, Sweden.

Fig 25.4 Reproduced with permission from Robert Heiduk, Germany.

Figs 27.1 A, B and 27.3 with permission from Performance Health.

Fig 30.1 Adapted from Sockol et al. (2007).

Fig 30.3 Adapted from Crompton, Vereecke and Thorpe, 2008.

Fig 33.2 Credit: Christian Puta.

Fig 33.3 Adapted from Benninghoff, 2008.

Fig 34.1 SiFu Pierre Yves Roqueferre.

Fig 34.2 Harumi Tribble, dancer and choreographer.

Fig 34.3 Master Li Jun Feng.

Fig 36.9 Reproduced with kind permission from Thomas Myers.

Fig 37.1 Reproduced with kind permission from: model, Helen Eadie; photographer, Amy Very; tube design/ styling, Joanne Avison.

Fig 37.2 Reproduced with kind permission from Shane McDermott (www.wildearthilluminations.com).

Fig 37.3 Model by Bruce Hamilton (see Further information).

Fig 37.4 Reproduced with kind permission from Katie Courts (www.yoga-nutco.uk).

Fig 37.5 Reproduced with kind permission from Art of Contemporary Yoga Ltd.

Fig 37.6 Reproduced with kind permission from Shane McDermott (www.wildearthilluminations.com).

PERMISSIONS

INDEX

INDEX